Pathophysiology

Reviews & Rationales

Mary Ann Hogan, RN, CS, MSN

Clinical Assistant Professor
University of Massachusetts, Amherst
Amherst, Massachusetts

Karen Hill, PhD, RN

Assistant Professor of Nursing
Southeastern Louisiana University
Hammond, Louisiana

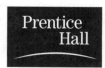

Prentice
Hall

Upper Saddle River, New Jersey 07458

Library of Congress Cataloging-in-Publication Data

Hogan, Mary Ann, MSN.
  Pathophysiology: reviews & rationales/Mary Ann Hogan,
Karen Hill.
      p. ; cm.—(Prentice Hall nursing reviews & rationales)
  Includes index.
      ISBN 0-13-030450-6
   1. Physiology, Pathological—Outlines, syllabi, etc. 2.
Nursing—Outlines, syllabi, etc.
      [DNLM: 1. Nursing Assessment—methods—Outlines. 2.
Pathology—Outlines. WY 18.2 H714p 2003] I. Hill, Karen,
RN. II. Title. III. Series.
      RB113 .H625 2003
      616.07—dc21
                                                        2002014480

Publisher: Julie Levin Alexander
Assistant to Publisher: Regina Bruno
Executive Editor: Maura Connor
Managing Development Editor: Marilyn Meserve
Development Editor: Jeanne Allison
Director of Production and Manufacturing: Bruce Johnson
Managing Production Editor: Patrick Walsh
Production Liaison: Danielle Newhouse
Production Editor: Jessica Balch, Pine Tree Composition
Manufacturing Buyer: Pat Brown
Design Director: Cheryl Asherman
Design Coordinator: Maria Guglielm

Interior Designer: Jill Little
Cover Designer: Joseph DePinho
Electronic Art Creation: Precision Graphics
Marketing Manager: Nicole Benson
Assistant Editor: Yesenia Kopperman
Editorial Assistant: Sladjana Repic
Production Information Manager: Rachele Strober
Manager of Media Production: Amy Peltier
New Media Project Manager: Stephen Hartner
Composition: Pine Tree Composition, Inc.
Printer/Binder: Courier/Westford
Cover Printer: Phoenix Color

Pearson Education Ltd., *London*
Pearson Education Australia Pty. Limited, *Sydney*
Pearson Education Singapore, Pte. Ltd.
Pearson Education North Asia Ltd., *Hong Kong*
Pearson Education Canada, Ltd., *Toronto*
Pearson Educación de Mexico, S.A. de C.V.
Pearson Education—Japan, *Tokyo*
Pearson Education Malaysia, Pte. Ltd.
Pearson Education, Upper Saddle River, New Jersey

10 9 8 7 6 5 4 3 2
ISBN 0-13-030450-6

Contents

Preface

INTRODUCTION

Welcome to the new Prentice Hall Reviews and Rationales Series! This 9-book series has been specifically designed to provide a clear and concentrated review of important nursing knowledge in the following content areas:

- Child Health Nursing
- Maternal-Newborn Nursing
- Mental Health Nursing
- Medical-Surgical Nursing
- Pathophysiology
- Pharmacology
- Fundamentals and Skills
- Nutrition and Diet Therapy
- Fluids, Electrolytes, & Acid-Base Balance

The books in this series have been designed for use either by current nursing students as a study aid for nursing course work or NCLEX-RN licensing exam preparation, or by practicing nurses seeking a comprehensive yet concise review of a nursing specialty or subject area.

This series is truly unique. One of its most special features is that it has been authored by a large team of nurse educators from across the United States and Canada to ensure that each chapter is written by a nurse expert in the content area under study. Prentice Hall Health representatives from across North America submitted names of nurse educators and/or clinicians who excel in their respective fields, and these authors were then invited to write a chapter in one or more books. The consulting editor for each book, who is also an expert in that specialty area, then reviewed all chapters submitted for comprehensiveness and accuracy. The series editor designed the overall series in collaboration with a core Prentice Hall team to take full advantage of Prentice Hall's cutting edge technology, and also reviewed the chapters in each book.

All books in the series are identical in their overall design for your convenience (further details follow at the end of this section). As an added value, each book comes with a comprehensive support package, including free CD-ROM, free companion website access, and a Nursing Notes card for quick clinical reference.

STUDY TIPS

Use of this review book should help simplify your study. To make the most of your valuable study time, also follow these simple but important suggestions:

- Use a weekly calendar to schedule study sessions.
  - Outline the timeframes for all of your activities (home, school, appointments, etc.) on a weekly calendar.
  - Find the "holes" in your calendar—the times in which you can plan to study. Add study sessions to the calendar at times when you can expect to be mentally alert and follow it!
- Create the optimal study environment.
  - Eliminate external sources of distraction, such as television, telephone, etc.
  - Eliminate internal sources of distraction, such as hunger, thirst, or dwelling on items or problems that cannot be worked on at the moment.
  - Take a break for 10 minutes or so after each hour of concentrated study both as a reward and an incentive to keep studying.
- Use pre-reading strategies to increase comprehension of chapter material.
  - Skim the headings in the chapter (because they identify chapter content).
  - Read the definitions of key terms, which will help you learn new words to comprehend chapter information.
  - Review all graphic aids (figures, tables, boxes) because they are often used to explain important points in the chapter.
- Read the chapter thoroughly but at a reasonable speed.
  - Comprehension and retention are actually enhanced by not reading too slowly.
  - Do take the time to reread any section that is unclear to you.
- Summarize what you have learned.
  - Use questions supplied with this book, CD-ROM, and companion website to test your recall of chapter content.
  - Review again any sections that correspond to questions you answered incorrectly or incompletely.

TEST TAKING STRATEGIES

Use the following strategies to increase your success on multiple-choice nursing tests or examinations:

- Get sufficient sleep and have something to eat before taking a test. Take deep breaths during the test as needed. Remember, the brain requires oxygen and glucose as fuel. Avoid concentrated sweets before a test, however, to avoid rapid upward and then downward surges in blood glucose levels.
- Read each question carefully, identifying the stem, the four options, and any key words or phrases in either the stem or options.
  - Key words in the stem such as "most important" indicate the need to set priorities, since more than one option is likely to contain a statement that is technically correct.
  - Remember that the presence of absolute words such as "never" or "only" in an option is more likely to make that option incorrect.

- Determine who is the client in the question; often this is the person with the health problem, but it may also be a significant other, relative, friend, or another nurse.
- Decide whether the stem is a true response stem or a false response stem. With a true response stem, the correct answer will be a true statement, and vice-versa.
- Determine what the question is really asking, sometimes referred to as the issue of the question. Evaluate all answer options in relation to this issue, and not strictly to the "correctness" of the statement in each individual option.
- Eliminate options that are obviously incorrect, then go back and reread the stem. Evaluate the remaining options against the stem once more.
- If two answers seem similar and correct, try to decide whether one of them is more global or comprehensive. If the global option includes the alternative option within it, it is likely that the more global response is the correct answer.

THE NCLEX-RN LICENSING EXAMINATION

The NCLEX-RN licensing examination is a Computer Adaptive Test (CAT) that ranges in length from 75 to 265 individual (stand-alone) test items, depending on individual performance during the examination. Upon graduation from a nursing program, successful completion of this exam is the gateway to your professional nursing practice. The blueprint for the exam is reviewed and revised every three years by the National Council of State Boards of Nursing according to the results of a job analysis study of new graduate nurses (practicing within the first six months after graduation). Each question on the exam is coded to one *Client Need Category* and one or more *Integrated Concepts and Processes.*

Client Need Categories

There are 4 categories of client needs, and each exam will contain a minimum and maximum percent of questions from each category. Each major category has subcategories within it. The *Client Need* categories according to the NCLEX-RN Test Plan effective April 2001 are as follows:

- Safe, Effective Care Environment
  - Management of Care (7–13%)
  - Safety and Infection Control (5–11%)
- Health Promotion and Maintenance
  - Growth and Development Throughout the Lifespan (7–13%)
  - Prevention and Early Detection of Disease (5–11%)
- Psychosocial Integrity
  - Coping and Adaptation (5–11%)
  - Psychosocial Adaptation (5–11%)
- Physiological Integrity
  - Basic Care and Comfort (7–13%)
  - Pharmacological and Parenteral Therapies (5–11%)
  - Reduction of Risk Potential (12–18%)
  - Physiological Adaptation (12–18%)

Integrated Concepts and Processes

The integrated concepts and processes identified on the NCLEX-RN Test Plan effective April 2001, with condensed definitions, are as follows:

- Nursing Process: a scientific problem-solving approach used in nursing practice; consisting of assessment, analysis, planning, implementation, and evaluation.

- Caring: client-nurse interaction(s) characterized by mutual respect and trust and directed toward achieving desired client outcomes.
- Communication and Documentation: verbal and/or nonverbal interactions between nurse and others (client, family, health care team); a written or electronic recording of activities or events that occur during client care.
- Cultural Awareness: knowledge and sensitivity to the client's beliefs/values and how these might impact on the client's healthcare experience.
- Self-Care: assisting clients to meet their health care needs, which may include maintaining health or restoring function.
- Teaching/Learning: facilitating client's acquisition of knowledge, skills, and attitudes that lead to behavior change.

More detailed information about this examination may be obtained by visiting the National Council of State Boards of Nursing website at http://www.ncsbn.org and viewing the *NCLEX-RN Examination Test Plan for the National Council Licensure Examination for Registered Nurses.* *

How to Get the Most Out of This Book

Chapter Organization

Each chapter has the following elements to guide you during review and study:

- Chapter Objectives: describe what you will be able to know or do after learning the material covered in the chapter.

Objectives

▌ Review basic principles of growth and development.

▌ Describe major physical expectations for each developmental age group.

▌ Identify developmental milestones for various age groups.

▌ Discuss the reactions to illness and hospitalization for children at various stages of development.

- Review at a Glance: contains a glossary of key terms used in the chapter, with definitions provided up-front and available at your fingertips, to help you stay focused and make the best use of your study time.

Review at a Glance

anticipatory guidance *the process of understanding upcoming developmental needs and then teaching caregivers to meet those needs*

cephalocaudal development *the process by which development proceeds from the head downward through the body and towards the feet*

chronological age *age in years*

critical periods *times when an individual is especially responsive to certain environmental effects, sometimes called sensitive periods*

development *an increase in capability or function; a more complex concept that*

is a continuous, orderly series of conditions that lead to activities, new motives for activities; and eventual patterns of behavior

developmental age *age based on functional behavior and ability to adapt to the environment; does not necessarily correspond to chronological age*

- Pretest: this 10-question multiple choice test provides a sample overview of content covered in the chapter and helps you decide what areas need the most—or the least—review.

Pretest

1 The nurse discusses dental care with the parents of a 3-year-old. The nurse explains that by the age of 3, their child should have:

(1) 5 "temporary" teeth.
(2) 10 "temporary" teeth.
(3) 15 "temporary" teeth.
(4) 20 "temporary" teeth.

2 The mother of a 6-month-old infant is concerned that the infant's anterior fontanel is still open. The nurse would inform the mother that further evaluation is needed if the anterior fontanel is open after:

(1) 6 months.
(2) 10 months.
(3) 18 months.
(4) 24 months.

- Practice to Pass questions: these are open-ended questions that stimulate critical thinking and reinforce mastery of the chapter content.

> **Practice to Pass**
>
> What would you explain as normal motor development for a 10-month old infant?

- NCLEX Alerts: the NCLEX icon identifies information or concepts that are likely to be tested on the NCLEX licensing examination. Be sure to learn the information flagged by this type of icon.

NCLEX!

- Case Study: found at the end of the chapter, it provides an opportunity for you to use your critical thinking and clinical reasoning skills to "put it all together;" it describes a true-to-life client case situation and asks you open-ended questions about how you would provide care for that client and/or family.

Case Study

A 6-month-old female infant is brought into the pediatric clinic for a well-baby visit. You as the pediatric nurse will be assigned to care for this family.

❶ Identify the primary growth and development expectations for a 6-month-old.

❷ What type common behavior is expected of this 6-month-old towards the nurse?

❸ What immunization(s) are recommended at this age to maintain health and wellness?

For suggested responses, see page 406.

- Posttest: a 10-question multiple-choice test at the end of the chapter provides new questions that are representative of chapter content, and provide you with feedback about mastery of that content following review and study. All pretest and posttest questions contain rationales for the correct answer, and are coded according to the phase of the nursing process used and the NCLEX category of client need (called the Test Plan). The Test plan codes are PHYS (Physiological Integrity), PSYC (Psychosocial Integrity), SECE (Safe Effective Care Environment), and HPM (Health Promotion and Maintenance).

Posttest

1 **When using the otoscope to examine the ears of a 2-year-old child, the nurse should:**

(1) Pull the pinna up and back.
(2) Pull the pinna down and back.
(3) Hold the pinna gently but firmly in its normal position.
(4) Hold the pinna against the skull.

2 **To assess the height of an 18-month-old child who is brought to the clinic for routine examination, the nurse should:**

(1) Measure arm span to estimate adult height.
(2) Use a tape measure.
(3) Use a horizontal measuring board.
(4) Have the child stand on an upright scale and use the measuring arm.

CD-ROM

For those who want to practice taking tests on a computer, the CD-ROM that accompanies the book contains the pretest and posttest questions found in all chapters of the book. In addition, it contains 10 NEW questions for each chapter to help you further evaluate your knowledge base and hone your test-taking skills. In several chapters, one of the questions will have embedded art to use in answering the question. Some of the newly developed NCLEX test items are also designed in this way, so these items will give you valuable practice with this type of question.

Companion Website (CW)

The companion website is a "virtual" reference for virtually all your needs! The CW contains the following:

- 50 NCLEX-style questions: 10 pretest, 10 posttest, 10 CD-ROM, and 20 additional new questions
- Definitions of key terms: the glossary is also stored on the companion website for ease of reference
- In Depth With NCLEX: features drawings or photos that are each accompanied by a one- to two-paragraph explanation. These are especially useful when describing something that is complex, technical (such as equipment), or difficult to mentally visualize.
- Suggested Answers to Practice to Pass and Case Study Questions: easily located on the website, these allow for timely feedback for those who answer chapter questions on the web.

Nursing Notes Clinical Reference Card

This laminated card provides a reference for frequently used facts and information related to the subject matter of the book. These are designed to be useful in the clinical setting, when quick and easy access to information is so important!

ABOUT THE PATHOPHYSIOLOGY BOOK

Chapters in this book cover "need-to-know" information about pathophysiology of a wide variety of health problems. They include health problems that relate to the respiratory, cardiovascular, neurological, musculoskeletal, gastrointestinal, endocrine, renal, reproductive, and integumentary systems. Others chapters address immunological, hematological, oncological, and infectious health problems. Finally, the last two chapters review two unique areas, genetically transmitted health problems and multisystem health problems. Mastery of the information in this book and effective use of the test-taking strategies described will help the student be confident and successful in testing situations, including the NCLEX-RN, and in actual clinical practice.

ACKNOWLEDGMENTS

This book is a monumental effort of collaboration. Without the contributions of many individuals, this first edition of *Pathophysiology: Reviews and Rationales* would not have been possible. We gratefully acknowledge all the contributors who devoted their time and talents to this book. Their chapters will surely assist both students and practicing nurses alike to extend their knowledge in the area of pathophysiology.

We owe a special debt of gratitude to the wonderful team at Prentice Hall Health for their enthusiasm for this project, as well as their good humor, expertise, and encouragement as the series developed. Maura Connor, Executive Editor for Nursing, was unending in her creativity, support, encouragement, and belief in the need for this series. Marilyn Meserve, Senior Managing Editor for Nursing, devoted many long hours to coordinating different facets of this project, and tirelessly and cheerfully encouraged our efforts as well. Her high standards and attention to detail contributed greatly to the final "look" of this series. Jeanne Allison, Developmental Editor, actively kept in communication with the different writers in this book and also facilitated getting the book itself into production. Editorial assistants, including Beth Ann Romph, Sladjana Repic, and others, helped to keep the project moving forward on a day-to-day basis, and we are grateful for their efforts as well. A very special thank you goes to the designers of the book and the production team, led by Danielle Newhouse, who brought our ideas and manuscript into final form.

Thank you to the team at Pine Tree Composition, led by Project Coordinator Jessica Balch, for the detail-oriented work of creating this book. We greatly appreciate their hard work, attention to detail, and spirit of collaboration. A special thanks also goes to Yesenia Kopperman, Assistant Editor for Nursing at Prentice Hall, and to Carlos Cooper, Lisa Donovan, and staff at the Pearson Education Development Group for designing and producing the *Nursing Notes* clinical reference card that accompanies this book.

Mary Ann Hogan acknowledges and gratefully thanks my husband Michael and children Mike Jr., Katie, Kristen, and Billy, who sacrificed hours of time that would have been spent with them, so that I could bring this book to publication. Your love and support kept me energized, motivated, and at times, even sane. I love you all!

Karen Yvonne Hill acknowledges my wonderful family Bobby, B.J., Kristopher, and Lindsey for their understanding and patience through this process. You were always supportive, encouraging and helped out whenever possible. I love each of you for being behind me in this effort. I dedicate this book to my husband, Bobby, who is my best friend, the best father, a wonderful husband, and willing to sacrifice so much for me. Thanks to you all!

---

*Reference: National Council of State Boards of Nursing, Inc. *NCLEX Examination Test Plan for National Council Licensure Examination for Registered Nurses.* Effective April, 2001. Retrieved from the World Wide Web September 5, 2001 at http://www.ncsbn.org/public/resources/res/NCSBNRNTestPlan Booklet.pdf.

Contributors

Julie A. Adkins, RN, MSN, FNP
Family Nurse Practitioner
West Frankfort, Illinois
Chapters 10 and 14

Jana G. Brannan, MN, RN, CNAA
Instructor
Southeastern Louisiana University
Hammond, Louisiana
Chapter 17

Carol D. Clark, MS, RN, ANP, GNPC
Associate Professor
Indiana Wesleyan University
Marion, Indiana
Chapter 8

Cathy Cormier, MN, RN, C
Instructor
Southeastern Louisiana University
Hammond, Louisiana
Chapter 5

Mical DeBrow, PhD, RN
Vice President/Healthcare Services
Gulf South Health Plans
Baton Rouge, Louisiana
Chapter 12

**Joseann Helmes DeWitt, MSN, RN, C,
    CLNC**
Assistant Professor
Alcorn State University School of Nursing
Natchez, Mississippi
Chapter 9

Lynn H. Doyle, RN, MS, CPNP
Assistant Professor Pediatrics
Marian College
Fond du Lac, Wisconsin
Chapter 16

Pam Hamre, RN, MS, CNM
Assistant Professor
College of St. Catherine
St. Paul, Minnesota
Chapter 11

Ann Harley, EdD, RN
Professor
Carson Newman College
Jefferson City, Tennessee
Chapter 3

Sherry Hendrickson, RN, PhD, CS
Assistant Professor of Clinical Nursing
The University of Texas at Austin
Austin, Texas
Chapter 4

Karen Hill, PhD, RN
Assistant Professor
Southern Louisiana University
Hammond, Louisiana
Chapter 1

Barbara Moffett, PhD, RN
Associate Professor
Southeastern Louisiana University
Hammond, Louisiana
Chapter 13

Patsy Rider, RN, MSN, CS
Instructor
The University of Texas at Austin
Austin, Texas
Chapter 4

Diane E. Smith, MSN, RN
Baton Rouge, Louisiana
Chapter 6

Susan K. Steele, MN, RN, AOCN
Oncology Clinical Nurse Specialist/Assistant
    Professor
Our Lady of the Lake College
Baton Rouge, Louisiana
Chapter 15

Betty Jane Sylvest, BSN, RN, MSN
Instructor
University of Southern Mississippi
Hattiesburg, Mississippi
Chapter 2

Eugenia H. Tickle, RN, MSN, EdD
Associate Professor
Midwestern State University
Wichita Falls, Texas
Chapter 7

Reviewers

Janie Butts, DSN, RN
Assistant Professor
University of Southern Mississippi
Hattiesburg, Mississippi

Christine A. Cannon, RN, PhD
Associate Professor
University of Delaware
Newark, Delaware

Linda Covington, PhD
Associate Professor
Middle Tennessee State University
Murfreesboro, Tennessee

Barbara Daniel, MEd, MS, CRNP
Professor
Cecil Community College
North East, Maryland

Ann M. Findley, PhD
Associate Professor
Department of Biology
University of Louisiana at Monroe
Monroe, Louisiana

Diane Ford, RN, MS, FNP, CS
Assistant Professor
Andrews University
Berrien Springs, Michigan

Wanda Gifford, RN, MSN, CS, FNP
Family Nurse Practitioner/Instructor
St. Josephs College
Rensselaer, Indiana

Sandra Smith Huddleston, RN, PhD
Associate Professor
Berea College
Berea, Kentucky

Robin Kirschner, RN, MA, CPAN
Professor
Scottsdale Community College
Scottsdale, Arizona

Jane Koeckeritz, RN, PhD
Professor
University of Northern Colorado
Greeley, Colorado

James A. Metcalf, PhD
Professor
George Mason University
Fairfax, Virginia

Mercy Mammah Popoola, RN, CNS, PhD
Assistant Professor
Georgia Southern University
Statesboro, Georgia

Elizabeth Ann Rettew, MSN, RN, FNP-BC
Associate Professor
Malone College
Canton, Ohio

Student Consultants

Alisa Beaulieu
Santa Fe Community College
Gainesville, Florida

Alison Cody
Germanna Community College
Locust Grove, Virginia

Daniel Dale
Valdosta State University
Valdosta, Georgia

Stephanie Hornby
George Mason University
Fairfax, Virginia

Amy Jeter
Ohio University-Chillicothe
Chillicothe, Ohio

Joan Lawrence
Auburn University
Auburn, Alabama

Lisa Marie Mays
Boise State University
Boise, Idaho

Shawn Shaughnessy
Santa Fe Community College
Gainesville, Florida

Phyllis Thieken
Ohio University-Chillicothe
Chillicothe, Ohio

Jenefer Thomas
Boise State University
Boise, Idaho

Gyleen Vickerman
Boise State University
Boise, Idaho

Carolyn Wilkinson
Auburn University
Auburn, Alabama

A Guide To
Prentice Hall's Reviews and Rationales Series

Each chapter has the following **feature elements** to guide you during review and study.

Chapter **Objectives** describe what you will be able to know or do after learning the material covered in the chapter.

Review at a Glance contains a glossary of key terms used in the chapter, with definitions provided up-front and available at your fingertips, to help you stay focused and make the best use of your study time.

The **Pretest** is a 10-question multiple choice test providing a sample overview of content covered in the chapter and helps you decide what areas need the most – or the least – review.

The **Practice to Pass** questions are open-ended questions that stimulate critical thinking and reinforce mastery of the chapter content.

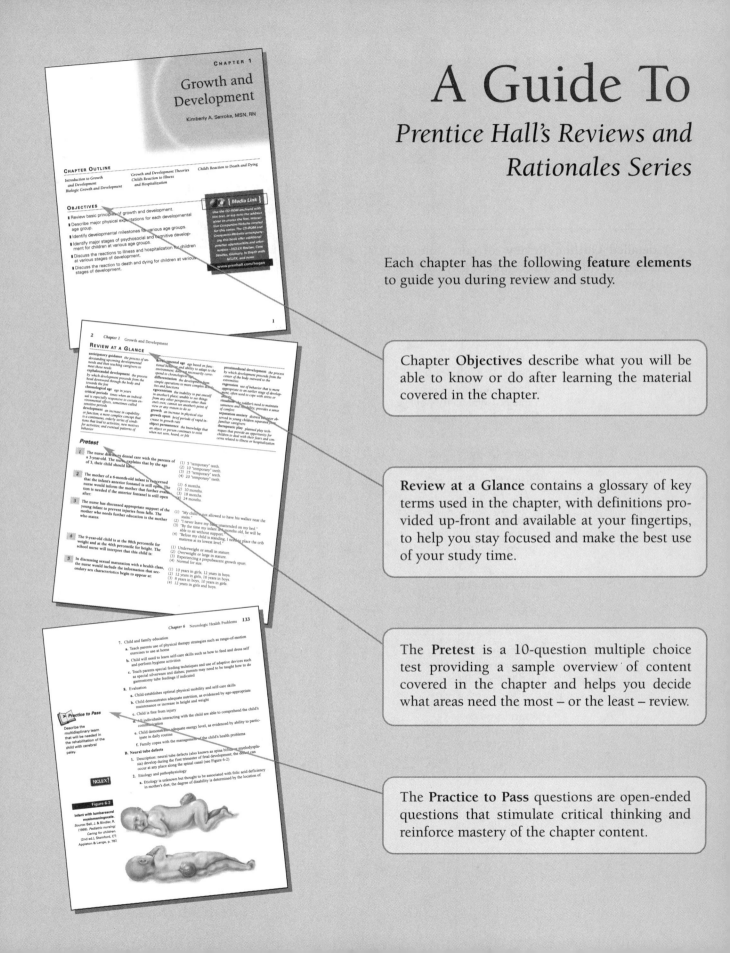

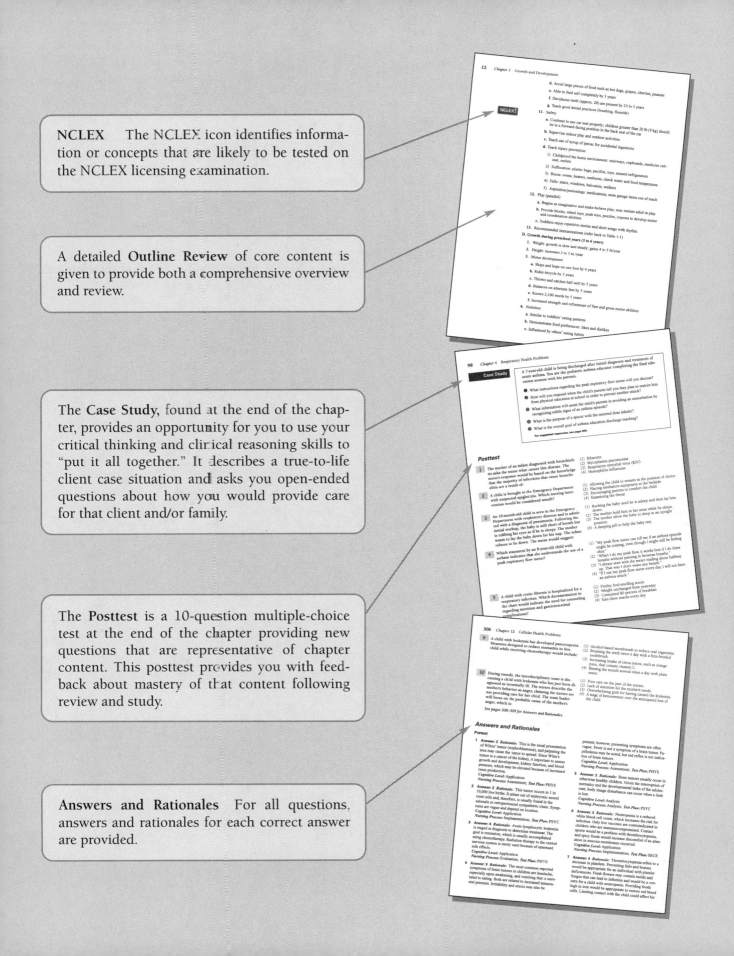

NCLEX The NCLEX icon identifies information or concepts that are likely to be tested on the NCLEX licensing examination.

A detailed **Outline Review** of core content is given to provide both a comprehensive overview and review.

The **Case Study**, found at the end of the chapter, provides an opportunity for you to use your critical thinking and clinical reasoning skills to "put it all together." It describes a true-to-life client case situation and asks you open-ended questions about how you would provide care for that client and/or family.

The **Posttest** is a 10-question multiple-choice test at the end of the chapter providing new questions that are representative of chapter content. This posttest provides you with feedback about mastery of that content following review and study.

Answers and Rationales For all questions, answers and rationales for each correct answer are provided.

CHAPTER 1

Respiratory Health Problems

Karen Hill, PhD, RN

CHAPTER OUTLINE

Risk Factors Associated with
  Respiratory Health Problems
Obstructive Pulmonary Disorders
Restrictive Pulmonary Disorders
Pneumonia

Pulmonary Tuberculosis (TB)
Pleural Effusion
Pleuritis (Pleurisy)
Pneumothorax/Hemothorax

Pulmonary Embolism (PE)
Pulmonary Hypertension
Lung Cancer
Respiratory Failure

OBJECTIVES

▌ Define key terms associated with respiratory health problems.

▌ Identify risk factors associated with the development of respiratory health problems.

▌ Discuss the common etiologies of respiratory health problems.

▌ Describe the pathophysiologic processes associated with specific respiratory health problems.

▌ Distinguish between normal and abnormal respiratory findings obtained from nursing assessment.

▌ Prioritize nursing interventions associated with specific respiratory health problems.

[**Media Link**]

Use the CD-ROM enclosed with this text, or log onto the address given to access the free, interactive Companion Website created for this series. The CD-ROM and Companion Website accompanying this book offer additional practice opportunities and infor-mation—NCLEX Review, Case Studies, Glossary, In Depth with NCLEX, and more.

www.prenhall.com/hogan

REVIEW AT A GLANCE

acute respiratory distress syndrome (ARDS) *a form of acute respiratory failure with respiratory insufficiency and inefficient gas exchange*

asthma *an obstructive airflow disorder where narrowing and inflammation of the airways cause respiratory distress*

atelectasis *collapse of a portion of the lung with limited gas exchange*

bronchiectasis *an irreversible state of bronchial dilation and destruction of the bronchial walls*

bronchitis *inflammation of the mucous membranes of the bronchial airways; another term for chronic bronchitis is "blue bloater" because of the hypoxemia that leads to cyanosis*

chronic obstructive pulmonary disease (COPD) *a group of pulmonary diseases involving obstruction of airflow that is chronic and recurrent, usually associated with asthma, emphysema, and bronchitis*

cor pulmonale *a disorder manifested by hypertrophy of the right ventricle caused by pulmonary hypertension; manifests as right heart failure*

cystic fibrosis (CF) *autosomal recessive disease of the exocrine glands that manifests itself in multiple organs, characterized by excess production of mucus and COPD in early childhood*

emphysema *a chronic disorder of the lungs resulting in overinflation of air spaces, loss of elasticity and decreased gas exchange; another term for chronic emphysema is "pink puffer" because the client does not become cyanotic until the end stages of the disease*

flail chest *instability of the chest wall usually caused by trauma or fractured ribs with a reverse in chest wall movement from normal; the chest wall contracts on inspiration and expands outward on expiration*

hemothorax *the collection of blood or fluid in the pleural space*

obstructive pulmonary disorders *any respiratory disorder where airflow is hindered to the lungs, may be chronic or acute*

pleural effusion *increased accumulation of fluid between the visceral and parietal pleura of the lung*

pleuritis *inflammation of the parietal space of the lungs, also known as pleuritis*

pneumonia *inflammation of the lungs caused by bacteria, viruses, fungi, or other pathogens*

pneumothorax *collapse of a portion or all of the lung due to trapping of air in the pleural space*

pulmonary embolus *blockage of a pulmonary artery by an embolus of fat, blood, or other foreign products*

pulmonary hypertension *a sustained elevation of the pulmonary artery pressure, greater than 20 mmHg*

restrictive pulmonary disorders *any disease that limits the expansion of the lungs or chest wall movement*

sleep apnea *having periods of delay or lack of breathing (usually longer than 10 seconds) during sleep*

status asthmaticus *an acute emergency of a prolonged or repetitive asthma attack*

tuberculosis (TB) *infection of the lung with an acid-fast bacillus, Mycobacterium tuberculosis*

Pretest

1 A client has chronic respiratory acidosis caused by end-stage chronic obstructive pulmonary disease (COPD). Oxygen is delivered at 1 L/min per nasal cannula. The nurse teaches the family that the reason for this precaution is to avoid respiratory depression, based on which of the following as the best explanation?

(1) COPD clients depend on a low oxygen level.
(2) COPD clients depend on a low carbon dioxide level.
(3) COPD clients tend to retain hydrogen ions if they are given high doses of oxygen.
(4) COPD clients thrive on a high oxygen level.

2 A client presents to the Emergency Department with acute respiratory distress and the following arterial blood gases (ABGs): pH 7.35, PCO_2 40 mmHg, PO_2 63 mmHg, HCO_3 23, oxygen saturation (Cal SO_2) 93 percent. Which of the following represents the best analysis of the etiology of these ABGs?

(1) Tuberculosis (TB)
(2) Pneumonia
(3) Pleural effusion
(4) Hypoxia

3 When assessing a client with early impairment of oxygen perfusion, such as in pulmonary embolus, the nurse would expect to find restlessness and which of the following symptoms?

(1) Warm, dry skin
(2) Bradycardia
(3) Tachycardia
(4) Eupnea

4 One day postoperative, the client complains of dyspnea, respiratory rate (RR) is 35, slightly labored, and there are no breath sounds in the lower-right base. The nurse would suspect:

(1) Cor pulmonale.
(2) Atelectasis.
(3) Pulmonary embolism.
(4) Cardiac tamponade.

5 A client with an acute case of pneumonia has a dry, hacking cough, elevated temperature, elevated white blood cell (WBC) count, decreased breath sounds, and pain upon deep inhalation or coughing. Which of the following would indicate positive results after a respiratory treatment of normal saline, acetylcysteine (Mucomyst), and metaproterenol (Alupent)?

(1) Crackles and moderate amount of productive sputum
(2) Absent breath sounds in bases and normal breath sounds in upper lobes
(3) Wheezing, nonproductive cough
(4) Diminished breath sounds with small amount of productive sputum

6 Which of the following needs *immediate* medical attention and emergency intervention? The client who:

(1) Complains of sharp pain upon taking a deep breath and excessive coughing.
(2) Exhibits yellow, productive sputum, low-grade fever, and crackles.
(3) Has a shift of the trachea to the left, with no breath sounds on the right.
(4) Has asthma and complains of inability to "catch her breath" after exercise.

7 A teenage client newly diagnosed with asthma is being discharged from the hospital after an episode of status asthmaticus. Discharge teaching should include which of the following?

(1) Incidence of status asthmaticus in children and teens
(2) The relationship of symptoms to a specific trigger such as physical exercise
(3) Limitations in sports that will be imposed by the illness
(4) Specific instructions on staying calm during an attack

8 A known cardiac client is experiencing angina at night only, excessive fatigue, and the spouse states that the client snores excessively. The physician orders a sleep apnea study with and without oxygen. The rationale for considering a pulmonary source rather than a cardiac source as the cause of the angina at this time is:

(1) Sleep apnea is an obstruction of the lower airway, which impedes airflow.
(2) Clients with sleep apnea have adequate amounts of REM sleep, but snoring contributes to the decrease in oxygen levels.
(3) Sleep apnea causes an increase in muscle tone during REM sleep in order to make breathing possible.
(4) Excess periods of apnea during sleep and severe drops in oxygen levels can contribute to the angina, which is occurring only at night.

9 Which of the following symptoms is most characteristic of a client with cancer of the lung?

(1) Exertional dyspnea
(2) Persistent changing cough
(3) Air hunger; dyspnea
(4) Cough with night sweats

10 A client is admitted to the unit after a traumatic encounter with a bull in a pasture that speared his right chest wall. The client is admitted with a flail chest and is treated accordingly. The nurse should be particularly observant to the sudden changes that may be evident of which of the following?

(1) Hypercapnia
(2) Sepsis
(3) Adult respiratory distress syndrome
(4) Metabolic acidosis

See page 37 for Answers and Rationales.

I. Risk Factors Associated with Respiratory Health Problems

A. Obstructive pulmonary disorders such as asthma, chronic obstructive pulmonary disease (COPD), cystic fibrosis, bronchitis

   1. Asthma: allergies, genetic disposition

   2. COPD: primarily smoking, exposure to lung irritants, immunological factors

    3. Cystic fibrosis: genetic transmission

    4. Bronchitis: smoking, exposure to pulmonary irritants, air pollution, exposure to infectious diseases

  B. Restrictive pulmonary disorders such as atelectasis, adult respiratory distress syndrome (ARDS), flail chest, pulmonary contusion, and sleep apnea

    1. Atelectasis: surgery, trauma, pneumonia or other respiratory disorders (COPD), prolonged bedrest, mechanical ventilation

    2. ARDS: shock, trauma, smoke inhalation

    3. Sleep apnea: obesity, COPD, smoking, aging process

  C. Pneumonia: aging process, compromised respiratory conditions, debilitating diseases

  D. Tuberculosis: individuals positive for human immunodeficiency virus (HIV), immigrants and disadvantaged groups, environment (overcrowding, poor ventilation, etc.)

  E. Pleural effusion: surgery, trauma, inflammation, malignancy, or other respiratory disorder

  F. Pleuritis: none, usually secondary to other respiratory conditions

  G. Pneumothorax: smoking, trauma, men (tall, young, thin chest), family history, underlying respiratory diseases (COPD, ARDS, cystic fibrosis, asthma)

  H. Pulmonary embolism: deep vein thrombosis (DVT) or blood clots in other areas, chronic bedrest, hypercoagulability, surgery, heart conditions (congestive heart failure [CHF], myocardial infarction [MI]), obesity, women taking oral estrogen, hormones, or contraceptives

  I. Pulmonary hypertension: young women in their 30s to 40s (primary); smoking, chronic lung disease, sleep apnea, obesity, neuromuscular disease, heart conditions leading to hypoxemia (secondary)

  J. Lung cancer: smoking, lung irritants, family history, air pollution

  K. Respiratory failure: other respiratory conditions or respiratory dysfunction (COPD, pneumonia)

II. Obstructive Pulmonary Disorders

  A. Overview

    1. Obstructive pulmonary disorders are defined as disorders that obstruct airflow out of the lung, primarily impeding expiration

    2. Disorders include asthma, COPD, cystic fibrosis, and bronchiectasis

    3. Causes include infection, air pollutants, allergies, smoke inhalation, or genetics

  B. Pathophysiology

    1. Asthma is a chronic inflammatory disorder of the airways resulting in reversible bronchoconstriction and air hunger in response to triggers from a variety of sources

      a. This disorder primarily affects the bronchial airways and causes mucosal edema, secretion of mucus, and inflammation of the airway

NCLEX!

NCLEX!

    b. When exposed to a trigger, the hyperactivity of the medium-sized bronchi causes the release of leukotrienes, histamine, and other substances from the mast cells of the lung; these agents intensify the inflammatory process and cause bronchospasm

    c. *Extrinsic asthma* is triggered by factors such as cold air, high altitude, strong odors, emotional stress, hormone changes, allergens, and exercise

    d. *Intrinsic asthma* is usually from an unknown cause

    e. **Status asthmaticus** is an emergency situation when an asthma attack is prolonged and not responding to the usual medications or the client is having one asthma attack after another; prompt treatment of this condition is needed to avoid respiratory failure

2. **Chronic obstructive pulmonary disease (COPD)** is a group of pulmonary diseases of a chronic nature characterized by increased resistance to airflow; the entity is made up of emphysema, bronchitis, and possibly asthma

    a. **Emphysema** is a break down of the elastin and fiber network of the alveoli where the alveoli enlarge or the walls are destroyed; the alveolar destruction leads to the formation of larger than normal air spaces

        1) There is loss of elastic recoil as a result of the destruction of the elastin and collagen fibers found in the lung; without this recoil, air is trapped in the lung and airways collapse

NCLEX!

        2) The trapping of air results in a hyperinflated lung, causing the "barrel chest" appearance

        3) The person has the ability to maintain blood gases by hyperventilating and keeps a pink appearance of the skin, thus known as a "pink puffer" early in the disease; cyanosis may develop in the late stages

    b. Chronic **bronchitis** is an inflammatory response in the small and large airways resulting in vasodilation, congestion, mucosal edema, and bronchospasm; a chronic cough and productive sputum for a minimum of 3 months in 1 year for at least 2 consecutive years is the usual method of diagnosing

        1) The bronchial mucosal glands hypertrophy and there is an increase in the number and size of goblet cells accompanied by inflammatory cell infiltration and edema of the bronchial mucosa

        2) As the bronchial walls thicken, airflow is impeded

        3) Unlike emphysema, the individual with bronchitis cannot increase breathing efforts to maintain blood gases

NCLEX!

        4) The presence of cyanosis and edema gives the bronchitis client the term "blue bloater"

        5) In the severe state of chronic hypoxia, the kidneys increase the production of red blood cells (RBCs) in an attempt to bring more oxygenated blood to the cells, causing polycythemia, increased blood viscosity, and a higher risk for blood clots

NCLEX!

    c. Hypercapnia is typical of a client with COPD along with hypoxemia

        1) Arterial blood gases (ABGs) reflect a high CO_2 and a low O_2

2) Therefore, hypoxia is the main stimulus for ventilation rather than the normal increase in PCO_2 as a stimulus to breathe

3) Clients with COPD cannot tolerate high levels of O_2

4) Hypoxia alone is usually indicated by PaO_2 less than 80 mmHg combined with a low oxygen saturation (Cal SO_2) (see Box 1-1)

    d. Nailbeds demonstrate clubbing (angle > 160°) or a more flattened appearance because of the chronic hypoxia

3. **Cystic fibrosis** (CF) is an autosomal-recessive disorder resulting in excessive production of mucus with chronic obstructive pulmonary disease in early childhood

    a. The lack of a necessary protein needed to transport chloride results in excess absorption of water and sodium

    b. The organs, primarily the lungs, in which this protein is absent, and the deficiency in transporting chloride results in thick, viscous mucous

    c. Because of the reabsorption of sodium, sweat will have high levels of sodium and chloride

    d. The excess mucus leads to atelectasis, infections, bronchiectasis, and eventually pulmonary hypertension, and **cor pulmonale** (right-sided heart failure due to pulmonary causes)

NCLEX!

    e. In older children, the pancreas fails to function properly leading to malabsorption problems and difficulty digesting foods because of a lack of pancreatic enzymes

4. **Bronchiectasis** is a permanent enlargement of the large bronchi, often associated with respiratory infections

    a. The combination of the infection and the airway obstruction from this disorder leads to atelectasis, abscesses, destruction, and necrosis of the bronchial wall

    b. Usually associated with cystic fibrosis, but can be related to tumors, foreign bodies, tuberculosis, or exposure to lung irritants

    c. Manifested by permanently deformed and dilated distal airways, damage to the cartilage and elastic tissue supporting the airways, and fibrosis

C. **Nursing assessment**

1. Asthma

NCLEX!

    a. Assessment includes complaints of air hunger and chest tightness, anxiety, use of accessory muscles, tachypnea (increased respiratory rate), tachycardia

Box 1-1		
Normal Adult Arterial Blood Gas Values	pH	7.35–7.45
	$PaCO_2$	35–45 mmHg
	PaO_2	80–100 mmHg
	HCO_3	21–28 mEq/L
	O_2 saturation	95–100 %

(increased heart rate), and lung sounds (wheezing, long expiratory effort, diminished breath sounds in lower airways)

   b. Diagnostic tests

     1) Pulmonary function studies (PFSs) will show the decreased expiratory flow of air: forced expiratory flow (FEV_1) indicates amount of expired air, which should be about 80 percent of the client's potential and less than 20 percent variation over time

     2) Peak expiratory flow (PEF) can be measured at home using a peak flow meter (PFM) to assess the amount of expired air before and after treatment

     3) Skin testing is often done to determine problems with allergies and a challenge test using an inhaled histamine or methacholine followed by a breathing treatment may be given

2. COPD

> **NCLEX!**

   a. Assessment includes cough (productive in bronchitis, dry in emphysema), dyspnea, pursed-lip breathing, use of accessory muscles, orthopnea, nasal flaring, cachectic appearance, adventitious breath sounds (wheezing, rhonchi, or crackles), increased A:P diameter (barrel-chest), prolonged expiration, skin color (pink if emphysema in early stage; cyanotic if later stage or with chronic bronchitis), emphysemic client may have quiet, distant breath sounds, air hunger, fever, chest pain, and tachypnea; symptoms of right-sided heart failure (cor pulmonale) may occur later in the disease process

   b. Diagnostic tests: arterial blood gases (ABGs) will usually show hypercapnia and hypoxemia, FEV_1 will be decreased, chest x-ray (CXR) will show flattening of diaphragm, complete blood count (CBC) will show polycythemia

3. Cystic fibrosis

> **NCLEX!**

   a. Assessment includes a complete history of the child with particular attention to whether the symptoms have changed as the child matures

     1) Frequent symptoms include delayed growth and development, frequent respiratory problems (pneumonia, cough with excess mucus production, inability to exercise), clubbing of the fingers and toes, barrel chest, crackles, and possibly right-sided heart failure symptoms

     2) Gastrointestinal symptoms include steatorrhea (excess fat in the stools), greasy foul-smelling stools, impaired digestion, and abdominal pain

     3) Diabetes mellitus and vitamin K deficiency (from malabsorption) may ensue

   b. Diagnostic tests: sweat chloride test indicates elevated sodium and chloride concentrations; ABGs show hypoxemia, PFSs show reduced air flow and forced vital capacity (FVC_1), CXR may show atelectasis or hyperinflation, stool specimen will show steatorrhea, pulse oximetry will be low

4. Bronchiectasis

   a. Assessment includes chronic productive cough (foul-smelling, purulent sputum), wheezing or crackles, hemoptysis, dyspnea, weight loss, recurrent respiratory infections, and often right-sided heart failure or cor pulmonale

    b. Diagnostic tests: CXR will show enlarged airways; ABGs will often show hypoxemia; PFS will be similar to bronchitis; CT scan may be used to determine the extent of the damage

D. Nursing management

   1. Asthma

      a. Medications

        1) Bronchodilators to maintain patency in the bronchi

          a) Methylxanthine: theophylline (Theo-Dur, Slophyllin, Slo-bid)

          b) Adrenergics: albuterol (Proventil, Ventolin), salmeterol (Serevent), terbutaline sulfate (Brethine), isoetharine HCL (Bronkosol)

          c) Anticholinergics: ipratropium bromide (Atrovent)

          d) Anti-inflammatory: cromolyn (Intal), nedocromil (Tilade)

        2) Steroids such as beclomethasone (Beclovent, Vanceril), dexamethasone (Decadron), fluticasone (Flonase), budesonide (Rhinocort) may be used on short-term basis when exacerbation of attacks occurs or as a maintenance inhaler to suppress the inflammatory process

        3) Nonsteroidal drugs are often used as maintenance inhalers especially in children

        4) Leukotriene modifiers: zafirlukast (Accolate), montelukast (Singulair)

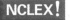

      b. Educate the client about the difference between rescue inhalers and maintenance inhalers

        1) Rescue inhalers (used for an acute attack) are drugs such as epinephrine (Adrenalin), isoproterenol solution (Isuprel), isoetharine inhalation (Bronkosol), albuterol (Ventolin, Proventil), metaproterenol (Alupent)

        2) Maintenance drugs/inhalers (used to prevent an attack) include ipratropium (Atrovent), leukotriene antagonists, salmeterol (Serevent), xanthine derivatives, cromolyn (Intal), nedocromil (Tilade)

      c. Client teaching about medications includes specific side effects and how to use metered dose inhalers (see Box 1-2)

        1) Attach canister to mouthpiece unit; shake for 3 to 5 seconds; place mouthpiece as shown (see Figure 1-1); exhale fully and slowly; press down on canister while inhaling fully through nose, *or* inhale with mouth open wide and canister in front of mouth; hold breath as long as possible; release canister and exhale; wait prescribed amount of time between inhalations (usually 30 seconds to 2 minutes) if two "puffs" ordered; rinse mouth (to reduce drying of mucous membranes and systemic absorption) and mouthpiece

        2) Teach children to use steroid inhalers before brushing their teeth to avoid oral infections

        3) Steroids can stunt the growth of children, especially under the age of 12, and may have many side effects if used on a long-term basis

Box 1-2

Using a Metered-Dose Inhaler

Purpose: To deliver a specific dose of aerosolized medication to be inhaled into the lungs for a local effect.

Rationale: Inhaled medications are easily deposited on the oral mucous membranes without reaching the lungs if a metered-dose inhaler is not used properly.

Expected Outcome: The client will correctly use an administration technique that results in the medication reaching the lungs.

Client Instructions

1. Insert the medicine canister into the inhaler unit and remove the cover from the mouthpiece. Shake the unit gently according to the manufacturer's recommendations.

2. Hold the inhaler ready for inspiration. Exhale slowly. (Do not breathe into the inhaler; that could clog the inhaler valve.)

3. Place the mouthpiece into your mouth and seal it with your lips. Tilt your head slightly back and keep your tongue away from the mouth of the inhaler.

4. Press the top of the canister at the same time as you breathe in through your mouth.

5. Remove the inhaler. Hold your breath for 2 to 3 seconds, then breathe out slowly through pursed lips.

6. Keep the cap in place between uses to prevent dirt from getting into the inhaler. To clean the inhaler, remove the metal canister and rinse the holder in warm water. Dry the holder thoroughly before using it again.

Source: Harkreader, H. (2000). *Fundamentals of nursing: Caring and clinical judgement.* Philadelphia: W. B. Saunders, p. 1071.

Figure 1-1

One method for using a metered-dose inhaler.

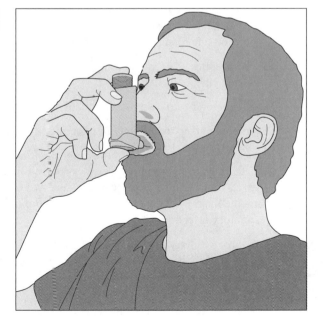

4) Theophylline preparations can reach toxic levels; monitor drug levels and report tremors or jitters to the physician

d. Teach client how to identify what triggers an attack and how to avoid these triggers

e. Educate the client on the disease process and how to avoid anxiety during an attack; immediate attention should be sought if the rescue inhaler does not work or status asthmaticus occurs

f. Teach children to carry their inhalers at all times; if an attack occurs and an inhaler is not available, drinking two regular caffeinated soda drinks may help until medications are available

g. Inhalers should be checked frequently for fullness; a convenient way to check a canister is to assess whether it floats (empty), sinks (full), or bobs halfway (half-full) when placed in water

h. Monitor VS and breath sounds, offering comfort until the medications take effect during an acute attack

i. Monitor peak flow readings, especially during allergy seasons

1) Peak flow readings may decrease as much as 24 hours prior to an attack

2) Effectiveness of the medicine used with an attack can be evaluated if the peak flow reading after use of the medicine is 80 percent of the potential for the client

2. COPD

a. Medications

1) Bronchodilators to maintain patent airways: anticholinergic agents, sympathomimetics, and methylxanthines

2) Steroids (or anti-inflammatory drugs) as needed during exacerbations; prednisone (orally) or inhalers similar to the client with asthma; monitor for side effects, especially fluid and sodium retention

3) Antibiotics as needed during acute infectious periods or prophylactically

4) Expectorants to help loosen mucus

b. Instruct clients to maintain their pneumonia and influenza vaccines

c. Educate the client about the following: smoking cessation, maintaining adequate hydration, breathing exercises (pursed-lip breathing to keep airways open by maintenance of positive pressure and abdominal breathing to expand the lungs), adequate nutrition, and avoiding other individuals with respiratory infections

d. Pulmonary toiletry may be necessary if secretions are thick: percussion (rhythmic clapping on the chest to loosen secretions), postural drainage, suctioning, and respiratory treatments

e. Use of low-flow oxygen to prevent depression of the respiratory drive

f. Evaluation of a low-profile exercise program

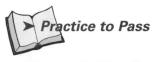

Practice to Pass

A 7-year-old child with asthma is placed on beclomethasone (Vanceril) as a maintenance inhaler. What is the major concern for a child taking this medication?

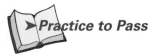

Practice to Pass

An elderly client with chronic obstructive pulmonary disease (COPD) also has a history of congestive heart failure (CHF). What is the major concern for placing this client on an oral dose of prednisone?

3. Cystic fibrosis

   a. Medications

      1) Bronchodilators if airway obstruction is problematic

      2) Antibiotics if an infection is present

      3) Dornase alfa recombinant: this drug hydrolyzes the DNA in the sputum of clients with CF; as a result, pulmonary function is improved and the number of respiratory infections is lessened

      4) Mucolytics in order to liquefy secretions as needed

NCLEX!

   b. Maintain adequate fluid, nutritional status (high in protein, fat, and calories), and electrolytes

   c. Monitor for signs and symptoms of infection closely

   d. Oxygen therapy may need to be initiated if hypoxemia is present

   e. Pulmonary toiletry may be needed to clear airways: postural drainage, positioning, suctioning, percussion, vibration, "huff" cough technique (a valved mask is used for 20 inhalations, followed by 3 to 4 huffs)

   f. Education includes respiratory care techniques, avoidance of respiratory irritants, medication administration, and dietary needs

4. Bronchiectasis: basically the same as for a client with COPD

   a. Medications include antibiotics as needed for infection; bronchodilators to maintain clear airway

   b. Pulmonary toiletry: suctioning as needed, oxygen therapy if hypoxic, percussion, and postural drainage

III. Restrictive Pulmonary Disorders

A. Overview

1. **Restrictive pulmonary disorders** are defined as disorders that limit the ability of the lung to expand normally in a respiratory cycle

2. This category includes many disorders

   a. Disorders discussed in this section: atelectasis, ARDS, flail chest, pulmonary contusion, sleep apnea

   b. Disorders discussed separately: pneumonia, pulmonary tuberculosis, pleural effusion, pneumothorax

   c. Other disorders: Pickwickian syndrome, pulmonary fibrosis, pulmonary edema

3. Causes include changes in hydrostatic or oncotic forces resulting in accumulation of fluid in the pleural spaces, trauma to the chest wall, fractured ribs, collapse of lung due to accumulation of air in the pleural sac, invasion of pathogens (bacterial, viral), reduced lung compliance, scarring and fibrosis of the parenchyma of the lung, musculoskeletal disorders, and neuromuscular disorders

B. Pathophysiology

1. **Atelectasis** is the collapse of a lung or an alveolus

   a. Perfusion occurs without ventilation because the collapsed alveoli do not participate in air exchange

   b. Without oxygen, little if any surfactant (the lipoprotein substance lining the alveoli) is produced; surfactant is needed to lower the surface tension, which lowers the resistance to expansion on inspiration and prevents collapse on expiration of the alveoli

   c. Blood flow is not interrupted, but the blood travels through airless alveoli; if a large enough area of the lung is affected, hypoxemia results

   d. *Primary atelectasis* is often associated with infants who are born with collapsed alveoli at birth; in premature births, a lack of surfactant can cause atelectasis

   e. *Secondary atelectasis* is a collapse of alveoli that were previously expanded and classified as three types

      1) *Compression atelectasis* is a result of crowding of the lung resulting in collapse and may be caused by fluid, tumor, puncture wound, or abdominal distention

      2) *Resorption atelectasis* is a result of blockage to the alveolus and can result from mucous buildup, pneumonia, cystic fibrosis, and surgery; the alveoli distal to the obstructed bronchus resorb the air and cause collapse of the alveolar wall

      3) *Contraction atelectasis* is the result of fibrosis of the lung or pleura and results in inadequate expansion of the lung

2. **Acute respiratory distress syndrome (ARDS)** is acute respiratory failure caused by many factors such as shock, trauma, burns, bacterial or viral pathogens, aspiration of fluids, and toxic injury

   a. Alveolar walls are severely impaired; pulmonary capillaries are injured or there is damage to the alveolar lining

   b. The result is increased permeability of the alveolar blood vessels, which allows fluid to accumulate in the alveolar spaces and the alveoli become airless; a tremendous strain is placed on the heart and cardiac complications are likely

   c. Fluid in the alveoli causes a decrease in surfactant and increased surface tension, leading to a loss of lung compliance, decreased ventilation, and hypoxia; the lungs become stiff and noncompliant because of the alveolar collapse

   d. As alveoli are damaged, hypoxia ensues and eventually cell injury and death occurs

      1) Inflammatory reactions can occur as the alveoli and capillaries are damaged

      2) The inflammation causes the release of cytokines that leads to damage of capillaries and alveoli nearby

3) Hyaline membranes form inside the alveoli and further hinder the exchange of oxygen and carbon dioxide

3. **Flail chest** and pulmonary contusion (bruising of lung tissue) are acute injuries of the chest wall that are usually caused by blunt trauma or penetrating objects; rib fractures and automobile accidents are a common source of chest wall injuries

   a. In flail chest, the injury results in instability of the chest wall

   b. The negative pressure created within the lung cavity upon inspiration causes the chest wall section to collapse

   c. Upon expiration, the positive pressure causes the chest wall section to expand outward

   d. Penetrating objects also affect the pressure within the lungs, which leads to collapse of portions or the entire lung

   e. Lack of proper lung expansion causes increased breathing effort, impaired gas exchange, reduced lung compliance, and pain

4. **Sleep apnea** is a lack of airflow in the upper airways for 10 seconds or more; three different forms exist:

   a. *Obstructive sleep apnea* is the most common and is caused by an obstruction to airflow while ventilatory efforts continue

      1) As many as 30 apnea periods per hour may occur while sleeping

      2) The normal pharyngeal muscle tone is lost, thus allowing the pharynx to collapse during inspiration

      3) Further obstruction occurs when the tongue falls against the posterior pharyngeal wall

      4) The individual attempts to breathe, but each effort shortens until the obstructive forces are reduced by movement or position change

   b. *Central apnea* is when the respiratory center of the brain is affected and the drive to breathe is inhibited

      1) There is no effort to breathe during the period of apnea

      2) This is thought to occur in sudden infant death syndrome (SIDS)

   c. *Mixed apnea* is a combination of both central and obstructive types of apnea

C. Nursing assessment

1. Atelectasis

   a. Assessment includes lung sounds (diminished, crackles or gurgles), tachypnea, depth and regularity of breathing, dyspnea, tachycardia, abnormal ABGs (hypoxia), temperature (if infection is suspected as the cause) and coughing

   b. Diagnostic tests: CXR that will usually reveal the area of collapsed lung, and ABGs that will show the strain the atelectasis is placing on the lung

NCLEX!

2. ARDS

a. Assessment includes respiratory distress (tachypnea, use of accessory muscles, marked dyspnea), lung sounds (crackles or rhonchi), abnormal ABGs (hypoxia and/or hypercapnia), cyanosis, retractions, agitation and confusion (late in stage)

b. Diagnostic tests: CXR (large, diffuse infiltrates or "white outs" with normal heart size), ABGs ($PaO_2 < 50$ mmHg and respiratory alkalosis), PFS (decreased lung compliance; reduced vital capacity, minute volume, and functional vital capacity), and pulmonary artery pressure monitoring for diagnostic purposes (normal pressures will be evident in ARDS versus elevated pressures in pulmonary edema)

3. Flail chest and pulmonary contusion

a. Assessment includes asymmetry of chest expansion and paradoxical chest movement, pain upon inspiration, dyspnea, tachypnea, lung sounds (diminished, rales, rhonchi), palpable crepitus (the sound of crackling cellophane when the skin is touched), and tachycardia

b. Specific symptoms for pulmonary contusion include the above symptoms plus copious (often blood-tinged) sputum, restlessness, and apprehension

c. Diagnostic tests: CXR, ABGs

4. Sleep apnea

a. Assessment includes changes in behavior and performance (irritability, daytime drowsiness, decreased ability to function, forgetfulness, lethargy), verbal complaints of feeling tired or listless, dark circles under eyes, frequent yawning, changes in posture, loud snoring, cardiac arrhythmias, angina at night, headaches due to hypercapnia, periods of apnea during sleep, impotence, and respiratory depression (related to certain medications used)

b. Diagnostic tests: electroencephalography (EEG) to identify stages of sleep, electrocardiogram (ECG) to identify arrhythmias, polysomnography (overnight sleep study—with and without oxygen); a CBC may be ordered to assess for erythrocytosis (or polycythemia) caused by oxygen needs, and a thyroid function study to rule out hypothyroidism

D. Nursing management

1. Atelectasis

a. Medications include antibiotics if an infection is suspected as the cause, bronchodilators, and analgesics as necessary

b. Administer oxygen to enhance oxygenation at the alveolar level and monitor oxygen saturation

c. Elevate the head of bed

d. Encourage turning, coughing, and deep breathing as often as every 2 hours

e. Encourage the use of the incentive spirometry every 1–2 hours

f. Encourage adequate fluid intake unless otherwise contraindicated

g. Encourage ambulation as ordered

NCLEX!

2. ARDS

    a. Medications

        1) Nitrous oxide for its analgesic effect or to dilate blood vessels and improve oxygenation

        2) Nonsteroidal anti-inflammatory drugs (NSAIDs), interleukin-1 receptor antagonists, neutrophil inhibitors, or corticosteroids to reduce inflammation

        3) Lung surfactants: beractant (Survanta) and calfactant (Beractant) to lower surface tension of the alveoli and prevent alveolar collapse; this action restores pulmonary compliance and oxygenation

        4) Antibiotics if an infection is suspected as the cause

        5) Heparin to prevent complication of ARDS such as thrombophlebitis, pulmonary embolus, or disseminated intravascular coagulation (DIC)

        6) Sedative agents or skeletal muscle relaxants such as pancuronium bromide (Tubocurarine) to control the agitation associated with mechanical ventilation

    b. Foremost therapy is to treat the cause

    c. Main form of therapy is endotracheal intubation and mechanical ventilation

        1) Continuous positive airway pressure (CPAP) or positive-end expiratory pressure (PEEP) is often used to open the airways and alveoli and to improve gas exchange

        2) PEEP has been associated with decreased cardiac output, lung injury caused by the high mechanical pressure to lung tissue known as barotrauma; vital signs (VS), especially a drop in blood pressure (BP), and lung sounds should be monitored

    d. Maintaining a prone position may improve oxygen perfusion

    e. Monitor pulmonary arterial pressure through use of a Swan-Ganz line

    f. Maintain adequate fluid and nutritional status

    g. Monitor oxygen saturation and signs of a pneumothorax, which is a complication of ARDS

3. Flail chest and pulmonary contusion

    a. Medications

        1) Analgesics to maintain control of pain, initially on a *scheduled dosing pattern* rather than as needed; continuous epidural analgesia or even intercostal nerve blocks may be recommended forms of analgesia

        2) Sedatives or neuromuscular blockers to control agitation while on mechanical ventilation

        3) Bronchodilators

        4) Antibiotics as a preventive measure

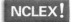

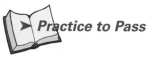

Practice to Pass

A client, who has suffered a large myocardial infarction (MI) and has had difficulty recuperating, suddenly goes into acute respiratory distress syndrome (ARDS). Why should treatment be aggressive in this situation?

    b. Administer oxygen as ordered

    c. Internal or external fixation of the flail area may be necessary

        1) Use of a sandbag for flail chest may help to stabilize the area through external fixation

        2) Endotracheal intubation and mechanical ventilation with PEEP may support ventilation and provide internal fixation

    d. Maintain adequate hydration while avoiding overhydration

    e. Turn, cough, and deep-breathe every 2 hours, yet restrict overall activity to reduce oxygen needs and plan for adequate rest periods

    f. Oral or nasal suctioning as needed

    g. Educate the client on using a pillow to splint the area during coughing

    h. Maintain the bed with the head in an elevated position

    i. Monitor VS, oxygen saturation, and level of consciousness (LOC)

    j. Chest tube insertion may be necessary for chest contusions

        1) For chest tubes, assess respiratory status every 2 to 4 hours, maintain a closed system, milk the chest tubes every 2 hours as needed if protocol present, check the water seal frequently (water level should fluctuate with inspiration and have periodic air bubbles), assess amount, color, consistency of drainage every 4 to 8 hours, and assess the water level

        2) Continuous air bubbles usually indicate an air leak and lack of fluctuation indicates inadequate function of the system

4. Sleep apnea

    a. Medications

        1) Medroxyprogesterone (Depo-Provera, Provera): stimulates respirations in obese clients who hypoventilate

        2) Theophylline: relaxes smooth muscle of bronchi

        3) Protriptyline (Vivactil): a tricyclic antidepressant

        4) Clonazepam (Klonopin): an anticonvulsant

        5) Fluoxetine hydrochloride (Prozac): an antidepressant

        6) Hypnotics, sedatives, androgens, and alcohol should be completely avoided because of their effects on the respiratory system

    b. Implementation of weight reduction plan

    c. Continuous positive airway pressure (CPAP) therapy is the most commonly prescribed treatment to force air into the back of the throat with the use of a compressor and reduce the airway occlusion experienced in sleep apnea; a humidifier is often recommended because of the drying effect of the oxygen treatment

    d. Nosebleeds and nasal congestion may occur while using the oxygen and CPAP secondary to dryness

    e. Oxygen supplementation may be recommended

f. Maintain adequate fluid intake

g. Surgery may be recommended including tonsillectomy, adenoidectomy, and uvulopalatopharyngoplasty, removal of tissue contributing to the obstruction from the soft palate, uvula and posterior pharyngeal wall

h. Oral/dental applications have been tried to reposition the mandible with success in some clients

IV. Pneumonia

A. Overview

1. Pneumonia is defined as inflammation of the bronchioles, alveoli, interstitial tissues, and on occasion the pleura as a result of infection

2. Pneumonia may be defined by the cause, location, or contributing factors

   a. Cause: bacteria, viruses, fungi, protozoa, or parasites

      1) Common bacteria include *Streptococcus pneumonia* (most common), *staphylococcus, Haemophilus influenzae* and *Pseudomonas* (Gram-negative)

      2) Fungi include *Aspergillus fumigatus, Candida albicans,* and *Pneumocystis carinii*

   b. Location: lobular pneumonia meaning involvement of the one lobe, lobar pneumonia meaning involvement of the entire lung, or bronchopneumonia meaning involvement of the lobes adjacent to the bronchi

   c. Contributing factors: aspiration pneumonia often occurs with tube feedings; postoperative pneumonia occurs following a surgical procedure; and hospital acquired pneumonia occurs after admittance into a hospital setting

NCLEX!

3. Atypical pneumonia is a type of pneumonia that does not present with the usual symptoms or evolve in the usual pattern; examples of two types of atypical pneumonia are pneumocystosis, caused by *pneumocystis carinii* (associated with immunosuppressed clients) or Legionnaires' disease (caused by *Legionella pneumophila*)

   a. Pneumocystosis is a type of pneumococci caused by the parasite *Pneumocystitis carinii;* most prominent in clients with AIDS, debilitated or immuno-suppressed individuals; symptoms include fever, cough, and dyspnea; has high mortality rate and is difficult to diagnose; treated with pentamidine isoethionate (Pentam 300)

   b. Legionnaires' disease is an acute bacterial pneumonia; flu-like symptoms occur followed by fever, chills, headache, and muscle aches; usually self-limiting and not highly contagious; treated with erythromycin

4. Organisms may enter the lung through accidental inhalation, close contact with an infected person, or introduction of the organism through an outside means such as suctioning, intubation, or through the blood

B. Pathophysiology

1. Although normal flora contains many bacteria, which are pathogens by nature, these organisms cause pneumonia when they invade the lower respiratory tract

2. Organisms such as *Escherichia coli* or *Pseudomonas aeruginosa* are common in the enteric flora but not a part of the upper respiratory tract; these organisms can contaminate the lungs by way of the circulatory system

3. The inflammation within the lung is similar to the inflammatory process anywhere within the body

   a. The introduction of the bacteria promotes an antigen-antibody response and endotoxins are released

   b. Air spaces of the alveoli become engorged with fluid and red blood cells and exudate forms

   c. The infiltration of lymphocytes, neutrophils, erythrocytes, and fibrin results in cellular infiltration and massive congestion

   d. The alveoli become airless because of the exudate and perfusion with poor ventilation results

   e. Consolidation of lung tissue results and presents on the CXR as white "patchy" infiltrate

   f. Damage may occur to the bronchial and alveolar mucous membranes

4. Signs and symptoms of pneumonia include coughing, fatigue, pleuritic pain, dyspnea, chills, fever, elevated white blood count (WBC), sputum production (rust-colored or purulent), crackles or rales, pleural rub, and tachypnea; elderly clients may present with less dramatic symptoms and may experience changes in mental status or be easily agitated

C. Nursing assessment

1. Assessment

   a. Subjective/objective: cough (productive or nonproductive; effectiveness of cough; if productive, color, amount, and odor); pain with inspiration or cough

   b. General symptoms: fever

   c. Inspect for dyspnea and tachycardia

   d. Auscultate lung sounds (rales, rhonchi)

2. Diagnostic tests: CXR (shows consolidation in affected lobe), CBC (elevated WBC), and culture and sensitivity (C&S) of sputum, possible gram stain, ABGs (expect to see $PaO_2 > 75$ mmHg), pulse oximetry (expect to see 95 percent or higher), and blood cultures

D. Nursing management

1. Medications

   a. Antibiotic therapy as indicated by culture and sensitivity; may begin with a broad-spectrum antibiotic such as one of the penicillins, erythromycins, or cephalosporins until results of culture and sensitivity (C&S) are available (see Chapter 13)

   b. Antipyretics

   c. Bronchodilators

      1) Sympathomimetic drugs such as albuterol sulfate (Proventil) or metaproterenol (Alupent)

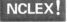

Practice to Pass

A client with pneumonia continues to run a temperature of 102 to 103°F even after taking an antibiotic for 3 days. What could account for this and what should be done?

2) Methylxanthines such as theophylline and aminophylline

    d. Drugs used to liquefy mucus, such as guaifenesin, acetylcysteine (Mucomyst)

2. Increase fluid intake to 2,500 to 3,000 cc/day to help liquefy secretions unless contraindicated due to a cardiac condition

3. Administer oxygen therapy as ordered

    a. Nasal cannula for delivering 24 to 45 percent oxygen concentration

    b. Face mask for delivering 40 to 60 percent oxygen concentration

    c. Nonrebreather mask for delivering up to 100 percent oxygen concentration

    d. Venturi mask for precise measurement of air flow

4. Chest physiotherapy including postural draining and percussion; in the initial stage, lung sounds may worsen and cough may become more productive after chest physiotherapy if the congestion is extremely consolidated and if the treatment is effective in loosening the secretions

5. Endotracheal suctioning if necessary

6. Monitor respiratory rate, depth, and use of accessory muscles

7. Instruct client how to splint the chest wall with a pillow to cough more effectively

8. Monitor for intolerance to exercise or need for assistance with activities of daily living (ADLs)

9. Encourage client to turn, cough, and deep-breathe

10. Encourage elderly and at-risk clients to have a pneumonia vaccine every 5 years

V. Pulmonary Tuberculosis (TB)

A. Overview

1. Tuberculosis (TB) is a type of pneumonia caused by the acid-fast bacillus, *Mycobacterium tuberculosis*

2. TB has been fairly controlled until recently; TB in the immunosuppressed population has aided in the development of resistant strains of the disease

3. The primary defense mechanism against the bacillus is a cell-mediated immune response instead of an acute inflammatory reaction

4. Two types exist: *primary infection,* which means someone who has not been previously exposed and *secondary tuberculosis,* which means reactivation of dormant bacilli has occurred

5. Although the organisms are contracted by airborne droplets from an individual with an active form of the disease and usually affect the lungs, the disease can lie dormant for many years and be reinactivated as well as invade other parts of the body

B. Pathophysiology

1. Organisms carried by airborne droplets enter the lungs and multiple in the pulmonary alveoli

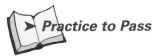

Practice to Pass

A female visits the Emergency Department because of symptoms of gonorrhea. She admits that she practices prostitution and has never been tested for human immunodeficiency virus (HIV). Why would a tuberculosis (TB) skin test be an appropriate order?

2. As the organisms multiply, they enter the lymphatic system and bloodstream, stimulating a cell-mediated response

3. Neutrophils and macrophages are immediately released to the lungs to assist in the attack on the bacilli

4. The bacilli cannot be destroyed, but can be isolated; as macrophages attack the organisms, a granuloma (or tubercle) is formed with inner areas of necrosis; the lymphocytes and macrophages form a giant cell known as Langerhans

5. If arrested, these granulomas scar or calcify (called Gohn's complex) and can be identified on a CXR; symptoms of the disease may not be present if the organisms are arrested early

6. In the event that the cell-mediated response by the body fails, organisms within a calcified granuloma can be reactivated; if the immune system is deficient or if the number of organisms is extremely large, damage to the lung tissue may occur

7. The *M. tuberculosis* is a rod-shaped bacteria that has a waxy capsule; the waxy capsule requires Gram-staining in order to turn the organism red, and is therefore called "acid-fast bacillus"

8. Major complications from the disease include diffusion of oxygen and carbon dioxide leading to decreased gas exchange, decreased surface area available for gas diffusion, abnormalities in ventilation-perfusion ratio, hypoxia, and pulmonary hypertension

9. Other complications

   a. Tuberculosis pneumonia, a massive lobular or lobar pneumonia

   b. Pleuritis

   c. Extrapulmonary tuberculosis: swallowed bacilli may cause tuberculosis in the GI tract (small intestines), liver, bones, joints, skin, and genitourinary tract; this type is often seen in individuals with HIV

   d. Miliary tuberculosis, spreading of the tubercle into the bloodstream

   e. Tuberculosis meningitis, spreading of the tuberculosis to the subarachnoid space

   f. Sepsis and respiratory failure

10. Signs and symptoms of tuberculosis include coughing (usually productive in active stage, dry in initial stage), fever in the afternoon or night (maybe low-grade), malaise, night sweats, anorexia, weight loss, chest pain, hemoptysis (blood in sputum), dyspnea, crackles, and enlarged, often painful lymph nodes

C. Nursing assessment

1. Assessment includes: symptom analysis of type and progression of symptoms; color, consistency, and amount of sputum; knowledge of the disease; weight pattern; vital signs; description of any pain; palpable lymph nodes; breath sounds; and activity tolerance

2. Diagnostic tests

   a. CXR (shows dense lesions in the upper lobes, enlarged lymph nodes, and formation of large cavities)

     b. CBC (presence of leukocytosis)

     c. Fiberoptic bronchoscopy and bronchial washing (for obtaining culture specimens)

     d. Tuberculin skin test (positive at 5 to 9 mm for clients with abnormal CXR or HIV; positive at 10 to 15mm for clients with high risk factors such as intravenous (IV) drug use, residence in a long-term facility, high-incidence country; positive at 15 mm for all other people)

     e. Three early morning sputum collections for acid-fast staining, culture and sensitivity positive for *M. tuberculosis;* results may take up to 10 days

D. Nursing management

    1. Medications include *single dose* treatment for prevention or exposure and *at least two* antibacterial medications for an active case of the disease or resistant strains

       a. Prevention of TB requires taking the medication for 6 to 12 months for exposure and at least 9 months for clients with HIV

       b. For resistant strains, three or more agents may be combined according to the sensitivity report

       c. Medications may be prescribed prophylactically even though symptoms are not present if a positive TB result was obtained

       d. Recommended anti-infective agents: isoniazid (INH), rifampin (Rifadin), ethambutol (EMB), streptomycin (SM), pyrazinamide (PZA)

       e. Secondary agents: para-aminosalicylic acid (PAS), cycloserine (Seromycin), capreomycin (Capastat), ethionamide (Trecator-SC)

    2. Hepatotoxicity is a common side effect for many of these agents and should be monitored closely

    3. Compliance is a common problem because of the length of time needed to administer the medications; instruct the client on the compliance needed with medication administration

    4. Clients should be informed of color changes in the urine with some of the agents like rifampin (Rifadin)

    5. Once positive, the purified protein derivative (PPD) will remain positive and should not be repeated; a CXR may be ordered to verify exposure versus active disease process

    6. Monitor vital signs, noting a pattern of late afternoon low-grade fever

    7. Suction as needed for productive cough

    8. Maintain adequate hydration and nutritional status; high-protein, high-carbohydrate diet recommended

    9. Monitor weight every day for loss

    10. Isolate clients (in negative-pressure room) with active cases until medication therapy has been initiated

    11. Initiate screening for all family members or close contacts

12. Assist client to turn, cough, and deep-breathe

13. Monitor breath sounds every 4 hours

14. Encourage frequent rest periods

VI. Pleural Effusion

A. Overview

1. **Pleural effusion** is defined as an excessive amount of fluid located in the pleural space between the visceral and parietal layers

2. Usually considered a secondary rather than primary disorder

3. Causes of pleural effusion are either systemic or local

   a. Systemic diseases

      1) Hydrothorax: heart failure, renal failure, liver failure

      2) Empyema (pus in the pleural cavity): infections, malignancies, connective tissue disorders

   b. Local diseases

      1) Hemothorax (blood in the cavity): chest wall injuries, surgery to the chest

      2) Chylothorax: trauma, inflammation (pneumonia, tuberculosis), or malignancy

B. Pathophysiology

1. A pleural effusion results from:

   a. An increase in hydrostatic pressure in the pleural capillaries or decreased colloid osmotic pressure in the circulatory system that can lead to excess pleural fluid (known as transudative)

   b. An increased capillary permeability as a result of inflammation, infection, or malignancy (known as exudative)

2. Regardless of the cause, the excess pressure exerted by the fluid in the pleural space compresses the lung and limits its ability to expand, thus compromising gas exchange

3. The amount of fluid in the pleural space can become so large as to displace lung tissue and result in a compression atelectasis

4. The decreased lung volume on the affected side results in diminished or absent breath sounds

5. Signs and symptoms include dyspnea, diminished or absent breath sounds on the affected side, pain, limited chest wall movement, and dull or flat sounds on percussion

C. Nursing assessment

1. Assessment includes symptom analysis of any pain experienced, c/o dyspnea, coughing, vital signs (elevated temperature), respiratory rate and status (shallow respirations, asymmetry), lung sounds (diminished), and percussion for flat or dull sound over area

2. Diagnostic tests: CXR ("white out"—opaque densities of area involved); thoracentesis (aspiration of fluid from pleural space); culture, sensitivity, and cytological examination of fluid if any removed; a CT scan and ultrasonography can determine pleural effusions if needed

D. Nursing management

1. Medications

   a. Antipyretics if fever or pain is present

   b. Antibiotics, parenterally or instillation into the pleural space for repeated effusions

NCLEX!

2. The goal of treatment should be to resolve the underlying disease process causing the problem and prevention of complications such as atelectasis or pneumothorax

3. Monitor VS, especially respiratory rate, rhythm, and use of accessory muscles

4. Monitor lung sounds and complaints of dyspnea

5. Manage pain if necessary along with bedrest

NCLEX!

6. Monitor for signs of changing status: tachycardia, hypotension, increasing shortness of breath (SOB)

VII. Pleuritis (Pleurisy)

A. Overview

1. **Pleuritis (pleurisy)** is an inflammation of the pleura and is often accompanied by abrupt onset of pain

2. Classifications

   a. Primary or secondary; secondary is typically a result of another respiratory illness such as pneumonia, pleural effusion, or trauma to the lung

   b. Unilateral, bilateral, or local; unilateral is most typical

   c. Acute or chronic; acute is most common

   d. Fibrinous or adhesive: fibrinous is characterized by typical symptoms of severe pain without any fluid return upon aspiration; adhesion occurs when the parietal pleura adhere to the visceral pleura and complete obliteration of the pleural space can occur

   e. Dry or with effusion (pleural effusion); dry is more painful and usually accompanies pneumonia; adhesions may form

B. Pathophysiology

1. The inner visceral layer that lies adjacent to the lung and the outer parietal layer that lies adjacent to the chest wall form a cavity with a thin layer of serous fluid known as the pleural cavity; the pressure in the pleural cavity is negative compared to the alveolar pressure in order to keep the lungs from collapsing

2. Introduction of an infectious process such as pneumonia or viral respiratory diseases can extend to the pleura and cause an inflammatory process in the pleural cavity

3. Signs and symptoms of pleurisy

   a. Abrupt pain that is usually unilateral and localized to a specific portion of the chest; the pain is sharp, stabbing and may radiate to the neck or shoulder; pressure changes caused by breathing, movement or coughing will intensify the pain

   b. Other symptoms may include fever, cough (dry, hacking), localized tenderness, diminished breath sounds, tachypnea, and pleural friction rub

C. **Nursing assessment**

1. Assessment includes symptom analysis of pain, vital signs, percussion, lung sounds, visual inspection for symmetry of chest wall during respirations

2. Diagnostic tests: CXR (diagnostic purposes only to rule out other pulmonary disorders) and ABGs

D. **Nursing management**

1. Medications include analgesics or NSAIDs for pain and fever; antibiotics; cough suppressant for nighttime such as codeine (this should be avoided, however, if a productive cough is present)

2. Encourage bedrest

3. Monitor VS, noting fever and respiratory rate

4. Assess respiratory status, percussion, and auscultation of lung sounds

5. Encourage deep breathing and coughing every 1–2 hours, splinting the chest wall when coughing

VIII. Pneumothorax/Hemothorax

A. **Overview**

1. **Pneumothorax** is defined as the entrance of air into the pleural cavity resulting in a complete or partial collapse of the affected lung

   a. *Spontaneous pneumothorax* is a sudden collapse of the lung due to leakage of air into the pleural cavity from within the lung or from an unknown cause; may occur in tall, thin young men who are healthy or secondary to other disease processes such as COPD, asthma, tuberculosis, emphysema, ARDS, cystic fibrosis, etc.; smoking and family history are thought to contribute to this type of pneumothorax

   b. *Traumatic pneumothorax* is usually caused by a traumatic injury to the chest wall causing blunt or penetrating trauma; is usually a result of a stabbing, gunshot wound, rib fracture, motor vehicle accident, or a severe fall; may be open or termed a "sucking chest" and is fatal due to the severe hypoventilation that occurs from the collapse of the lung

   c. *Tension pneumothorax* is a dangerous complication and a medical emergency where the entering air cannot escape by the same route and pressure within the pleural cavity increases resulting in complete collapse of the lung; a mediastinal shift to the unaffected side and a downward displacement of the diaphragm can be observed

   d. *Iatrogenic pneumothorax* is defined as a pneumothorax resulting from a medical intervention, i.e., placement of a catheter, biopsy procedures, cardiopulmonary resuscitation (CPR), mechanical ventilation, or anesthesia

2. **Hemothorax** is defined as the presence of blood in the pleural cavity

3. The symptoms, diagnosis, and treatment for all are similar; the severity, type, and size of the pneumothorax determine the degree of symptoms experienced by the client

B. Pathophysiology

1. The pleural cavity surrounding the lungs maintains an airtight seal and has pressure less than that within the lungs in order for the lungs to remain expanded, known as "negative" pressure; if this negative pressure is lost due to any opening of the pleural cavity, the lung collapses because of the natural contraction of the elastic tissue of the lung; the rupture of the pleural cavity allows air to flow in and out of the space, thus affecting the expansion and recoil of the lung (see Figure 1-2)

NCLEX!

2. In a tension pneumothorax, an added complication hinders the lungs even further

   a. The air enters the pleural space on inspiration as seen with a pneumothorax

   b. On expiration, the rising pressure in the pleural space closes the tear or rupture and air is trapped

   c. Each consecutive breath forces more air into the pleural cavity and the lung collapses completely because of the force of the pressure being exerted

   d. Pressure is exerted on the opposite lung and venous return to the heart is affected; his condition can be fatal if not treated promptly (refer again to Figure 1-2)

NCLEX!

3. Signs and symptoms of a pneumothorax/hemothorax are severe shortness of breath, sharp, intense pain on the affected side which may be worse on inspiration, tympanic resonance, absence of breath sounds on affected side, distention

Figure 1-2   **Pneumothorax. A. A spontaneous pneumothorax with an air leak from the lung into the pleural space. B. A traumatic or open pneumothorax (sucking chest wound) in which air enters the pleural space through a wound in the chest wall. C. A tension pneumothorax. Air enters the pleural space during inspiration but is unable to exit during expiration, resulting in rapid lung collapse and a shift of mediastinal structures toward the unaffected side.**

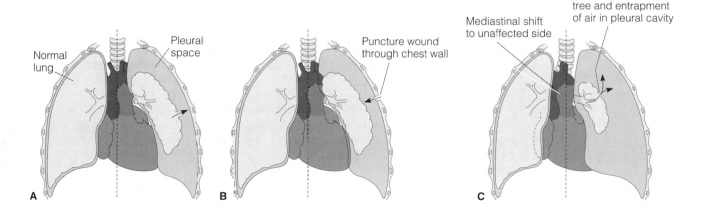

on one side of chest, tachypnea, distended neck veins due to the pressure in the thorax, subcutaneous emphysema (crepitus), hypoxemia, cyanosis, anxiety, and diaphoresis; a shift of the mediastinum to the unaffected side may be visibly seen in a tension pneumothorax

C. Nursing assessment

1. Assessment includes description of pain and onset, visual inspection (asymmetry of lungs, shift of trachea, and use of accessory muscles), percussion over affected area, auscultation of lung sounds bilaterally, vital signs (tachycardia, hypotension, tachypnea), signs of hypoxemia (ABGs, pulse oximetry, color)

2. Diagnostic tests: CXR (asymmetry of lung expansion, shift in diaphragm or mediastinum, air in pleural cavity), ABGs (decreased PaO_2, decreased pH, increased $PaCO_2$), pulse oximetry (saturation of less than or equal to 92 percent), and CBC if hemothorax suspected; thoracentesis may be indicated to assess for fluid in the pleural cavity as a treatment or diagnostic tool

D. Nursing management

1. Medications include analgesics and antibiotics (if fluid is present and chest tube is inserted)

NCLEX!

2. Administer oxygen as indicated, monitoring pulse oximetry

NCLEX!

3. Assist with insertion of and maintenance of chest tube, noting fluid drainage, color, consistency, and amount; monitor that water-seal is maintained and that tubing is not kinked; monitor insertion site for signs of infection

4. Administer blood transfusion as indicated by orders

5. Assist with thoracentesis (insertion of a needle to withdraw air)

6. Monitor lung sounds and vital sounds

NCLEX!

7. Maintain high Fowler's position for ease in breathing

8. Turn and ambulate client, allowing for frequent rest periods

IX. Pulmonary Embolism (PE)

A. Overview

1. **Pulmonary embolism** is defined as blockage of a pulmonary artery by an embolus or blood clot that has often traveled from a lower extremity

2. This disorder is often a major complication of a deep vein thrombosis (DVT), therefore maintenance heparin therapy is recommended to prevent the dislodging of an embolus

3. Although the lower extremity is the usual source of the emboli, other sources include a thromboembolism from the systemic venous system entering the right side of the heart, a tumor, or other substances such as fat, air, amniotic fluid, or pieces of tissue

4. The disorder may manifest itself as several tiny clots, one large clot, or a multitude of showered clots in the lung

5. Contributing factors for a pulmonary embolus include venous stasis often associated with prolonged bedrest or surgery, hypercoagulability, obesity, childbirth, use of birth control pills, cardiac diseases, and trauma

B. Pathophysiology

1. A portion of a thrombus dislodges and travels (as an embolus) through the venous circulation to the right side of the heart and enters the pulmonary artery, typically lodging there

2. The blocked pulmonary artery causes a decreased blood flow to the lung and can result in infarction to the lung tissue

   a. The lung does have two other sources of oxygen however to compensate: air from the bronchi and oxygen from the blood flow from the bronchial artery arising from the descending portion of the aorta

   b. Death can occur if the infarcted section of the lung is large enough

3. The clot may block the entire main pulmonary artery (known as a *saddle embolus,* which is lethal) or may block smaller branches of the pulmonary circulation, causing pulmonary infarcts (can be asymptomatic or cause pleuritic pain due to the irritation on the pleura); the fibrinolytic action in the body often destroys smaller clots

4. The result of an embolus to the lung is ventilation without perfusion, which alters the oxygenation of body tissues; with pulmonary embolism, alveolar dead space (the alveoli not participating in gas exchange) is increased

5. As a result of the blockage of the pulmonary artery, the right side of the heart is unable to pump blood sufficiently and distends as does the proximal portion of the pulmonary artery (prior to the obstruction)

6. This decrease in oxygenation of blood results in less blood flow to the left side of the heart and consequently to the brain and other vital organs

7. Complications of a pulmonary embolus include pulmonary edema, atelectasis, severe hypoxia, shock, and elevated pulmonary circulation pressures

8. Signs and symptoms include tachypnea, tachycardia, hypotension, sudden acute dyspnea with extreme anxiety, chest or pleuritic pain (sharp, localized), abnormal lung sounds (wheezing, decreased breath sounds or crackles), hypoxemia, respiratory alkalosis, friction rub, diaphoresis, and coughing; large clots or more complicated situations include pulmonary hypertension, shock, right heart failure, or sudden respiratory arrest

9. Suspect PE whenever a client presents with *sudden onset* of pleuritic pain, SOB, and extreme anxiety while recovering from a lower extremity surgery, childbirth, major surgery, DVT, or on prolonged bedrest; the anxiety is often described as a feeling of doom, impeding death, and is associated with fear of suffocating

C. Nursing assessment

1. Assessment includes analysis of type of pain (increased with inspiration), anxiety level, color (cyanosis), LOC, respiratory status, vital signs, symptoms of DVT (warmth, tenderness, swelling or lower leg or calf), and auscultation of lung sounds

2. Diagnostic tests

   a. CXR: wedge-shaped density (infarcted area), elevated diaphragms, atelectasis, or pleural effusions

   b. ABGs: decreased PaO_2, $PaCO_2$, and elevated pH—respiratory alkalosis

   c. Electrocardiogram (ECG): ST-T wave changes, right axis deviation; done also to rule out a myocardial infarcion

   d. Ventilation-perfusion lung scan or radioisotope lung scan: by injecting radioisotope, peripherally blocked areas will show no blood flow; does not actually diagnose an embolus

   e. Pulmonary angiography: direct visualization of pulmonary artery and branches for a definite diagnosis

   f. Ultrasound of legs

   g. CT scan

   h. Lab work: decreased partial thromboplastin time (PTT) or prothombin time (PT), elevated bilirubin, elevated lactic dehydrogenase (LDH), elevated fibrin degradation tests

   i. The partial thromboplastin time (PTT) and prothrombin time (PT) will be used for monitoring anticoagulant therapy once started and should be 1.5 to 2.0 times the control value for a therapeutic level; monitor closely for signs of bleeding while on the heparin; an international normalized ratio (INR) may be used to monitor oral anticoagulant therapy (2.0–3.0 therapeutic)

D. Nursing management

1. Medications

   a. Anticoagulants: heparin followed by sodium warfarin (Coumadin) for confirmed PE; low molecular weight heparin (LMWH) for prevention after surgery, particularly hip surgery

   b. Thrombolytic therapy if the clot is excessively large or needs to be dissolved immediately (tissue plasminogen activator [t-PA], streptokinase)

   c. Analgesics for discomfort or anxiety

   d. Vasopressors if needed for hypotension

2. Administer parenteral fluids as indicated

3. Maintain bed rest to reduce oxygen needs and a high Fowler's position if indicated

4. Reassure client often to reduce anxiety

5. Administer oxygen as ordered

6. Apply antiembolism stockings

7. Prevention includes early ambulation after surgery and leg exercises

8. Monitor ECG for cardiac arrhythmias

9. Monitor pulmonary artery wedge pressures and cardiac output

10. Monitor vital signs, respiratory assessment, LOC, skin color, and mental status

11. Auscultate heart and lung sounds

12. Monitor lab values and signs of bleeding if on anticoagulant therapy (hematuria, oozing from venipuncture sites or IV lines, bleeding from gums or incisions, excessive bruising)

13. PT or PTT values are not recommended during LMWH therapy

X. Pulmonary Hypertension

A. Overview

1. **Pulmonary hypertension** is defined as elevated pressures in the pulmonary artery usually resulting from pulmonary or cardiac disease

2. Pulmonary artery pressure is normally 12 to 15 mmHg (25 systolic/8 diastolic), a resting mean pressure greater than 20 mmHg constitutes an elevation

3. Usually classified as primary or secondary

   a. *Primary pulmonary hypertension* (PPH) is not related to any known cause, has a higher incidence in young women 20 to 30 years of age, is highly uncommon, and can lead to death in 3 to 5 years

   b. *Secondary pulmonary hypertension* is caused by a pulmonary or cardiac disease process including hypoxia, congenital cardiac disease, emboli, COPD, sleep apnea, mitral stenosis, left ventricular failure, and pulmonary emboli

   c. Cor pulmonale, right ventricular hypertrophy and failure result from long-term pulmonary hypertension

B. Pathophysiology

1. Narrowing of the pulmonary vascular bed from major cardiac or pulmonary diseases is the common cause of pulmonary hypertension; vessel destruction, vasoconstriction, or obstruction may all contribute to the narrowing of the pulmonary bed

2. The medial (muscular) layer of the pulmonary vasculature thickens and extensive intimal fibrosis may occur in severe cases

3. The pulmonary vascular system usually has low pressure, high blood flow, and low resistance

4. Pulmonary hypertension can be caused by any condition that results in an exaggerated blood flow in the pulmonary bed, a higher resistance to the blood flow, or a blockage of the blood flow

5. Complications of pulmonary hypertension include cor pulmonale or pulmonary edema due to the inability of the pressures in the pulmonary artery to be lowered

6. Signs and symptoms of pulmonary hypertension may not be detected until a significant rise in the pulmonary artery pressure occurs and is reflected in a rise in the systolic pressure

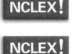

7. Clinical manifestations may include fatigue, angina, dyspnea (on exertion and at rest), tachypnea, abnormal breath sounds (distant, decreased, crackles), cyanosis, and dizziness especially upon exertion; in addition, there may be signs of the underlying condition that can mask the symptoms of pulmonary hypertension

C. Nursing assessment

1. Assessment includes symptom analysis of any physical complaints, skin color, signs of edema, vital signs, use of accessory respiratory muscles, breath sounds, and heart sounds

2. Diagnostic tests: CBC (may show polycythemia), ABGs (hypoxemia), CXR (enlarged right ventricle, dilated pulmonary arteries), ECG (right ventricular hypertrophy, right axis deviation, right bundle branch block), echocardiogram (enlarged right atrium, decreased wall motion), cardiac catheterization (elevated pulmonary artery pressures, decreased cardiac output)

D. Nursing management

1. Medications

   a. Calcium channel blockers: nifedipine (Procardia), diltiazem (Cardizem) to lower pulmonary vascular resistance

   b. Direct vasodilators: adenosine (Adenocard), inhaled nitric oxide, hydralazine (Apresoline) to decrease afterload

   c. Angiotensin converting enzyme (ACE) inhibitors

   d. Diuretics and digitalis in the event cor pulmonale occurs

2. Secondary pulmonary hypertension is aimed at treating the underlying disease

3. Administer oxygen as ordered to assist in treating hypoxemia

4. Phlebotomy is recommended if polycythemia is present

5. Treatment of cor pulmonale includes fluid restriction, limited salt, and diuretics

6. Monitor activity if intolerance to physical exertion is severe, plan rest periods, and assist with ADLs

7. Monitor vital signs, lung sounds, and heart sounds

8. Assist the client in high Fowler's position if needed

9. Encourage coughing and deep-breathing

10. Educate client and family on signs of cor pulmonale and pulmonary edema

XI. Lung Cancer

A. Overview

1. Lung cancer is termed *bronchogenic carcinoma* because the tumor usually stems from the bronchial mucosa and is defined as cancer of the epithelial lining of the lung or the lung parenchyma

2. It is still the leading cancer of an internal organ, closely linked to cigarette smoking, and carries a poor prognosis

3. Classification of lung cancer

   a. Non–small-cell lung cancer (NSCLC): squamous cell carcinomas, large cell carcinomas, adenocarcinoma

   b. Small-cell lung cancer (SCLC): oat cell carcinoma

B. Pathophysiology

1. Various chemicals and irritants act as carcinogens in the lung, primarily those from tobacco smoke

2. The polycyclic hydrocarbons in cigarette smoke are mutagenic and can transform normal cells into malignant ones; the direct effect of these carcinogens on cellular DNA may explain why some individuals who smoke get lung cancer and others do not

3. The combined action of several of the carcinogens in tobacco may account for the rapid neoplasia that can occur

4. Another theory is that the bronchial epithelium undergoes metaplasia, which is a reversible state initially; in the presence of carcinogenic stimuli, metaplasia progresses to carcinoma

5. Some tumors of lung cancer are highly invasive and may extend into the mediastinum or spread into the pleural cavity; because of the highly vascular network of the lung, invasion into the lymphatic system occurs early, contributing to metastasis in other areas; distant metastasis may occur in the liver, brain, bones, kidneys, and adrenals

6. Complications include pneumonia, pleural effusions, Cushing's disease, hypercalcemia, anemia, disseminated intravascular coagulopathy (DIC), syndrome of inappropriate antidiuretic hormone (SIADH), and airway obstruction

7. Signs and symptoms initially may not be present until the tumor is large enough to interfere with airway function and the cancer is then well advanced

8. Clinical manifestations will then include a persistent productive cough, hemoptysis, frequent lower respiratory tract infections, abnormal breath sounds (wheezing), angina, pleuritic pain (if pleura is involved), hoarseness and dysphagia (due to pressure from the tumor)

9. In advanced stages with metastasis, weight loss, extreme dyspnea, fatigue, bone pain, and various endocrine, neurological, and cardiovascular symptoms are usually present

C. Nursing assessment

1. Assessment includes symptom analysis of any pain being experienced, changes in respiratory function or illnesses, lung sounds, sputum assessment (red or rust color), palpation of lymph nodes or enlarged liver, and weight loss analysis

2. A persistent cough that changes in character is common with lung cancer

3. Diagnostic tests: CXR, magnetic resonance imaging (MRI), CT scan of lung, brain or bone, bronchoscopy, sputum cytology, and lab tests (CBC, liver function, electrolytes, and coagulation studies)

D. Nursing management

1. Medications

   a. Combination chemotherapy: alkylating agents such as mechlorethamine (Mustargen), antibiotics such as doxorubicin (Adriamycin) or other drugs such as cisplatin (Platinol)

   b. Bronchodilators

   c. Antibiotics if an infection is present

   d. Analgesics: opioids, NSAIDs, non-opioids

2. Radiation (use of high-energy radioactive particles for palliative treatment) or surgery (lobectomy—removal of a lobe; pneumonectomy—removal of entire lung; or thoracotomy—incision of chest wall) are also treatment protocols; radiation therapy may be used to decrease the tumor size prior to surgery

3. Administer oxygen therapy as ordered

4. Assess respiratory status and vital signs

5. Auscultate lung and heart sounds

6. Manage pain (around-the-clock) and educate family how to treat pain, especially if client is being discharged; palliative care is essential especially in the end stages

7. Assist the client to turn, cough, and deep-breathe; placing the bed in a high Fowler's position may be helpful

8. Provide chest physiotherapy with percussion and postural drainage, suctioning as needed

9. Plan rest periods, especially immediately following an analgesic

10. Assist the client and family in the grieving process

XII. Respiratory Failure

A. Overview

1. Respiratory failure is defined as the inability of the lungs to maintain adequate oxygenation and usually manifested by hypoxemia, hypercapnia, and respiratory acidosis

2. ABGs reveal a PaO_2 less than 50 mmHg, $PaCO_2$ greater than 50 mmHg and pH less than 7.35; it is not a disease process, but a sign of severe dysfunction of the respiratory system

3. In the COPD client, a drop of 10 to 15 mmHg O_2 from *previous levels* indicates respiratory failure

4. Classification

   a. *Acute* (ARF): develops suddenly and can be life threatening; causes can be pulmonary diseases, cardiac diseases, or non-pulmonary disorders (infections, injuries); ARF can develop in individuals with normal lungs

   b. *Chronic* (CRF): develops slowly or more gradually and is usually a result of chronic bronchitis or emphysema

5. Can also be classified by whether there is impairment of ventilation or diffusion

   a. Impaired ventilation can be caused by airway obstruction (from laryngospasm, foreign body aspiration, or laryngeal/tracheal edema), respiratory diseases (asthma or COPD), neurologic disorders (spinal cord injury, stroke, and neuromuscular diseases), or chest trauma (pneumothorax, flail chest)

   b. Impaired diffusion can be caused by disorders affecting the alveoli (pneumonitis, pneumonia), pulmonary edema (near-drowning, ARDS, cardiac failure), or ventilation-perfusion mismatch (pulmonary embolus)

6. Types include Type I, hypoxemia only; Type II, hypoxemia with hypercapnia; or Type III, hypercapnia caused by hypoventilation

B. Pathophysiology

1. The lungs are unable to remove CO_2 and there is inadequate oxygen inhalation; severe hypoventilation of the lung causes a rise in the CO_2 level and respiratory acidosis

2. In chronic respiratory disorders such as emphysema and COPD, breathing becomes more labored, respiratory muscles weaken, and airway resistance is increased

3. Clients with respiratory failure become extremely exhausted and lose the energy to breathe; ventilation, diffusion, or perfusion problems may cause respiratory failure (see Figure 1-3)

4. Respiratory failure is a cycle that can end in death; as breathing difficulty increases, less oxygen is brought to the alveoli resulting in less production of surfactant, thus an increased resistance to expansion

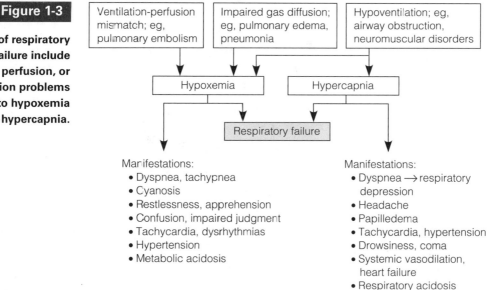

Figure 1-3

Causes of respiratory failure include ventilation, perfusion, or diffusion problems leading to hypoxemia and/or hypercapnia.

5. If the client is hyperventilating, the pCO_2 may be low; if the client is hypoxic only, the pH will be less than 7.35 and the pCO_2 will be normal; if the bicarbonate levels are low, metabolic acidosis can occur

6. Complications include ARDS, cardiac dysrhythmias, and cardiac failure

7. Signs and symptoms include those of the underlying disease process along with hypoxemia, hypercapnia, dyspnea, neurological changes (restlessness, apprehension, impaired judgment and motor skills), cyanosis, diaphoresis, cool skin, and initial vital sign changes (tachycardia, hypertension, tachypnea)

8. As fatigue develops and hypoxemia worsens, cardiac output decreases, cardiac arrhythmias may develop, and vital signs decrease (bradycardia, bradypnea, and hypotension)

C. Nursing assessment

1. Assessment includes: LOC, neurovascular assessment, skin color, vital signs, use of accessory respiratory muscles, auscultation of breath sounds, and ECG pattern

2. Diagnostic tests: ABGs (mild hypoxia is PaO_2 of less than 80 mmHg; moderate hypoxia is PaO_2 of less than 60 mmHg; and severe hypoxia is PaO_2 of less than 40 mmHg), CXR (shows that of the underlying disease process), ECG (dysrhythmias), hemodynamic monitoring, sputum for C & S

D. Nursing management

NCLEX!

1. Medications

   a. Bronchodilators: methylxanthines (theophylline derivatives)

   b. Sympathomimetic or anticholinergic drugs in aerosol form for bronchodilation

   c. Corticosteroids

   d. Antibiotics if an infection exists

   e. Sedatives and analgesia while on mechanical ventilation

   f. Benzodiazepines: diazepam (Valium), lorazepam (Ativan), or midazolam (Versed) to decrease the respiratory drive

   g. Neuromuscular blocking agents: pancuronium bromide (Pavulon) or vecuronium (Norcuron) to suppress the client's ability to breathe while on a ventilator

NCLEX!

2. Administer oxygen therapy as ordered (usually low levels) or maintain mechanical ventilation with PEEP; high oxygen levels may cause hypoventilation

NCLEX!

3. Administer parenteral therapy, monitor fluid and electrolyte status

4. Administer nebulized inhalation, chest physiotherapy, and suctioning as needed

5. Auscultate breath and lung sounds

6. Assess vital signs, respiratory status, nasal flaring, and use of accessory muscles

7. Assess ECG and hemodynamic monitoring

8. Maintain nutritional support

9. Monitor pulse oximetry

| **Case Study** | A 10-year-old boy has just been diagnosed with asthma related to allergies. The nurse working in the clinic is responsible for discharging the child on montelukast (Singulair) 1 tablet every day, albuterol (Ventolin) inhaler as needed for an asthma attack, nedocromil (Tilade) inhaler once a day, and albuterol (Ventolin) drops with saline for use with a nebulizer in the event the rescue inhaler does not work. |

❶ What discharge instructions should the nurse give the mother about the child's medications?

❷ What explanation should the nurse give the mother about asthma?

❸ What instructions should the nurse give the mother about when to seek immediate medical attention?

❹ What should the child know about an asthma attack?

❺ What are triggers and how do they affect asthma?

For suggested responses, see page 564.

Posttest

1 A client was involved in a motor vehicle accident (MVA) in which the seat belt was not worn. The client is exhibiting crepitus, decreased breath sounds on the left, complains of shortness of breath (SOB), and has a respiratory rate of 34/min. Which of the following assessment findings would concern the nurse the most?

(1) Temperature of 102°F and a productive cough
(2) Arterial blood gases (ABGs) with a PaO_2 of 92 and $PaCO_2$ of 40 mmHg
(3) Trachea deviating to the right
(4) Barrel-chested appearance

2 A nurse is teaching a client newly diagnosed with emphysema about the disease process. Which of the following statements best explains the problems associated with emphysema and could be adapted for use in the nurse's discussion with the client?

(1) Hyperactivity of the medium-sized bronchi caused by an inflammatory response leads to wheezing and tightness in the chest.
(2) Larger than normal air spaces and loss of elastic recoil cause air to be trapped in the lung and collapse airways.
(3) Vasodilation, congestion, and mucosal edema cause a chronic cough and sputum production.
(4) Chloride is not being transported properly, producing excess absorption of water and sodium, and thick, viscous mucus.

3 A sweat test, arterial blood gases (ABGs) and chest x-ray (CXR) are ordered for a child with symptoms suggestive of cystic fibrosis (CF). Which of the following results would be consistent with this diagnosis?

(1) Sodium 140 mEq/L, PaO_2 of 82 mmHg, and atelectasis in the lower lobe
(2) Sodium 132 mEq/L, PaO_2 of 95 mmHg, and hypoinflation of the lungs
(3) Sodium 150 mEq/L, PaO_2 of 90 mmHg, and whiteout of the lungs
(4) Sodium 155 mEq/L, PaO_2 of 70 mmHg, and hyperinflation of the lungs

4 A middle-aged man who suffered a large myocardial infarction develops adult respiratory distress syndrome (ARDS) as a complication. The client is intubated and placed on positive end expiratory pressure (PEEP). Which of the following is a finding of concern while on the PEEP?

(1) Sinus tachycardia of 125 beats/min
(2) Anxiety
(3) Blood pressure (BP) of 88/52
(4) Temperature 100.5°F

5 A client admitted to the medical nursing unit has classic symptoms of tuberculosis (TB) and tests positive on the purified protein derivative (PPD) skin test. Several months later, the nurse who cared for the client also tests positive on an annual TB skin test for work. The most likely course of treatment if the chest x-ray (CXR) is negative is to:

(1) Repeat a TB skin test in 6 months.
(2) Treat the nurse with an antiinfective agent for 6 months.
(3) Monitor for signs and symptoms within the next year.
(4) Follow up in 1 year at the next annual physical with a CXR only.

6 Clients with severe sleep apnea who are members of a support group should be educated to plan frequent rest periods and activities around how well they feel in order to maximize energy because they may complain of which of the following during the day?

(1) Cardiac arrhythmias
(2) Fatigue
(3) Jaw pain
(4) Productive cough

7 A client who has a known history of cardiac problems and is still smoking, enters the clinic complaining of sudden onset of sharp, stabbing pain that intensifies with a deep breath. The pain is occurring on only one side and can be isolated upon general assessment. The nurse concludes that this description is most likely caused by:

(1) Pleurisy.
(2) Pleural effusion.
(3) Atelectasis.
(4) Tuberculosis.

8 The nurse is delivering post-mortem care to a client who died from a large pulmonary embolus (PE). While thinking about the client's death, the nurse concludes that it was most likely caused by which of the following?

(1) Decreased blood flow
(2) Decreased alveolar dead space
(3) Inefficiency of the heart to pump adequately
(4) Infarction of the lung tissue

9 An elderly client recuperating from hip surgery will most likely be placed on which of the following in order to prevent a pulmonary embolism (PE)?

(1) Tissue plasminogen activator (t-PA)
(2) Warfarin (Coumadin)
(3) Low molecular weight heparin (LMWH)
(4) Heparin

10 A 50-year-old chronic obstructive pulmonary disease (COPD) client who has smoked two packs of cigarettes a day is being cared for in an intensive care unit for an acute exacerbation of the disease. Which of the following should alert the nurse to the possibility of pulmonary hypertension?

(1) Pulmonary artery pressure of 30 mmHg
(2) Rust-colored sputum
(3) Thick, viscous mucus
(4) Absent breath sounds

See pages 37–38 for Answers and Rationales.

Answers and Rationales

Pretest

1 Answer: 1 *Rationale:* COPD clients have low oxygen and high carbon dioxide levels. Therefore, hypoxia is the main stimulus for ventilation in persons with chronic hypercapnia. Increasing the level of oxygen would decrease the stimulus to breathe.
Cognitive Level: Application
Nursing Process: Analysis; *Test Plan:* SECE

2 Answer: 4 *Rationale:* A combined low PO_2 and low Cal SO_2 represents hypoxia. The pH, PCO_2, and HCO_3 are normal. ABGs will not necessarily be altered in TB or pleural effusion. Initially, in pneumonia, both the PO_2 and PCO_2 are usually low because the hypoxia leads to hyperventilation.
Cognitive Level: Analysis
Nursing Process: Analysis; *Test Plan:* PHYS

3 Answer: 3 *Rationale:* The cardinal signs of respiratory problems and hypoxia are restlessness, diaphoresis, tachycardia, and cool skin. Bradycardia might occur much later in the process when the condition is severe. Eupnea is normal respirations in rate and depth.
Cognitive Level: Application
Nursing Process: Assessment; *Test Plan:* PHYS

4 Answer: 2 *Rationale:* The first three symptoms could be indicative of any of the conditions. The distinguishing symptom is the lack of breath sounds in the lower-right base when a portion of the lung has collapsed.
Cognitive Level: Analysis
Nursing Process: Analysis; *Test Plan:* PHYS

5 Answer: 1 *Rationale:* The effects of the respiratory treatment should break up the congestion and cause bronchodilation; thus the change in lung sounds and more productive the cough effort. As the pneumonia resolves, the lungs should begin to clear and the cough diminish. Notice that the question asks about an *acute case;* be careful to note the situation in the stem.
Cognitive Level: Analysis
Nursing Process: Evaluation; *Test Plan:* PHYS

6 Answer: 3 *Rationale:* Option 3 is indicative of a tension pneumothorax, which is considered a medical emergency. The respiration system is severely compromised and venous return to the heart is also affected. The mediastinal shift is to the unaffected side. Option 1 contains symptoms of pleurisy, and option 2 lists symptoms of bronchitis; neither are emergencies.

The client in option 4 should expect difficulty breathing after exercise when asthma is an existing condition and may need immediate attention if the rescue inhaler is ineffective.
Cognitive Level: Analysis
Nursing Process: Assessment; *Test Plan:* SECE

7 Answer: 2 *Rationale:* A young person needs to know the triggers of asthma. Physical exercise in school and as a part of life will be ever-present, and prevention of an attack before exercise is essential at this time in the client's life. Sports do not have to be limited in all asthmatic people. Living a productive, normal life should be stressed. The client may have to use preventative medications before a sport of his/her choice. The fear associated with asthma is common and may take awhile to overcome. Instructions on identifying triggers and using the rescue inhalers needs to be taught and the fear will eventually subside.
Cognitive Level: Application
Nursing Process: Planning; *Test Plan:* HPM

8 Answer: 4 *Rationale:* As the upper airflow obstruction occurs in sleep apnea, the CO_2 rises and cardiac arrhythmias and angina can occur because of the lack of oxygenated blood to the heart. Clients with sleep apnea do not get adequate amounts of REM sleep and are often awakened frequently during the night in order to make breathing possible.
Cognitive Level: Analysis
Nursing Process: Analysis; *Test Plan:* PHYS

9 Answer: 2 *Rationale:* The most common sign of cancer of the lung is a persistent cough that changes. Other signs are dyspnea, bloody sputum, and long-term pulmonary infection. Option 1 is common with chronic obstructive pulmonary disease (COPD); option 3 is common with asthma, and option 4 is common with tuberculosis.
Cognitive Level: Application
Nursing Process: Assessment; *Test Plan:* PHYS

10 Answer: 3 *Rationale:* Adult respiratory distress syndrome is common after a trauma or shock situation. Clients will often become hypoxic and alkalotic with pulmonary edema.
Cognitive Level: Analysis
Nursing Process: Analysis; *Test Plan:* PHYS

Posttest

1 Answer: 3 *Rationale:* A mediastinal shift is indicative of a tension pneumothorax along with the other

symptoms in the question. Since the individual was involved in a MVA, assessment would be targeted at acute traumatic injuries to the lungs, heart, or chest wall rather than other conditions indicated in the other answers. Option 1 is common with pneumonia; values in option 2 are not alarming; and option 4 is typical of someone with chronic obstructive pulmonary disease (COPD).
Cognitive Level: Analysis
Nursing Process: Analysis; *Test Plan:* PHYS

2 **Answer: 2** *Rationale:* Option 2 is the pathophysiology behind emphysema. Option 1 explains asthma; option 3 explains bronchitis; and option 4 explains cystic fibrosis.
Cognitive Level: Application
Nursing Process: Analysis; *Test Plan:* PHYS

3 **Answer: 4** *Rationale:* CF is diagnosed with a high chloride level (normal is 135 to 148 mEq/L) on the sweat test, hypoxemia on the ABGs, and atelectasis or hyperinflation on the CXR.
Cognitive Level: Application
Nursing Process: Assessment; *Test Plan:* PHYS

4 **Answer: 3** *Rationale:* Barotrauma (decreased cardiac output and damage to lung tissue) is a common complication of PEEP. A drop in BP is associated with a decreased cardiac output. The sinus tachycardia may be a compensatory mechanism to raise the BP or a response to the ARDS. Anxiety is to be expected with intubation and a small rise in temperature may or may not indicate an infectious process.
Cognitive Level: Analysis
Nursing Process: Analysis; *Test Plan:* PHYS

5 **Answer: 2** *Rationale:* Exposure with a positive TB skin test usually requires 6 months of prophylactic treatment unless contraindicated. The TB skin test should not be repeated; the results will always be positive. A CXR is usually not required annually in the event that the skin test was positive.
Cognitive Level: Application
Nursing Process: Implementation; *Test Plan:* HPM

6 **Answer: 2** *Rationale:* The deprivation of oxygen during the night often leaves individuals tired during the day. Any activity increases the need for oxygen, which is already limited in a client with this disorder.
Cognitive Level: Application
Nursing Process: Planning; *Test Plan:* SECE

7 **Answer: 1** *Rationale:* Pleuritic pain is typically sharp and stabbing; pleural effusion (option 2) and atelectasis (option 3) can cause pain but usually have other symptoms like dyspnea and diminished or absent breath sounds. Pleurisy is common with smokers. Tuberculosis (option 4) causes chest pain along with other symptoms.
Cognitive Level: Application
Nursing Process: Analysis; *Test Plan:* PHYS

8 **Answer: 4** *Rationale:* If the blockage is large enough and blood flow is hindered to the lung, the tissue will die. This usually occurs when a large clot blocks the entire main pulmonary artery. Option 1 is rather vague because blood flow is decreased to the heart, lung, brain, and other vital organs because of the blockage but the amount of decrease can be variable. Option 2 is incorrect; dead space is increased with PE. Option 3 is correct in pulmonary embolism but is usually not the reason for death.
Cognitive Level: Application
Nursing Process: Analysis; *Test Plan:* PHYS

9 **Answer: 3** *Rationale:* Without any evidence of a blood clot or PE, LMWH is usually used for prevention purposes, especially since the client is elderly and will be on bedrest for a period of time. Heparin and Coumadin are used when a confirmed clot exists. Thrombolytics are used when a clot needs to be immediately dissolved.
Cognitive Level: Application
Nursing Process: Implementation; *Test Plan:* HPM

10 **Answer: 1** *Rationale:* A sustained elevation in the resting mean pressure above 20 mmHg from a pulmonary artery is defined as pulmonary hypertension, which could be caused by the COPD. Rust-colored sputum is usually indicative of lung cancer; thick mucus can be significant in a number of disorders; and absent breath sounds are indicative of many pulmonary disorders, not pulmonary hypertension.
Cognitive Level: Application
Nursing Process: Assessment; *Test Plan:* PHYS

References

Bullock, B. A. & Henze, R. L. (2000). *Focus on pathophysiology.* Philadelphia: Lippincott, pp. 527–586.

Corbett, J. V. (2000). *Laboratory tests and diagnostic procedures* (5th ed.). Upper Saddle River, NJ: Prentice Hall, pp. 157–160.

Corwin, E. (2000). *Handbook of pathophysiology* (2nd ed.). Philadelphia: Lippincott Williams & Wilkins, pp. 412–458.

Cronin, S. & Miracle, K. (2001). Management of clients with lower airway and pulmonary vessel disorders. In J. Black, J. Hawks, & A. Keane (Eds.), *Medical–surgical nursing: Clinical management for positive outcomes* (6th ed.). Philadelphia: W.B. Saunders.

Crowley, L. (2001). *An introduction to human disease: Pathology and pathophysiology correlations* (5th ed.). Sudbury, MA: Jones and Bartlett. pp. 369–403.

Damjanov, I. (2000). *Pathology for the health-related professions* (2nd ed.). Philadelphia: W.B. Saunders, pp. 173–207.

LeMone, P. & Burke, K. (2000). *Medical-surgical nursing: Critical thinking in client care* (2nd ed.). Upper Saddle River, NJ: Prentice Hall, pp. 207–208, 1326–1507.

McKenry, L. M. & Salerno, E. (2001). *Mosby's pharmacology in nursing* (21st ed.). St. Louis, MO: Mosby.

Neighbors, M. & Tannehille-Jones, R. (2000). *Human diseases.* Albany, NY: Delmar.

Porth, C. (2002). *Pathophysiology: Concepts of altered health states* (6th ed.). Philadelphia: Lippincott, pp. 475–562.

Tucker, S., Canobbio, M., Paquette, E., & Wells, M. (2000). *Client care standards: collaborative planning & nursing interventions* (7th ed.). St. Louis, MO: Mosby.

Venes, D. (Ed.). (2001). *Taber's cyclopedic medical dictionary* (19th ed.). Philadelphia: F. A. Davis.

Verst, A. (2001). Assessment of the respiratory system. In J. Black, J. Hawks, & A. Keane (Eds.), *Medical-surgical nursing: Clinical management for positive outcome* (6th ed.). Philadelphia: W.B. Saunders.

Wilson, B., Shannon, M., & Stang, C. (2001). *Nursing drug guide 2001.* Upper Saddle River, NJ: Prentice Hall.

York, N. (2001). Management of clients with parenchymal and pleural disorders. In J. Black, J. Hawks, & A. Keane (Eds.), *Medical-surgical nursing: Clinical management for positive outcomes* (6th ed.). Philadelphia: W.B. Saunders.

Youngkin, E., Sawin, K., Kinninger, J., & Israel, D. (1999). *Pharmacotherapeutics: A primary care clinical guide.* Stamford, CT: Appleton & Lange.

CHAPTER 2

Cardiac Health Problems

Betty Jane Sylvest, BSN, RN, MSN

CHAPTER OUTLINE

Risk Factors Associated with
  Cardiac Health Problems
Coronary Artery Disease (CAD)
Angina Pectoris
Myocardial Infarction (MI)

Congestive Heart Failure (CHF)
Cardiac Dysrhythmias
Inflammatory Diseases of the Heart
Valvular Heart Disease

OBJECTIVES

▮ Define key terms associated with cardiac health problems.

▮ Identify risk factors associated with the development of cardiac health problems.

▮ Discuss the common etiologies of cardiac health problems.

▮ Describe the pathophysiologic processes associated with specific cardiac health problems.

▮ Distinguish between normal and abnormal cardiac findings obtained from nursing assessment.

▮ Prioritize nursing interventions associated with specific cardiac health problems.

[Media Link]

Use the CD-ROM enclosed with this text, or log onto the address given to access the free, interactive Companion Website created for this series. The CD-ROM and Companion Website accompanying this book offer additional practice opportunities and information—NCLEX Review, Case Studies, Glossary, In Depth with NCLEX, and more.

www.prenhall.com/hogan

Review at a Glance

afterload *pressure the heart must pump against*

angina pectoris *chest pain associated with anaerobic metabolism from decreased oxygen supply to the myocardium*

automaticity *the ability of a cardiac cell in the muscle to contract independently, without stimulation*

cardiac output *amount of blood pumped out of the left ventricle each minute; determined by HR × stroke volume*

collateral circulation *additional outgrowth of tiny vessels that supply the heart muscle with oxygenated blood*

congestive heart failure (CHF) *inability of the heart to pump sufficient blood to maintain adequate oxygen and nutrients to the tissue*

coronary artery disease (CAD) *atherosclerotic plaque deposits lining the walls of the coronary arteries narrowing the vessel causing decreased oxygen supply to the myocardium*

electrocardiogram (ECG) *graphic representation of the electrical activity of the heart*

intermittent claudication *cramping in lower extremities, especially when walking or with exercise*

ischemia *insufficient blood flow that may lead to decreased oxygen supply to the tissue causing anaerobic cellular metabolism rather than aerobic metabolism*

mitral valve prolapse *the mitral valve prolapses back into the atrium causing regurgitation of blood from ventricle to atrium*

myocardial infarction (MI) *death of tissue of the myocardium caused by lack of oxygen supply*

myocarditis *an inflammatory disorder of the heart muscle that is unrelated to coronary artery disease or myocardial infarction*

pericarditis *inflammation of the pericardium and/or pericardial sac surrounding the heart*

preload *volume of blood returning to the heart, creating the "stretch" or tension of the myocardial fibers at end diastole*

reentry phenomena *the blockage of an impulse through one of the bundle branches, causing the impulse to retrograde backwards, reenter the other side and cause a premature contraction*

regurgitation *blood flowing backward through a valve that should be closed but cannot close completely because of damage or disease*

stenosis *the valves of the heart become hardened and blood does not flow through them adequately*

stroke volume *amount of blood ejected from the left ventricle with each heartbeat*

ventricular fibrillation *chaotic, irregular quivering of the ventricles; a lethal dysrhythmia requiring immediate defibrillation*

Pretest

1 The client complains of chest pain after mowing the lawn. This pain is most likely the result of which of the following?

(1) Pericardial effusion of fluid
(2) Pulmonary edema
(3) Myocardial ischemia
(4) Pulmonary emboli

2 The client who has peripheral edema during the day states he wakes up in bed at night having difficulty breathing. Which of the following is he most likely experiencing?

(1) Angina pectoris
(2) Orthopnea caused by recumbent position
(3) Sinus infection
(4) Sleep apnea

3 The client is experiencing shortness of breath, productive cough, tachycardia, and orthopnea. The nurse concludes that these are frequently noted as signs and symptoms of:

(1) Hypertension (HTN).
(2) Left ventricular failure.
(3) Coronary artery disease (CAD).
(4) Peripheral vascular disease.

4 The client has S-T segment depression on his 12-lead electrocardiogram (ECG). The nurse determines that this would be indicative of:

(1) Necrosis.
(2) Injury.
(3) Ischemia.
(4) Nothing significant.

5 The early stage of left ventricular failure would most likely result in which of the following changes in the client?

(1) Right ventricular failure
(2) Diminished left atrial pressures
(3) Higher pulmonary pressures
(4) Low pulmonary pressure

6   The client on a telemetry monitor has a heart rate
    of 54 bpm. The nurse knows that this rate would
    probably not increase oxygen demand for the my-
    ocardium, but the rate is indicative of:

(1) Tachycardia.
(2) Ventricular hypertrophy.
(3) Hypertension.
(4) Bradycardia.

7   The client demonstrates significant Q waves on the
    electrocardiogram (ECG). The nurse should notify
    the physician because this is indicative of:

(1) Gangrene.
(2) Ischemia.
(3) Infection.
(4) Infarction.

8   The client in the Emergency Department was diag-
    nosed with acute myocardial infarction (MI). He
    asks the nurse to explain what this is to him. The
    nurse should tell him that an MI usually results
    from which of the following?

(1) Obstruction of a coronary artery with death of tissue
    distal to the blockage
(2) Spasm of a coronary artery causing temporary de-
    creased blood supply
(3) A slow heart rate leading to decreased blood supply
    to myocardium
(4) Dilation of the ventricular wall causing decreased
    blood supply

9   The nurse teaching the client about behavioral
    changes, which can affect development of athero-
    sclerosis, should discuss which of the following as
    a nonmodifiable risk factor for atherosclerosis?

(1) Female over 55 years of age
(2) Hyperlipidemia
(3) Cigarette smoking
(4) Sedentary lifestyle and obesity

10 The client is in the clinic for a follow-up visit fol-
    lowing new onset of stable angina. The nurse
    should teach the client precipitating causes of
    angina such as exercise and stress. Which of the
    following should also be taught as a way to handle
    these precipitating causes?

(1) Avoid these activities
(2) Perform such activities anyway
(3) Lead a sedentary lifestyle
(4) Use a nitroglycerin (NTG) tablet before the activity

See pages 81–82 for Answers and Rationales.

I. Risk Factors Associated with Cardiac Health Problems

NCLEX!

A. Coronary artery disease (CAD), angina, and myocardial infarction (MI):
smoking, alcohol intake, obesity, sedentary life style, diabetes mellitus, hypercholesterolemia (total cholesterol over 240 mg/dL), hyperlipidemia (LDL over 160
mg/dL); nonmodifiable risk factors include age (over 45 for male and over 55 for
female), male gender, family history, hypertension, stress, race, personality type,
elevated triglycerides

B. Congestive heart failure (CHF): anyone with cardiac conditions such as CAD,
MI, hypertension (HTN), diabetes mellitus (DM), pericarditis; clients with pulmonary conditions such as chronic obstructive pulmonary disease (COPD), pulmonary HTN, post coronary bypass clients

C. Cardiac dysrhythmias: clients with known cardiac diseases (CAD, MI, CHF);
elderly; electrolyte disturbances; any condition that creates stress on the body
(fever, hypoxia, etc.)

D. Inflammatory disease: environmental and economic factors, damp weather,
crowded living conditions, malnutrition, immunodeficiency, decreased access to
health care, other illnesses involving the development of streptococcal infections

or severe stress/trauma to the heart; may have genetic tendency; risk factor for myocarditis can be alcohol use, stress, age, and ionizing radiation

E. **Valvular heart disease:** aging process, diseases such as MI, congenital heart defects

F. **Control of risk factors** by effective screening and public education can reduce cardiac morbidity and mortality

II. Coronary Artery Disease (CAD)

A. **Overview**

1. **Coronary artery disease (CAD)** is defined as narrowing of the arteries causing a decreased lumen and decreased blood flow through the coronary arteries

2. Coronary atherosclerosis is the most common cause of CAD

    a. Defined as narrowing of vessel wall by atherosclerotic plaques

    b. The following factors speed the development of plaque, which in turn impedes blood flow to myocardium, thereby decreasing oxygen availability to tissue

        1) Elevated cholesterol and triglyceride levels

        2) Elevated blood pressure (BP) by damaging lining

        3) Infection that initiates the inflammatory response

        4) Elevated iron levels carry free radicals that cause damage to the lining

        5) Elevated homocysteine levels (clients often have vascular disease also)

B. **Pathophysiology**

1. Injury to the lining of the artery occurs, resulting in increased permeability of the endothelial cells, allowing components of the plasma to enter

2. An inflammatory reaction occurs to the injury, bringing macrophages and platelets

3. Hemorrhage into the plaque produces thrombi; thrombus formation within the lumen of the artery is initiated by platelet aggregation

4. Embolization of a thrombus or plaque fragment can occur

5. Cholesterol, fat, and thrombi develop into a plaque formation

6. Progressive narrowing of lumen by plaque enlargement results in **ischemia** (insufficient blood flow leading to decreased oxygen supply to myocardium) due to narrowing of the artery lumen

    a. ECG changes (inverted T wave; depressed S-T segment) occur during an acute or severe episode of ischemia (Figure 2-1)

    b. Chest pain or angina pectoris occurs

7. Cholesterol and triglycerides are circulated in the blood as lipoproteins

    a. High-density lipoprotein (HDL), known as "good cholesterol" is protective against coronary heart disease (CHD) by taking fats away for breakdown

**S-T depression
suggesting ischemia.**

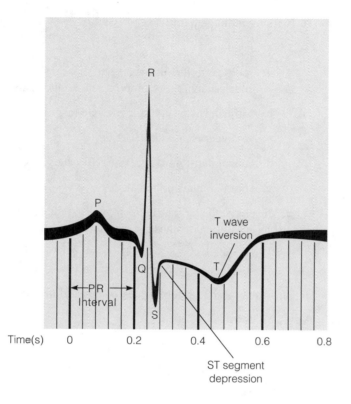

ST segment
depression

b. Low-density lipoprotein (LDL) and very low density lipoprotein (VLDL) helps fat remain in cells, known as "bad cholesterol"

8. Signs and symptoms include chest pain, hypertension, increased pulse, increased respirations, pallor of skin, diminished peripheral pulses occasionally; the comparable symptom of atherosclerosis in the legs is called **intermittent claudication** (cramping in the lower extremities, especially when walking or with exercise)

C. Nursing assessment

 1. Assessment

 a. Pain

   1) Location: midsternal, arms, jaw, abdomen, back

   2) Description: heaviness, tightness

   3) Duration: more than 3 minutes

   4) Quantity: pain scale of 1 to 10

 b. Other: assess vital signs, heart sounds, exercise tolerance, peripheral pulses, skin color

 2. Potentiating factors: exercise, stress, cold temperature, anemia, substance abuse, thyrotoxicosis, hyperthyroidism

 3. Relieving factors: rest, remove stressors

 4. Diagnostic tests: cholesterol level (HDL [highest], VLDL [lowest], LDL [lower than HDL]), triglyceride level, radiographic studies of arteries (arteriogram, angiogram), ECG

D. Nursing management

1. Medications

   a. Antihyperlipidemic agents and those that lower triglycerides: HMG-COA reductase inhibitors, atorvastatin (Lipitor), cerivastatin (Baycol)

   b. Antiplatelets: acetylsalicylic acid (aspirin)

   c. Antihypertensives if necessary

   d. Antianginals: nitroglycerine (Nitrostat; NTG)

   e. Antimicrobials if indicated

2. Teach risk factor management: low-fat diet, regular exercise, regular check-ups, cessation of smoking, stress management

3. Teach person to recognize signs and symptoms of CAD: shortness of breath, chest pain, and dyspnea on exertion

4. Teach person to stop and rest at onset of discomfort

III. Angina Pectoris

A. Overview

1. **Angina pectoris** is defined as chest pain caused by myocardial ischemia from:

   a. Reduced blood flow

   b. Reduced oxygen supply for demand of myocardium

   c. Temporary or reversible cause

2. Classified as stable, unstable, or Prinzmetal's angina

3. Causes include CAD, coronary spasms, thrombi or any condition that creates an imbalance between oxygen supply and demand of myocardium

B. Pathophysiology

1. When there is decreased blood flow (oxygen supply) to myocardium (ischemia) and/or increased demand for oxygen that cannot be met, angina occurs; this is the body's way of communicating that there isn't enough oxygenated blood; angina is a forewarning that a myocardial infarction (MI) or heart attack may occur

   a. *Reduced oxygen supply* causes a switch from aerobic metabolism to anaerobic metabolism

      1) Anaerobic metabolism causes lactic acid build-up

      2) Anaerobic metabolism affects cell membrane permeability releasing histamine, bradykinins, and specific enzymes that stimulate terminal nerve fibers in myocardium sending pain impulses to CNS

      3) Congestive heart failure, congenital heart defects, pulmonary hypertension, left ventricular hypertrophy, and cardiomyopathy also cause decreased oxygen supply to myocardium

      4) Silent ischemia: caused by decreased oxygen supply, just without warning signs of pain

> **▶ Practice to Pass**
>
> A client who is diagnosed with coronary artery disease (CAD) states that she did not know she had experienced a heart attack. What should the nurse's response be?

5) Coronary artery spasm: another form of occlusion and cause of ischemia, occurs from an unknown etiology; causes temporary narrowing of coronary arteries and angina

b. *Increased oxygen demand* of myocardium results in angina and can be caused by anemia, exercise, thyrotoxicosis, substance abuse (cocaine), hyperthyroidism, and emotional stress

2. Types of angina

NCLEX!

a. Stable angina (most common type)

1) Caused by specific amount of activity; rather predictable

2) Relieved with rest and nitrates

3) No change in cause, amount, or duration of pain over time

NCLEX!

b. Unstable angina (more concerning)

1) Pain occurring with increasing frequency, severity, and duration over time

2) Unpredictable and occurs with decreasing levels of activity or stress

3) May occur at rest

4) High risk for myocardial infarction

c. Prinzmetal's (variant) angina

1) Atypical form occurring without identified precipitating cause

2) May occur at same time each day or awaken client from sleep

3) May intensify or worsen over years but does not carry same concern as unstable angina

4) Usual cause is coronary artery spasm, therefore making it difficult to control

NCLEX!

3. Signs and symptoms include pressure or heaviness in chest, which the client may describe in other terms; may be accompanied by sweating, light-headedness, hypotension, pulse changes (low or high), or indigestion; pain may radiate to arms, jaw, abdomen, or back; depressed S-T segment on electrocardiogram

C. Nursing assessment

1. Assessment includes symptom analysis of pain (location, duration, precipitating factors and relieving factors); vital signs; dyspnea; respiratory pattern; color (pallor); anxiety; heart sounds

2. Diagnostic tests: **electrocardiogram** (**ECG** or **EKG**) graphic representation of the electrical activity of the heart, stress test (with and without contrast), radiographic study (angiogram), muga scan, creatinine phosphinase (CK or CPK) lactic dehydrogenase (LDH) (with isoenzymes), troponin to rule out MI, tests for gastric esophageal reflux disease (GERD) may be ordered to rule out gastric causes

D. Nursing management

1. Medications

NCLEX!

a. Antianginals: nitroglycerin (Nitrostat, NTG)

b. Antiplatelet agents

c. Beta blockers

d. Calcium channel blockers to decrease **afterload** (pressure the heart must pump against) and spasms

e. Analgesics for headache (common side effect of NTG)

f. Thrombolytic therapy if thrombi identified as cause

g. Stool softeners

h. Class I-B antiarrhythmics may be given prophylactically if premature ventricular contractions (PVCs) occur

2. Goal is to reduce oxygen demand and improve blood and oxygen supply; primary nursing care is related to education of the client

a. Educate on signs and symptoms of angina pectoris

b. Use of NTG: take one tablet every 5 minutes for 3 times, report to physician if no relief

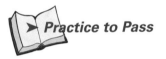

c. NTG can be used prior to activities that may cause angina (such as sexual activity, work-related activities that cannot be modified, etc.)

3. Administer oxygen as needed

Practice to Pass

The client presents with history of stable angina and asks the nurse "Does this mean I will have a heart attack?" How should the nurse respond?

4. Treatment may consist of percutaneous transluminal coronary angioplasty (PTCA) or coronary artery bypass graft (CABG) surgery to prevent a MI; client should be instructed on these procedures

5. Monitor vital signs (VS); heart sounds

6. Monitor EKG pattern, heart rate (HR) may increase as a response of the sympathetic nervous system (SNS) if blood pressure (BP) drops

7. Instruct client not to strain for bowel movement (BM) or create excess pressure by bending; administer stool softener as needed

8. Help client identify known stressors

9. Begin cardiac exercise program

10. Pulse should be monitored before beta blockers and held if pulse is less than 60 bpm; also assess BP as hypotension can occur

11. BP should be checked before each NTG tablet and recorded since NTG can cause drastic hypotension; morphine sulfate (MS) may be administered in small doses if BP is below 100 systolic

12. BP should be carefully assessed during the administration of calcium channel blockers

IV. **Myocardial Infarction (MI)**

A. **Overview**

1. **Myocardial infarction (MI)** is defined as death of cells in the myocardium usually related to prolonged or severe ischemia to that area

2. Many MIs are caused by sudden onset of ventricular fibrillation

3. Other causes include embolus, thrombosis, atherosclerotic occlusion, prolonged vasospasm

B. Pathophysiology

1. Cellular injury occurs because of a lack of oxygen over time (ischemia); prolonged (20 to 45 minutes) ischemia can lead to cell death (necrosis)

2. Coronary artery occlusion results in cell death distal to occlusion

3. Scar replaces muscle, but does not contract or conduct an impulse

4. Damage begins at subendocardial layer and progresses to epicardium within 1 to 6 hours

5. Damaged cells cause a decrease in myocardial contractility resulting in:

   a. Decreased **stroke volume** (volume of blood ejected by left ventricle with each heartbeat)

   b. Decreased **cardiac output** (volume of blood from left ventricle each minute)

   c. Decreased blood pressure

   d. Decreased tissue perfusion

6. Prolonged ischemia may lead to development of **collateral circulation** (additional outgrowth of tiny vessels), which provide additional pathways for delivery of oxygen and nutrients to the area of ischemia

7. MIs are described by:

   a. Location

      1) Anterior: usually occurring in area supplied by left anterior descending coronary artery (LAD)

      2) Posterior: usually occurring in area supplied by the right coronary artery (RCA)

      3) Lateral: occurring in area supplied by the left circumflex

   b. Myocardial surface

      1) Transmural infarct: endocardium to epicardium

      2) Subendocardial: endocardial surface into myocardial muscle

      3) Intramural infarction: patchy areas of myocardium

8. Signs and symptoms associated with myocardial infarction

   NCLEX!

   a. Pain (typical): midsternal, radiating to jaw, arms, abdomen, or shoulder; tightness, crushing feeling; lasting 15 to 20 minutes; and not relieved with NTG or by rest

   b. May be pain-free (silent MI)

   c. Duration of pain important in distinguishing from angina pectoris

   d. Sudden onset of pain, usually not associated with activity, may awaken in middle of night

   e. Tachycardia related to pain, increased need of tissue for oxygen

Figure 2-2

S-T segment suggesting myocardial injury. A. S-T segment elevation. B. Presence of Q wave.

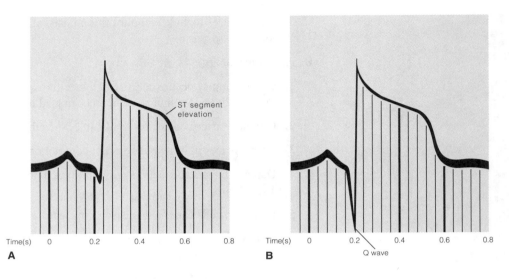

ST segment elevation

Time(s) 0   0.2   0.4   0.6   0.8

A

Time(s) 0   0.2   0.4   0.6   0.8

Q wave

B

f. Diaphoresis

g. Tachypnea, dyspnea

h. Change in level of consciousness, anxiety, feelings of impending doom

i. Nausea/vomiting

j. ECG changes: depressed or *elevated S-T segment* (most common), inverted T wave, formation of Q waves (Figure 2-2)

k. Elevated cardiac enzymes: enzymes are normally present in the muscle fiber of the body and are not elevated in the serum unless injury to the muscle occurs; when any muscle is injured, the enzymes are released into the blood stream as a response to the injury; isoenzymes are a breakdown of the total exzyme level and when elevated give an indication of which particular muscle has been damaged (Table 2-1)

1) Creatinine phosphokinase (CK or CPK): the isoenzymes are CPK I (BB) present in brain tissue and smooth muscle; CPK II (MB) present in heart tissue; and CPK III (MM) present in muscle tissue; therefore, when the total CPK level is elevated, the nurse should assess for an elevated CPK II or MB isoenzyme to determine if a MI has occurred

2) Lactic dehydrogenase (LDH): the isoenzymes are LDH I present in cardiac muscle; LDH II present in the reticuloendothelial system; LDH III present in lungs and other tissue; LDH IV present in the placenta, kidney, and pancreas; and LDH V present in the liver and striated muscle; normally LDH I is less than LDH II, however in an MI, LDH I is greater than II (termed a "flipped ratio"); therefore, when the total LDH level is elevated, the nurse should assess for an elevated LDH I isoenzyme to determine if an MI has occurred

l. Elevated temperature

m. Leukocytosis

n. Cardiac arrhythmias: premature ventricular contractions (PVCs), ventricular tachycardia caused by irritability

9. The most common reaction to an MI is to deny the symptoms and delay health care

Table 2-1	Enzyme Changes in MI					
Marker	**Normal Level**	**Primary Tissue Location**	**Significance of Elevation**	**Appears**	**Peaks**	**Duration**
CK (CPK)	Male: 12 to 80 U/L Female: 10 to 70 U/L	Cardiac muscle, skeletal muscle, brain	Injury to muscle cells	3 to 6 hours	12 to 24 hours	24 to 48 hours
CK-MB	0% to 3% of total CK	Cardiac muscle	MI, cardiac ischemia, myocarditis, cardiac contusion, defibrillation	4 to 8 hours	18 to 24 hours	72 hours
cT_nT	<0.2 mcg/L	Cardiac muscle	Acute MI, unstable angina	2 to 4 hours	24 to 36 hours	10 to 14 days
cT_nI	<3.1 mcg/L	Cardiac muscle	Acute MI, unstable angina	2 to 4 hours	24 to 36 hours	7 to 10 days
LDH	45 to 90 U/L	Heart, liver, kidneys, skeletal muscle, brain, RBCs, lungs	MI; pulmonary, liver, renal, RBC, or skeletal muscle disease; CVA; intestinal ischemia; others	24 to 72 hours	3 to 4 days	10 to 14 days

Source: LeMone, P. & Burke, K. (2000). *Medical-surgical nursing: Critical thinking in client care* (2nd ed.). Upper Saddle River, NJ: Prentice Hall, p. 1106.

C. Nursing assessment

NCLEX!

1. Assessment includes symptom analysis of chest pain (location, duration, radiation, quality); associated symptomatology (diaphoresis, nausea/vomiting); vital signs; auscultate heart sounds (murmur, friction rub, gallop [S_3 or S_4]); assess cardiac rhythm; nonverbal cues of discomfort

2. Diagnostic tests: CPK and LDH with isoenzymes, troponin Level, 12-lead ECG, chest x-ray (CXR), angiogram, echocardiogram, stress tests, muga scan, arterial blood gases (ABGs), electrolytes, complete blood count (CBC), obtain pulse oximetry for quick reference of Sa O_2

D. Nursing management

NCLEX!

1. Medications

   a. Antianginals: nitroglycerin (Nitrostat, NTG) for vasodilation; anticipate use of sublingual/topical spray, Nitrol drip, and/or Nitrol paste

   b. Analgesics as needed for pain relief; morphine sulfate (MS) if BP too low or pain unrelieved by nitrostat

   c. Stool softener

   d. Electrolyte replacement as necessary

   e. Calcium channel blockers

   f. Beta blockers

   g. Antihypertensives

   h. Anticoagulants such as heparin, warfarin (Coumadin) or low molecular weight heparin (LMWH) such as enoxaparin (Lovenox)

        i. Antiarrhythmics may be given prophylactically

          1) Lidocaine (Xylocaine): ventricular antidysrhythmics such as PVCs

          2) Atropine: treatment of bradydysrhythmias

          3) Adenosine: treatment of tachydysrhythmias

        j. Thrombolytics as indicated

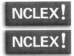

2. Supplement oxygen via nasal canula at 2 to 5 L/min

3. Elevate head of bed for respiratory comfort

4. Maintain intravenous (IV) access site

5. Monitor bowel movements, encourage client not to strain, and offer stool softener as needed

6. Provide for physical and psychological rest

7. Provide emotional support for the client and the family

8. Reassess client frequently for pain relief or continued pain; use pain scale to assess quality of pain

9. Teach client and family when they are ready to listen and absorb the information

10. Monitor VS and record with administration of nitrates, beta blockers, and calcium channel blockers: hold if pulse less than 60 bpm or BP less than 100 systolic (see Angina, Section D)

11. Begin cardiac rehabilitation program for education and exercise as ordered

12. Monitor for major side effects of medications: hypotension, bradycardia, bleeding, constipation, and depression

V. Congestive Heart Failure (CHF)

A. Overview

1. Congestive heart failure (CHF) is defined as the inability of the heart to pump sufficiently to meet the metabolic needs of the body, causing decreased tissue perfusion as a result of decreased cardiac output

2. May be acute (pulmonary edema or cardiogenic shock) or chronic (heart failure); left-sided, right-sided, or both

3. Causes include diseases such as MI, HTN, CAD, kidney failure; cardiomyopathies; valve disorders; inflammatory conditions; water intoxication; side effects of medications such as corticosteroids (Table 2-2)

4. Prognosis determined by effectiveness of therapeutic regime

B. Pathophysiology

1. The heart pumps blood to the pulmonary and systemic vascular systems in order to maintain an adequate oxygenated blood supply to the heart and produce a sufficient cardiac output (CO)

2. Cardiac output is regulated by metabolic needs of the body

3. Damage to the pump (heart) regardless of cause leads to decreased cardiac output and decreased tissue perfusion

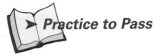

Practice to Pass

The client arrives in the Emergency Department with complaints of midsternal chest pain, diaphoresis, and nausea. The client states "I'm dying." How should the nurse respond?

Table 2-2	Causes of Heart Failure				
Excess Volume Load	**Excess Pressure Load**	**Increased Metabolic Demand**	**Acute Conditions**	**Altered Function**	**Filling Disorders**

Volume overload
Valve regurgitation
Left-to-right shunts
	Hypertension
	Aortic stenosis
	Hypertrophic
	  cardiomyopathy
	Coarctation of
	  the aorta
		Anemias
		Thyrotoxicosis
		Pregnancy
		Infection
		Fever
		Physical, emotional,
		  or environmental
		  stressors
			Acute
			  hypertensive
			  crisis
			Aortic valve
			  rupture
			Massive
			  pulmonary
			  embolism
				Cardiomyopathy
				Myocarditis
				Rheumatic fever
				Infective
				  endocarditis
				Coronary heart
				  disease
				Dysrhythmias
				Toxic disorders
					Valve stenosis
					  (mitral or tricuspid)
					Cardiac tamponade
					Restrictive
					  pericarditis

Source: LeMone, P. & Burke, K. (2000). *Medical-surgical nursing: Critical thinking in client care* (2nd ed.). Upper Saddle River, NJ: Prentice Hall, p. 1119.

4. Two dysfunctions that contribute to CHF

   a. *Diastolic dysfunction:* when ventricle pumps against an extremely high afterload as in primary HTN; this effect leads to a decrease in the ventricles ability to comply, decreases filling of ventricles (preload), which leads to decreased stroke volume; hypotension can manifest

   b. *Systolic dysfunction:* when ventricle experiences damage as in a MI and the ventricle cannot contract effectively; the stroke volume decreases, leading to an increased **preload** (volume of blood returning to the heart creating the "stretch" or tension of the myocardial fibers at end of diastole) and the ventricle becomes distended; signs of decreased cardiac output can manifest

5. Compensatory mechanisms for heart failure (Table 2-3)

   a. Frank-Starling mechanism: force of contraction determined by amount of stretch

   b. Neuroendocrine responses

      1) Sympathetic nervous system (SNS) activation: increase in HR

      2) Renin: angiotensin-aldosterone mechanism activation

   c. Myocardial hypertrophy

6. Decreased CO stimulates aortic baroreceptors, causing the release of norepinephrine to increase heart rate and contractility; this causes vasoconstriction, thereby increasing blood return to the heart and increasing CO

7. Decreased cardiac output leads to decreased renal perfusion; remember the kidneys need blood in order to function properly

   a. Decreased renal perfusion leads to release of renin from juxtoglomerular cells

   b. Activation of renin-angiotensin-aldosterone mechanism

      1) Causes vasoconstriction

      2) Stimulates adrenal cortex to produce aldosterone and anti-diuretic hormone (ADH) from posterior pituitary

         a) Aldosterone causes sodium reabsorption and water retention, thus increasing the BP

NCLEX!

Table 2-3	Compensatory Mechanisms of Heart Failure		
Mechanism	**Pathophysiology**	**Effect on Body Systems**	**Complications**
Frank-Starling mechanism	The greater the stretch of cardiac muscle fibers, the greater the force of contraction.	Increased contractile force leading to increased CO	Increased myocardial oxygen demand
Neuroendocrine response	Decreased CO causes sympathetic nervous system stimulation and catecholamine release.	Increased HR, BP, and contractility Increased vascular resistance Increased venous return	Tachycardia with decreased filling time and decreased CO Increased vascular resistance Increased myocardial work and oxygen demand
	Decreased CO and decreased renal perfusion stimulate renin-angiotensin system.	Vasoconstriction and increased BP	Increased myocardial work Renal vasoconstriction and decreased renal perfusion
	Angiotensin stimulates aldosterone release from adrenal cortex.	Salt and water retention by the kidneys Increased vascular volume	Increased preload and afterload Pulmonary congestion
	ADH is released from posterior pituitary	Water excretion inhibited	Fluid retention and increased preload and afterload Pulmonary congestion
	Atrial natriuretic factor is released.	Increased sodium excretion Diuresis	
	Blood flow is redistributed to vital organs (heart and brain).	Decreased perfusion of other organ systems Decreased perfusion of skin and muscles	Renal failure Anaerobic metabolism and lactic acidosis
Ventricular hypertrophy	Increased cardiac workload causes myocardial muscle to hypertrophy and ventricles to dilate.	Increased contractile force to maintain CO	Increased myocardial oxygen demand Cellular enlargement

Source: LeMone, P. & Burke, K. (2000). *Medical-surgical nursing: Critical thinking in client care* (2nd ed.). Upper Saddle River, NJ: Prentice Hall, p. 1121.

      b) ADH inhibits water excretion in distal tubules and causes vasoconstriction, thus increasing vascular volume and raising BP

8. Vasoconstriction causes increased blood return to the heart (preload), causing greater stretch (Frank-Starling law), and therefore increases cardiac output

9. Atrial stretch stimulates release of atrial natriuretic factor (ANF) or atriopeptin that balances effects of renin and aldosterone, promotes sodium and water excretion and inhibits norepinephrine, renin, and ADH

10. Ventricular hypertrophy results from excess fluid volume and pressure causing cells to enlarge, stiffen, thereby decreasing force of contraction

11. The compensatory mechanisms hasten the deterioration of cardiac function and the onset of heart failure

      a. Increased heart rate decreases diastolic filling time, compromises coronary artery perfusion, and increases myocardial oxygen demand; the resulting ischemia leads to decreased cardiac output

    b. Beta-receptors in the heart become less sensitive to SNS stimulation, thereby decreasing heart rate and contractility

    c. Alpha receptors on peripheral blood vessels are increased in sensitivity, which promotes vasoconstriction, thereby increasing afterload and therefore cardiac work load

12. Chronic ventricular dilation leads to ventricular wall thinning, degeneration, and loss of effective contractility

13. Chronic atrial dilation leads to depletion of ANF leaving renin, aldosterone, and norepinephrine to continue unabated; causes increased preload, afterload, and further deterioration of heart failure, thereby decreasing the oxygen supply to the tissue, leading to further ischemia and tissue death (infarction)

14. Left-sided heart failure (see Figure 2-3)

    a. Left side affected more often than right side

    b. Results from left ventricular wall damage or dilatation

    c. Left ventricular and atrial end-diastolic pressures increase and cardiac output decreases

Figure 2-3

Pathophysiology of left-sided heart failure.

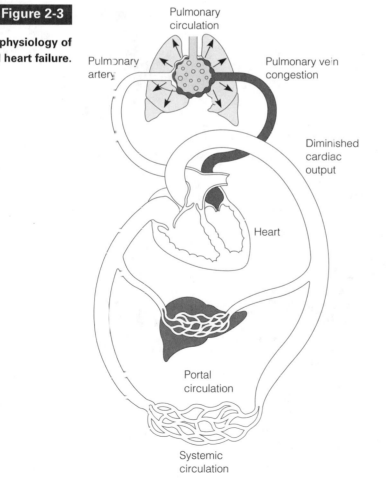

Pulmonary circulation

Pulmonary artery

Pulmonary vein congestion

Diminished cardiac output

Heart

Portal circulation

Systemic circulation

d. Impaired left ventricular filling results in congestion and increased pulmonary vascular pressures; remember "**L**"eft and "**L**"ung, the fluid "backs up" to the lungs

   1) Increased pulmonary vascular pressure causes shifting of fluid interstitially, leading to alveolar congestion and pulmonary edema

   2) Increased pulmonary artery pressures as measured by a pulmonary artery catheter (normal PA pressure 25/10 mmHg)

e. Signs and symptoms of left heart failure: fatigue, activity intolerance, dizziness, syncope, dyspnea, shortness of breath, cough, orthopnea, pulmonary crackles on auscultation, S_3 heart sound, tachycardia with possible atrial dysrhythmia, and decreased urine output

15. Right-sided heart failure (see Figure 2-4)

a. Right heart failure caused by pulmonary hypertension (cor pulmonale) and left heart failure

b. Right ventricular infarction can cause right-sided heart failure

Figure 2-4

Pathophysiology of right-sided heart failure.

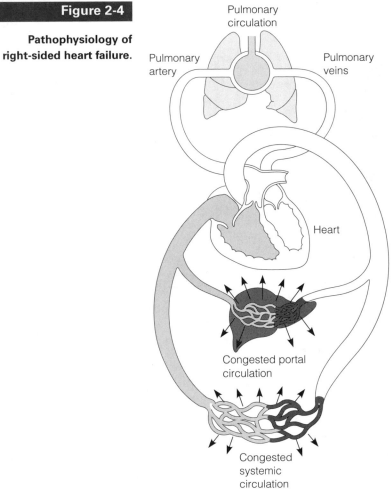

        c. Pulmonary hypertension causes increased pressure the right ventricle must pump against so right ventricle cannot empty; hypertrophy and dilation results

        d. Right ventricular distention leads to blood accumulation in the systemic venous system; remember "**R**"ight and "**R**"est of the body, the fluid "backs up" to the rest of the body

        e. Increased venous pressure causes abdominal organ congestion and peripheral edema

           1) Lower extremity edema occurs in the client who is ambulatory

           2) The bedridden client will experience sacral edema

           3) Liver engorgement will lead to right upper quadrant pain

           4) Anorexia and nausea occur with gastrointestinal venous congestion

        f. Jugular venous distention occurs

    16. Biventricular failure; both ventricles fail

        a. Client experiences signs and symptoms of both left and right failure

        b. Paroxysmal nocturnal dyspnea (PND) occurs as peripheral edema is reabsorbed into circulation when client goes to bed and feet are elevated causing fluid overload and pulmonary congestion

        c. Severe heart failure predisposes the client to dyspnea at rest

        d. S_3 and S_4 heart sounds may be heard

        e. Hepatomegaly and splenomegaly result from abdominal engorgement or congestion: increased abdominal pressure, ascites, gastrointestinal problems (anorexia, nausea, and vomiting), decreased digestion and absorption of nutrients

        f. Dysrhythmias may develop from myocardial distention causing interference with conduction and lowering cardiac output

        g. Cardiogenic shock or acute pulmonary edema may develop as cardiac function deteriorates

C. Nursing assessment

    1. Assessment includes VS; cardiac monitor; heart rhythm; pulse quality (full, bounding, thready); respiratory status (dyspnea, shortness of breath, tachypnea); lung sounds (crackles, rhonchi, wheezes); heart sounds (S_3 or S_4, murmur or rub); jugular neck vein distention; abdominal assessment (palpation, distention, ascites); edema; activity tolerance

    2. Diagnostic tests

        a. Electrocardiogram

           1) Signs of ischemia: depressed S-T segment, inverted T wave

           2) Signs of injury: elevated S-T segment, Q wave development

        b. Other: electrolytes, liver function test, ABG analysis, chest x-ray, echocardiogram, pulse oximetry

        c. Tests to rule out an MI may be done if client is having chest pain also

D. Nursing management

1. Medications

    NCLEX!

    NCLEX!

    a. Diuretics: furosemide (Lasix)

    b. Positive inotropic agents: dopamine (Inotropin)—increases urinary output, systemic vasoconstrictor; dobutamine (Dobutex)

    c. Analgesics to decrease stress and discomfort and allow decreased oxygen needs

    d. Antihypertensives

    e. ACE inhibitors

    f. Direct vasodilators

    g. Beta blockers

    h. Antidysrhythmics as needed

    NCLEX!

    i. Cardiac glycosides: digitalis (Lanoxin)

    j. Nitrates

2. Primary goal is to reduce oxygen demand of the myocardium: physical and psychological rest

3. Manage prescribed medication for reducing cardiac workload, improving contractility, and management of symptoms

4. Management of decreased cardiac output

    a. Monitor and record vital signs

    1) Decreased CO stimulates SNS to increase HR and increase diastolic blood pressure, as the heart's pumping action deteriorates, BP decreases

    2) Assessment of subtle changes in vital signs may lead to early intervention

    b. Auscultate heart and lung sounds

    1) S_1 and S_2 may be diminished as cardiac function fails

    2) S_3 is an early sign of heart failure (ventricular gallop)

    3) S_4 may also be present (atrial gallop)

    4) Basilar crackles may be heard

    5) Increasing crackles and dyspnea mean worsening of condition

    c. Note level of consciousness (LOC)

    NCLEX!

    1) Mental changes occur as blood flow to the brain decreases

    2) SaO_2 changes may also lead to changes in LOC

    NCLEX!

    d. Note urine output (UO)

    1) Decreased blood flow to kidney leads to decreased output

    2) Assessing output assists in evaluating the effectiveness of some medications used to treat heart failure such as diuretics and positive inotropic agents

    e. Note color and temperature of skin

        1) Cool, clammy skin frequently present in acute phase of heart failure

        2) Pale, cyanotic coloring is often seen in later stages as cardiac pumping action deteriorates

    f. Monitor client for cardiac dysrhythmias

        1) Sinus tachycardia is usually present

        2) Atrial dysrhythmias are frequently seen in heart failure: atrial fibrillation, atrial flutter, premature atrial contractions (PACs), and atrial tachycardia

        3) Ventricular dysrhythmias will be seen as ventricular hypertrophy and dilation occurs

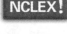

    g. Supplemental oxygen is given to decrease the effects of hypoxia and ischemia

    h. Place client at rest with head of bed elevated to improve respiratory function and reduce cardiac workload

        1) Assist with personal care needs

        2) Use bedside commode to reduce effort necessary in placing on bed pan

        3) Instruct client to avoid Valsalva maneuver

        4) Avoid isometric exercises

    i. Promote psychological rest and minimize anxiety to reduce oxygen consumption and improve cardiac function: maintain quiet environment, allow expression of fear, explain procedures to client's satisfaction

5. Management of fluid volume excess

    a. Assess respiratory status; declining respiratory status indicates worsening left heart failure—shortness of breath, dyspnea, cough, orthopnea, paroxysmal nocturnal dyspnea

    b. Acute pulmonary edema can develop rapidly

        1) Air hunger develops

        2) Client begins to panic

        3) Overwhelming sense of impending doom

        4) Tachypnea

        5) Need to sit straight up in bed

        6) Productive cough with large amounts of pink, frothy sputum occurs

    c. Monitor urinary output closely

        1) Notify physician if output is equal to or less than 30 cc/hr

        2) Use of diuretics reduces circulating volume producing hypovolemia even in the presence of peripheral edema

        3) Decreased urinary output could indicate decreased cardiac output and renal ischemia

    d. Weigh the client daily

       1) Weight provides objective measure of fluid status

       2) 1 liter of fluid is equal to 2.2 pounds of weight

    e. Assess and record abdominal girth every shift

       1) Venous congestion leads to development of ascites and may produce gastrointestinal complaints: nausea, loss of appetite, abdominal discomfort

       2) Increasing girth means increased ascites production

    f. Keep client on bedrest with head of bed elevated 45 degrees to improve lung expansion and reduce cardiac workload

    g. Assess for signs of deteriorating condition

    h. Monitor hemodynamics (if pulmonary artery catheter in place)

       1) Monitor pulmonary capillary wedge pressures

       2) Monitor pulmonary artery pressure (normal 25/10 mmHg)

       3) Monitor right atrial pressure (CVP)

       4) Systemic vascular resistance

       5) Cardiac output

       6) Cardiac index

    i. Restrict fluids if ordered to decrease fluid overload

6. Management of activity intolerance: minimal or no cardiac reserve for increased activity leads to self-care deficits

    a. Allow adequate rest periods prior to activity

    b. Assess for signs of decreasing activity intolerance

    c. Assist with activities of daily living allowing client to do as much as possible to provide some control to the client and reduce feelings of helplessness

    d. Provide passive and active range-of-motion (ROM) to progressively promote improved cardiac function

    e. Teach the client regarding discharge instructions

       1) Low sodium diet

       2) Perform activities as independently as possible

       3) Space meals and activities

       4) Allow time for rest and relaxation

       5) Stop any activity that causes chest pain or shortness of breath

       6) Avoid straining

       7) Begin slowly progressive exercise program

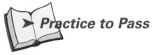

Practice to Pass

The client is being discharged tomorrow after a 6-day hospitalization for heart failure. The client asks when he can return to work. How should the nurse explain the recovery phase?

7. Close monitoring and recording of drug therapy should be done by the nurse

   a. Monitor apical pulse for one minute prior to administering digoxin (Lanoxin); hold if pulse is less than 60 bpm

   b. Monitor VS and intake and output (I&O) carefully while administering dopamine (Intropin)

   1) Low doses: renal perfusion

   2) Moderate to high doses: elevate BP

   c. Close monitoring of I & O with furosemide (Lasix), avoid intravenous push (IVP) too rapidly—ototoxicity can occur

VI. Cardiac Dysrhythmias

A. Overview

1. Electrical stimulation of the normal heart causes depolarization of the myocardium; this depolarization produces a synchronized, rhythmic contraction of the myocardium producing a beat; propelling the blood through the arteries and capillaries

2. Cardiac dysrhythmias are defined as alterations in this stimulation, which can affect the synchronized pattern of contractions and affect the efficiency of the heart

3. Normal sinus rhythm conduction progresses from the sinoatrial (SA) node → atrioventricular (AV) node → bundle of HIS → bundle branches (right bundle branch and left bundle branch) simultaneously → Purkinje fibers, causing contraction of the atria and ventricles

4. Cardiac dysrhythmias

   a. May be benign or lethal

   b. Caused by many factors (see Table 2-4)

   c. Any dysrhythmia can affect cardiac function, regardless of cause

   d. Client's response to the rhythm determines urgency of treatment

5. Dysrhythmias originate as sinus, atrial, junctional, ventricular, or heart blocks

B. Pathophysiology

1. Altered electrical activity may cause alterations in cardiac function

2. Dysrhythmias may result from internal or external forces

   a. Internal forces

   1) Hypoxia

   2) Electrolyte disturbances

   3) Acidosis

   4) Diseases of the myocardium

   5) Atherosclerotic processes

Table 2-4

Causes of Cardiac
Dysrhythmias

Dysrhythmia	Common Causes
Sinus arrhythmia	Increase in vagal tone, digitalis toxicity or morphine administration
Sinus tachycardia (ST)	Normal response to any condition that increases the body's need for more oxygen and nutrients: fever, stress, exercise, hypoxia, hypovolemia, anemia, hyperthyroidism, myocardial infarction, heart failure, cardiogenic shock
Sinus bradycardia (SB)	Increased vagal tone; depressed automaticity; may be normal in athletic heart syndrome or during sleep; other causes include pain, increased intracranial pressure, sinus node disease, myocardial infarction, hypothermia, acidosis, certain drugs such as digoxin (Lanoxin), beta blockers, calcium channel blockers
Sick sinus syndrome (SSS)	Injury during surgery, ischemia, infarct, fibrosis of conduction fibers associated with aging, drugs such as digitalis (Lanoxin), beta blockers, and calcium channel blockers
Premature atrial contractions (PAC)	Strong emotions, excessive alcohol intake, tobacco, adrenergic stimulants (caffeine), myocardial infarction, heart failure, pericarditis, valvular disorders, hypoxemia, pulmonary embolism, digitalis toxicity, hypokalemia, hypomagnesemia, metabolic alkalosis
Atrial tachycardia or paroxysmal supraventricular tachycardia	Sympathetic nervous system stimulation, fever, sepsis, hyperthyroidism, heart disease, myocardial infarction, rheumatic heart disease, myocarditis, acute pericarditis
Atrial flutter	Sympathetic nervous system stimulation, anxiety, caffeine, alcohol intake, thyrotoxicosis, coronary artery disease, myocardial infarction, pulmonary embolism, abnormal conduction syndromes, elderly persons with rheumatic heart disease or valvular disease
Atrial fibrillation (A-fib)	Congestive heart failure, mitral valve disease, rheumatic heart disease, coronary artery disease, hypertension, hyperthyroidism, thyrotoxicosis
Junctional rhythm	Digitalis toxicity, quinidine reaction, overdose on beta blockers or calcium channel blockers, hypoxemia, hyperkalemia, increased vagal tone, damage to the AV node, myocardial infarct, congestive heart failure
Premature ventricular contractions (PVC)	Anxiety or stress, tobacco, alcohol, caffeine use, hypoxia, acidosis, electrolyte imbalances, sympathomimetic drugs, ischemic heart disease, coronary artery disease, myocardial infarct, congestive heart failure, mechanical stimulation of the heart, reperfusion after thrombolytic therapy
Ventricular tachycardia (V-tach)	Myocardial infarct, ischemia, valvular disease, rheumatic heart disease, cardiomyopathy, anorexia nervosa, metabolic disorders, drug toxicity
Ventricular fibrillation (V-fib)	Myocardial infarct, ischemia
First-degree heart block	Myocardial infarct, digitalis toxicity, complications from cardiac surgery, chronic heart disease, effects of certain drugs
Second-degree heart block, type I, Wenckebach	Myocardial infarction, electrolyte imbalance, acute rheumatic infections, myocarditis, drug toxicity: digitalis (Lanoxin), procainamide (Procan), quinidine sulfate (Quinidine), propranolol (Inderal), verapamil (Isoptin)
Second-degree heart block, type II, Classical	Myocardial infarction, electrolyte imbalance, acute rheumatic infections, myocarditis, progressive from Type I drug toxicity myocardial infarction, digitalis, procainamide (Procan), quinidine sulfate (Quinidine), propranolol (Inderal), verapamil (Isoptin)
Third-degree or complete heart block	Ischemia or damage to AV node, frequently associated with inferior or anteroseptal myocardial infarction, degenerative conduction system disease, damage to conduction system during surgery, acute myocarditis, increased vagal tone, digitalis (Lanoxin) or propranolol (Inderal) toxicity, electrolyte imbalance, progression from Type II

    b. External forces

        1) Stress

        2) Exercise

        3) Pain

        4) Anemia

        5) Hypovolemia

3. Cardiac muscle cells have the capability of **automaticity** (ability to fire without stimulation), allowing the cell to serve as a pacemaker or cause premature beats

4. Each heartbeat creates distinctive wave forms: P, QRS, and T (see Table 2-5); each QRS should correspond to the pulse

Table 2-5	Wave Formations on an EKG	
Configuration	**Wave Form**	**Characteristics**
	P wave	First upright, positive wave; normally smooth, round configuration; one should proceed each QRS; demonstrates atrial contraction
	QRS—Q wave	First negative deflection
	QRS—R wave	First positive deflection after the Q
	QRS—S wave	Next negative deflection after R wave; called the QRS regardless of the presence of all three waveforms; demonstrates ventricular contraction
	T wave	Large wave form after QRS, upright, positive, round; demonstrates ventricular relaxation
	P-R interval	From beginning of P wave to beginning of Q wave; length of time it takes the impulse to travel from SA node through the bundle of HIS; normally 0.12 to 0.20 sec
	QRS interval	Beginning of Q wave to end of S wave; length of time it takes the impulse to travel from bundle of HIS to Purkinje fibers; ventricular contraction (depolarization) and beginning of repolarization (resting); normally 0.04 to 0.12 sec
	S-T segment	Should be a straight line between the S wave and beginning of T wave (isoelectric); demonstrates beginning and end of ventricular repolarization

5. An action potential is the electrical activity that occurs in a cell by the movement of ions across cell membranes

   a. During the resting state, the cell is *polarized,* with positive and negative ions equal on either side of the membrane; maintained by the sodium (Na)-potassium (K) pump

   b. Depolarization (contraction) requires a change from a negative to positive state; Na ions enter rapidly, opening the Na channels; Calcium (Ca) is allowed in, K is not allowed to cross

   c. A threshold potential is reached when the cell becomes less negative, creating an action potential; which depolarizes cardiac muscle cells; Ca enters the cell and causes contraction of the cardiac muscle

   d. Repolarization then occurs in order to return the cell to a polarized state, Na channels close, the cell begins to gain negative charge; the Na-K pump restores the ions to proper concentration

   e. The sequence is repeated for each heartbeat

6. A refractory period is a certain stage in the conduction cycle where there is resistance to stimulation

   a. *Absolute refractory period:* from beginning of Q to middle of T wave; no stimulus of any size can cause another impulse to occur

   b. *Relative refractory period:* from middle of T to end of T wave; a stimulus that is larger than the usual stimulus to create an impulse can stimulate the muscle cells to contract; an example is when a PVC occurs directly at the same time as a T wave, resulting in ventricular tachycardia or ventricular fibrillation

7. Two major categories of dysrhythmias

   a. Alteration in impulse formation

      1) Rate: tachycardia or bradycardia

      2) Rhythm: regular or irregular

      3) Ectopic beats (extra impulse)

         a) Premature atrial contractions (PAC)

         b) Premature junctional contractions (PJC)

         c) Junctional escape beats

         d) Premature ventricular contractions (PVC)

   b. Alteration in conductivity

      1) Heart blocks

      2) **Reentry phenomena** is the blockage of an impulse through one of the bundle branches, causing the impulse to retrograde backwards, reentering the other bundle branch and causing a premature beat

8. Cardiac rhythms are classified according to the site of impulse formation or the site and degree of conduction block (see Table 2-6)

a. Sinus rhythms

1) Normal sinus rhythm (NSR): impulse originates at the SA node, travels normal pathway; no delays; wave forms are uniform; all waveforms are of a fixed duration; P wave present representing atrial depolarization and the waveform is normal, smooth, and upright

2) Sinus arrhythmia: sinus rhythm that varies in rate during inspiration (faster) and during expiration (slower); common in very young and the very old

3) Sinus tachycardia (ST)

a) Same configuration as normal sinus rhythm except rate is greater than 100 bpm

b) Can be an early warning sign of cardiac dysfunction, such as heart failure

c) Client may be asymptomatic; symptoms experienced may be "racing" feeling, syncope, dyspnea

4) Sinus bradycardia (SB)

a) Same configuration as normal sinus rhythm except rate is less than 60 bpm

b) Clients may be asymptomatic; if not tolerating the bradycardia, may experience decreased level of consciousness, syncope, hypotension

5) Sinus arrest or sinus block

a) All configurations are normal; drop one or more complete complexes

b) Sinus block: measurement of R-R will be exact, even with missing complex

c) Sinus arrest: measurement of R-R will not be exact with missing complex

d) Symptoms may not be present unless pause is great enough to decrease cardiac output; client will experience same signs and symptoms as bradycardia

6) Sick sinus syndrome (SSS)

a) From diseases that affect the SA node; often found in older clients

b) Dysfunctions that cause problems with formation, transmission, or conduction of the impulse

c) Electrocardiographic characteristics of SSS are changes in the type of rhythm, pacemaker site and/or rate; the client may alter between: sinus bradycardia or sinus arrhythmia; sinus pauses or sinus arrest; atrial tachydysrhythmias such as atrial fibrillation, atrial flutter, or atrial tachycardia; brady-tachy syndrome (alternating periods of bradycardia and tachycardia)

d) Signs and symptoms of SSS: dizziness, light-headedness, syncope, fatigue or other signs of decreased cardiac output

| Table 2-6 | ECG Characteristics of Selected Cardiac Rhythms and Dysrhythmias | |

Rhythm/ECG Appearance	ECG Characteristics	Management

Supraventricular Rhythms

Normal sinus rhythm (NSR)

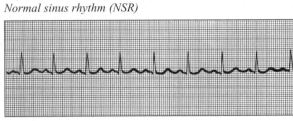

Rate: 60 to 100 bpm
Rhythm: Regular
P:QRS: 1:1
PR interval: 0.12 to 0.20 sec
QRS complex: 0.06 to 0.10 sec

None; normal heart rhythm.

Sinus arrhythmia

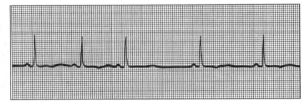

Rate: 60 to 100 bpm
Rhythm: Irregular, varying with respirations
P:QRS: 1:1
PR interval: 0.12 to 0.20 sec
QRS complex: 0.06 to 0.10 sec

Generally none; considered a normal rhythm in the very young and very old.

Sinus tachycardia

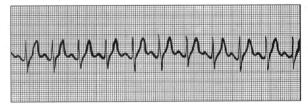

Rate: 101 to 150 bpm
Rhythm: Regular
P:QRS: 1:1 (With very fast rates, P wave may be hidden in preceding T wave)
PR interval: 0.12 to 0.20 sec
QRS complex: 0.06 to 0.10 sec

Treated only if the client is experiencing symptoms or is at risk for myocardial damage.
Treat underlying cause (e.g., hypovolemia, fever, pain).
Beta blockers or verapamil may be used.

Sinus bradycardia

Rate:< 60 bpm
Rhythm: Regular
P:QRS: 1:1
PR interval: 0.12 to 0.20 sec
QRS complex: 0.06 to 0.10 sec

Treated only if the client is experiencing symptoms. Intravenous atropine and/or pacemaker therapy may be used.

Premature atrial contractions (PAC)

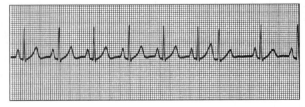

Rate: Variable
Rhythm: Irregular, with normal rhythm interrrupted by early beats arising in the atria
P:QRS: 1:1
PR interval: 0.12 to 0.20 sec, but may be prolonged
QRS complex: 0.6 to 0.10 sec

Usually require no treatment. Advise client to reduce alcohol and caffeine intake, to reduce stress, and to stop smoking.

Paroxysmal supraventricular tachycardia (PSVT)

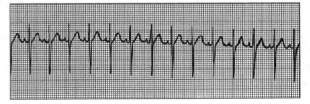

Rate: 100 to 280 bpm (usually 150 to 200 bpm)
Rhythm: Regular
P:QRS: P waves often not identifiable
PR interval: Not measured
QRS complex: 0.06 to 0.10 sec

Treat if client is experiencing symptoms. Treatment may include vagal manuevers (Valsalva, carotid sinus massage); oxygen therapy; adenosine, verapamil, procainamide, propranolol, and esmolol; and synchronized cardioversion.

Table 2-6	ECG Characteristics of Selected Cardiac Rhythms and Dysrhythmias (*cont.*)

Rhythm/ECG Appearance	**ECG Characteristics**	**Management**
Atrial flutter 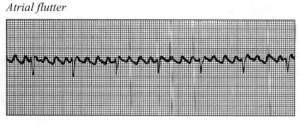	Rate: Atrial 240 to 360 bpm; ventricular rate depends on degree of AV block and usually is < 150 bpm Rhythm: Atrial regular, ventricular usually regular P:QRS: 2:1, 4:1, 6:1; may vary PR interval: Not measured QRS complex: 0.06 to 0.10 sec	Synchronized cardioversion; medications to slow ventricular response such as a beta blocker or calcium channel blocker (verapamil), followed by quinidine, procainamide, flecainide, or amiodarone.
Atrial fibrillation 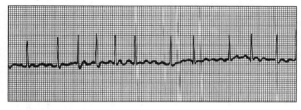	Rate: Atrial 300 to 600 bpm (too rapid to count); ventricular 100 to 180 bpm in untreated clients Rhythm: Irregularly irregular P:QRS: Variable PR interval: Not measured QRS complex: 0.06 to 0.10 sec	Synchronized cardioversion; medications to reduce ventricular response rate: verapamil, propranolol, digoxin, anticoagulant therapy to reduce risk of clot formation and stroke.
Junctional escape rhythm 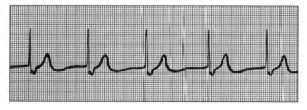	Rate: 40 to 60 bpm; junctional tachycardia 60 to 140 bpm Rhythm: Regular P:QRS: P waves may be absent, inverted and immediately preceding or succeeding QRS complex, or hidden in QRS complex PR interval: < 0.10 sec if P wave is prior to QRS complex QRS complex: 0.06 to 0.10 sec	Treat cause if client is experiencing symptoms.
Ventricular Rhythms *Premature ventricular contractions (PVC)* 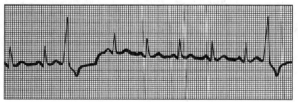	Rate: Variable Rhythm: Irregular, with PVC interrupting underlying rhythm and followed by a compensatory pause P:QRS: No P wave noted before PVC PR interval: Absent with PVC QRS complex: Wide (> 0.12 sec) and bizarre in appearance; differs from normal QRS complex	Treat if client is experiencing symptoms. Advise against stimulant use (caffeine, nicotine). Drug therapy includes intravenous lidocaine, procainamide, quinidine, propranolol, phenytoin, bretylium.
Ventricular tachycardia (VT or V tach) 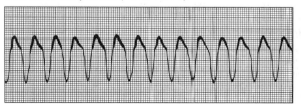	Rate: 100 to 250 bpm Rhythm: Regular P:QRS: P waves usually not identifiable PR interval: Not measured QRS complex: 0.12 sec or greater; bizarre shape	Treat if VT is sustained or if the client is experiencing symptoms. Treatment includes intravenous procainamide or lidocaine and/or immediate defibrillation if the client is unconscious or unstable.

Table 2-6	ECG Characteristics of Selected Cardiac Rhythms and Dysrhythmias (*cont.*)	
Rhythm/ECG Appearance	**ECG Characteristics**	**Management**
Ventricular fibrillation (VF, V fib) 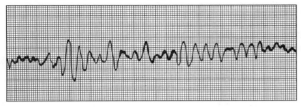	Rate: Too rapid to count Rhythm: Grossly irregular P:QRS: No identifiable P waves PR interval: None QRS: Bizarre, varying in shape and direction	Immediate defibrillation.
Atrioventricular Conduction Blocks *First-degree AV block* 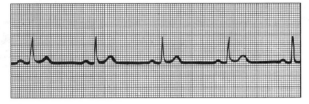	Rate: Usually 60 to 100 bpm Rhythm: Regular P:QRS: 1:1 PR interval: > 0.20 sec QRS complex: 0.06 to 0.10 sec	None required.
Second-degree AV block, type I (Mobitz I, Wenckebach) 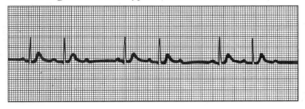	Rate: 60 to 100 bpm Rhythm: Atrial regular; ventricular irregular P:QRS: 1:1 until P wave blocked with no subsequent QRS complex PR interval: Progressively lengthens in a regular pattern QRS complex: 0.06 to 0.10 sec; sudden absence of QRS complex	Monitoring and observation; atropine or isoproterenol if client is experiencing symptoms.
Second-degree AV block, type II (Mobitz II) 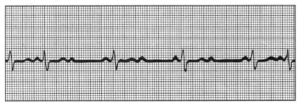	Rate: Atrial 60 to 100 bpm; ventricular < 60 bpm Rhythm: Atrial regular; ventricular irregular P:QRS: Typically 2:1, may vary PR interval: Constant PR interval for each conducted QRS complex QRS complex: 0.06 to 0.10 sec	Atropine or isoproterenol; pacemaker therapy.
Third-degree AV block (Complete heart block) 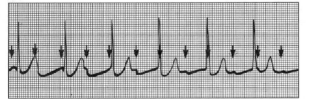	Rate: Atrial 60 to 100 bpm; ventricular 15 to 60 bpm Rhythm: Atrial regular; ventricular regular P:QRS: No relationship between P waves and QRS complexes; independent rhythms PR interval: Not measured QRS complex: 0.06 to 0.10 sec if junctional escape rhythm; > 0.12 sec if ventricular escape rhythm	Immediate pacemaker therapy.

b. Atrial dysrhythmias

1) Impulse originates in the atrial tissue (ectopic) outside the normal conduction system (SA node)

2) Premature atrial contractions (PAC)

a) Ectopic beat that comes early in the cycle with the same configuration as normal beats

b) Usually asymptomatic and benign

3) Atrial tachycardia (AT) or paroxysmal supraventricular tachycardia (PST)

a) Fast rate with unidentifiable, normal P wave or P wave with a different configuration

b) Sudden onset, sudden termination

c) Usually related to reentry mechanism around AV node

d) Seen more often in females

NCLEX!

e) Signs and symptoms: palpitations, "racing" heart, anxiety, dizziness, dyspnea, angina pain, diaphoresis, extreme fatigue, polyuria

4) Atrial flutter

a) Usually regular rhythm (but may be irregular) with saw-toothed waves instead of P waves

b) Thought to be result of intra-atrial reentry mechanism

NCLEX!

c) Signs and symptoms: may be asymptomatic, palpitations or "fluttering" in chest, if rapid ventricular response is present, signs of decreased cardiac output are present because of the loss of "atrial kick" and decreased ventricular filling time

5) Atrial fibrillation (A-fib)

a) Chaotic atrial activity causing the atria to quiver instead of contract normally

b) Rapid impulse firing from atrial wall bombards the AV node, resulting in a wavy baseline between R-R, no visible consistent P waves, and an irregular ventricular response pattern

c) May be intermittent or a chronic rhythm disturbance

d) Clinical signs and symptoms depends on ventricular response: signs and symptoms of decreased cardiac output, hypotension, shortness of breath, fatigue, angina, syncope, heart failure; peripheral pulses will be irregular and variable in quality

NCLEX!

e) High risk for thromboemboli formation due to pooling of blood in atria and absence of "atrial kick"

c. Junctional dysrhythmias

1) Premature junctional contraction (PJC)

a) Early impulse in the cycle, originates in the AV node with P wave that may fall before, during, or after the QRS but is *always* inverted

b) Usually asymptomatic

2) Junctional rhythm

    a) Impulse originates in AV node, rate slower (40-60 bpm)

    b) Failsafe mechanism when SA node does not fire; but should not remain as dominant pacemaker

    c) Depolarization of atria is through retrograde conduction (backward) so any visible P wave would be inverted on the ECG strip; P wave may be absent or inverted before or behind the QRS

    d) Signs and symptoms of decreased cardiac output from absence of "atrial kick" and decreased myocardial tissue perfusion leading to ischemia may lead to signs of heart failure

3) Accelerated junctional rhythm and junctional tachycardia

    a) Same characteristics as junctional rhythm; rate distinguishes the two arrhythmias

    b) Accelerated junctional rhythm (60–100), faster than the normal rate of the A-V node

    c) Junctional tachycardia (greater than 100)

d. Ventricular dysrhythmias

1) Originate in the ventricles (idioventricular rhythm); inherent rate 20 to 40 bpm

2) Denoted by wide and bizarre QRS complexes that are greater than 0.12 second in duration with an increased amplitude, abnormal S-T segment, and a T wave that has an opposite deflection from the QRS complex

3) P wave will have no relationship to the QRS complex

4) Premature ventricular contraction (PVC)

    a) Most common dysrhythmia

    b) Comes early in the cycle

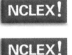

    c) Frequent, recurrent, or multifocal PVCs indicate myocardial irritability; may precipitate lethal dysrhythmias

    d) Incidence greatest following myocardial ischemia, infarction, hypertrophy, or infection

    e) Common and usually clinically insignificant in older adults

    f) May be unifocal (coming from one site); multifocal (coming from different sites in the ventricular wall)

    g) May come in patterns: bigeminy—every other beat is a PVC; trigeminy—every third beat is PVC; couplets—two beats together; triplets—three beats together; salvo—three to six beats in a row

    h) Signs and symptoms: may be asymptomatic; feeling "skipped beats"; chest discomfort, dyspnea, hypotension, dizziness

5) Ventricular tachycardia (V-tach or VT)

    a) Rapid ventricular rhythm disturbance defined as three or more consecutive PVCs; can be short burst or sustained rhythm; usually regular with a rate greater than 100 bpm

    b) Reentry mechanism usual cause

    c) Signs and symptoms: fluttering in chest, palpitations, shortness of breath, signs of decreased cardiac output, hypotension, loss of consciousness, no palpable pulses, may soon deteriorate into lethal rhythm

6) **Ventricular fibrillation (V-fib)**

    a) Rapid chaotic ventricular rhythm causing the ventricles to quiver; heart does not pump; cardiac arrest occurs

    b) Without effective treatment death occurs

    c) Effective treatment: defibrillation and cardiopulmonary resuscitation (CPR)

    d) ECG shows chaotic irregular bizarre complexes with no discernable rate or rhythm

7) Idioventricular rhythm

    a) Normal complexes are not present; P waves, if present, are not associated with QRS; QRS wide and bizarre like a PVC; overall rate slow (20 to 40)

    b) Lethal arrhythmia, may follow defibrillation, V-fib or V-tach

    c) Signs and symptoms: decreased cardiac output, usually unconscious

e. Atrioventricular conduction blocks (heart blocks)

1) Conduction defects that delay or block transmission of the sinus impulse through the AV node

    a) May be from injured or diseased SA node or AV node area

    b) May be from increased vagal tone

    c) May be benign or severe

    d) Should be monitored for progression to a more severe level of block

2) First-degree AV block

    a) Benign condition and is not considered a true block

    b) Prolonged but constant PR interval (greater than 0.20 sec.) in duration, otherwise normal sinus rhythm (see Table 2-7)

    c) Usually asymptomatic; can progress to higher level block

3) Second-degree AV block: Type I

    a) Also called Mobitz I or Wenckebach (tip to remember: "W"encke-back and "w"eird pattern)

    b) Cyclic pattern of complexes with a progressively prolonging PR interval until one QRS is totally blocked or dropped (see Table 2-7)

       c) Signs and symptoms: asymptomatic; if rate drops, then signs and symptoms of decreased cardiac output would be observed

   4) Second-degree AV block: Type II

       a) Also called Mobitz II or Classical

       b) Usually seen in coronary artery disease and anterior wall MI

       c) Nonconducted impulses usually occurring in a regular manner

       d) Must have more than one P wave to every QRS complex (can have several Ps to each QRS)

       e) PR interval is constant (see Table 2-7)

       f) Signs and symptoms depend on ventricular rate

   5) Third-degree AV block

       a) Also called complete heart block

       b) SA node fires, P waves are regular but do not conduct through to AV node; ventricular rhythm (QRS) will be regular but in no way related to the P wave

       c) No relationship between P waves and QRS complexes; may or may not have more Ps than QRS complexes

       d) PR interval constantly varies (see Table 2-7)

NCLEX!

       e) Signs and symptoms associated with bradycardia and decreased cardiac output: light-headedness, confusion, syncope

       f) Requires intervention, can be life-threatening

   6) Bundle branch blocks

       a) Right or left bundle branch block can occur

       b) Impulse conducted slowly through the ventricles causing a widened QRS complex (greater than 0.12 second) and rabbit ear configuration occurs on QRS

       c) Usually a benign process without symptoms, unless coupled with an AV block

F. Other

   1) Wandering pacemaker

       a) Origination of impulse changes sites, from SA node, atrial cell, and AV node

Table 2-7	**PR Interval Is Constant**	**PR Interval Is NOT Constant**
Determining the Type of Heart Block	First-degree heart block—PR interval > 0.20	Second-degree heart block—Type I, Mobitz I, Wenckebach
	Second-degree heart block—Type II, Mobitz II, Classical	Third-degree heart block

      b) ECG shows variation: normal Ps, no Ps, inverted Ps

      c) May be benign unless ventricular rate is slow or fast; client would experience symptoms of bradycardia or tachycardia

  2) Permanent pacemakers

      a) Can be atrial (pace atrium), ventricular (pace ventricle) or A-V sequential (pace both)

      b) Demand pacemaker most common: set at a rate that is individualized for each client; should begin to fire when clients own HR drops to or below set rate

      c) Types: atrial pacemaker: (spike occurs before each P wave while in demand mode); ventricular pacemaker: (spike occurs before each QRS wave while in demand mode); A-V sequential: (two spikes occur while in demand mode; one before the P wave and one before QRS)

      d) Problems encountered: failure to sense (pacemaker does not sense clients own rhythm and continues to send an impulse; ECG will show spike at regular intervals throughout clients regular rhythm); failure to pace (pacemaker fails to begin firing when the HR drops below set rate; ECG may show whatever rhythm occurred that caused the need for the pacer); failure to capture (pacemaker fires in a regular pattern but the ventricle does not depolarize; ECG shows spikes without any QRS)

C. Nursing assessment

  1. Nursing assessment includes VS, symptoms of decreased cardiac output; analysis of monitor pattern for rate, rhythm, assessment of P wave morphology, calculation of intervals; assessment of S-T segment, determination of rhythm

  2. Diagnostic tests: 12-lead ECG; single-lead telemetry (usually lead II); electrophysiologic studies

    a. No specific laboratory test for cardiac dysrhythmias

    b. Laboratory tests may be helpful in determining the cause of dysrhythmia

      1) Hypoxia

      2) Electrolyte imbalances

      3) Acid-base imbalances

      4) Drug levels

D. Nursing management

  1. Medications: antidysrhythmic drugs (see Table 2-8)

  2. Recognition of normal sinus rhythm as well as knowledge of dysrhythmias

  3. Observation of monitoring system and rapid decision making process

  4. Collaborative care between nurse and physician; standing orders needed for lethal arrhythmias

  5. Administer oxygen as necessary

NCLEX!

Table 2-8		Antidysrhythmic Drug Classifications	
Class	**Group**	**Action**	**Common Drugs**
I	Class I-A	Prolong action potential	Quinidine sulfate (Quinidine), procainamide hydrochloride (Pronestyl), disopyramide phosphate (Norpace), moricizine (Ethmozine)
	Class I-B	Decrease refractory period	Xylocaine hydrochloride (Lidocaine), mexiletine hydrochloride (Mexitil), ocainide hydrochloride (Tonocard)
	Class I-C	Decrease automaticity and conduction through the AV node	Flecainide (Tambocor), encainide hydrochloride (Enkaid), propafenone hydrochloride (Rythmol)
II	Beta blockers	Decrease automaticity and conduction through the AV node	Esmolol hydrochloride (Brevibloc), propranolol hydrochloride (Inderal), acebutolol hydrochloride (Brivibloc)
III		Prolong repolarization and refractory period and decreases intraventricular conduction	Sotalol (Betapace), amiodarone hydrochloride (Cordarone), ibutilide fumarate (Corvert)
IV	Calcium channel blockers	Blocks calcium influx across the myocardial cell; negative dromotropic effect	Verapamil hydrochloride (Isoptin), nifedipine (Procardia) diltiazem (Cardizem)

6. Countershock

   a. Used to interrupt cardiac rhythms that compromise cardiac output

   b. Causes total depolarization of all cardiac cells wiping out the dysrhythmia and allowing the SA node to resume its normal rhythm

   c. Two types of countershock

      1) Defibrillation: emergency treatment for ventricular fibrillation; the quicker the delivery of the shock, the higher the survival rate; place paddles or pads at base and apex of heart

      2) Synchronized cardioversion: countershock synchronized with the R wave so that heart is totally depolarized to allow SA node to resume sinus rhythm and to avoid repolarization phase of the cells; also used as an electric procedure for treatment of tachydysrhythmias (atrial fibrillation, atrial flutter, supraventricular tachycardia, stable ventricular tachycardia)

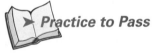

Practice to Pass

The client is on telemetry monitoring showing a normal sinus rhythm with a rate of 82 bpm. The alarm sounds and the monitor shows chaotic activity on the screen. What should the nurse's actions include?

VII. Inflammatory Diseases of the Heart

A. Overview

1. Inflammatory diseases of the heart are defined as inflammation of any layer of cardiac tissue (endocardium, myocardium, pericardium) that can damage the valves, muscle, or pericardial lining

2. Conditions include rheumatic heart disease, endocarditis, myocarditis, and pericarditis

3. Causes

   a. Rheumatic heart disease: a *Beta-hemolytic streptococcus* bacteria

   b. Infective endocarditis: bacterial infection or abnormal immunological reaction

      c. Myocarditis: viral, bacterial, or fungal infection, often *Coxsackievirus*

      d. Pericarditis: cardiac trauma, MI, infection, neoplasm, kidney disease, rheumatic fever

B. Pathophysiology

  1. Rheumatic heart disease (RHD)

NCLEX!

    a. A chronic condition characterized by valvular deformity, which slowly progresses; follows an acute or repeated episode of rheumatic fever (inflammatory disease from a *Beta-hemolytic streptococcus*)

    b. In acute stage, valves become red, swollen and inflamed with lesions developing on the leaflets

    c. In chronic stage, scar tissue develops, leaflets become rigid and deformed; stenosis or regurgitation may develop

    d. Left heart valves are affected more often; mitral valve most often

    e. Signs and symptoms

NCLEX!

      1) Precordial chest discomfort

      2) Tachycardia

      3) Evidence of heart failure

      4) Pericardial friction rub

      5) S_3 (atrial gallop) or S_4 (ventricular gallop)

      6) Murmur from mitral or aortic regurgitation may be noted

      7) Cardiomegaly

      8) Pericardial effusion

  2. Infective endocarditis

    a. Defined as inflammation of the lining of the heart; involves any part of endothelial lining of the heart, most often the mitral valve

    b. *Staphylococcus aureus* usual infective organism

    c. Acute and subacute classifications

    d. Begins with platelet–fibrin vegetation on healthy valves (acute) and on damaged valves or endocardial tissue (subacute)

    e. Signs and symptoms of infective endocarditis: murmur, cough, shortness of breath, anorexia, abdominal pain, anemia, splenomegaly, fever (greater than 101.5°F), chills, night sweats, flu-like symptoms, joint pain, and petechiae

  3. Myocarditis

    a. Defined as an inflammatory disorder of the heart muscle that is unrelated to CAD or MI

    b. Infection can be caused by viruses, bacteria, or protozoa; immunologic response can be due to effects of radiation, chemical poisons, drugs, burns, or *Coxsackie B enterovirus* (most common in United States)

    c. Inflammatory process causing local or diffuse swelling and damage to the cells of the myocardium; abscesses in interstitial tissue from infectious agents; pinpoint hemorrhage in layers of the heart

    d. If condition deteriorates, could lead to dilated cardiomyopathy

    e. Results in weakening of heart muscle and decreased contractility

    f. Signs and symptoms depend on the degree of cardiac damage

        1) May be asymptomatic at first

        2) Signs of inflammation: fever, chills, fatigue, malaise, dyspnea, palpitations, arthralgias

        3) Signs of heart failure: tachycardia, dysrhythmias, S_3 or S_4 gallop, systolic murmur, transient pericardial friction rub, cardiomegaly, and ECG abnormalities

  4. Pericarditis

    a. Defined as an inflammation of the pericardium (fluid-filled sac surrounding the heart)

    b. May be primary or secondary to other disease processes; usually viral; affects more men than women

    c. Frequent complication of end stage renal failure; frequently seen after MI or following open heart surgery

    d. When inflammatory mediators are released, vasodilatation occurs causing hyperemia (increased blood flow) and edema

    e. Increased capillary permeability allows plasma proteins and fibrinogen to gather in the pericardial space

    f. Exudate is formed that may contain red blood cells or be purulent if infective

    g. Fibrosis and scarring may restrict the heart's ability to function effectively; pericardial effusions may develop

    h. Chest pain occurs due to inflammation of nerve fibers in pericardium

    i. Acute pericarditis lasts 2 to 6 weeks

    j. Signs and symptoms

        1) Sharp chest pain (rapid onset) worsening with deep breath, cough or change in position; pain improves if elevated or sits up

        2) Dyspnea

        3) Dry cough

        4) Fever (low grade)

        5) Pericardial friction rub (leathery, grating sound) heard most commonly on expiration

    k. Complications include cardiac tamponade or pericardial effusions

C. Nursing assessment

   1. Assessment

     a. Rheumatic fever: VS, lung sounds, heart sounds, apical pulse, symptom analysis of any chest discomfort

     b. Infective endocarditis: VS, symptom analysis of complaints, nutritional status, palpate spleen, skin assessment for bleeding; heart sounds, peripheral pulses, capillary refill

     c. Myocarditis: VS, symptom analysis of complaints and pain, ECG pattern, heart sounds

     d. Pericarditis: VS, symptom analysis of pain and what worsens or relieves it, lung sounds, respiratory status

   2. Diagnostic tests

     a. Rheumatic fever: CBC, C-reactive protein (show inflammation), erythrocyte sedimentation rate (ESR), antistreptolysin titer (ASO) titer

     b. Infective endocarditis: CBC, immune testing, blood cultures, urine (increased creatinine, hematuria and increased protein), ECG

     c. Myocarditis: ESR, CBC, antiviral antibodies, ECG, heart catheterization with biopsy of heart muscle, serum immunoglobulins, cultures

     d. Pericarditis: ESR, ECG, echocardiogram, hemodynamic monitoring, CXR, CT scan, and MRI

D. Nursing management

   1. Medications

     a. Rheumatic fever: antibiotics (penicillin, erythromycin [EES], clindamycin [Cleocin], amoxicillin [Amoxil]); salicylates (Aspirin); or corticosteroids for inflammation and joint pain

     b. Infective endocarditis: antibiotics (may use multiple drugs—oxacillin [Bactocill], penicillin, ampicillin [Ampicin], gentamycin sulfate [Gentamycin], cefazolin sodium [Ancef], vancomycin hydrochloride [Vancocin]); antipyretics, antiinflammatory agents

     c. Myocarditis: antipyretics, antidysrhythmics, anticoagulants, digoxin (Lanoxin) if heart failure occurs, corticosteroids or immunosuppressive drugs, antimicrobial agents

     d. Pericarditis: non-narcotic analgesics, NSAIDs, antipyretics, corticosteroids

   2. Provide supportive care, emotional rest

   3. Prevent complications and future recurrences; IV therapy if indicated

   4. Monitor VS, heart sounds, ECG pattern, respiratory status

   5. Priorities of nursing care

     a. Assess and treat pain

     b. Assist with activities of daily living; allow rest periods

    c. Provide diversional activity

    d. Monitor for signs of infection

    e. Monitor for signs of decreased cardiac output

    f. Teach client importance of compliance and taking antibiotics until completed

    g. Teach client effective coping mechanisms

6. With myocarditis, client needs to decrease workload and increase oxygen supply to the heart

7. Pericarditis may require a pericardiocentesis (removal of fluid) or surgery

8. Administer oxygen as needed

VIII. Valvular Heart Disease

A. Overview

1. Valvular heart disease is defined as diseases or conditions that interfere with unidirectional blood flow within the heart

2. Can be acquired from either acute (endocarditis or calcium deposits) or chronic (rheumatic heart disease) conditions

3. Occurs as **stenosis** (inability of leaflets to open and close properly) or **regurgitation** (backflow of blood through a valve that cannot close properly due to damage or disease)

4. Other causes include MI, congenital heart defects

B. Pathophysiology

1. Stenosis

    a. Involves fusion of valve leaflets producing a narrow opening and rigidity

    b. The fusion may result from scarring of valves caused by:

        1) Endocarditis

        2) Myocardial infarction

        3) Calcification

    c. Blood flow is impeded resulting in decreased cardiac output, impaired ventricular filling, ejection fraction and stroke volume

    d. Can affect mitral, tricuspid, aortic, or pulmonary valve

2. Regurgitation

    a. Caused by insufficient or incompetent valves causing incomplete closure, allowing backflow of blood

    b. Result from deformity or erosion of valve by vegetative lesions of bacterial endocarditis; scarring or tearing from MI; cardiac dilation—as heart enlarges, valves stretch; leaflets no longer meet causing regurgitation

3. Hemodynamic changes occur

    a. Blood volume and pressure are reduced in front of affected valve

    b. Volume and pressure increase behind the affected valve

4. Chambers behind the affected valve hypertrophy due to increased pressure of the blood flow; cardiac output falls as compensatory mechanisms become ineffective; heart begins to fail

    a. Increased muscle size leads to increased oxygen demand

    b. Decreased blood supply to the enlarged muscle leads to heart failure

    c. Infarction occurs and loss of functional muscle

5. Affect aortic and mitral valve; **mitral valve prolapse** is when the mitral valve prolapses back into the atrium causing regurgitation of blood from ventricle to atrium

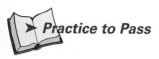

6. Signs and symptoms

    a. Stenosis: pulmonary congestion, dyspnea, pulmonary HTN, dizziness, fatigue, tachycardia, murmur or rub, S_3 or S_4 heart sound, angina; pulmonary stenosis may cause venous distention and swelling of the ankles

    b. Regurgitation

        1) Mitral: dyspnea, pulmonary HTN, decreased cardiac output, dizziness and fatigue, tachycardia, angina, murmur or rub, S_3 or S_4 heart sound

        2) Aortic: wide pulse pressure, hyperkinetic (strong, bounding) peripheral pulses, signs and symptoms of CHF, angina

C. Nursing assessment

1. Assessment includes: vital signs, heart sounds, lung sounds, symptom analysis of complaints and pain, respiratory status, exercise tolerance, presence of edema, peripheral pulses

2. Diagnostic tests: ECG, echocardiogram, CXR, cardiac catheterization

D. Nursing management

1. Medications include digitalis (Lanoxin), diuretics, Class I or III antidysrhythmic, prophylactic antibiotics prior to invasive procedures

2. Close observation for progression of disease, angina that might occur

3. Monitor prophylactic therapy to prevent infection of the diseased valves

4. Observe for signs and symptoms of congestive heart failure; treat as necessary

5. Pre- and postoperative teaching when medical treatment no longer effective and surgical intervention necessary

6. Teach client not to abruptly stop taking beta blockers or symptoms may return

7. Prepare client for and monitor following percutaneous balloon valvuloplasty

Practice to Pass

The client has been diagnosed with mitral prolapse. What should the nurse teach the client regarding treatment plans?

Case Study

M. J. presents to the emergency department with complaints of substernal crushing chest pain radiating to his left arm. He is a 58-year-old executive. He was having dinner with a client when the pain began. He states the pain started 2 hours ago and has been increasing in intensity since that time.

❶   What type of assessment should the nurse do?

❷   What parts of his past medical history would be important?

❸   What diagnostic studies should the nurse anticipate the physician ordering?

❹   What medications should the nurse anticipate being ordered for his chest pain?

❺   What ECG changes should the nurse look for?

For suggested responses, see pages 564–565.

Posttest

1   The client on a telemetry unit exhibits regular ECG complexes of normal duration and a heart rate of 82 bpm. The nurse assesses the client and notes that for each complex there is a corresponding palpable pulse. The nurse knows that for each pulse to be palpable what had to occur?

(1) Ventricular contraction
(2) Ventricular relaxation
(3) Fibrillation
(4) Cardiac standstill (asystole)

2   The client arrives in the Emergency Department with a heart rate of 130 bpm. The client appears anxious and is tachypneic. What part of the central nervous system is most likely responsible for this increased heart rate?

(1) Parasympathetic nervous system (PSNS)
(2) Sympathetic nervous system (SNS)
(3) Acetylcholine-cholinesterase feedback
(4) Vagus nerve

3   The client appears in the Emergency Department with distended neck veins, large round abdomen, palpable liver edges, and peripheral edema. These signs are suggestive of which of the following?

(1) Congestive heart failure
(2) Acute liver dysfunction
(3) Chronic liver disease
(4) Restrictive lung disease

4   A client with chest pain is given nitroglycerin (NTG) 1/150 sublingual for complaint of angina pectoris. Prior to the NTG, his blood pressure was 110/78. After 5 minutes, he says the chest pain is better but not gone. The nurse should first:

(1) Give another NTG.
(2) Check the pulse rate.
(3) Give morphine sulfate instead of NTG.
(4) Check the blood pressure (BP).

5   A client with congestive heart failure has digoxin (Lanoxin) ordered every day. Prior to giving the medicine, the nurse checks the digoxin level which is therapeutic and auscultates an apical pulse. The apical pulse is 62 bpm for 1 full minute. The nurse should:

(1) Hold the Lanoxin.
(2) Give half the dose now, wait an hour and then give the other half.
(3) Call the physician.
(4) Give the Lanoxin as ordered.

6   Which of the following clients is at high risk for developing coronary artery disease (CAD) that may not be responsive to diet and exercise alone? A client who:

(1) Has diabetes.
(2) Has a strong family history for cardiovascular disease.
(3) Is overweight and 55 years old.
(4) Had a stroke at age 40.

7   The client presents to the emergency room with substernal chest pain and is diagnosed with a subendocardial infarction. The client asks the nurse what that means. The nurse should tell him that the damage is:

(1) On the anterior wall of the left ventricle.
(2) On the posterior wall of the left ventricle.
(3) Involving the full thickness of the wall.
(4) Involving the inner layer of the heart.

8   The client is admitted to the coronary care unit with a diagnosis of left-sided heart failure. When listening to the lung sounds, the nurse hears crackles bilaterally. The nurse anticipates this because left ventricular failure leads to:

(1) Increased coronary artery perfusion.
(2) Pulmonary emboli.
(3) Increased peripheral resistance.
(4) Pulmonary congestion.

9   The client with a diagnosis of anterior myocardial infarction begins to show dysrhythmias on the monitor. Which of these most likely predisposes to dysrhythmia development with a myocardial infarction (MI)?

(1) Respiratory alkalosis
(2) Tissue ischemia
(3) Hypokalemia
(4) Digitalis toxicity

10   The client is being discharged from the hospital and needs discharge teaching. Some important measures the nurse should teach the client to prevent reinfarction following a myocardial infarction (MI) would include:

(1) Thrombolytic therapy.
(2) Heavy exercise such as high-intensity aerobics.
(3) Low-fat, low-sodium diet.
(4) Reduction in cigarette smoking.

See pages 82–83 for Answers and Rationales.

Answers and Rationales

Pretest

1   **Answer: 3** *Rationale:* Angina pectoris is the term for chest pain related to myocardial ischemia (not enough oxygen supply to the tissue for the demand). Any activity that increases the need for oxygen without an adequate available supply can cause angina. Pain from a pulmonary embolus would be abrupt onset and not necessarily related to activity. *Cognitive Level:* Application *Nursing Process:* Assessment; *Test Plan:* PHYS

2   **Answer: 2** *Rationale:* Orthopnea is shortness of breath caused by the movement of fluid back into the vasculature when the client lies down. He may have beginning signs of congestive heart failure and should be checked. Sleep apnea may cause orthopnea, but not

edema; angina doesn't necessarily cause edema either but should be accompanied by chest pain. *Cognitive Level:* Application *Nursing Process:* Assessment; *Test Plan:* PHYS

3   **Answer: 2** *Rationale:* Left heart failure causes pulmonary congestion and increased pressure in the lungs, which leads to tachycardia. Remember "L"eft and "L"ung; the two Ls go together; two of the symptoms deal with respiratory symptoms and none of the other answers are related to a diagnosis affecting the lungs. *Cognitive Level:* Application *Nursing Process:* Assessment; *Test Plan:* PHYS

4 Answer: 3 *Rationale:* Depressed S-T segment and inverted T-waves represent myocardial ischemia. Injury usually has a S-T segment elevation.
Cognitive Level: Application
Nursing Process: Assessment; *Test Plan:* PHYS

5 Answer: 3 *Rationale:* Left ventricular failure results in inability to empty the pulmonary vascular system leading to increased pulmonary pressures.
Cognitive Level: Application
Nursing Process: Analysis; *Test Plan:* PHYS

6 Answer: 4 *Rationale:* Bradycardia decreases the myocardium's demand for oxygen by decreasing workload of the heart. Heart rates less than 60 bpm are considered bradycardia. If, however, the heart rate is too low, blood supply is decreased and oxygen supply may be hindered.
Cognitive Level: Application
Nursing Process: Analysis; *Test Plan:* PHYS

7 Answer: 4 *Rationale:* Infarction (or heart attack) is the term for tissue that has been deprived of oxygen until the cells have died. Immediate attention should be given to the client who has just had a myocardial infarction (MI), which is noted by Q waves on an ECG.
Cognitive Level: Application
Nursing Process: Assessment; *Test Plan:* PHYS

8 Answer: 1 *Rationale:* Occlusion of a coronary artery blocks the blood flow and prevents oxygen getting to the myocardium. Option 2 is ischemia; option 3 could be bradycardia or a block; option 4 could be hypertrophy.
Cognitive Level: Application
Nursing Process: Analysis; *Test Plan:* PHYS

9 Answer: 1 *Rationale:* Lifestyles, cigarette smoking, and hyperlipidemia can be changed by changing behaviors. These risk factors should be stressed and plans made for how to change them.
Cognitive Level: Application
Nursing Process: Implementation; *Test Plan:* HPM

10 Answer: 4 *Rationale:* NTG can be used as a preventive to activities that trigger angina. This is especially helpful with sexual activity or work-related activities that may need to be continued. Modifying such activities may be necessary, but cardiac clients should not become crippled by their condition and lead sedentary lifestyles.
Cognitive Level: Application
Nursing Process: Planning; *Test Plan:* PHYS

Posttest

1 Answer: 1 *Rationale:* Depolarization of the myocardium results in contraction (systole) and that produces the palpable pulse and the corresponding QRS complex on the electrocardiogram.
Cognitive Level: Comprehension
Nursing Process: Analysis; *Test Plan:* PHYS

2 Answer: 2 *Rationale:* Stimulation of the SNS increases heart rate and respiratory rate. Remember "fight-or-flight" syndrome is a response by the SNS and heart rate increases.
Cognitive Level: Application
Nursing Process: Analysis; *Test Plan:* PHYS

3 Answer: 1 *Rationale:* Right-sided heart failure leads to backward venous congestion resulting in jugular vein distention, portal hypertension, and abdominal venous congestion resulting in ascites. Remember "R"ight means "R"est of the body whereas "L"eft means "L"ung in identifying where fluids stagnate.
Cognitive Level: Application
Nursing Process: Assessment; *Test Plan:* PHYS

4 Answer: 4 *Rationale:* The client does need another NTG if the chest pain is still present; however, a BP should be assessed *first*. If the systolic is greater than 100, another NTG can be given. If the systolic is less than 100, the physician should be consulted. Morphine sulfate is often given in this case.
Cognitive Level: Analysis
Nursing Process: Implementation; *Test Plan:* SECE

5 Answer: 4 *Rationale:* The Lanoxin should be held for a pulse rate less than 60 bpm. Nurses cannot arbitrarily give half of a dose without a physician's order. Unless specific parameters are given concerning pulse rate, most resources identify 60 as the reference pulse.
Cognitive Level: Application
Nursing Process: Implementation; *Test Plan:* SECE

6 Answer: 2 *Rationale:* Family history is a nonmodifiable risk factor. Although diet and exercise should be encouraged, this may not be sufficient to lower cholesterol and prevent CAD.
Cognitive Level: Analysis
Nursing Process: Analysis; *Test Plan:* HPM

7 Answer: 4 *Rationale:* The inner layer of the myocardium is referred to as the endocardium.
Cognitive Level: Application
Nursing Process: Analysis; *Test Plan:* PHYS

8 **Answer: 4** *Rationale:* Left ventricular failure leads to pulmonary congestion. When the left side cannot pump the blood out adequately, congestion occurs in the lungs where the blood backs up from the left ventricle.
Cognitive Level: Application
Nursing Process: Analysis; *Test Plan:* PHYS

9 **Answer: 2** *Rationale:* The ischemia that causes the MI can also cause the heart muscle to become irritable and irritated cells fire early, causing dysrhythmias. Although options 3 and 4 are true, nothing in the stem indicates these are specific to this client. Acidosis is usually the shift with MI, if one occurs.
Cognitive Level: Analysis
Nursing Process: Assessment; *Test Plan:* PHYS

10 **Answer: 3** *Rationale:* A low-fat, low-sodium diet aids in the reduction of cholesterol and/or triglycerides which could have caused the MI. A client having had a MI should not participate in heavy exercise this soon; a moderate exercise program with daily walking would be sufficient. Anticoagulant therapy with aspirin may be recommended, not thrombolytics, and clients with a MI should stop smoking all together.
Cognitive Level: Application
Nursing Process: Implementation; *Test Plan:* PHYS

Chapter References

Bullock, B. A. & Henze, R. L. (2000). *Focus on pathophysiology.* Philadelphia: Lippincott.

Corwin, E. J. (2000). *Handbook of pathophysiology* (2nd ed.). Philadelphia: Lippincott.

LeMone, P. & Burke, K. M. (2000). *Medical-surgical nursing: Critical thinking in client care* (2nd ed.). Upper Saddle River, NJ: Prentice Hall Health, pp. 1017–1171.

Price, S. A. & Wilson, L. M. (1997). *Pathophysiology: Clinical concepts of disease processes* (5th ed.). St. Louis, MO: Mosby, pp. 409–527.

Thomas, C. L. (Ed.). (1997). *Taber's cyclopedic medical dictionary* (19th ed.). Philadelphia: F. A. Davis.

Walraven, G. (1999). *Rapid EKG interpretation* (5th ed.). Upper Saddle River, NJ: Prentice Hall Health.

Wilson, B. A., Shannon, M. T., & Stang, C. L. (2001). *Nursing drug guide: 2001.* Upper Saddle River, NJ: Prentice Hall Health.

CHAPTER 3

Vascular Health Problems

Ann Harley, EdD, RN

CHAPTER OUTLINE

*Risk Factors Associated
  with Vascular Health Problems*
Hypertension
Peripheral Vascular Disease
Aneurysms

Thrombophlebitis
Varicose Veins
*Arteriospastic Disease (Raynaud's
  Disease)*

*Thromboangiitis Obliterans
  (Buerger's Disease)*

OBJECTIVES

▪ Define key terms associated with vascular problems.

▪ Identify risk factors associated with the development of a
vascular health problem.

▪ Discuss the common etiologies of vascular health problems.

▪ Describe pathophysiologic responses associated with specific
vascular health problems.

▪ Distinguish between abnormal and normal vascular findings
obtained from nursing assessment.

▪ Prioritize nursing interventions associated with specific
vascular health problems.

[*Media Link*]

*Use the CD-ROM enclosed with
this text, or log onto the address
given to access the free, interactive Companion Website created
for this series. The CD-ROM and
Companion Website accompanying this book offer additional
practice opportunities and information—NCLEX Review, Case
Studies, Glossary, In Depth with
NCLEX, and more.*

www.prenhall.com/hogan

REVIEW AT A GLANCE

aneurysm *a dilatation or an outpouching of the wall of an artery or vein that can occur anywhere in the body*

arterial steal *this phenomenon occurs when the arterioles are maximally dilated because of hypoxia; in order to meet the metabolic needs of the tissue, these arterioles steal from cutaneous and peripheral vessels, which causes the client to be aware of a "pins and needles" sensation in the affected area(s)*

chronic venous insufficiency *chronic failure of the venous valves to function, resulting in interference with the venous blood return to the heart and the production of generalized systemic edema*

diastolic *the pressure of the blood against the arterial walls when the ventricles of the heart are at rest*

embolus *a foreign object such as a piece of a thrombus floating in the bloodstream until such time as it becomes trapped in vessel*

hemodynamics *a study of the movement of blood within the body*

hypertension *a blood pressure that is greater than normal, usually greater than 140 systolic and 90 diastolic*

ischemia *a deficiency in the supply of oxygenated blood caused by a circulatory obstruction to a body part; the client will experience considerable pain in the affected part*

orthostatic hypotension *syncope or dizziness with sudden position changes, usually from supine to upright position, because of a drop in blood pressure*

peripherial vascular resistance *the sum of all resistances that the body has within the vascular system*

pheochromocytoma *this tumor originates in the neural crest cells of the sympathetic nervous system and is responsible for about 0.1 to 2.0 percent of hypertension; the tumor cells release catecholamines that cause episodic and sustained palpitations of the heart, sweating, headaches, fainting, and hypertensive emergencies*

primary hypertension *also known as idiopathic hypertension or essential hypertension; it is an elevated blood pressure from unknown causes that occurs in about 95 percent of diagnosed hypertensive clients*

primary varicose veins *superficial veins; seldom involves communicating veins; if valvular breakdown occurs, it is caused by hereditary factors*

pulse pressure *the difference between the systolic and the diastolic blood pressure readings; the range of difference is 30 to 40 mmHg*

secondary hypertension *an elevated blood pressure associated with pulmonary, circulatory, endocrine, and renal diseases such as hyperaldosteronism, pheochromocytoma, Cushing's syndrome, diabetes mellitus, coarctation of the aorta, and hyperthryroidism*

secondary varicose veins *characterized by venous status and chronic venous insufficiency of the deep and communicating veins*

systolic *the pressure of the blood against the arterial walls when the ventricles of the heart are contracted*

thrombophlebitis *inflammation of the vein with a clot formation within the vein*

thrombus *a collection of fibrin, platelets, clotting factors, and cellular elements of the blood that attach to the interior wall of the artery or vein; sometimes, the thrombus will occlude the vessel*

vasospasm *a spasm or constriction of the blood vessel*

white coat phenomenon *hypertension that occurs in a normotensive client when a healthcare professional approaches to take his or her blood pressure; differentiation between white coat hypertension and secondary hypertension is essential for effective therapy to begin*

Pretest

1 A client is at the local health clinic and the nurse takes and records a systolic blood pressure of greater than 160 mmHg. The nurse tells the client that it could be caused by:

(1) An increase in the electrical activity, causing hypertrophy of the left ventricle.
(2) Failure of the elastic tissue or the side effects of hypertension medications.
(3) Use of over-the-counter medications, renal stenosis, or increased ingestion of salt.
(4) Anaphylactic shock or increased electrical activity of the heart causing hypertrophy of the heart muscle.

2 The nurse should assess the client's pulse and blood pressure as part of the administration of which of the following drugs?

(1) Sulfinpyrazone (Anturane) and calcitonin (Calcimar)
(2) Propranolol (Inderal) and clonidine (Catapres)
(3) Glucogon (GlucaGen) and pyridostigmine bromide (Regonol)
(4) Hydroxyzine (Vistaril) and prazosin hydrochloride (Minipress)

3 The nurse should discuss which of the following as non-modifiable risk factors influencing hypertension?

(1) Ethnicity and stress
(2) Obesity and substance abuse
(3) Nutrition and occupation
(4) Family history and gender

4 In the process of a physical examination of an adult client with a possible diagnosis of hypertension, the nurse should gather data through the use of which method?

(1) Blood pressure from one arm only
(2) Orthostatic blood pressure with 2 minutes between each reading
(3) Blood pressure from both arms taken 5 minutes apart
(4) Cuff and Doppler blood pressure in both arms

5 Priority teaching for a client with Buerger's disease would include which of the following?

(1) Wear gloves if the extremities are cold and painful.
(2) Avoid wearing flat-heeled shoes.
(3) Report severe pain that may require opioid analgesics.
(4) Cessation of smoking

6 One of the largest concerns with the hypertensive client is non-adherence to the care regimen. Non-compliance is most likely influenced by which of the following factors?

(1) Medications are not working as indicated by the client statement, "I don't feel any different."
(2) A health professional reportedly stating, "Take it easy and stop worrying about taking those medications."
(3) The many lifestyle changes needed in diet, exercise, and smoking patterns seem overwhelming.
(4) The client has a lack of support persons to assist the client with different therapies.

7 Which of the following clients has the greatest risk of developing a thromboembolism?

(1) A 20-year-old client
(2) A client with a cardiac disease
(3) A female client who is Jewish
(4) A client with known kidney disease

8 The nursing management for a client with thrombophlebitis would include:

(1) The use of anticoagulant therapy to inhibit the clotting factors.
(2) Keeping the client's legs in a position of comfort.
(3) Using low molecular weight heparin (LMWH) once a confirmed diagnosis exists.
(4) Elevating the head of the bed 6 inches on wooden blocks.

9 An elderly gentleman enters the Emergency Department with complaints of back pain and feeling fatigued. Upon examination, his blood pressure is 200/110, pulse is 120, and hematocrit and hemoglobin are both low. The nurse palpates the abdomen which is soft, nontender, and auscultates an abdominal pulse. The most likely diagnosis is:

(1) Secondary hypertension.
(2) An aneurysm.
(3) Congestive heart failure (CHF).
(4) Buerger's disease.

10 When caring for a client with Raynaud's disease, which of the following outcomes concerning medication regimen is of highest priority?

(1) Relaxing smooth muscle to avoid vasospasms
(2) Controlling the pain once vasospasms occur
(3) Avoiding lesions on the feet
(4) Preventing major disabilities that may occur

See pages 110–111 for Answers and Rationales.

I. Risk Factors Associated with Vascular Health Problems

A. Hypertension

1. Risk factors that cannot be modified

   a. Family history

      1) Multifactorial and multiple genes may be involved

      2) Family incidence of elevation of the intracellular sodium levels with an associated lower potassium-sodium ratio

      3) Clients with parent(s) with hypertension are at higher risk at a younger age

   b. Age

      1) Primary hypertension: usually appears between the ages of 30 and 50 years

      2) Clients over 50 years of age have a higher incidence of hypertension; clients over 60 years of age have a 50 percent to 60 percent chance of having blood pressure over 140/90

      3) Blood pressure readings are a good predictor for potential stroke, coronary heart disease, heart failure, and renal disease

   c. Mortality caused by hypertension according to ethnicity

      1) White females—4.7%

      2) White males—6.3%

      3) Black males—22.5%

      4) Black females—29.3%

   d. Gender

      1) Men have a higher incidence of hypertension until about age 55 years

      2) Men and women are approximately equal between the age of 55 and 74 years

      3) After 74 years of age, women are at greater risk for hypertension

2. Factors responding to physiological modification

   a. Stress

      1) Environmental stressors, such as noise, heat, and cold

      2) Personality characteristics, such as responses to life events and/or life-changing events

      3) Physiological events, such as pain, decrease in blood oxygen concentration, drugs, and obesity

      4) Food choices

         a) High sodium intake may induce high amounts of natriuretic hormone to be released, suggesting a possible link to increasing the blood pressure

b) Low intake of potassium, calcium, and magnesium

c) Overweight: the distribution of fat, particularly in the upper body

d) High consumption of alcohol, legal and illegal drugs

e) Smoking: nicotine from cigarette smoking immediately raises the blood pressure

5) Caffeine consumption: coffee, soda with caffeine, and chocolate are stimulants and are associated with a rise in blood pressure

B. Peripheral vascular disease

1. Arterial

   a. Diseases such as atherosclerosis, autoimmunity

   b. Clotting problems: **embolus** (a foreign object such as a piece of a thrombus floating in the bloodstream), **thrombus** (collection of fibrin, platelets, clotting factors, and cellular elements of the blood that attach to the interior wall of the artery or vein)

   c. Trauma, inflammation

   d. Vasospasm (spasm or constriction of the blood vessel)

   e. Obesity

2. Venous

   a. Over the age of 40 years

   b. Surgery longer than 30 minutes using general anesthesia, spinal anesthesia, or epidural anesthesia

   c. Venous stasis caused by prolonged travel, bedrest, cerebral vascular accident (CVA)

   d. History of previous deep vein thrombosis (DVT), family history of blood clotting disorder

   e. Cardiac disease such as heart failure, myocardial infarction, cardiomyopathy, malignancy

   f. Pregnancy, estrogen therapy, and oral contraceptives

   g. Obesity

C. Aneurysms: clients with hypertension and/or atherosclerosis

D. Thrombophlebitis: diseases causing venous stasis, surgery, oral contraceptives, varicose veins, obesity, pregnancy, prolonged immobility

E. Raynaud's disease: gender (female, 18 to 40); heredity

F. Buerger's disease: smoking, gender (more prominent in males)

II. **Hypertension (HTN)**

A. Overview

1. **Hypertension (HTN)** is defined as a sustained blood pressure (BP) that is greater than normal, usually greater than 140 mmHg **systolic** (the pressure of the blood against the arterial walls when the ventricles of the heart are

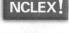

contracted) and 90 mmHg **diastolic** (the pressure of the blood against the arterial walls when the ventricles of the heart are at rest); however age specifics need to be considered

2. Two types

   a. **Primary hypertension,** also known as *idiopathic hypertension* or *essential hypertension* (an elevated blood pressure from unknown causes, which occurs in about 95 percent of diagnosed hypertensive clients)

   b. **Secondary hypertension** (an elevated pressure associated with a disease process or an abnormality)

      1) Cause can usually be identified: pulmonary, circulatory, endocrine, renal diseases, medicines such as volume expanders, increased sodium (Na) intake

      2) Examples: hyperaldosteronism, **pheochromocytoma** (tumor that releases catecholamines and causes hypertensive emergencies), Cushing's syndrome, diabetes mellitus, hyperthyroidism

3. **White coat phenomenon:** client is normotensive except when the blood pressure is measured by a health professional

4. Isolated systolic hypertension: a systolic blood pressure over 140 mmHg and a diastolic blood pressure of less than 90 mmHg; this phenomena has a higher incidence with advancing age

5. Labile HTN is extreme elevation of BP at one time with a normal BP later without other noted causes; limited physiological changes; changes do occur over time in the heart, brain, and kidneys; should be closely monitored

6. Pregnancy-induced hypertension: a complication of pregnancy with increasing blood pressure, proteinuria, and edema

   NCLEX!

   a. The diagnosis is made if the pressure increase is 30 mmHg systolic and 15 mmHg diastolic over the baseline blood pressure on two assessments with a minimum of 6 hours between readings; and the confirmed presence of proteinuria and edema

   b. This condition is most frequently present in the third trimester of pregnancy and must be treated promptly; if untreated, the condition may quickly become critical

   NCLEX!

7. Malignant hypertension is a progressive, rapidly developing HTN that causes vascular damage and possibly death; persistent severe diastolic hypertension of over 110 to 120 mmHg; often occurs after anesthetic drugs are given

8. HTN is called the "silent killer" because many clients do not have symptoms

   NCLEX!

9. Diagnosis should be made after three or more consistent BP readings are taken after a 5-minute period of rest because BP can vary from day to day, within different periods of the same day, and because of many factors

B. **Pathophysiology**

1. Regulation of blood pressure

   a. Is continually influenced by cardiac output and **peripheral vascular resistance** (PVR) (the sum of all resistances that the body has within the vascular system)

    b. Regulated by the management of the arterioles, venules, heart, and kidneys

    c. Blood Pressure = Cardiac Output × Peripheral Vascular Resistance (BP = CO × PVR)

    d. Regulation of cardiac output

        1) Autonomic nervous system (ANS)

        2) Heart rate and stroke volume

        3) Fluid volume, which is influenced by mineralocorticoids, sodium, and water

    e. Peripheral resistance

        1) A smaller diameter of the vessel will cause changes in the vascular resistance, causing the blood pressure to rise

        2) A decrease in the vascular resistance will cause the blood pressure to fall

        3) Increases in peripheral resistance may be caused by increased activity of the sympathetic nervous system, angiotensin and catecholamines (elements controlling autoregulation), and thickening of the blood vessel walls from artherosclerosis

    f. Neurohormonal mediators

        1) Arterial baroreceptor: monitors arterial pressure

        2) Baroreceptors are located in the carotid sinuses and the wall of the left ventricle, which monitors the level of arterial blood pressure and counteracts rising pressure by vasodilation through the stimulation of the vagus nerve

        3) Chemoreceptors: are located in the medulla and carotid and aortic body

            a) Sensitive to the changes in the blood pH produced by variations in the concentrations of carbon dioxide, oxygen levels, and hydrogen ions

            b) A major reflex response is caused by changes in the body's oxygen saturation, but to a lesser extent changes in the blood pH and the carbon dioxide concentration

    g. Body fluid volume

        1) Excess concentration of sodium and water: as the systemic fluid volume increases, the result is an increase in the blood pressure and rise in the kidney filtration pressure, causing diuresis

        2) Blood pressure is altered through the loss of salt and water and an over production of sodium-retaining hormone

    h. Increased activity of the renin/angiotensin/aldoserone (RAA) system

        1) Renin: is released under the control of the central neural influence; a decrease blood flow to the kidney; a fall in blood pressure; and a decreased concentration of tubular sodium

2) Angiotensin I combines with renin to form a nonpressor form of angiotensin I

    a) It is converted in the lungs to angiotension II (a potent vasoconstrictor) by angiotensin converting enzyme, which because of its potency can elevate the BP

    b) Angiotensin II causes a release of aldosterone, leading to reabsorption of Na and water, leading to hypertension

3) Additional explanations concerning hypertension

    a) Inability of the kidneys to increase the excretion of sodium in response to an elevated systolic pressure

    b) Failure of the normal sodium-potassium or sodium-calcium transport mechanism within the intracellular space

  i. Vascular autoregulation

1) Blood viscosity: blood flow resistance increases as the blood becomes thicker, and the blood flow resistance decreases as viscosity decreases

2) Autoregulation is aided through kinins by:

    a) Relaxing the arteriolar smooth muscle, which increases capillary permeability as well as the constriction of the venules

    b) Prostaglandins producing either vasoconstriction or vasodilation

2. Primary hypertension

  a. Primarily caused by an increased peripheral vascular resistance (PVR)

  b. PVR results from vasoconstriction or narrowed peripheral blood vessels

  c. In HTN, the left ventricle must work harder to overcome the resistance met when emptying (afterload); a constant increased workload and more pressure within the left ventricle leads to hypertrophy (known as left ventricular hypertrophy or LVH)

  d. Initially, LVH is a compensatory mechanism by the heart to regulate BP; later LVH is a complication in that more oxygen and blood flow is needed for the muscle to meet the workload

  e. Initially, the arterioles increase resistance to blood flow, leading to increased PVR and hypertension

  f. Later, the kidneys are involved by activating the RAA system

3. Secondary hypertension

  a. Multiple system involvement with direct or indirect impact on the renal system

  b. Aldosterone, cortisol, and catecholamines in excess

  c. Chronic stress: prolonged excess of catecholamines

4. Signs and symptoms

  a. May be asymptomatic

    b. Headache is the most common

    c. Severe HTN: dizziness, nausea, vomiting, confusion (can signify encephalopathy), visual disturbances, renal insufficiency, aortic dissection, HTN crisis

  5. Complications include cerebral vascular accident (CVA), congestive heart failure (CHF), ventricular hypertrophy, damage to retina, renal insufficiency, aortic dissection, hypertensive crisis

C. Nursing assessment

  1. Assessment

    a. Complete health, nutritional, medication, and social history

    b. An assessment of the client's understanding concerning the plan of care

    c. Assess for the following

      1) Occipital headache (HA) in the morning and length of time HA occurs

      2) Periods of dizziness: frequency, when does it occur, and what is the duration, and is it related to any activity

      3) Tinnitus: have client describe the characteristics of this phenomenon

      4) Pounding in the chest: frequency, duration, and when it last happened

      5) Assess the client's blood pressure: a blood pressure is obtained in each arm using three positions—lying down, sitting, standing (orthostatic BP)

        a) Record the findings, identifying the client's position for each reading

        b) An average amount of time between each reading should be 2 minutes

        c) When the client is seated, the arm is supported at the level of the heart

        d) Note the **pulse pressure** (the difference between the systolic and the diastolic pressure reading; the range of difference is 30 to 40 mmHg)

      6) A physical examination, with emphasis on the cardiovascular and associated systems

        a) Abdominal masses: may be pulsating, describe the location and the size

        b) Bruits: where are they found and are they bilateral or unilateral

        c) Characteristics of Cushing's syndrome

        d) Signs of pheochromocytoma

        e) Funduscopic examination

        f) Cardiac, vascular, and extremity examination

        g) Pulmonary examination

2. Diagnostic tests

   a. Urinalysis including tests for renin, cortisol, urine catecholamines

   b. Blood chemistries (potassium, sodium, fasting glucose, complete blood count [CBC], and blood urea nitrogen [BUN], creatinine, and lipid profile), serum calcium, and magnesium

   c. Other: electrocardiogram (ECG), echocardiogram, and possible vascular studies to determine the significance of end-organ involvement

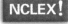

   d. Measurement of BP with appropriate cuff size for a week

D. Nursing management

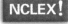

1. A change in lifestyle is always recommended *first*: diet control, weight loss, increased activity, and decreasing stress

2. Medications include diuretics, beta blockers, calcium channel blockers, ACE inhibitors, centrally acting sympatholytics, and direct-acting vasodilators

   a. Clients are usually started on diuretics or beta blockers initially; if managed on one drug, no further action is taken

   b. Clients not responding to one drug may have another added; ACE inhibitors are being combined with many drugs successfully

   c. Stepped approach may involve adding drugs in the order listed above

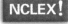

3. Discuss the nutritional needs of the client

   a. Assess amount of sodium consumption and recommend 2 to 6 g of sodium

   b. Blood cholesterol of less than 200 mg/dL

   c. Reduction of calories and weight: the body mass index (BMI) should be less than 25; otherwise a weight reduction plan should be investigated

4. Monitor vital signs (VS) and intake and output (I&O); test for edema

5. Monitor weight daily

6. Emphasize compliance with food, medications, and risk involved in not keeping BP in appropriate range; factors to be considered include:

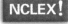

   a. High cost of the medication(s); unpleasant side effects; interference with lifestyle; does not understand the need to take medications when feeling well

   b. Hypertension being an asymptomatic disease, the seriousness of the condition is underestimated by the client and the significant others

   c. Some of the lifestyle changes prescribed for the client are difficult to accept and implement; support groups may be of assistance

7. Teach client how to check own BP at home

   a. Help the client plan a realistic schedule for taking the BP and recording the findings

   b. Teach the client and the significant others when it is necessary to call the healthcare professional because of an unusually high or low reading

8. Monitor heart rate (HR) and BP prior to administration of antihypertensives

   a. Hold if systolic is less than 100 mmHg and HR is less than 50 BPM

   b. Always check BP and pulse before taking beta blockers

   c. Monitor for **orthostatic hypotension** (syncope or dizziness with sudden position changes because of a drop in BP)

9. Discuss the importance of medical follow-up for a lifetime

10. Discuss the over-the-counter medications the client is taking; educate about avoiding cold remedies that can increase the BP

11. Health maintenance program should include an individualized aerobic exercise program; monitored by using a self-reporting system or within an organized club

    a. The client reports the following: the heart rate during exercise, sensations of reduced physical and emotional stress, and reduction in the systematic blood pressure

    b. Guidelines for aerobic exercise indicate that 20 to 30 minutes, three times per week are dependent on the age and physical condition of the client

    c. Maximal heart rate is determined by subtracting the client's age from 220

    d. Prior to beginning the rehabilitation, an exercise physiologist must conduct a detailed performance evaluation

12. Avoid smoking cigarettes or cigars

13. Monitor drugs' effectiveness, especially in elderly who may experience fluid shifts, which can change distribution

III. Peripheral Vascular Disease

A. Overview

1. Peripheral vascular disease is defined as those conditions resulting in interference in blood flow to or from the extremities

2. Can be arterial or venous in orgin (Table 3-1)

   a. Peripheral arterial occlusive disorders: partial stenosis or complete occlusion

   b. Venous disorders

      1) Acute, such as thromboembolism

      2) Chronic, such as **varicose veins** (superficial veins) and **chronic venous insufficiency** (chronic failure of the venous valves to function, resulting in interference with the venous blood return to the heart)

3. Causes include cardiovascular disease, thrombi, prolonged immobility, excess standing, pulmonary diseases

B. Pathophysiology

1. Arteriole

   a. Any alteration of blood supply compromises the oxygen supply and alters the demand

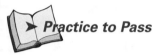

NCLEX!

▶ Practice to Pass

A client was diagnosed 3 months ago with essential hypertension. The client states to the nurse, "It doesn't matter if I forget to take my medicine. I just take the make-up dose at the next medication time." How should the nurse answer?

Table 3-1		Arterial	Venous
Comparison of Arterial and Venous Insufficiency	**Description of Pain**	Intermittent claudication; relieved by dependent position	Aching; cramping; relieved by elevation
	Pulse Assessment	Diminished or absent	Present
	Ulcer Characteristics	Deep, pale; located on toes, feet or other area of skin	Superficial, pink; over inner or outer ankle
	Skin Characteristics	Dependent rubor; pallor upon elevation; dry, shiny skin; cool or cold temperature; edema mild if present at all	Thick and tough; brawny pigment; skin normal temperature; may have edema
	Complications	Gangrene	Poor healing

b. Prolonged change in the blood flow or decreased blood perfusion to large areas will start a sequence of vasodilatation; this in turn will promote the development of collateral arterial pathways, as well as the use of anaerobic mechanisms to met the oxygen demands of the cells

c. The vasodilatation has a limited effect, as the arteries deprived of oxygen become maximally dilated and **arterial steal** occurs (when arterioles are maximally dilated because of hypoxia, they steal from cutaneous and peripheral vessels which causes the client to be aware of a "pins and needles" sensation in the affected area)

d. A concern is the potential for the development of tissue acidosis; this occurs when large amounts of lactic acid and pyruvic acid build up quickly; these acids are very toxic to the body

e. If the compensatory mechanisms prove inadequate, the client will experience pain called intermittent claudication

   1) The symptoms occur when a muscle is forced to contract without an adequate amount of blood supply to meet the activity needs

   2) All muscles of the body may claudicate, however, this often refers to the lower extremities

f. The lower limbs are most susceptible to arterial occlusive disorders and atherosclerosis because of limitation in the collateral circulation

g. Signs and symptoms

   1) Intermittent claudication

   2) Dusky, purplish discoloration when feet are dependent

   3) White, pale color when legs are elevated

   4) Thickened toenails

   5) Ulcers on legs (see Table 3-1)

   6) Venous refilling when the foot is dependent

   7) Decreased or absent pedal pulse

   8) Numbness and cold, tingling feeling in the extremity

    h. The progression of symptoms from onset is slow, being from 20 to 40 years; some of these clients have an associated severe coronary artery disease (CAD) and the symptoms are influenced by the body's use and speed of oxygen of consumption in the legs

2. Venous

    a. Blockage within the venous system may occur in the system of superficial veins or the deep veins

    b. Causes of thrombus formation

        1) Venous stasis from immobility, prolonged travel, obesity, pregnancy, and heart disease

        2) Hypercoagulability from conditions causing dehydration and blood dyscrasias may cause platelet counts to rise, decrease fibrolysis, increase clotting factors, thus changing the blood viscosity; in addition, oral contraceptives and hematologic disorders may increase blood coagulability

        3) Injury to the vessel wall may be caused by trauma of an intravenous infusion, fractures, contusions, and chemical injury from sclerosing agents and from Buerger's disease (thromboangiitis obliterans)

            a) The injury to the venous wall attracts platelets and debris gathers

            b) With the low blood flow, a hypercoagulable state occurs with the result being the formation of a thrombus

    c. Signs and symptoms

        1) Discoloration of lower extremities

        2) Edema over the tibia

        3) Ulcers (see Table 3-1)

        4) Tenderness in the legs

        5) Positive Homan's sign

C. Nursing assessment

  1. Assessment

    a. Arterial

        1) Symptom analysis of the reason for seeking medical help

        2) Assess activity tolerance and presence of pain

        3) Assessment of skin color

        4) Use a Doppler for pulses

        5) Other circulatory assessment: capillary refill, temperature and the presence of venous refilling

        6) Observe the sitting position of the client for the crossing of the legs at the knees, use of garters or knee stockings, and foot, leg, or ankle edema

    b. Venous

        1) Identify clients who are at high risk for thrombophlebitis

NCLEX!

NCLEX!

2) Assess the legs of the client for discoloration, edema, and tenderness

3) Measure the leg circumference

4) Determine the amount of discomfort the client is experiencing through asking about the location, intensity, and duration

5) Assess for Homan's sign

2. Diagnostic tests

   a. Cholesterol and lipid panel

   b. Arteriogram

   c. Doppler ultrasonic flow study to identify blood flow through arteries

   d. Digital subtraction angiography to identify arteries in specific areas

   e. Oscillometry to determine the volume of a pulse

   f. Stress testing

   g. Coagulation studies: partial thromboplastin time (PTT) for heparin; prothrombin time (PT) for warfarin (Coumadin)

D. Nursing management

1. Medication

   a. Pentoxifylline (Trental) to decrease blood viscosity and increase microcirculation

   b. Vasodilator prostaglandins

   c. Anticoagulant or thrombolytic therapy for a thrombus

   d. Antiplatelet drugs: cilostazol (Pletal)

2. Risk reduction through the management of body weight of the overweight client using a low-fat, low-cholesterol diet with fruits and vegetables

3. Risk reduction through physical exercise: clients are encouraged to walk 30 to 60 minutes each day if no skin alterations are present; clients need to have individualized physical exercises modified for them

4. Educate on cessation of smoking: client must be educated to the actions of nicotine, and be referred to a support group

5. If the client has hyperlipidemia, the reduction of total calorie intake, total fat intake, and other sources of cholesterol must be evaluated; in some cases, the only management is a pharmacological regime

6. Discuss with the client the reason to avoid standing in one spot for a long period of time; if intermittent claudication occurs, stop, rest and then continue the activity

7. Recommend to the client to wear light warm clothing in order to prevent vasoconstriction of the vessels of the lower legs

8. Inform the client to avoid crossing the legs or ankles because it will decrease the rate of perfusion and to elevate the legs when sitting in a chair or when in bed

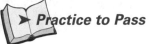

Practice to Pass

A client with a peripheral vascular disease (PVD) asks the nurse why it is essential to follow the healthcare provider's plan of care to reduce his cardiovascular risk. What should the nurse tell this individual?

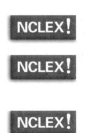

NCLEX!

NCLEX!

NCLEX!

IV. Aneurysms

A. Overview

1. An **aneurysm** is defined as a permanent dilatation of an artery or an out-pouching of the wall of an artery

2. Most aortic aneurysms are situated below the renal arteries; other sites are at the bifurcation of the aorta or within the structure of an artery or vein anywhere in the body

3. Classified as true or false aneurysm

   a. *True aneurysm* is a result of weakening of the vessel wall over time and is usually a result of high pressure or atherosclerosis

   b. *False aneurym* is usually a result of a traumatic break in the vascular wall instead of the weakening seen in a true form

4. Aneurysms vary in pathophysiology, clinical findings, and treatment depending on where the aneurysm is located

5. They may occur in either artery or vein

6. Causes of aneurysms include hypertension, trauma, atherosclerosis, infections

B. Pathophysiology

1. Morphology

   a. Fusiform aneurysm is cylindrical and involves the entire circumference of the vessel

   b. Saccular aneurysm is an outpouching of a sac on the vessel; example: berry aneurysm

   c. Pseudoaneurysm: the wall of the aneurysm is not the original wall of the aorta; the mass is made up of connective tissue and the structures surrounding extravasated blood

2. Etiology: aneurysms may be classified according to cause

   a. Atherosclerotic aneurysm: caused by atherosclerosis

   b. Mycotic aneurysm: caused by bacterial infection

   c. Luetic aneurysm: caused by syphilis

3. Location: the type of aneurysm is determined by its location

   a. Thoracic aorta

      1) Progresses rapidly and often ruptures

      2) Symptoms include pain in back, neck and substernal areas; respiratory problems (stridor, dyspnea, cough); hoarseness

   b. Superior vena cava: accompanied by distended neck veins, facial edema

   c. Abdominal aorta

      1) Most develop below level of renal arteries; are most frequent

NCLEX**!**

    2) Often asymptomatic with audible pulsation in abdomen or pulsating mass in abdomen

    3) Other symptoms can include: mild to severe abdominal and back pain, cool extremities, claudication

  d. Dissecting aneurysms

    1) A medical emergency

    2) Hemorrhage occurs because of a tear in the aorta intima

    3) Often occurs in high pressure areas such as ascending aorta

    4) Symptoms include pain (abrupt, severe), elevated BP, undetectable pulses, syncope, heart failure

  4. An aneurysm of 5 cm may be palpable in a non-obese client

  5. Treatment of an abdominal aneurysm is surgery (Figure 3-1)

C. Nursing assessment

  1. Assessment includes characteristics of the client's pain (intense pain in the abdomen, back, flank, and scrotum); auscultation of abdomen; palpation (rigid because of the accumulation of blood); VS; signs of hemorrhagic shock

  2. Diagnostic tests

    a. Ultrasonography

    b. CT scan or MRI

    c. Chest x-ray (CXR)

    d. Renal function studies

Figure 3-1

**A. Clamping of aorta and visualization of clot within the vessel.
B. Graft within the vessel used for repair.**

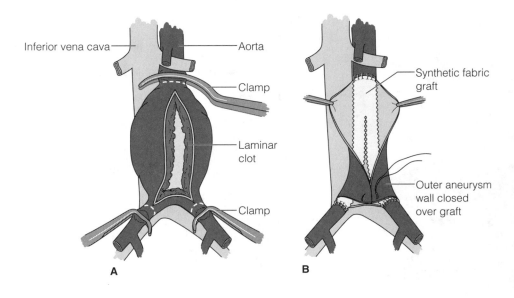

D. **Nursing management**

1. Medications

   a. Antihypertensives

   b. Beta adrenergic blockers

   c. Anticoagulants and antibiotics postsurgery

   d. Analgesics

2. Monitor for complications following a major surgical procedure

   a. Underlying coronary artery disease and chronic obstructive pulmonary disease

   b. Postoperative atelectasis

   c. Decreased toleration of changes in **hemodynamics** (movement of blood within the body) such as low blood volume and fluid shifts

   d. Myocardial infarction

   e. Kidney function: reflects the integrity of the cardiovascular system

   f. Emboli

3. Postoperative care

   a. Monitor for fluid volume deficit to prevent hemorrhagic shock

   b. Monitor client for increasing pulse rate, decreasing blood pressure, clammy skin, anxiety, changing levels of consciousness (LOC), oliguria, pallor, and thirst

4. Educate the client on compliance with hypertension control

V. **Thrombophlebitis**

A. **Overview**

1. **Thrombophlebitis** is defined as an inflammation of the vein with a clot formation made up of various elements in the blood supply trapped in a fibrin mesh

2. Causes are usually associated with Virchow's triad

   a. Injury to the vessel wall: mechanical trauma, thermal injury, septic states, or an autoimmune problem

   b. Blood stasis: thrombus forms in the area of the static blood flow and in the valve cusps of the vein

   c. Hypercoagulability, change in the blood concentration, or the blood coagulation factors; deficiency of naturally occurring antithrombins; and factors that assist in increasing the blood viscosity

B. **Pathophysiology**

1. Injury to the intimal lining of the vein causes a decrease in circulation and stimulates the aggregation of platelets as well as other inflammatory mediators

2. A protrusion from this site begins to occlude the vessel and may partially or completely block blood flow

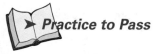

Practice to Pass

A 70-year-old client with an abdominal aortic aneurysm needs an MRI every 6 months. The aneurysm currently measures 4.5 cm. The physician tells the family surgery is usually not done until it is greater than 5 cm, as long as there is no evidence of growth or hemorrhage. The family asks the nurse why surgery can't be performed now. How should the nurse respond?

3. The inflammatory mediators (leukocytes, lymphocytes, and fibroblasts) gather, causing congestion within the vessel wall

4. Thrombi may occur in any vessel, but are more prominent in veins because blood flow is more sluggish than in an artery

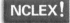

5. Emboli can break away from thrombi and travel to different parts of the body, most commonly the pulmonary circulation

6. Signs and symptoms

   a. Small- and medium-sized veins may produce no symptoms

   b. Larger vessels: temperature (102°F)

   c. Superficial veins: redness, pain, tenderness, and swelling

   d. Deep vein thrombosis (DVT): calf pain, tenderness in calf muscle, positive Homan's sign

   e. Iliofemoral vein: thigh and/or groin pain, edema (may be pitting), cyanotic appearance to leg, fever, tachycardia; brawny edema (skin is thick, hard, has "orange-peel" appearance, and edema)

C. **Nursing assessment**

1. Assessment includes blood perfusion to the affected part (capillary refill, temperature, pulses, sensation, color of skin); VS; symptom analysis of pain; positive Homan's sign

2. Diagnostic tests

   a. Blood cultures and CBC

   b. Phlebography (assess location of clot through use of contract medium)

   c. Doppler ultrasound

   d. Venous pressure measurement

   e. Plethysmography (measure changes in fluid volume passing through a vessel)

D. **Nursing management**

1. Medications include anticoagulants, low-molecular weight heparin (LMWH), antiplatelets, anti-inflammatory agents, thrombolytics, and antibiotics

2. Elevate the foot of the bed 6 to 8 inches on blocks or elevate the affected part

3. Maintain the client on bedrest

4. Administer moist heat to the involved extremity; if warm moist soaks are prescribed to the affected area, the frequency prescribed is usually every 4 to 6 hours for 30 minutes; an aquathermia pad may be applied over a moist towel

5. Listen to the client's concerns; use community referrals as needed

6. Monitor intravenous infusions carefully

7. Encourage the client to rest the affected part

8. Monitor the effect of medications and treatments used; teach the client about the effect of medications and potential side effects

VI. Varicose Veins

1. Overview

2. Varicose veins are defined as a superficial vein that is twisted and enlarged

3. May involve any part of the body but occurs most often in the lower extremities and esophagus

4. Types

   a. Primary: involving superficial veins and not communicating veins

   b. Secondary: involve deep communicating veins

5. Causes

   a. Primary varicose veins frequently are familial and predispose the client to the loss of elasticity of the vein wall and incompetent valves

   b. Secondary varicose veins occur with trauma, deep vein thrombosis, and inflammation/damaged valves

B. Pathophysiology

NCLEX!

1. Chronic venous insufficiency results from incompetent valves that cause:

   a. Reduction in the venous return

   b. Increase in the venous pressure

   c. Venous stasis

2. Excessive dilation of the vein causes the spreading of the valve cusps

3. This causes valvular incompetency and produces a reflux of blood from the superficial veins to enter the deep veins by the muscular pump

NCLEX!

4. Signs and symptoms appear after the veins have been chronically engorged and tortuous

   a. Distended veins that may be bluish in color and bulging

   b. Pain in feet and ankles; heaviness or feeling of heat in legs

   c. Swelling of lower extremities

   d. Stasis ulcers

   e. Itching over affected extremity

C. Nursing assessment

NCLEX!

1. Assessment includes inspection of the lower extremities for edema, discoloration, tenderness or discomfort (location and intensity), positive Homan's sign, signs of pulmonary embolism (anxiety, dyspnea, increased respiratory rate, "air hunger," tachycardia, diaphoresis, chest pain); bowel habits for constipation

2. Diagnostic tests

   a. Tourniquet tests: determine the location of incompetent valves

   b. Doppler ultrasonic flow tests

  c. Angiographic studies

  d. Plethysmography

D. Nursing management

1. Medications are not recommended unless over-the-counter (OTC) analgesics are needed

2. If the client is a smoker, discuss the value and need to stop smoking; possible referral of the client to a support group

3. Encourage the client not to stand in one position for a long period of time; to take a walk each day for 30 to 60 minutes; and to rest if intermittent claudication occurs

4. A referral to the Bureau of Vocational Rehabilitation would be helpful if the client's position can not be accommodated by the employer

5. Suggest to the client that light warm clothing is essential to prevent a vasoconstriction of the blood vessels in the lower extremities

6. Assist the client in learning about not crossing his or her legs or ankles when sitting and to elevate legs when in a supine position

7. Prevent constipation or straining

VII. Arteriospastic Disease: Raynaud's Syndrome

A. Overview

1. Arteriospastic disease: Raynaud's syndrome is defined as a condition of small arteries and arterioles of the fingers and skin that constrict in response to cold or emotional upsets (Table 3-2)

Table 3-2	**Comparison of Raynaud's Disease and Buerger's Disease**	
	Raynaud's Disease	**Buerger's Disease**
Definition	Condition of small arteries and arterioles of the fingers and skin; constriction in response to cold or emotional upsets	An inflammatory occlusive vascular disease involving the medium-sized arteries and veins
Causative Factors	Autoimmune disorders such as systemic lupus erythematosus; genetic tendency; unknown etiology	Genetic disposition; smoking; tobacco allergy; autoimmune response
Population Affected	Primarily affects young women	Primarily men of Asian and Jewish descent, less than 40 years of age; history of heavy smoking
Pathophysiology	Causative stimuli leads to color changes in hands; digital artery spasm; tissue hypoxia causes arteries to dilate; rubor occurs when spasms cease	Thrombi develop; vessel is blocked; lesion becomes fibrotic; vasospasms obstruct flow of blood
Signs and Symptoms	Red-white-blue syndrome of digits; pallor or cyanosis that is bilateral or unilateral; normal pulse; sensory changes in extremities; pain	Pain at rest; intermittent claudication; decreased or absent pulses; rubor and cyanosis of extremities; signs of decreased circulation
Characteristics	Triggers include exercise, long-term exposure to cold, stress; lesions can progress to gangrene	Triggered by smoking, cold, and emotional stress Most commonly affects hands and feet; upper extremities may be affected also; has periods of exacerbations and remissions; gangrene is a complication

2. Raynaud's syndrome is termed Raynaud's disease if the symptoms are persistent for 3 years with intermittent attacks

3. May be associated with autoimmune disorders, such as systemic lupus erythematosus; genetic tendency; unknown cause

4. Primarily a disease of young women

B. Pathophysiology

NCLEX!

1. Raynaud's syndrome causes color changes in the hands when the hands are exposed to causative stimuli

2. The digital arteries go into spasm, and the hands change color, becoming very pale

3. This may occur after exercise

4. Tissue hypoxia occurs causing the arteries to dilate slightly

5. The fingers will appear bluish because they are now carrying mostly deoxygenated blood; this may occur in one or both hands

6. A rubor (redness) will occur when the arterial spasms have stopped

7. One digit may demonstrate severe **ischemia** (deficiency in the supply of oxygenated blood) with the other digits demonstrating good blood flow

8. Stenosis may cause an absence of pulse and a localized bruit

9. Main difference between Raynaud's disease and Raynaud's syndrome is that the amount of involvement is less in Raynaud's syndrome

NCLEX!

10. Stimuli triggering an attack include exercise, long-term exposure to cold, and stress

11. Signs and symptoms

NCLEX!

a. Raynaud's disease: known as blue-red-white disease (digits turn blue, then white, then red as spasms resolve)

b. Other: pallor or cyanosis that is bilateral or unilateral; normal pulse; sensory changes (tingling, stiffness, pain, decreased sensation)

c. Long-term: fingertips thicken because of lack of oxygen and nails become brittle; gangrene is a serious complication

C. Nursing assessment

1. Assessment

a. Complete a careful history from a client that is presenting with hand(s) that are demonstrating changes in color and discomfort

b. Palpate distal pulses bilaterally noting the rate and volume

c. Assess the pain levels, noting the frequency of pain, its duration, intensity, location and treatment selected to control this pain; determine if the present medication management is sufficient to control the pain

d. Assess all extremities for edema, lesions, and gangrene

e. If lesions are present, measure the circumference of each extremity; measure and document location of any lesion

  f. Assess the client's use of medications

  g. Assess if the client is continuing to smoke

 2. Diagnostic tests: diagnosis is determined by symptoms and ruling out other causes of decreased circulation

D. Nursing management

 1. Medications include: vasodilators; a low-dose calcium channel blocker such as nifedipine (Procardia); nitrates (transdermal nitroglycerine or long-acting oral forms); analgesics for pain

 2. If the client is a smoker, discuss the importance of quitting; consider a referral to a smoker support group or to a healthcare provider for nicotine patches or other medications

 3. Clothing must be loose and warm to aid in the maintenance of circulation: warm gloves, wool or heavy socks, comfortable, supportive shoes, and a warm hat

 4. Teach the client techniques of relaxation

VIII. Thromboangiitis Obliterans: Buerger's Disease

A. Overview

 1. Buerger's disease is defined as an inflammatory occlusive vascular disease involving the medium-sized arteries and veins (see Table 3-2)

 2. The primary clients are men (Asian and Jewish) who are less than 40 years of age and have a history of heavy smoking

 3. Commonly affects the legs and feet, but may affect the upper extremities as well

 4. Known for periods of exacerbations and remissions; long-term effects include more intense and longer episodes with ulcerations and gangrene as complications

 5. Causes include genetic disposition; smoking (primary); tobacco allergy; autoimmune response

B. Pathophysiology

 1. Characteristic problems in this disease are the development of panarteritis (inflammation of the coats of an artery) and panphlebitis (inflammation of the veins)

 2. Thrombi develop on the vessel wall, which subsequently block the vessel, and the lesion becomes fibrotic; arteriosclerosis is not noted in the lesion

 3. Vasospams occur commonly and may obstruct the flow of blood

 4. Primary result is arterial occlusion but the veins may become involved

 5. Signs and symptoms

  a. Pain (most common) at rest or intermittent claudication; may be triggered by smoking, cold, emotional stress

  b. Intolerance to cold

  c. Decreased pulses (even absent), cool or cold temperature in feet

  d. Rubor and cyanosis of extremities

  e. Loss of hair and thin shiny skin in extremities

    f. Thick nails

    g. Signs of decreased circulation in the extremities; changes with position changes

C. Nursing assessment

1. Symptom analysis of pain including the toes and forefoot when the client is at rest

2. Assess the lower extremities and foot muscles for claudication

3. Assess for migratory thrombophlebitis in a variety of veins

4. Assess for the development of gangrene in the foot or feet

5. Assess the foot for fulminating digital ischemia (temperature, capillary refill, pulses)

D. Nursing management

1. Medications

    a. To offer some relief: antibiotics, corticosteriods, vasodilators, and anticoagulants

    b. Calcium channel blockers: diltiazem (Cardizem) and verapamil (Isoptin)

    c. Antiplatelets: pentoxifylline (Trental)

2. Non-surgical treatment of a client with Buerger's disease is to stop smoking; if smoking is stopped, symptom relief is expected

3. Surgical treatment of a client with Buerger's disease is amputation of the affected limb

4. Educate the client to avoid drugs that decrease circulation or diminish blood supply to the extremities

5. Educate the client on the triggers and to avoid extreme temperature changes

6. Instruct client to inspect the feet frequently; keep clean and dry and use soft padding if necessary

7. Avoid standing in one position for long periods of time and avoid tight or restrictive clothing/shoes

8. Use of a bedcradle to relieve pressure from linens may be necessary

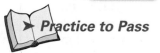

Practice to Pass

How should the nurse explain to a client the difference between Raynaud's syndrome and Buerger's disease?

NCLEX!

NCLEX!

Case Study

M. N., a 65-year-old female, has been diagnosed with essential hypertension. She attends the local Council on Aging (COA) and sees a different doctor at a local clinic whenever necessary. She has her blood pressure (BP) monitored at the COA once a month by a volunteer nurse. She has been maintained on a beta blocker and a diuretic, and her BP ranges from 130–140/70–90. She is compliant with her diet, doesn't smoke, and watches her weight. During the fall of the year, she has a few colds and begins to experience an increase in her blood pressure, ranging from 190–210/100–120. The COA arranges for her BP to be checked more frequently, and she is referred to her physician. The dose of her beta blocker and diuretic are increased, and she continues to have high BP readings. Concerned about a stroke, her family is notified and a copy of her BP readings over the month is given to the family. She is again referred by the nurse to a physician, who places her on an ACE inhibitor.

❶ What information should the healthcare provider gather concerning the client's present state of health and history data?

❷ What education does the family need?

❸ What is the essential information for clients to know concerning self-administration of their pharmacological regime?

❹ What are the nursing priorities of care for this client? What is the plan for the implementation of this client's care?

❺ How should the nurse explain the diagnosis of essential hypertension to the client and family?

For suggested responses, see page 565.

Posttest

1 In teaching a group of middle-aged men concerned about hypertension, the nurse should emphasize which of the following?

(1) Adequate intake of dietary calcium, magnesium, and potassium
(2) Alcohol consumption should not exceed 5 ounces per day
(3) Jogging 3 miles per day
(4) Use of herbal therapy containing licorice

2 Secondary hypertension (HTN) is an elevated blood pressure caused by a number of underlying physiological processes. Which of the following statements about secondary HTN is correct?

(1) A nonsystematic short-term use of contraceptives containing estrogen can cause HTN.
(2) Coarctation of the aorta has little to no relationship with the renin-angiotension-aldosterone system of the kidney.
(3) Hypertension in pregnancy is a frequent cause for maternal and fetal morbidity and mortality.
(4) Hypertension with an endocrine disorder accounts for a large population of clients.

3 The pathophysiology of hypertension is related to which of the following monitoring systems?

(1) Baroreceptors only
(2) Regulation of the amount of body fluid volume
(3) Endocrine system
(4) Underproduction of sodium retaining substances

4 Laboratory tests are usually ordered to complete the assessment of the client with hypertension (HTN). Which laboratory values are essential in the diagnosis?

(1) Serum sodium, serum potassium, and a bone density scan.
(2) Hemoglobin, hematocrit, and a glucose tolerance test.
(3) Stress test, prothrombin time, and urine analysis.
(4) Serum cholesterol, complete blood count, and serum creatinine.

5 Which of the following clients is at high risk for thrombophlebitis?

(1) 25-year-old male smoker with hypertension
(2) 67-year-old overweight female recovering from a hip replacement (1st day post-op)
(3) 22-year-old female with a history of Raynaud's disease in the family
(4) 72-year-old male with a history of arthritis and by-pass surgery

6 A male client is seen in the clinic complaining of pain when he tries to walk in order to exercise three times a week. Upon examination, his feet are noted to be dusky and purplish while dangling from the stretcher. The pedal pulse is palpable but diminished, and he states his feet "tingle on occasion." The nurse has him be supine on the stretcher with the foot of the stretcher elevated for about 30 minutes, after which his feet show pallor. The client is probably suffering from:

(1) Varicose veins.
(2) Thrombophlebitis.
(3) Raynaud's disease.
(4) Peripheral vascular disease (PVD).

7 The client with intermittent claudication is at risk for activity intolerance and possible tissue breakdown. If tissue breakdown occurs, the plan of care would consist of:

(1) Limited exercise.
(2) Bed rest.
(3) Range of motion exercises.
(4) Walking in comfortable light slippers.

8 The most common cause of a thrombus is:

(1) Arterial stasis, hypocoagulability, and arterial wall injury.
(2) Myocardial infarction, stroke, and prolonged sitting.
(3) Venous stasis, hypercoagulability, and venous wall injury.
(4) Motor vehicle accident and prolonged bed rest.

9 Assessment of a client with possible thrombophlebitis to the left leg and a deep vein thrombosis is done by pulling up on the toes while gently holding down on the knee. The client complains of extreme pain in the calf. This should be documented as:

(1) Positive tourniquet test.
(2) Positive Homan's sign.
(3) Negative Homan's sign.
(4) Negative tourniquet test.

10 Effective teaching for a client with Raynaud's disease is evident in which of the following statements?

(1) "I will decrease my smoking to 6 cigarettes per day."
(2) "I will try to learn to relax, but I can't promise anything."
(3) "I will wear gloves and socks to bed at night."
(4) "I will try to eat a healthier diet."

See pages 111–112 for Answers and Rationales.

Answers and Rationales

Pretest

1 Answer: 3 *Rationale:* Systolic hypertension over 150 mmHg may occur after the use of over-the-counter (OTC) cold remedies. A warning is placed on OTC medications, cautioning clients with hypertension to consult a physician first. Renal diseases contribute to hypertension, and salt causes fluid volume retention, which increases the blood pressure. Increases in the electrical activity of the heart will cause a variety of arrhythmias, not systolic hypertension (option 1). The failure of the elastic tissue is frequently seen in the skin of elderly and side effects of antihypertensives would most likely cause systolic hypotension (option 2). Anaphylactic shock or an increased electrical activity of the heart would cause a state of systolic hypotension (option 4).
Cognitive Level: Application
Nursing Process: Analysis; *Test Plan:* PHYS

2 Answer: 2 *Rationale:* When administering propranolol (Inderal), the client's apical pulse and blood pressure must be assessed. Propranolol is a beta blocker used to treat hypertension and tachycardia. The drug should not be given if the apical pulse is below 60 beats per minute (bpm), if there has been a significant drop in the blood pressure, or if the systolic pressure is below 100 mmHg. Side effects include bradycardia, congestive heart failure, pulmonary edema, hypotension and edema, depression, memory loss, insomnia, drowsiness, and dizziness. Clonidine (Catapres) is an alpha blocker prescribed to control mild to moderate hypertension. Side effects are drowsiness, nightmares, nervousness, depression, hypotension, and bradycardia. Sulfinpyrazone (Anturane) is a medication used to manage long-term gout, while calcitonin (Calcimar) is used in the treatment of Paget's disease by decreasing the rate of bone destruction (option 1). Glucagon (GlucaGen) is a specific medication for the management of hypoglycemia when glucose is not appropriate (option 3). Hydroxyzine (Vistaril) is used in the treatment of anxiety, pruritus caused by allergies, psychiatric and emotional emergencies, nausea and vomiting (excluding the nausea and vomiting of pregnancy), as a preoperative and postoperative sedation, and as a prepartum and postpartum adjunct therapy (option 4).
Cognitive Level: Application
Nursing Process: Assessment; *Test Plan:* SECE

3 Answer: 4 *Rationale:* Family history and gender cannot be modified as risk factors in any form of hypertension. Current research suggests there are several genes influencing the development of hypertension. Ethnicity is a non-modifiable risk factor; however, stress can be modified if the interruption of the stressor is undertaken (option 1). Obesity and substance abuse are risk factors that may be managed through behavioral modification and support groups (option 2). Nutrition and occupation are both modifiable with assistance (option 3).
Cognitive Level: Application
Nursing Process: Implementation; *Test Plan:* HPM

4 Answer: 2 *Rationale:* Blood pressure readings from three different positions are helpful in ruling out the presence of hypertension. The difference between each of these readings should be less than 5 mmHg. If the reading difference is higher, repeat readings should be within the follow-up plan for this client. Options 1, 3, and 4 will not provide enough data to determine if a problem exists.
Cognitive Level: Application
Nursing Process: Implementation; *Test Plan:* PHYS

5 Answer: 4 *Rationale:* Smoking is the primary etiological factor identified with clients diagnosed with Buerger's disease. Emphasis should be placed on cessation of smoking, use of nicotine (Nicoderm™) patches, and support groups. Option 1 is usually required with clients with Raynaud's disease, although clients with Buerger's should protect the extremities from cold injury as well. Clients with Buerger's disease should wear comfortable shoes that will not cause blisters or sores, but they do not necessarily have to be flat (option 2). Although pain is present, the use of opioids is usually not indicated (option 3).
Cognitive Level: Analysis
Nursing Process: Implementation; *Test Plan:* HPM

6 Answer: 3 *Rationale:* Frequently, clients perceive and become helpless when confronted with multiple lifestyle changes. The healthcare team and the client need to determine the most significant lifestyle modification needed and begin to work with this one. The other modifications are started as the client is able to incorporate them. The major focus is to establish and maintain a partnership with this client. Many times the therapeutic action of the medication will not cause the client to feel or perceive any difference in their well-being (option 1); however, client education can help to enlighten a client about the need for life-long therapy. Option 4 may or may not be true for

some clients, and option 2 is not a plausible response by healthcare workers.
Cognitive Level: Application
Nursing Process: Implementation; *Test Plan:* HPM

7 Answer: 2 *Rationale:* Cardiac diseases such as congestive heart failure, myocardial infarction, and cardiomyopathy are conditions that coexist with thromboembolism. Each of these conditions creates the possibility of thrombus occurring because of ineffective emptying of the heart during its pumping action. Thromboembolism generally occurs in clients over the age of 40. Gender usually does not play a role in embolism; a male who is Jewish and over the age of 40 is more prone to Buerger's disease (option 3). Kidney disease has not been identified as a cause of emboli (option 4).
Cognitive Level: Analysis
Nursing Process: Assessment; *Test Plan:* HPM

8 Answer: 1 *Rationale:* Part of the medical regime will include anticoagulant therapy. The rationale for this is to prevent the development or extension of thrombi by inhibiting the synthesis of the clotting factors or through deactivation of the mechanism. The client's legs need to remain in an elevated position for comfort and to facilitate venous circulation to prevent the development of emboli and thrombi in the lower extremities (option 2). Low molecular weight heparin (LMWH) is usually used as a preventative agent in clients prone to thrombophlebitis, not as a treatment with a confirmed diagnosis (option 3). The treatment is usually to raise the foot of the bed 6 inches off the floor (Trendelenburg's position). The knee lever needs to remain in this position 24 hours per day until the healthcare team considers the need for elevation of the legs no longer exists (option 4). The head of the bed may be elevated for activities such as eating and bathing.
Cognitive Level: Application
Nursing Process: Implementation; *Test Plan:* PHYS

9 Answer: 2 *Rationale:* The symptoms exhibited by the client are typical of an abdominal aortic aneurysm. The most significant sign is the audible pulse in the abdominal area. If hemorrhage were present, the abdomen would be tender and firm. There isn't enough information to determine if the hypertension is secondary or essential (option 1). There is no evidence of congestive heart failure (CHF) in the scenario (option 3). Signs of Buerger's disease involve the extremities (option 4).
Cognitive Level: Analysis
Nursing Process: Analysis; *Test Plan:* PHYS

10 Answer: 1 *Rationale:* The major task of the healthcare team is to medicate the client with drugs that produce smooth muscle relaxation, which will decrease the vasospasm and increase the arterial flow to the affected part. The drugs used are calcium antagonists. Frequently, the client will be medicated during the cool to cold months when vasoconstriction is a physiological response to the environmental temperature. Options 2 and 3 are a concern, but the highest priority is reducing spasms. If the medicines work, pain will be reduced and blood flow maintained (thus lesions prevented). Raynaud's disease does not usually cause major disabilities (option 4). A client may develop gangrene of the skin of the tips of the digits, but these are in the upper extremities (option 3).
Cognitive Level: Analysis
Nursing Process: Implementation: *Test Plan:* PHYS

Posttest

1 Answer: 1 *Rationale:* The healthcare provider must be sure that the client is aware of the need to eat sufficient amounts of calcium, magnesium, and potassium. Foods high in magnesium include green leafy vegetables, seafood, wheat bran, milk, legumes, bananas, oranges, grapefruit, and chocolate. Foods high in calcium include milk, cottage cheese, cheese, yogurt, rhubarb, broccoli, collard greens, spinach, tofu, canned sardines, and salmon. Potassium-rich foods include fruits and fruit juices, vegetables and vegetable juices, meats, and milk products. These food products are best if they are fresh and not processed. The consumption of alcohol is limited to 1 ounce per day; however, with some anti-hypertensive medications, the recommendation is the client not consume any alcohol (option 2). Jogging is a good activity in moderation, i.e., 1 mile per week (option 3). Herbal therapies containing licorice cannot be safely used by a hypertensive client. Licorice causes the blood pressure to rise (option 4).
Cognitive Level: Application
Nursing Process: Implementation; *Test Plan:* HPM

2 Answer: 3 *Rationale:* By definition, secondary hypertension has some underlying cause. Approximately 10 percent of all pregnant women develop this condition. The criteria are that the systolic blood pressure rises 30 mmHg and the diastolic blood pressure rises 15 mmHg prior to the 20th week of gestation. Diagnostic tests are conducted to confirm the diagnosis and rule out polycythemia, hyperaldosteronism, and pheochromocytoma. The systematic long-term use of contraceptives containing estrogen may contribute to secondary hypertension (option 1).

Coarctation of the aorta is rare; when it occurs, it interferes with the renal blood flow, which stimulates the renin-angiotension-aldosterone system of the kidney (option 2). Endocrine disorders and hypertension are rare and involve the adrenal medullary system (option 4).
Cognitive Level: Knowledge
Nursing Process: Analysis; *Test Plan:* PHYS

3 **Answer: 2** *Rationale:* One of the factors that regulates blood pressure is the amount of fluid volume within the body system. Excess concentration of sodium and water increases the blood pressure and the pressure in the kidney filtration, resulting in diuresis. The baroreceptors respond to the activity of the receptors as well as pressure and chemical composition within the vascular system. Arterial receptors are also involved (option 1). The endocrine system is usually not involved (option 3). Hypertension causes an increased production of sodium and water releasing hormone (option 4).
Cognitive Level: Comprehension
Nursing Process: Analysis; *Test Plan:* PHYS

4 **Answer: 4** *Rationale:* These laboratory studies would be the most helpful and give an estimate of the degree of vascular involvement as well as the degree of damage. An elevated cholesterol level would suggest HTN related to atherosclerosis. Creatinine is the most specific test of kidney function (a cause of HTN) and is not affected by foods as is the blood urea nitrogen (BUN). A hematocrit will be helpful in determining fluid problems, which could account for HTN also. Bone scan (option 1), glucose tolerance (option 2), and prothrombin time (option 3) are not essential tests for diagnosing HTN.
Cognitive Level: Application
Nursing Process: Assessment; *Test Plan:* PHYS

5 **Answer: 2** *Rationale:* An overweight client on bed rest from a hip surgery is at higher risk because of the two risk factors (obesity and immobility). Even though the client will be ambulated and progressively increase weight-bearing, the potential exists because of the immobility. HTN does not increase the risk, nor does smoking (option 1). Raynaud's is not a factor (option 3); option 4 is vague about the cardiac history and further information is needed.
Cognitive Level: Analysis
Nursing Process: Analysis; *Test Plan:* PHYS

6 **Answer: 4** *Rationale:* These are signs and symptoms of PVD; the diagnosis is supported by the pallor noted when the feet are elevated for 30 minutes. The

pulse is diminished because it is arterial occlusion and not venous. Pain and itching are usually felt with varicose veins (option 1). Thrombophlebitis is associated with redness, warmth, and swelling of an extremity (option 2). Raynaud's is more involved with the digits of both the hands and feet (option 3).
Cognitive Level: Application
Nursing Process: Assessment; *Test Plan:* PHYS

7 **Answer: 2** *Rationale:* Whenever there is tissue breakdown associated with intermittent claudication, the client will be confined to bed in order to be able to meet the oxygen requirements for the damaged tissues. Activity (options 1, 3, and 4) raises the amount of oxygen required to sustain both healthy and diseased tissues to a point where deficits will occur and healing will be stalled. At the time the client is to be ambulated, the shoe of choice is a supportive, comfortable shoe.
Cognitive Level: Application
Nursing Process: Implementation; *Test Plan:* PHYS

8 **Answer: 3** *Rationale:* These are known as Virchow's triad and are the most commonly associated reasons for a blood clot. A thrombus usually involves the venous, not arterial, system (option 1). Situations that contribute to venous stasis are myocardial infarction and prolonged sitting; however, a stroke is not classified in this manner (option 2). Injury may or may not cause thrombi, while continued bed rest can contribute (option 4).
Cognitive Level: Knowledge
Nursing Process: Assessment; *Test Plan:* PHYS

9 **Answer: 2** *Rationale:* Pain felt in the calf while pulling up on the toes is abnormal and indicates a positive test. If the client feels nothing or just feels like the calf muscle is stretching, it is considered negative (option 3). A tourniquet test (options 1 and 4) is used to measure for varicose veins.
Cognitive Level: Knowledge
Nursing Process: Assessment; *Test Plan:* PHYS

10 **Answer: 3** *Rationale:* A client with Raynaud's disease needs to be taught to protect the digits from extreme cold by using warm clothing, gloves, and socks. Use of gloves is essential anytime the digits may be cold (such as at night). Smoking should be stopped completely (option 1). Relaxation and stress management are essential (option 2). Diet is not associated with Raynaud's disease (option 4).
Cognitive Level: Analysis
Nursing Process: Evaluation; *Test Plan:* HPM

References

Barkauskas, V. H., Bauman, L. C., & Darling-Fisher, C. (2001). *Health and physical assessment* (3rd ed). St. Louis, MO: Mosby.

Black, J., Hawks, J. H., & Keene, A. M. (2001). *Medical surgical nursing* (6th ed.). Philadelphia: W. B. Saunders.

Brashers, V. L. (2001). *Clinical applications of pathophysiology: Assessment, diagnostic reasoning and management* (2nd ed.). St. Louis: Mosby.

Burrel, G. & Pless, B. S. (1998). *Adult nursing: Acute and community care* (2nd ed.). Upper Saddle River, NJ: Prentice Hall.

Guyton, A. & Hall, J. E. (2001). *Textbook of medical physiology* (10th ed.). Philadelphia: W. B. Saunders.

Huether, S. E. & McCance, K. L. (2000). *Understanding pathophysiology* (2nd ed.). St. Louis Mosby.

Kelly-Powell, M. L. (1997). Personalizing choices: Client's making treatment decisions. *Research in Nursing and Health, 20:* 219–227.

Kozier, B., Erb, G., Berman, A. J. & Burke, K. (2000). *Fundamentals of nursing* (6th ed.). Upper Saddle River, NJ: Prentice Hall.

Leao de Aquino, E., Magalhaes, L., Araujo, M. J., Chagas de Almeida, M. da C., & Leto, J. P. (200_). Hypertension in female nursing staff—pattern of occurrence, diagnosis, and treatment. San Paulo. *Arquivos Brasileiros de Cardiologia.* (http://www.scielo.br/cgi-bin/fbpebtext?pid=S0066782X2001000300003)

LeMone, P. & Burke, K. M. (2000). *Medical surgical nursing: Critical thinking in client care* (2nd ed.). Upper Saddle River, NJ: Prentice Hall.

NHLBI, "Issues New Clinical Advisory on Systolic Blood Pressure." From: National Institutes of Health. May 4, 2000. (http://www. nhlbi.nih.gov/new/press/may04-00.htm)

NHLBI, "Stops part of study—High blood pressure drug performs no better than standard treatment." From: National Institutes of Health, Wednesday, March 8, 2000. (http://www. nhlbi.nih.gov/new/press/mar08-00.htm)

NHLBI, "Study shows association between sleep apnea and hypertension." From: National Institutes of Health. April 11, 2000. (http://www.nhlbi.nih.gov/new/ press/ apr11-00.htm)

Phillips, R. A. (1999). Hypertension: What's new in diagnosis? *Consultant 39*(5): 2337.

Rankin-Box, D. (2001). *The nurse's handbook of complementary therapies* (2nd ed.). Edinburgh: Bailliere Tindall.

Springhouse (2000). *Nurse's drug guide* (3rd ed.). Springhouse, PA.: Springhouse Corporation.

vanWissen, K., Litchfield, M., & Maling, T. (1998). Living with high blood pressure. *Journal of Advanced Nursing, 27:* 567–574.

Walker, B. R., McConnachie, A., Noon, J. P., Webb, D. J., & Watt, G. C. M. (1998). Contribution of parental blood pressures to association between low birth weight and adult high blood pressure: cross sectional study. *British Medical Journal 316*(4): 834.

CHAPTER 4

Neurological Health Problems

Patsy Rider, RN, MSN, CS
Sherry Hendrickson, RN, PhD, CS

CHAPTER OUTLINE

OBJECTIVES

▮ Define key terms associated with neurologic health problems.

▮ Identify risk factors associated with the development of neurologic health problems.

▮ Discuss the common etiologies of neurologic health problems.

▮ Describe the pathophysiologic processes associated with specific neurologic health problems.

▮ Distinguish between normal and abnormal neurologic findings obtained from the nursing assessment.

▮ Prioritize nursing interventions associated with specific neurologic health problems

▮ Describe the pathophysiology of pain.

▮ Prioritize nursing interventions used to treat pain.

[**Media Link**]

Use the CD-ROM enclosed with this text, or log onto the address given to access the free, interactive Companion Website created for this series. The CD-ROM and Companion Website accompanying this book offer additional practice opportunities and information—NCLEX Review, Case Studies, Glossary, In Depth with NCLEX, and more.

www.prenhall.com/hogan

REVIEW AT A GLANCE

anterior cord syndrome *complete paralysis below level of lesion; hyperaesthesia below level of lesion; hypalgesia below level of lesion; preservation of touch, position, pressure and vibration*

automatism *automatic action or behavior without conscious knowledge; repetitive, semi-purposeful, patterned movement such as lip smacking*

autonomic dysreflexia *a life-threatening involuntary sympathetic response of the central nervous system to a noxious stimulus with injury above T6*

Brown-Séquard's syndrome *hemi-section of the cord; ipsilateral motor loss below level of lesion; ipsilateral loss of position and vibration sense below level of lesion; contralateral loss of pain and temperature senses below level of lesion*

Brudzinski's sign *flexion of neck causes neck pain and the hip and knee to flex*

bulbocavernous reflex *contraction of bulbocavernosis muscle on percussing dorsum of penis*

central cord syndrome *greatest percentage of incomplete injuries; motor loss in upper extremities greater than loss in lower extremities; spasticity in lower extremities; variable degree of sensory loss; variable degree of bladder dysfunction*

"cogwheel" rigidity *manual manipulation of body parts may take on the feel of a cogwheel*

decerebrate *extensor posturing indicating brainstem injury*

decorticate *flexor posturing indicating corticospinal tract lesions*

diplopia *double vision*

equianalgesic chart *shows pain relief obtained with different drugs, dose, and route*

hematomyelia *hemorrhage within the cord*

hydrocephalus *brain substance expanded into a watery sac protruding through a cleft in the cranium*

Kernig's sign *flexion of the hip and knee and then extension of the leg causes hamstring pain*

lead-pipe rigidity *cataleptic condition during which limbs remain in any position in which placed; smooth, stiff movement*

Monro-Kellie hypothesis *as volume of one brain component increases, volume of another decreases, to a limit*

nuchal rigidity *muscle contraction to the nape of the neck*

neurogenic pulmonary edema *an extremely rapid discharge of nerve impulses from a cerebral injury disrupting vascular permeability*

phantom pain *the sensation that pain exists in the removed part*

spinal shock *a neurophysiologic cessation of all or nearly all reflexes below level of injury*

status epilepticus *intense, repetitive seizures with very short periods of calm between them*

Pretest

1 The priority in preparing the room for a client with a C7 level spinal cord is having:

(1) The special kinetic bed.
(2) The halo brace device.
(3) A ventilator on stand-by.
(4) A catheterization tray.

2 Upon return of the closed-head injury client from CT scan, the head of the bed is maintained at 30 degrees, and the client is positioned on his side with a towel roll placed vertically under the pillow. This unique positioning facilitates:

(1) Prevention of pulmonary embolism.
(2) Venous drainage from the brain.
(3) Airway management.
(4) Intracranial pressure (ICP) readings.

3 After regaining consciousness, a client reports a tremendous headache as he was taken from the site of a motorcycle crash by ambulance. His wife is unprepared when arriving at the hospital to find he had become comatose. The nurse explains the cause as which of the following?

(1) An expanding epidural hematoma
(2) A reticular activating system concussion
(3) A diffuse axonal injury
(4) An expanding pericardial hematoma

4 Following a grand mal seizure, the client is unconscious and unresponsive when the nurse tries to awaken the client. The nurse takes which of the following actions?

(1) Calls a code
(2) Notifies the physician
(3) Reduces the Dilantin
(4) Allows gradual awakening

5 The nurse assesses the client's understanding of discharge needs and goals after experiencing a cerebral vascular accident (CVA). Which of the following statements indicates further information and teaching will be necessary?

(1) "I'm getting a lifetime supply of adult diapers."
(2) "I worry about those scary transient ischemic attacks."
(3) "I've got to find a walking buddy."
(4) "I'm getting a rail installed in my tub."

6 The major focus for nursing care of the client with meningitis will be to:

(1) Enhance coping skills.
(2) Provide cognitive stimulation.
(3) Assess risk for injury and prevent complications.
(4) Increase cardiac output.

7 The client comes to the Emergency Department with weakness that has been progressing upward in both legs for a couple of days. The nurse, suspecting Guillain-Barré syndrome, begins care by:

(1) Taking medical history, noting recent viral influenza.
(2) Giving the client orange juice for fatigue and low blood sugar.
(3) Instructing on tests for myasthenia gravis.
(4) Evaluating for petit mal seizures.

8 The teaching plan for a client with myasthenia gravis should include which of the following as a priority instruction?

(1) Exercise to increase peripheral circulation.
(2) Plan important activities for late afternoon.
(3) Identify signs of and action during crisis.
(4) Eat three well-balanced meals a day.

9 The client with Parkinson's disease finds the resting tremor he is experiencing in his right hand very frustrating. The nurse advises him to:

(1) Practice deep-breathing.
(2) Take a warm bath.
(3) Hold an object in that hand.
(4) Take diazepam (Valium) as needed.

10 A client on the first day after abdominal surgery ranks his pain as 9 on a scale of 0 to 10, 0 being no pain and 10 being the most pain possible. He is laughing and talking with visitors at this time. The client has defined a pain level of 5 as his comfort level goal. He has an order for analgesics every 1 to 2 hours. His last dose was the maximum ordered 2 hours ago. He had no untoward effects. The nurse should do which of the following?

(1) Record his pain level at 5.
(2) Administer the maximum dose of the analgesic.
(3) Administer half the maximum dose of the analgesic.
(4) Take his vital signs in 30 minutes.

See page 164 for Answers and Rationales.

I. Risk Factors Associated with Neurological Health Problems

A. Increased intracranial pressure: stroke, tumor, head trauma, inflammation, and neurological conditions such as meningitis

B. Intracranial hematomas: males (adolescent to young adulthood), injury, radiation, jobs or incidents where electrocution is a possibility, outside employment where weather can be severe or falls are a high probability

C. Stroke: diseases (hypertension [HTN], sickle cell anemia, polycythemia, atherosclerosis, cardiac valvular disease, diabetes), valve and organ replacement, anticoagulant therapy, atrial fibrillation, cardioversion, oral contraceptives, drug abuse, smoking, high salt or alcohol intake, sedentary lifestyle

D. **Spinal cord injury:** athletes, drug and/or alcohol abuse, employment where falls are a high probability, diseases such as tumors, syringomyelia, degenerative diseases

E. **Encephalitis:** populations living with an abundance of mosquitoes, especially if cattle and horses are close by; individuals drinking goat's milk; exposure to ticks; metal poisonings; recent immunizations and illnesses such as German measles or chickenpox

F. **Meningitis:** impaired immune function as in the very old or very young, clients with human immunodeficiency virus (HIV), those on chemotherapy, otitis media, sinusitis, basal skull fracture, neurosurgery, systemic sepsis, crowded living conditions (college dorms, military institutions, and prisons)

G. **Seizures:** brain tumors, family history, head injury or neurological disorders

H. **Guillain-Barré Syndrome:** viral infections, recent immunizations

I. **Myasthenia gravis (MG):** family or previous history of autoimmune diseases

J. **Parkinson's disease (proposed theories only):** cerebral anoxia, advancing age, genetic factors, and factors toxic to dopaminergic cells

K. **Multiple sclerosis (MS):** individuals living in colder climates; genetic or family history of MS or autoimmune illnesses; age

L. **Amyotrophic lateral sclerosis (ALS):** possibly genetics

M. **Pain:** work requiring strenuous lifting or bending, individuals with poor posture, stage of life factors, chronic diseases, arterial or ischemic wounds

N. **Alzheimer's disease:** aging, head trauma, family history, trauma, presence of the risk gene, apoE4

II. Increased Intracranial Pressure (IICP)

A. **Overview**

1. Defined as a rise in the pressure of the cerebrospinal fluid that maintains the subarachnoid space between the skull and the brain; nondistendable bone and meninges surround the brain; a balance among volumes of content (brain 80 percent, blood 10 percent, cereberal spinal fluid [CSF] 10 percent) of cranial vault usually exists

2. IICP is an intracranial pressure (ICP) greater than 15 mmHg

3. A significant increase is termed intracranial hypertension

4. Causes:

a. Increases in tissue volume

1) Neoplasm

2) Cerebral edema: interstitial; vasogenic seen in tumor, trauma; cytotoxic in hypoxic-ischemic injury; infarction; and infection or other disease state

b. Abscess

c. Increases in blood volume: hemorrhage and hematoma formation, increased arterial inflow, and decreased venous return

d. Increases in CSF volume

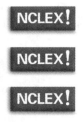

   1) Obstruction of CSF pathways produces **hydrocephalus** (brain substance expanded into a watery sac)

   2) Deficient CSF absorption: usually caused by blockage of arachnoid villi or idiopathic as in normal pressure hydrocephalus

   3) Overproduction of CSF

e. Other causes: congenital or developmental, metabolic, or pseudotumor cerebri (benign intracranial hypertension)

B. Pathophysiology

1. **Monro-Kellie hypothesis:** as volume of one component (brain tissue, blood, CSF) increases, volume of another decreases, to a limit

   a. Controlled by autoregulation: cerebral arterioles change diameter to maintain blood flow when ICP increases

   b. Brain tissue unable to compensate (decrease volume)

2. Maximal compensation occurs after volume increases; ICP begins to increase

3. ICP values

   a. ICP value alone is not a reliable measure of brain's compliance: ICP may be in normal range (< 15 mmHg); but client is still in danger of herniation because of poor compliance

   b. Changes in ICP in response to stimuli may be predictive of compliance; decreased compliance indicated by: sustained increases in ICP in response to stimuli; large increases in response to non-noxious stimuli

4. Physiology

   a. Cerebral blood flow (CBF): normally 750 mL/min

   1) Hypercarbia: $PaCO_2$ greater than 45 mmHg produces vasodilation; increases ICP by increasing volume

   2) Hypocarbia: $PaCO_2$ less than 25 mmHg produces rebound cerebral vasodilation, loss of autoregulation

   b. Cerebral perfusion pressure (CPP)

   1) Normal CPP ranges from 60 to 100 mmHg; determines CBF

   2) Hyperperfusion and increased intracranial pressure (IICP) occur with CPP greater than 100 mmHg

   3) Hypoperfusion and cerebral ischemia: with CPP 40 to 60 mmHg

   4) Irreversible ischemia and infarction: with CPP less than 40 mmHg

   5) Brain death: with CPP 0–40 mm Hg

5. Compensatory mechanisms

   a. Activated when increase in ICP occurs to balance volumes within cranial vault to protect brain

   b. Dependent upon rate of expansion of brain volume

NCLEX!

NCLEX!

NCLEX!

NCLEX!

NCLEX!

c. Rapidly increasing volume prevents activation of compensatory mechanisms

d. Compensatory mechanisms involve CSF changes

   1) Normal shunting of CSF into spinal subarachnoid space to reduce pressure (most common)

   2) Increased absorption of CSF

   3) Decreased secretion of CSF

e. Venous blood may also be shunted to allow more room for expansion

NCLEX!

6. Failure of compensatory mechanisms causes ischemia, hypoxia, herniation, and brain death

   a. As ICP approaches systemic arterial pressure, CPP and CBF decrease

   b. When ICP equals systemic arterial pressure, CBF ceases and brain death ensues

   c. Elevated range

      1) Moderate: 20 to 40 mmHg

      2) Severe: greater than 40 mmHg

      3) Effect of elevation on circulation determined by CPP with mean arterial pressure (MAP) a primary influence; MAP is the average pressure in the arteries during a cardiac cycle (influenced by elasticity of arterial walls and mean volume of arterial blood)

7. Signs and symptoms

   a. Gastrointestinal: ulceration and bleeding

   b. Cardiovascular: elevation or depression of S-T segments; large positive or negative U waves; prolonged Q-T or Q-U intervals; Q waves in both standard and precordial leads; deeply inverted or tall spiky upright T waves; dysrhythmias

NCLEX!

   c. Cushing's triad/response

      1) A response involving three classic signs: widening pulse pressure, elevated systolic pressure, and bradycardia

      2) The brainstem reflects the final effort to maintain cerebral perfusion

      3) Caused by rapidly expanding lesions as epidural hematoma or lesion in posterior fossa

      4) Seen when ICP is greater than 45 mmHg or when ICP approaches systemic diastolic blood pressure

      5) Pressure on brainstem causes ischemia of vasomotor center of medulla

      6) Systolic blood pressure increases while diastolic remains the same causing widened pulse pressure

      7) Increased blood pressure: sensed in baroreceptors of carotid arteries and aortic arch; causes vagal response of bradycardia

    d. Neurogenic pulmonary edema is an extremely rapid discharge of nerve impulses from the injured brain disrupting vascular permeability

    e. Intracranial effects

      1) Increase in ICP decreases microvascular CBF leading to tissue hypoxia and causing respiratory center dysfunction

      2) Hypoventilation develops causing increased $PaCO_2$ and decreased blood pH

      3) Hypercarbia causes cerebral vessel vasodilation and edema

      4) ICP increases resulting in herniation, cerebral ischemia, and brain death

8. Herniation syndromes occur, which are displacement of a portion of the brain through or around linings of brain or openings within the intracranial cavity

    a. Mechanism categorized as supratentorial, infratentorial, or extracranial

      1) Caused by increased pressure in one or all compartments; usually occurs when difference exists in pressure between supratentorial and infratentorial (posterior fossa) compartments

      2) Supratentorial herniation syndromes: herniation of structures normally lying above tentorium cerebelli; cingulated herniation; uncal herniation; and transtentorial or central herniation

      3) Infratentorial herniation syndrome: herniation of structures lying below tentorium cerebelli; upward transtentorial herniation; and downward cerebellar or tonsillar herniation

      4) Extracranial herniation syndrome: occurs when opening in skull allows intracranial contents under pressure to herniate outward; may occur through open wound, surgical incision, ICP monitor site or through fractures of ear or nose; resulting decrease in volume lowers ICP and possibly prevents intracranial herniation

    b. Results: compression, laceration, distortion or necrosis of brain structures; vascular compromise; blocked flow of CSF; brain compression and death

C. Nursing assessment of increased intracranial pressure

    1. Assessment

      a. Airway patency and breathing patterns: central nervous system dysfunction is associated with decreased level of consciousness (LOC), hypercapnia, and potential for pulmonary edema

NCLEX!

      b. Changes in vital signs: Cushing's triad of increased systolic pressure, bradycardia, and an irregular respiratory pattern is seen with sustained and elevated ICP; fever is possible as compensatory measures fail

NCLEX!

      c. Pupillary dysfunction: compression of the oculomotor nerve (CN III) results in dilatation of the ipsilateral pupil, sluggish or no response to light, with inability to move the eye upward, and ptosis (drooping) of the eyelid; a nonreactive, dilated pupil is a neurological emergency heralding transtentorial brain herniation

      d. Visual abnormalities: decreased or blurred vision or extraocular movements

e. Papilledema: swelling of the optic disc, as seen with an ophthalmoscope; indicative of long-standing IICP

f. Motor function: contralateral hemiparesis or hemiplegia may be seen; no movement or flaccidity is the least favorable sign; localization to a painful stimulus may result in an effort to produce movement

1) **Decorticate:** flexor posturing indicating corticospinal tract lesions (see Figure 4-1A)

2) **Decerebrate:** extensor posturing indicating brainstem injury (see Figure 4-1B)

g. Headache: unusual, seen with slowly increasing ICP, worse with straining and position changes, especially on awakening

h. Emesis: projectile vomiting without nausea

2. Diagnostic tests: arterial blood gases (ABGs), complete blood count (CBC), CSF cultures, CT scan, serum osmolality

D. Nursing management

1. Medications include: stool softeners, diuretics (osmotics, loop), corticosteroids: dexamethasone (Decadron), antipyretics: acetaminophen (Tylenol), H_2 receptor antagonists, anticonvulsants if seizures occur

2. Secure airway patency and clearance

a. Hyperventilate and oxygenate at 100 percent using sigh mode on ventilator prior to suctioning; avoid suctioning for longer than 10 seconds

b. Auscultate lungs and clear any secretions

c. Position client side to side to decrease aspiration risk in case of emesis

d. Promote normal breathing pattern: monitor arterial carbon dioxide pressure ($PaCO_2$) to stay within 25 to 30 mmHg, avoiding cerebral vasodilation

Figure 4-1

Abnormal posturing
seen in head injuries.
A. Decorticate.
B. Decerebrate.

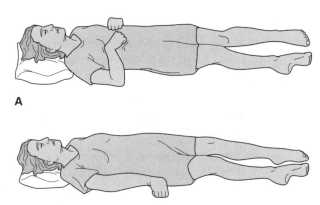

A

B

3. Optimize cerebral perfusion

   a. Monitor signs and symptoms of pulmonary edema including: increasing restlessness, anxiety, dyspnea, weak and rapid pulse, and blood-tinged, frothy fluid

   b. Position client to avoid extreme rotation or flexion of neck resulting in raising jugular venous pressure and ICP; a neutral or midline position aids cerebral venous drainage

   c. Avoid or greatly reduce extreme hip flexion causing an increase in intra-abdominal and intrathoracic pressure, producing IICP

   d. Provide high-fiber diet to decrease use of the valsalva maneuver; assist with bowel movements using bedpan

   e. Avoid physiological and environmental stimuli

   f. Monitor nursing care to keep ICP below 25 mmHg and to promote return to baseline levels within five minutes

4. Monitor for symptoms prior to herniation

   a. Report and treat per protocol signs of acutely increasing ICP: decreasing Glasgow Coma Scale (GCS) score, behavioral changes, disorientation, difficulty in following simple commands, speech changes, less purposeful response to painful stimuli, posturing movements, loss of or abnormal (i.e., positive Babinski) reflexes

   b. Notify the physician and follow unit protocol for pupil and eye changes: blurred vision, **diplopia** (double vision), extraocular movement (EOM) abnormalities, and nystagmus

5. Prevent infection

   a. Adhere to written protocols for care of the client with an intracranial pressure monitoring device

   b. Monitor indicators of infection: white blood cell (WBC) counts, positive cultures, fever, chills, nuchal rigidity and changes in vital signs

   c. Inspect ICP monitoring site and connections for leaking cerebrospinal fluid or drainage

6. Avoid administration of medications such as narcotics that can mimic signs of IICP

7. Support family: encourage family to visit the client; provide information to optimize decision making when clients are unable to make treatment choices; anticipate grieving and identify sources of community support

III. Intracranial Hematomas

A. Overview

1. Defined as a break in a blood vessel within the cranium or skull that leads to swelling caused by hemorrhage

2. Peak occurrence during evening and night hours on weekends

3. Pathological mechanisms

   a. Direct impact

      1) Acceleration: rapidly moving object strikes relatively stationary head

      2) Deceleration: coming to a sudden, abrupt stop, as when head strikes an immobile object/static surface (more severe damage because of the effects on brain stem)

      3) Rotation: lateral blow rotates brain, contusing the brain stem and disrupting the white matter

   b. Indirect stresses: trauma not to head but involves brain; rotational displacement of head on extreme motion of the neck causes shear, tensile strains and compressive forces transmitted to the brain; landing on buttocks or feet from a height transmits force through the spinal column to the base of the brain

   c. Systemic: chronic alcoholism, cerebral atrophy, anticoagulants, long history of hypertension

4. Mechanisms of injury: blunt (closed, non-penetrating); penetrating (open); and compression: skull compressed between two forces causing a crush effect on brain

5. Types of injury

   a. Scalp injuries

   b. Skull fractures

   c. Dural integrity

      1) Open: dura torn by laceration; compound, depressed fractures, penetrating objects

      2) Closed: dural continuity maintained; simple, linear fracture may be present

6. Intracranial hemorrhage classified as epidural, subdural, or intracerebral

7. Common causes: vehicular accidents (automobiles, motorcycles), falls, violence, sports-related injuries, ingestion of alcohol and/or drugs, other (intrauterine and birth injury, radiation, electrocution, heat stroke, lightning)

B. Pathophysiology

1. *Epidural* hematoma: cerebral artery bleed above the dura mater; usually in middle fossa caused by laceration of the middle meningeal artery; 2 to 6 percent of head injuries

   a. Signs of brain stem compression usually occur within 24 hours

   b. Signs and symptoms

      1) Short period of unconsciousness followed by a lucid interval

      2) Lucid interval followed by progressive depression of consciousness

      3) Focal signs: ipsilateral pupil dilation, weakness of contralateral extremities

NCLEX!

2. *Subdural* hematoma: bleeding into subdural space of the brain with disruption of cortical veins; most often over parietal areas; 29 percent of head injuries

    a. Acute: symptomatic within 24 to 72 hours

        1) Majority of clients deteriorate quickly, become deeply comatose, with brain unable to compensate from rapid compression; often associated with severe brain trauma and high mortality; may mimic epidural

        2) Signs and symptoms include depressed LOC, usually from the time of injury; ipsilateral pupil dilation and contralateral weakness

    b. Subacute: symptomatic within 2 to 10 days

        1) Better prognosis than acute, still 25 to 35 percent mortality

        2) Signs and symptoms include headaches; decreased LOC and focal signs of compression; failure to show improvement

    c. Chronic: symptomatic occurring after 10 days (elusive, nonspecific, and fluctuating)

        1) Gradual clot formation allows brain time to accommodate; traumatic etiology may be unclear, minor, forgotten; prognosis good (mortality rates 10 percent); may reaccumulate

        2) Signs and symptoms include slowly progressive change in behavior (apathy) or personality, headaches; variable LOC; lethargy, confusion, motor weakness with loss of upward gaze, dysphasia, urinary or bowel incontinence

3. *Intracerebral* hematoma: bleeding from the small arteries or veins in subcortical white matter

    a. Lucid interval followed by decreased LOC

    b. Focal signs based on location

    c. Signs and symptoms include possible headache, hemiplegia, ipsilateral pupil dilation, progressing ICP with potential for herniation; petechiae common, usually seen with contusion, edema; majority occur in frontal and temporal lobes; signs and symptoms according to location

4. Subarachnoid hemorrhage

    a. Bleeding between the pia mater of the covering of the brain and spinal cord and the arachnoid membrane

    b. Signs and symptoms include severe headache and restlessness; **nuchal rigidity** (muscle contraction to the nape of the neck), fever, and a positive **Kernig's sign** (flexion of the hip and knee and then extension of the leg causes hamstring pain)(see Figure 4-2); positive Babinski sign (dorsiflexion of great toe upon stimulating sole of feet)

C. Nursing assessment

1. Assessment

    a. Airway and breathing pattern

    b. Assess vital signs (VS), level of consciousness, pupils, and motor responses; document baseline and monitor for subtle, sudden changes

Figure 4-2

Kernig's sign.

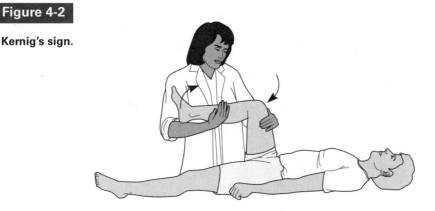

NCLEX!

    c. Observe for clinical indications of expanding lesions

        1) Localized/focal signs: hemiplegia, visual field defect, eye deviation, cerebellar signs, cranial nerve signs

        2) Generalized signs of IICP: headache, restlessness, irritability

    d. Gather data about traumatic event from family, witnesses including: details and time of injury; change in consciousness (lucid period, duration of unresponsiveness); and seizure activity

    e. Assess signs and symptoms of IICP, which may increase suddenly, resulting in tentorial herniation and sudden respiratory arrest

  2. Diagnostic tests: CT scan, MRI, ABGs, CBC

D. Nursing management

  1. Surgical intervention is the recommended treatment; no specific medications are recommended

NCLEX!

  2. Maintain adequate airway and cerebral perfusion: monitor respiratory pattern, breath sounds, cyanosis, restlessness, and use of accessory muscles; monitor ICP readings; prepare for oxygen administration, intubation or tracheostomy; prepare for possible cranial surgery if unable to maintain perfusion

  3. Advocate for client rest periods between frequent vital sign and neurological assessments

NCLEX!

  4. Provide seizure precautions due to risk secondary to IICP

  5. Support client and family in understanding assessment and management issues

IV. Cerebrovascular Accident (CVA)/Stroke

A. Overview

  1. Defined as an abrupt loss of consciousness with resulting paralysis that may be temporary or permanent

2. Often preceded by transient ischemic attacks (TIAs) or mini-strokes, which mimic a stroke for a few seconds to a few hours without permanent paralysis; cause is a temporary interference in cerebral blood flow

3. Causes of stroke include thrombus, embolus, and hemorrhage

B. Pathophysiology

1. Cellular level changes begin four to five minutes after blood flow and oxygenation of neurons are reduced

2. The sodium pump and neurotransmitters fail as a result of anaerobic glycolysis, resulting in cerebral edema as sodium draws water into brain

3. Cerebral blood vessel walls swell, circulation is compromised, and vasospasm combined with blood viscosity reduces cerebral perfusion

4. Outcomes of decreased cerebral perfusion: cerebral anoxia caused by interruption of blood supply to brain; cerebral infarction if anoxia lasts longer than 10 minutes resulting in irreversible changes; cerebral edema causing secondary damage; contralateral deficits when stroke is in cerebral hemisphere; permanent deficit reflecting locality of stroke

NCLEX!

5. Signs and symptoms include altered consciousness or unconsciousness, stertorous breathing, unequal pupils (larger pupil noted on same side as stroke), paralysis of one side, perspiration, aphasia (abnormal or absent speech), blank stare, dysphagia, inability to make decisions, loss of memory, and gait instability

C. Nursing assessment

1. Assessment

   a. Nursing history: interview client and family; history of risk factors; client and family's understanding of illness

   b. Assessment: airway obstruction and hypoxia if decreased level of consciousness; neurological deficits; vital sign stability; urine output; fluid and caloric needs; visual impairment (corneal abrasions, eye discomfort, diplopia); loss of sensation and functional ability of mouth, face and swallowing ability; bowel and bladder function; immobility issues; communication; perceptual deficits; psychosocial needs; and understanding of therapeutic regimen

2. Diagnostic tests: electrolytes, CT scan, MRI, ABGs, arteriography, ultrasound of carotid arteries, lumbar puncture, coagulation studies; prothrombin time (PT), partial thromboplastin time (PTT), international normalized ratio (INR)

D. Nursing management

NCLEX!

1. Medications include stool softeners, anticoagulants or thrombolytics, antiplatelets, calcium channel blockers, diuretics (if IICP exists), anticonvulsants if seizures occur; monitor effects of drugs

NCLEX!

2. Monitor neurological status

   a. Hyperthermia: maintain temperature within normal limits

   b. Neglect syndrome: provide care around perceptual deficits

   c. Seizures: promote safety and cerebral perfusion

   d. Agnosia: support recognition of previously known subject

       e. Communication deficits: consult with speech therapist, use communication board

       f. Visual: provide care with recognition of hemianopia, diplopia, or decreased acuity; placing a patch over one eye reduces double vision

       g. Cognitive changes: create plan of care with health care team to address memory loss, poor attention span, distractibility, judgment, problem solving difficulty, and disorientation

       h. Behavioral changes: educate family as to causes and approaches to use with labiality, loss of inhibitions, fear, anger, and depression

       i. Increased intracranial pressure: monitor closely for any changes in LOC

3. Respiratory status

       a. Brainstem damage: test for decerebrate posturing as a response to noxious stimuli as one indicator of brainstem involvement

       b. Airway obstruction: suction per assessment, after oxygenating and with goal of preventing IICP; monitor blood gases

       c. Poor cough and gag reflexes: intermittent positive pressure breathing (IPPB) therapy and position client on side to decrease risk of aspirating own secretions

       d. Pulmonary emboli: mobilize client as soon as tolerated; administer anticoagulant therapy, monitoring appropriate lab values

4. Monitor gastrointestinal system

       a. Dysphagia (difficulty swallowing): provide swallow evaluation before instituting feeding

       b. Constipation: provide stool softeners and bowel routine

       c. Stool impaction: encourage roughage, high fiber, and mobility to prevent impaction; increase fluid intake; remove any fecal impaction and document

5. Monitor genitourinary system

       a. Incontinence: evaluate behavioral, pharmacological, and supportive devices to create a plan with client for long-term maintenance but discourage dependency on adult diapers early in stroke phase

       b. Urgency: offer bedpan, urinal, or commode use every two hours; avoid caffeine

       c. Retention: avoid in-dwelling catheters; catheterize for post-void residuals or develop intermittent catheterization schedule; use bladder scan device

       d. Renal calculi: keep urine dilute (at least 2000 cc per day), prevent urinary stasis and infection; teach clients a prevention diet low in oxalate-rich foods and purines; monitor fluid and nutritional status

6. Monitor musculoskeletal system

       a. Hemiplegia: apply pneumatic compression device or elastic hose to reduce deep vein thrombosis; instruct family on range-of-motion exercises of joints from the shoulder down to ankle; initiate physical therapy for gait training

b. Contractures: create positioning schedule of two hours on unaffected side, 30 minutes on affected side, 30 minutes prone, indicating schedule in charting; use high top tennis shoes or therapeutic boot to prevent foot drop

c. Atrophy: begin range-of-motion exercises early, combined with stretching at least 4 times a day, instructing family as able

d. Dysarthria (difficulty and defective speech caused by impairment of the tongue or other muscles essential to speech): use communication board, avoid frustration; keep communication simple; consult with speech pathology for motor relearning plan

e. Osteoporosis: facilitate weight-bearing activity, screen for progression of condition

f. Sensory deprivation: create plan to optimize balance in sensory stimulation; provide appropriate repetition for learning

g. Self-image: provide positive feedback; encourage grooming and street attire; begin rehabilitation as soon as tolerated

h. Sexual dysfunction: encourage open communication among partners; inform client/partner of options; introduce topic before discharge from acute care

7. Monitor safety: explore what life will be like in home setting with new deficits; provide safety assessment for home setting, identifying areas to modify based on fall risk; create plan with client and family to optimize return to community, to identify support services, to recognize warning signs of another stroke event

V. Spinal Cord Injuries

A. Overview

1. Defined as a fracture or injury (twisting, compression, pulling) of the bones of the spinal column; damage may involve part of or all of the spinal cord

2. Incidence is more prominent in young males (18 to 30); is increasing in young females; increases with use of alcohol and/or drugs

3. Types of injury

a. Level of injury: cervical (most common site); thoracic (least common site); and lumbar

b. Upper and lower motor neuron damage (see Table 4-1)

1) Upper motor neurons (UMN) drive voluntary movement; UMNs originate in cerebral cortex and end at anterior horn cell of cord resulting in spastic paralysis and reflexes

2) Lower motor neuron (LMN) begins at the anterior horn cell; LMNs become part of the peripheral nerve to muscle, motor side of reflex arc; usually present in cauda equina injuries; areflexia results in flaccid paralysis; these neurons are responsible for innervation and contraction of skeletal muscles

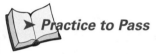

Practice to Pass

A stroke client is preparing for transfer to a rehabilitation setting. What would support the client and family's transition?

Table 4-1	Degrees of Motor and Sensory Loss in Spinal Cord Injury
Level of Lesion	**Degree of Motor and/or Sensory Loss**
Central cord syndrome, greatest percentage of incomplete injuries	Motor loss in upper extremities greater than loss in lower extremities; spasticity of lower extremities Variable degree of sensory loss Variable degree of bladder dysfunction Associated with hyperextension injuries of cervical spine, especially in osteoarthritis of spine
Anterior cord syndrome, associated with flexion injuries of cervical spine	Complete paralysis below level of lesion Hyperesthesia below level of lesion Hypalgesia below level of lesion Preservation of touch, position, pressure, and vibration **Paresthesia** (sensation of numbness, tingling, and heightened sensitivity) may be present
Brown-Sequard's syndrome, (hemi-section of the cord) associated with open penetrating wounds to the cord	Ipsilateral motor loss below level of lesion Ipsilateral loss of position and vibration sense below level of lesion Contralateral loss of pain and temperature senses below level of lesion
Posterior cord syndrome (rare)	Loss of light touch and proprioception below level of lesion Motor function of extremities, pain, and temperature remain intact Associated with cervical hyperextension
Sacral sparing	Preservation of sensation in genitals and saddle area (S_3–S_5) Can occur in presence of profound motor and sensory loss Characteristic of central and anterior cord syndromes
Cauda equina lesions	Sparing of function unpredictable: unilateral or bilateral, motor, sensory, or both Indirect trauma to peripheral nerves associated with fractures Potential for re-growth and recover

4. Mechanism of injury: hyperextension (usually with rotation), hyperflexion (usually with rotation), vertical compression (axial loading), cord contusion without vertebral disruption (fracture, dislocation), and penetrating wounds

5. Types of vertebral injury

   a. Fractures: spinous, lateral and/or articular processes, body, pedicles

      1) Odontoid fractures: Types I, II, III

      2) Hangman's fracture: bilateral arches of axis, with or without dislocation of axis on C3

      3) Jefferson: burst fracture of atlas

      4) Occiput-atlanto dislocation

   b. Dislocation: unilateral or bilateral facets, vertebral body

   c. Subluxation: facets

   d. Compression: burst or wedge fractures

   e. Fracture: dislocation

6. Common causes: motor vehicle crashes; falls and falling objects; athletics (diving, football, skiing, boating); penetrating wounds: gunshot, stabbing

B. Pathophysiology

1. Influencing factors

   a. Spinal cord is located in a relatively small space

   b. Peculiarities of spine: canal space varies

      1) Wider in children: fewer children with traumatic cervical injuries become quadriplegic; wide canal allows cord more space to move without compression

      2) Narrower with congenital anomalies, cervical spondylosis, age, osteoarthritic changes

   c. Variability of vascular supply

   d. Presence of osteophytes

2. Mechanisms

   a. Concussion: pressure waves propagated through cord, resulting in transient loss of function with immediate flaccid paralysis and complete recovery in minutes to hours

   b. Compression: bone, ligaments, extruded disc material and hematoma

   c. Contusion: results in edema, petechial hemorrhages, neuronal changes, inflammation

   d. Hematomyelia: hemorrhage within the cord

   e. Transection: actual (rare) or functional

   f. Overstretching: causing disruption of tissue

   g. Edema: produces further impairment of capillary circulation and venous return

   h. Ischemia: interruption of blood flow of anterior or posterior arterial system by compression

3. Necrosis of spinal cord substance

   a. Vascular pathology: ischemia is implicated as causing reduction or interruption of blood supply, leading to necrosis

      1) Injury to spinal cord causes increase in permeability of blood vessels which leads to edema formation, causing a decrease in blood flow to the area

      2) Further ischemia leads to necrosis with vascular stasis, causing thrombosis, which leads to further decrease in blood flow and the vicious cycle continues, leading eventually to traumatic hemorrhagic necrosis of gray matter (within 4 to 48 hours)

   b. Neuronal pathology

      1) Injury alters the electrophysiology of the neuron cell, causing sodium leakage to the cell, creating a negative resting potential

      2) This results in spinal shock stage, where there is a neurophysiologic cessation of all or nearly all reflexes below level of injury

NCLEX!

NCLEX!

    c. Biochemical pathology

        1) Accumulated vasoactive amines (norepinephrine, serotonin, dopamine, histamine) are released or transported to the wounded tissue after injury

        2) Induces maximal toxic vasospasm, impedes microcirculation, diminishes local oxygenation, and produces necrosis of vessels and neurons

    d. Disintegration of myelin sheath and axis cylinder

    e. Spinal cord may liquefy in severe disruption

4. Hematomyelia and edema of the cord may ascend above the level of initial injury; syringomyelia (progressive, chronic spinal cord disease) may develop as a result

5. Degree of functional impairment of the spinal cord

    a. Complete: total sensory/motor loss and autonomic disruption below level of lesion, reflecting irreversible spinal cord damage

        1) Tetraplegia or quadriplegia: occurs in cervical region; loss of leg function with variable loss of arm function depending on level of injury

        2) Paraplegia: occurs in thoracic region and lumbar 1 and 2 region; loss of leg function

    b. Incomplete and variable degrees of motor an/or sensory loss below level of lesion, reflecting sparing of certain tracts

6. Horner's syndrome

    a. Incomplete cord transection involving cervical sympathetic nerves

    b. Ipsilateral ptosis of eyelid, constricted pupil, and lack of facial sweating (anhidrosis)

NCLEX!

7. Spinal cord segmental level: functional loss depends on degree of spinal cord damage, may not correspond to vertebral level, particularly in thoracolumbar and sacral level (see Table 4-2)

NCLEX!

8. Spinal shock: loss of all reflex activity below level of injury

    a. Duration: two days to several months

    b. Associated with hypotension and bradycardia

    c. Bulbocavernous reflex (contraction of the bulbocavernous muscle on percussing dorsum of penis) is early sign of resolving spinal shock: absence of this spinal reflex arc implies there is no physiological continuity between the lower spinal cord and supraspinal centers

    d. Appearance of involuntary spastic movement indicates spinal shock has resolved

9. Degree of functional loss: depends on level and amount of damage to spinal cord; myelopathy refers to cord damage; radiculopathy refers to dysfunction of nerve roots; may have some sparing or eventual return, as part of the peripheral nervous system

Table 4-2	Functional Loss According to Spinal Cord Segmental Level	
Spinal Column	**Vertebrae**	**Functional Loss**
Cervical	C 1–2	Total tetraplegia and respiratory paralysis
	C 3–4	Total tetraplegia, weak diaphragm, absent intercostals
	C 5–6	Tetraplegia with gross arm movements; diaphragm may be impaired initially
	C 6–7	Tetraplegia with biceps and deltoid function; no triceps
	C 7–8	Tetraplegia with triceps function; no intrinsic hand function
Thoracic	T 1–5	Paraplegia often with diaphragmatic breathing; arm function intact; loss of leg function, bladder, bowels; sensation present down to nipple line
	T 6–12	Paraplegia with no abdominal reflexes present at T12; usually spastic paralysis of lower limbs; at level of T12, sensation is present down to groin area
Below T12	Conus medullaris	Bowel and bladder sphincter dysfunction; may have lower leg weakness; sacral dermatome hyperaesthesia or anesthesia, back pain
	Cauda equina	Asymmetric, atrophic, areflexic paralysis (lower motor neuron); sensory root loss; outer aspect legs, ankles, posterior lower limbs, and saddle area; sphincter dysfunction
Sacral	S 1–5	Loss of bladder, bowel, sex function; some foot displacement may be present; no paralysis of leg muscle from S3 to S5; loss of sensation involves saddle area, scrotum, perineum, penis, anal area, and upper third of posterior aspect of thigh

10. Early intervention (within first few hours after injury) reduces or minimizes cellular damage leading to better prognosis for function

11. Prognosis for degree of bladder, bowel, and sexual function varies with level of lesion: related to upper or lower motor neuron lesion; if sacral nerve roots are damaged prognosis for any reflex activity of these functions is very poor

12. Late stage: spinal cord may become fibrotic, and pathological changes may extend above and below damaged segment

NCLEX!

13. Signs and symptoms include hypotension, loss of motor control and sensation below level of injury, decreased or absent reflexes, urinary retention, stool and urinary incontinence, neurogenic bladder, impotence, muscle spasms, muscle atrophy, paraplegia, tetraplegia, decreased chest expansion, decreased cough reflex, hypercalcemia, cardiac dysrhythmias, pain (note: manifestations will depend on the level of the injury)

NCLEX!

14. Complications from a spinal cord injury: stress ulcers, paralytic ileus, decubitus, stool impaction, decreased venous return, pathologic fractures caused by bone demineralization and joint contractions

C. **Nursing assessment**

1. Assessment

   a. Emergency assessment at scene or in emergency department

      1) Suspect cervical spine injury until proven otherwise

      2) Maintain airway, breathing, and circulation

NCLEX!

    3) Maintain neck in neutral position, palpate cervical spine region

    4) Assess movement and sensation in extremities: if *conscious*, ask client to move toes, feet, legs, fingers, hands, arms; ask if client can feel touch on toes, feet, legs, fingers, hands, arms; test for reflex withdrawal; if *unconscious*, observe any spontaneous movements by client; use stimuli to elicit more purposeful voluntary movements or reflex withdrawal

  b. Physical examination

    1) Precise level of motor and sensory findings include sacral sparing, voluntary toe flexion

    2) Presence/absence of all deep tendon and superficial reflexes

    3) Tenderness or gaps between spinous processes

    4) Deformities, swelling, limitation of movement particularly in neck

    5) Evidence of other trauma: head, chest, abdomen, extremities

NCLEX!

  c. Establish early, accurate baseline: motor and sensory function of all extremities; breathing pattern; presence of sweating; subjective reports of pain; bladder function, distention, voiding reflex; presence of bowel sounds, anal reflex; vital signs; neuro exam, including cognition level; and sexuality

  d. Assess abdomen for distention; ileus is common

  e. Assess for trauma to other systems; note lacerations, abrasions, etc.

  f. Collect pertinent data to assist in formulation of care plan: previous health problems, allergies; health programs (include medications, treatments); and psychosocial data (include previous hospital experience)

NCLEX!

  g. Assess for **autonomic dysreflexia** (a life-threatening involuntary sympathetic response of the central nervous system to a noxious stimuli) with injury above T6

    1) Occurs after spinal shock is resolved

    2) Precipitated by bowel or bladder distention or other noxious stimuli

    3) Symptoms: hypertension, bradycardia, headache, profuse sweating above level of injury and pale, cold, dry skin below injury

  h. History: type of accident; speed, site of impact; symptoms at time of injury (drugs/alcohol, hypoxia, hypotension, arrest)

  2. Diagnostic tests

    a. Multiple spine films specific to area of suspected injury

    b. Cervical spine films to rule out fracture

      1) C7 to T1 difficult to view; may need "swimmer's" view

      2) May need flexion-extension views (with caution)

    c. Computerized tomography, with or without contrast (metrizamide)

    d. Laminar tomography, useful to identify injuries at cervicothoracic junctions

    e. Myelography, especially if progression of deficit

f. Head injury clients generally require cervical spine films

g. Lab: CBC, electrolytes, ABGs

D. Nursing management

1. Medications include: stool softeners, H_2 antagonists or antacids, low-dose anticoagulant therapy, vasopressor drugs if hypotensive, topical antibiotics if halo brace applied, corticosteroids, antispasmodics, a non-steroidal antinflamatory drug (NSAID) analgesic, tricyclic antidepressants

2. Emergency management at scene or in emergency department: secure an airway without flexing, extending or rotating the neck; immobilize the neck before moving the client, transport supine with forehead taped to stretcher to prevent movement; administer oxygen or place on ventilator, and monitor cardiovascular stability

3. Promote optimal breathing

   a. Observe client, consult with healthcare team to treat decreasing vital capacity and arterial blood gases

   b. Suction bronchial and pharyngeal secretions with care to avoid vagal nerve irritation leading to bradycardia and potential cardiac arrest

   c. Provide percussion or appropriate chest physiotherapy for weak cough

   d. Plan routine breathing exercises with the client to support accessory muscles of inspiration

   e. Hydrate client and ensure humidification to thin pulmonary secretions

   f. Create cough during exhalation by pushing in and up between umbilicus and xiphoid process

NCLEX!

4. Prevent and treat autonomic dysreflexia

   a. Prevent fecal impaction, bladder distention, or other triggering stimuli

   b. Raise the head of the bed and remove compression stocking to decrease venous return, and assess blood pressure

   c. Catheterize immediately; remove impaction after antihypertensive medication given

   d. Continue to assess blood pressure while medicating, until stable

   e. Assess client's knowledge of prevention and management

5. Report any deterioration in neuro function; do not turn until treatment plan has been established; monitor level of consciousness, pupillary reaction, possibility of head injury; note affect, reaction to information and events

6. Check motor and sensory level hourly or as ordered; sensory level may be marked on client's skin

7. Monitor cardiovascular function: interruption of sympathetic function leads to wide fluctuations of blood pressure, hypotension, dysrhythmias

8. Prevent hazards of immobility

   a. Maintain dorsal or supine body alignment until placement of halo brace if appropriate

    b. Reposition and turn every 2 hours, monitoring clients with mid-thoracic lesions or higher for hypotension

    c. Provide client with passive range-of-motion exercises and instruct family members how to assist in preventing contractures and atrophy within 48 to 72 hours after injury

    d. Initiate deep vein thrombosis and pulmonary embolism precautions: low-dose anticoagulation therapy and pneumatic compression devices

    e. Reduce hypotensive episodes: slowly change positions, use abdominal corset before sitting upright, thigh-high elastic stockings and vasopressor drugs

9. Maintain skin integrity: inspect the skin, pad or lubricate bony prominences and reposition every 2 hours, using circular motion massage to increase circulation; apply skin barrier ointment/spray to perineum before irritation begins; teach and encourage client and family to prevent pressure ulcers

10. Promote urinary elimination

    a. Involve client and family in intermittent catheterization routine addressing prevention of distension and infection

    b. Encourage client and family to track fluid intake to assure adequate fluids, assess voiding pattern and characteristics of urine

    c. Teach client to practice trigger voiding technique prior to straight catheterization: stroking inner thigh, pulling pubic hair, tapping on the abdomen over the bladder, and pouring warm water over the perineal area in female clients

    d. Explain that successful stimulation of the parasympathetic nerve fibers causes reflex activity; this triggered voiding should be followed by catheterization for residual urine during bladder retraining; less than 80 cc of residual urine is acceptable

11. Optimize bowel function

    a. Check for residual amounts of tube feeding, and client tolerance of gastric feedings after bowel sounds resume

> NCLEX!

    b. Offer a high-calorie, high-protein, high-fiber diet, gradually increasing oral amounts as tolerated

    c. Institute a bowel retraining program; use stool softeners, rectal suppositories with digital stimulation as needed after meals

    d. Manual removal of stool on a routine timetable may be required for the client with LMN injury lacking the defecation reflex

12. Halo brace care

> NCLEX!

    a. Prevent infection at pin sites by shaving hair around pins to facilitate inspection; clean with 1/2-strength peroxide, normal saline, and topical antibiotic ointment

    b. Maintain integrity of halo device by inspecting pins and traction bars for tightness, reporting loosened parts to physician

    c. Cleanse client's skin under the vest's sheepskin liner per protocol; do not use powder or allow vest to become wet

    d. Change sheepskin vest when soiled and per protocol

    e. Maintain positioning so that back of head is free of pressure point, massaging with care not to move the neck

13. Provide sexuality information: offer accurate information on sexual function; discuss alternatives to intercourse if not physically possible and strategies for initiating or maintaining a sexual relationship; secure sexual counseling for client as needed

14. Support optimal self-esteem: open communication lines, encouraging client self-awareness; encourage decision making and progressive self-care; identify with the client strategies to address goals; refer to support groups and family counseling

15. Prepare for discharge

    a. Reassess and update baseline data in terms of self-care

    b. Explore mobility issues

    c. Facilitate preparation of home setting

    d. Plan for ongoing psychological support

    e. Identify community resources

    f. Evaluate client and family's knowledge of medications, activities of daily living, use of assistive devices, and caregiver respite

VI. Encephalitis

A. Overview

1. Defined as a central nervous system disorder with inflammation of the brain; if both the brain and the meninges are affected, it is termed meningoencephalitis

2. Viral encephalitis is more serious than meningitis, can be fatal or cause long-term neurologic disability

3. Termed as: Western equine encephalitis (occurs in West and in horses); Eastern equine encephalitis (occurs in East and in horses); St. Louis and California encephalitis (not limited to those geographic areas); herpes encephalitis (usually fatal); Japanese encephalitis (similar to St. Louis); Russian spring-summer encephalitis (tick-borne)

4. Outbreaks are usually in the summer and fall when mosquito (vector) is most active

5. Causes include transfer of arthropod-borne virus (arbovirus) from animals (particularly horses) to humans by mosquitoes; following diseases (rabies, German measles, chickenpox, herpes virus, smallpox); post-vaccination; can be caused by viruses, bacteria, rickettsia, parasites, and fungi; exposure to toxins such as lead poisoning

B. Pathophysiology

1. Organism (usually virus) enters the body and makes its way to the central nervous system (CNS) through the cerebral capillaries and choroid plexus, then affecting specific cells and producing a wide variety of effects

2. Damage to the CNS results in invasion and lysis of cells, demyelination and selective lysis, an immune response to the viral antigens; and destruction of the cells without inflammation

3. Effects of viral encephalitis vary with the age of the individual and may include general symptoms, focal impairment, movement limitations, brainstem involvement, mental and personality changes, cerebral edema, hemorrhage, and even coma

4. Signs and symptoms include cerebral edema, headache, high fever (always present), confusion, convulsions, restlessness, hemiparesis, asymmetry of reflexes, positive Babinski's sign, ataxia, difficulty in speaking or understanding, facial weakness, ocular palsies, mental deterioration, muscle stiffness, malaise, sore throat, upper respiratory tract problems, nuchal rigidity, projectile vomiting, pupil irregularities, changes in vital signs, ptosis, diplopia, strabismus, and abnormal sleep patterns

C. Nursing assessment

1. Assessment includes neurovascular assessment, fluid status, symptom analysis of pain or discomfort, reflexes, ambulation, coordination, vital signs, cranial nerves

2. Diagnostic tests: lumbar puncture for CSF (increased pressure, increased proteins, normal glucose and chloride); CBC, electrolytes, MRI, CT scan

D. Nursing management

1. Medications include antipyretics, antiviral agents, corticosteroids, anticonvulsants if seizures occur, sedatives, analgesics, stool softeners

2. Monitor fluid balance, measure intake and output (I & O)

3. Monitor nutritional status, measure weight

4. Monitor for signs of increasing intracranial pressure

5. Keep the environment conducive to rest and decrease stimulation (lights low, limit visitors)

6. Protect the environment in the event seizures occur

7. Reposition the client frequently, positioning the neck for comfort and to decrease joint stiffness

8. Physical therapy should be initiated for range-of-motion (ROM) activities

9. Offer assurance to the client and family, especially if a child is involved

VII. Meningitis

A. Overview

1. Meningitis is defined as an inflammation of the meninges (pia mater and arachnoid membrane) surrounding the brain and spinal cord

2. Classifications

    a. Viral meningitis (aseptic meningitis) is usually self-limiting with complete recovery

    b. Bacterial meningitis (septic) may leave residual effects

3. Higher incidence occurs in the fall, winter, early spring with children more susceptible because they have more upper respiratory tract infections

4. Causes include bacterial or viral infection, often after an upper respiratory tract infection; fungi or toxins may also be causes

B. Pathophysiology

1. Infection occurs when the pathogen crosses the blood-brain barrier and migrates throughout the CNS

    a. Bacterial meningitis is most often preceded by *Neisseria meningitis* (meninogococcal), *Streptococcus pneumoniae,* or *Haemophilus influenzae*

    b. Viral meningitis often occurs after mumps or herpes zoster, herpes simplex, or cytomegalovirus (CMV) infection

2. The inflammatory response causes increased CSF, as well as pressure and purulent exudate that spreads quickly throughout the brain and spinal cord in bacterial meningitis

3. Signs and symptoms

    a. Acute infection with inflammation: high fever, nausea, vomiting, chills, malaise, tachycardia

    b. Irritated meninges (nuchal rigidity)

        1) Stiff/sore neck

        2) Positive Kernig's sign (refer back to Figure 4-2)

        3) Positive Brudzinski's sign: flexion of neck causes neck pain and the hip and knee to flex (Figure 4-3)

    c. Signs of increased intracranial pressure (ICP)

NCLEX!

Figure 4-3

Brudzinski's sign.

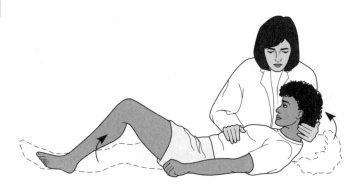

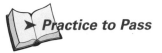

    d. Vascular problems

        1) Thrombophlebitis of cerebral vessels may lead to infarction, seizures, and stroke

        2) Septic emboli may block small vessels of the hand and feet leading to gangrene

        3) Fibrinolysis occurring in bacteremia may lead to disseminated intravascular coagulopathy (DIC), a generalized response to injury associated with septic shock with simultaneous bleeding and clotting

C. Nursing assessment

    1. Assessment includes pain (especially neck); reflexes (Brudzinski's, Kernig's sign); mental assessment (LOC, neurovascular); vital signs (VS), peripheral neurovascular status of all extremities (cool pale to cyanotic extremities with decreased pulses and sensation may indicate emboli); fluid status, respiratory status, nutritional status

    2. Diagnostic tests: lumbar puncture with CSF analysis (high protein, low glucose, positive for bacteria); culture & sensitivity of CSF; CT scan, magnetic resonance imaging (MRI) (swelling and sites of necrosis), blood urea nitrogen (BUN), creatinine (CR), electrolytes, ABGs, C & S of throat, blood, urine, sputum; urine specific gravity

D. Nursing management

    1. Medications include broad-spectrum antibiotics (penicillins, third-generation cephalosporins) until cultures return, analgesics, antipyretics, antiemetics if nausea occurs, anticonvulsants if seizures occur, diuretics for cerebral edema

    2. Essential to nursing management of the client with meningitis is careful assessment and supportive intervention as needed for acute infection, irritated meninges and increased intracranial pressure; elderly clients should receive their pneumonia and flu vaccines regularly

    3. Administer medications as prescribed and monitor for client's response; avoid narcotics such as opioids that further depress the CNS and mask changes in symptoms; clients should be instructed to take all of the antibiotics to avoid relapse

    4. Carefully monitor vital signs, neurological and peripheral neurovascular status for changes

        a. Signs of increasing ICP (changes in LOC, widening pulse pressure, bradycardia, bounding pulse)

        b. Signs of peripheral vascular compromise: cool, pale, decreased sensation, faint to absent pulses

        c. Severe headache

        d. Seizures

        e. Cranial nerve dysfunction

5. Carefully monitor fluid and electrolyte status: strict intake and output, daily weights, condition of mucous membranes, skin turgor, urine specific gravity

6. Promote effective airway clearance and exchange: monitor oxygen saturation levels, ABGs; turn every 2 hours, perform chest physiotherapy; suction if needed; elevate head of bed to 30 degrees

7. Relieve hyperthermia; apply cooling blanket or tepid sponge baths as needed

8. Relieve pain: maintain a quiet, dark environment, administer analgesic medications as ordered, encourage gentle ROM, back rub and massage, arrange care/visitors to promote periods of rest

9. Protect from injury: have oral airway, oxygen and suction equipment available; keep side rails up, bed in low position; rails padded; record seizure: event, length, head and eye deviations, interventions, postictal state; monitor for generalized bleeding

10. Maintain adequate nutrition via nasogastric tube feeding if needed, high protein, high calorie, in small frequent feedings

11. Promote health maintenance: instruct client in all medications; instruct to take all antibiotics until completion as ordered; instruct client and close contacts to seek exposure care for fever, headache, irritability, neck stiffness and prophylactic antibiotic therapy; refer as needed for rehabilitation of residual effects

VIII. Seizures

A. Overview

1. Seizures are defined as uncontrolled discharge of neurons of cerebral cortex that interferes with normal function; may be associated with involuntary muscle contractions; may originate as aura or sensory experience before clinical signs are evident

2. **Status epilepticus** can develop during seizure activity; seizures become continuous with very short periods of calm between intense, repetitive seizures; the cumulative effect is life-threatening

3. Epilepsy is defined as recurrent paroxysmal disorder of cerebral function characterized by sudden, brief attacks of altered consciousness, motor activity, or sensory phenomena

4. Classifications of seizures

   a. Generalized: tonic-clonic (grand mal) or absence (petit mal)

   b. Tonic-clonic: simple or Jacksonian, complex

5. Causes

   a. Genetic tendency/chromosomal abnormalities

   b. Structural factors: head trauma, infections (encephalitis, meningitis, brain abscess, opportunistic lesions from acquired immunodeficiency syndrome [AIDS]); cerebrovascular disorders: hemorrhage, embolism, ischemia; space-occupying lesions: primary and metastatic tumors, neurofibromatosis, arteriovenous malformation (AVM), subdural hematoma

c. Metabolic-nutritional factors

   1) Electrolyte and water imbalance, hyponatremia, hypocalcemia, hypocapnia, hypoglycemia

   2) Hypoxia

   3) Acidosis

   4) Pyridoxine deficiency

   5) Fat and amino acid metabolism disorder

   6) Toxins and toxic factors: heavy metals

   7) Systemic disorders: uremia, toxemia

   8) Drugs: "street" drugs, theophylline overdose

   9) Withdrawal: alcohol, barbiturates, antiepileptic drugs, diazepam (Valium)

d. Idiopathic: no known etiology, possible genetic tendency

B. Pathophysiology

1. Excessive synchronous discharge of neurons

2. Neurons in epileptogenic focus recruit other neurons to fire synchronously in adjacent and more distant areas

3. Abnormal electrical discharge may occur without clinical manifestations

4. Clinical manifestations occur when sufficient number of neurons are excited

5. Resulting clinical manifestations depend upon part of brain from which discharge originates and path of spread

6. Classification and clinical characteristics

a. *Partial seizures* (involve part of brain)

   1) Simple partial seizures (consciousness not impaired), with motor symptoms: "Jacksonian" march, spread topographically (systematically); limited to one part of body

   2) Simple partial seizures, with sensory or somatosensory symptoms: may be somatic sensory phenomena only, e.g., tingling, numbness of body part; may have visual, auditory, olfactory or taste symptoms only; dizzy spells may be seizure manifestations

   3) Complex partial seizures (impaired consciousness): begin as simple partial and progress to impairment of consciousness; impairment of consciousness at onset: most commonly involves **automatisms** (automatic actions or behavior without conscious knowledge; repetitive, semi-purposeful, patterned movements such as lip smacking); may include antisocial or aggressive behavior especially if forcefully restrain

   4) Partial seizures secondarily generalized: may spread from original discharge site to other parts of brain and become generalized; generalized seizure preceded by specific aura is partial seizure that becomes generalized

    b. *Generalized seizures* (involving whole brain at onset) are classified as tonic-clonic, tonic, absence, myoclonic, tonic, or infantile spasms

        1) Absence—simple (petit mal): staring spell; usually lasts less than 15 seconds, during which client is unaware of surroundings; diagnosed by a three cycle/second (C/S) spike and wave on electroencephalogram (EEG); usually present only in children

        2) Absence—atypical: staring spell accompanied by myoclonic jerks and automatisms such as chewing and smacking of lips; atypical spike wave pattern on EEG

        3) Myoclonic—single jerk of one or more muscle groups; lasting only a second

        4) Atonic—drop attack; sometimes associated with myoclonic seizure

        5) Clonic—jerking of muscle groups

        6) Tonic—stiffening of muscle groups

NCLEX!

        7) Tonic clonic (grand mal): starts with tonic or stiffening phase followed by clonic or jerking phase, unconsciousness, possible bowel and bladder incontinence, may have only tonic or only clonic phase, may bite tongue, reduced consciousness during postictal recovery

        8) Metabolic or toxin induced seizure activity—usually generalized; usually does not recur as long as underlying cause remains corrected

    c. Status epilepticus: continuing or immediately recurring seizures, recovery between attacks incomplete, usually lasts 30 minutes or more

  7. Precipitating factors (unique for each individual)

    a. Physical: specific sensory stimuli (flashing lights and certain sounds); fever (children under 5 years of age at risk); injury; physical exhaustion; sleep deprivation; inadequate nutrition; drugs, alcohol, other addictive substances; and hyperventilation

    b. Psychosocial: family and environmental stress, coping, shock

NCLEX!

  8. Signs and symptoms include partial or complete loss of consciousness, falling, incontinence of bowel and bladder, aura before event, muscular contractions, tonic-clonic convulsions of all extremities, facial movements, tongue biting, salivation, a postictal stage (decreased LOC, decreased VS), headache, and fatigue

C. Nursing assessment

  1. Assessment

    a. History: description of seizure from client or witness; antecedent events; precipitating factors and postictal events; frequency and duration; past history of illness, trauma, infection; alcohol or drug use; family history of seizures; perinatal history, growth and development

NCLEX!

    b. Physical and neurological examination: seizure activity (length, progression of jerking, time started), presence of oral bleeding, postictal stages, vital signs, posturing

    c. Assess client's knowledge of lifestyle and factors that may trigger seizures

2. Diagnostic tests

   a. Serum electrolytes: hyponatremia, hypocalcemia (especially in children), hypoglycemia

   b. BUN

   c. Arterial blood gases (ABG): hypoxia and acidosis

   d. Cerebrospinal fluid (CSF) analysis: infection and/or hemorrhage

   e. Drug screen: toxicity of sedatives, hypnotics, heavy metals, drug interactions, "street" drugs, theophylline, and anticonvulsant drug levels

   f. EEG

      1) May be normal between seizures

      2) Activation techniques may elicit epileptic discharge: hyperventilation, photo stimulation, or sleep deprivation

      3) Nasopharyngeal or sphenoidal leads used to localize temporal lobe focus

   g. Initial studies may include computed tomography (CT) scan or magnetic resonance imaging (MRI)

D. Nursing management

  1. Medications

   a. Anticonvulsants: phenytoin (Dilantin), carbamazepine (Tegretol), valproic acid (Depakene), ethosuximide (Zarontin), clonazepam (Klonopin), gabapentin (neurontin)

   b. Diazepam (Valium) or phenobarbital for status epilepticus

  2. Document details of seizure: date, time of onset, duration of seizure; activity of client at time of onset; precipitating factors, if any; aura; seizure activity (body parts involved and sequence); character of movements (tonic, clonic, head or eye deviation, behavior)

  3. Monitor autonomic signs: pupil size and reactivity, respirations, cyanosis, diaphoresis, incontinence, salivation

  4. Record and evaluate LOC during and after seizure: arousability, duration of reduced consciousness, awareness of and memory for event

  5. Monitor postictal state (period immediately following termination of a seizure; usually lasts 30 to 90 minutes): confusion, exhaustion, sleepiness, difficulty to arouse, muscle soreness, headache, weakness, aphasia, inability to maintain airway if not arousable, partial paralysis

  6. Inspect for presence of injury, especially head or tongue: lacerations or bruises

  7. Provide safety management during seizure

   a. Protect from injury

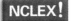

   b. Do not force hard object between teeth

   c. Do not restrain

   d. Turn to side to keep airway open

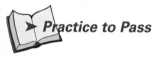

Practice to Pass

How will the nurse prepare a client who is newly diagnosed with seezures for his first EEG?

8. Monitor serum drug levels to determine if antiepileptic drug (AED) in therapeutic range; dosage depends on pharmacokinetics, individual metabolism and degree of seizure control; clarify that the AED must be taken on a continuous basis; if adverse effects occur, dose is lowered or different drug tried

9. Control precipitating factors

10. Surgical intervention may be a treatment option: cortical resection of epileptic focus may be indicated if criteria met

11. Maintain large vein access while hospitalized for treatment of status epilepticus

IX. Guillain-Barré Syndrome

A. Overview

1. Defined as an acute (sudden onset), rapidly progressing inflammation of peripheral motor and sensory nerves characterized by:

   a. Variable motor weakness and paralysis

   b. Paralysis that ascends symmetrically from lower extremities in most cases

   c. With excellent care, has a 96 percent complete recovery

2. Occurs most commonly in persons between the ages of 30 to 50 years, equally in both genders

3. Causes include unknown etiology; autoimmune attack, common after viral infections, immunizations, febrile illness, injury or surgery

B. Pathophysiology

1. A cell-mediated immune reaction is triggered by a viral illness or immunization

2. Instead of the normal antibody role of preventing the invading organism from having a harmful effect, the antibody formed has a damaging effect on peripheral nerve myelin; an IgM antimyelin antibody exists, lymphocytes are sensitized and aid in damaging the myelin

3. With demyelination, nerve impulses are slowed or stopped and muscles lose innervation and begin to waste without exercise

4. During recovery, remyelination occurs in descending order over a period of a few months to a couple of years

5. Signs and symptoms include weakness/paresis (partial paralysis), paralysis progressing upward from lower extremities to total paralysis requiring ventilatory support; paresthesias (numbness and tingling) and pain; muscle aches, cramping and nighttime pain; respiratory compromise and/or failure: dyspnea, diminished vital capacity, breath sounds, decreasing O_2 saturation, abnormal blood gases; cranial nerve involvement: extraocular eye movement difficulties, dysphagia, diplopia, difficulty speaking; and autonomic dysfunction: orthostatic hypotension (lowered BP and dizziness with sudden position changes), hypertension, change in heart rate (bradycardia, heart block, asystole or tachycardia), bowel and bladder dysfunction, flushing and diaphoresis

C. Nursing assessment

1. Assessment includes onset and chronology of symptoms including any illnesses in previous 1 to 8 weeks; head to toe muscle strength testing (see Tables 4-3 and 4-4); head-to-toe sensory assessment; cranial nerve involvement, respiratory status, fluid balance, skin integrity, bladder and bowel control

2. Diagnostic tests: electrolytes, ABGs, nerve conduction tests, lumbar puncture for CSF (elevated protein)

D. Nursing management

1. Medications and treatment

   a. IV immunoglobulins: may cause low-grade fever, muscle aches, headache to rare acute renal failure, retinal necrosis

   b. Plasmapheresis: plasma is removed and separated from whole blood and blood cells are returned without the plasma to remove antibodies responsible for disease; monitor for complications

      1) Loss of clotting factors, bleeding

      2) Fluid and electrolyte imbalance

   c. Adrenocorticoid hormone (ACTH) and corticosteroids or antiinflammatory drugs

   d. Other: stool softeners, antacids or H_2-receptor antagonists, analgesics

NCLEX!

2. Care is supportive with attention to function of all systems, especially respiratory and cardiac

   a. Monitor respiratory status: rate, depth, breath sounds, vital capacity, note secretions and check gag, cough, and swallowing reflexes

   b. Monitor cardiac status: heart rate, blood pressure (BP), dysrhythmias

3. Administer chest physiotherapy and pulmonary hygiene measures

4. Maintain adequate nutrition as appropriate: administer tube feeding, parenteral nutrition or assisted small frequent feedings of soft foods; weigh client weekly; check electrolyte status, give mouth care every two hours

5. Monitor bowel and bladder function: assess bowel sounds and frequency, amount, color of bowel movements; offer bed pan; check for distention and residuals in client who cannot void spontaneously; perform intermittent catheterization as needed; encourage fluid intake to 3,500 cc/day

Table 4-3		
Muscle Strength Scale	0	No visible muscle contraction: paralysis
	1	Trace: slight contraction but no movement
	2	Poor: ROM with gravity eliminated
	3	Fair: ROM against gravity
	4	Good: ROM against gravity with some resistance
	5	Normal: full ROM and full resistance

Table 4-4	Ocular and lids	Close eyes tightly
	Facial	Puff cheeks, stick out tongue
Head to Toe Muscle Strength Testing	Neck	Bend head forward and back
	Deltoid	Hold arms up
	Biceps	Flex arm
	Triceps	Extend arm
	Wrists	Flex and extend
	Finger	Grip examiner's crossed plexor and second finger
	Hip	Raise straight leg from supine
	Gluteal and leg	Cross legs
	Ankle and foot	Flex and extend

NCLEX!

6. Prevent complications of immobility

   a. Encourage use of weak extremities as able

   b. Work with physical therapy to plan passive and active ROM to all extremities

   c. Protect immobile extremities with use of:

      1) Air mattress or special bed

      2) Elbow and heel protectors

   d. Turn and position in good body alignment

   e. Elevate extremities to prevent dependent edema

   f. Use antiembolic compression devices/stockings

NCLEX!

7. Provide eye care for the client with inability to close eyelids completely: instill artificial tears, cleanse eyes as needed, use eye shields and tape eyes closed as needed

8. Provide comfort and analgesics as needed: assess pain with vital signs; administer analgesics before painful activities; log roll and move client gently; use imagery, relaxation, distraction, humor, music as appropriate

9. Promote communication, encouragement, and support to client and family

   a. If client is on ventilator or is unable to communicate because of weak speech muscles, collaborate with speech therapist to develop a communication system

   b. Explain all care with rationale and provide information about the progression of the disease

   c. Encourage client and family to express feelings and participate in care as much as possible

10. Begin to plan for discharge needs upon admission to acute care setting

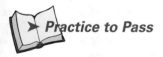

Practice to Pass

List nursing diagnoses in order of priority for the client with Guillain-Barré syndrome who is in the acute phase experiencing tetraplegia (quadriplegia).

X. Myasthenia Gravis

A. Overview

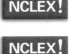

1. Myasthenia gravis is a chronic progressive disorder of the peripheral nervous system affecting transmission of nerve impulses to voluntary muscles, causing muscle weakness and fatigue that increases with exertion and improves with rest; eventually leads to fatigue without relief from rest

2. Varies from mild disturbance of eye and eyelid movement to respiratory failure from weakness of the diaphragm and muscles of respiration

3. Characterized by unpredictable remissions and exacerbations

4. Affects women three times more than men until after age 50 with onset usually between the ages of 20 and 30 years of age

5. Causes include unknown etiology, family history of autoimmune disorders, thyroid tumors

B. Pathophysiology

1. An autoimmune process triggers the formation of autoantibodies that decrease the number of acetylcholine receptors and widen the gap between the axon ending and the muscle fiber in the neuromuscular junction; muscle contraction is hindered because the IgG autoantibodies prevent acetylcholine from binding with the receptors; destruction of the receptors at the neuromuscular junction occur

2. Associated with continued production of autoantibodies by the thymus gland in 75 percent of cases

3. Onset is usually slow but can be precipitated by emotional stress, hormonal disturbance (pregnancy, menses, thyroid disorders), infections/vaccinations, trauma and surgery, temperature extremes, excessive exercise, drugs that block or decrease neuromuscular transmission (opioids, sedatives, barbiturates, alcohol, quinidine, anesthetics), and thymus tumor

4. Signs and symptoms include: mild diplopia (double vision) and unilateral ptosis (eyelid drooping) caused by weakness in the extraocular muscles; may also involve the face, jaw, neck, and hip; complications arise when severe weakness affects the muscles of swallowing, chewing, and respiration; respiratory distress manifested by tachypnea, decreased depth, abnormal ABGs, O_2 saturation less than 92 percent, decreased breath sounds; bowel and bladder incontinence, paresthesias, and pain in weak muscles

5. Myasthenic crisis: sudden motor weakness; risk of respiratory failure and aspiration; most often caused by not enough medication or an infection

6. Cholinergic crisis: severe muscle weakness; caused by overmedication; signs are cramps, diarrhea, bradycardia, and bronchial spasm with increased pulmonary secretions and risk of respiratory compromise

C. Nursing assessment

1. Assessment

   a. Progression and severity of fatigue; which body parts are affected; effect on ADLs; adequacy of coping skills

    b. Cranial nerve dysfunction

      1) Ocular: diplopia and ptosis; test for ptosis by asking client to look upward for 2 to 3 minutes; eyelid droop will increase so that eye can hardly be held open; after rest, eyes can open

      2) Facial: smile may be a snarl, jaw may need to be propped closed

      3) Laryngeal and pharyngeal: voice may be weak with a nasal twang, may have dysphagia (difficulty swallowing), and difficulty chewing with some choking

    c. Other muscle weakness

      1) Test all muscle groups (see Table 4-3): flexors of the neck, shoulder and hip may be affected: difficulty holding head up, difficulty climbing stairs, lifting, raising arms over head, difficulty holding, sitting, standing posture

      2) Bowel and bladder incontinence

    d. Respiratory distress from weakness of diaphragm and respiratory muscles and difficulty swallowing secretions; lung sounds, respiratory rate (RR) and depth

  2. Diagnostic tests: ABGs, pulmonary function tests

    a. Electromyography (EMG) shows decreased amplitude when motor neurons are stimulated

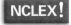

    b. Confirmation of the clinical diagnosis can be made by IV administration of edrophonium chloride (Tensilon), which allows voluntary muscle contraction; Tensilon allows acetylcholine to bind with its receptors, which temporarily improves symptoms; weakness returns after the effects of Tensilon are discontinued

D. Nursing management

  1. Medications and treatment

    a. Anticholinesterases: neostigmine (Prostigmin), pyridostigmine (Mestinon)

    b. Immunosuppressants: corticosteroids, azathioprine (Imuran), cyclosporine (Cytoxan)

    c. Anti-inflammatory drugs

    d. Thymectomy (removal of the thymus gland)

    e. Plasmapheresis: removes IgG antibodies

    f. Atropine sulfate (Atropine) for cholinergic crisis

  2. Monitor client response and side effects to medications; give medications on time to maintain blood levels and thus muscle strength during essential activities and eating

  3. Maintain effective breathing pattern and airway clearance

    a. Thoroughly assess for respiratory distress

    b. Monitor meals and teach client to bend head slightly forward while eating/drinking

    c. Teach client to avoid exposure to infections, especially respiratory

      d. Teach client effective coughing, use chest physiotherapy and incentive spirometry

      e. Have oral suction available, teach client how to use it

      f. Have intubation equipment on hand

    4. Provide adequate nutrition

NCLEX!

      a. Schedule medications 30 to 45 minutes before eating for peak muscle strength while eating

      b. Offer food frequently in small amounts that are easy to chew and swallow; soft or semisolid as needed

      c. Administer IV fluids and nasogastric tube feedings if client is unable to swallow

    5. Instruct in alternative methods of communication if needed: eye blink, finger wiggle for yes or no; flash cards, communication board; teach to support lower jaw with hands to assist with speech

    6. Promote improved physical mobility

      a. Refer to physical therapy/occupational therapy

NCLEX!

      b. Instruct client to plan rest periods and to conserve energy

        1) Plan major activities early in day

        2) Schedule activities during peak medication effect

      c. Passive and active ROM

NCLEX!

      d. Instruct client to avoid extremes of hot and cold, exposure to infections, emotional stress and medications that may worsen or precipitate an exacerbation (alcohol, sedatives, local anesthetics)

      e. Instruct client in signs of crisis

      f. Encourage client to wear a Medic alert bracelet

    7. Provide eye care: instill artificial tears, use a patch over one eye for double vision; wear sunglasses to protect eyes from bright lights

    8. Promote positive body image and coping skills

      a. Encourage participation in treatment plan

      b. Set aside time for active listening and encourage client to express feelings

      c. Reinforce progress and explain all care

      d. Provide low energy diversional activities

      e. Refer to myasthenia gravis self-help group

XI. Parkinson's Disease

  A. Overview

    1. Defined as a progressive gradual neurological degenerative disorder of the brain characterized by: "resting" (non-intentional) tremors; bradykinesia (slow, sometimes frozen movement); and muscle rigidity or stiffness

    2. Affects mostly older adults between the ages of 50 and 60

3. Classified as primary or secondary (caused by other disorders)

4. Causes: primary—unknown; secondary—linked to infection; neoplasms; encephalitis; intoxication with carbon monoxide, manganese, and mercury; use of some drugs (reserpine, methyldopa, haloperidol, phenothiazines); and hypoxia and cerebral ischemia

B. Pathophysiology

1. Affects brain centers that control and regulate movement

2. Neurons in the substantia nigra and corpus striatum in the midbrain degenerate and become deficient in production and storage of the neurotransmitter dopamine

3. When dopamine levels that inhibit motor activity deplete, acetylcholine is not inhibited allowing increased excitation that is the basis for symptoms of Parkinson's disease

4. Signs and symptoms include weight loss, constipation, dysphagia, depression, and dementia

   a. Tremors

      1) Mild "pill-rolling": nonintentional tremor of thumb and first finger as if rotating a small object

      2) May begin in one hand with tremor spreading to the arm, then the other arm, and later the head

      3) Usually lessens with purposeful movement

   b. Bradykinesia and loss of automatic movement characterized by: mask-like face with staring gaze; soft, monotone voice; drooling of saliva; impaired balance and loss of righting reflex (correcting posture when changing positions); stooped posture; difficulty initiating movement; and unsteady shuffling propulsive gait

   c. Rigidity

      1) **Cogwheel:** manual manipulation of the body parts may take on the feel of a cogwheel; increased resistance to passive range of motion with jerky catches when joint is moved

      2) **Lead pipe:** cataleptic condition during which limbs remain in any position in which placed; smooth, stiff movement

   d. Autonomic dysfunction: insomnia, oily skin, sweating, heat intolerance, orthostatic hypotension

C. Nursing assessment

1. Assessment includes onset and progression of disease; changes in function throughout the day and in response to medication (difficulty dressing, eating, walking, writing); movement (tremors, bradykinesia, rigidity), bowel function, nutritional status, mental status (forgetfulness, long-term and short-term memory), reflexes, and memory

2. Diagnostic tests: no specific tests are diagnostic, based on signs and symptoms; glucose may be tested because of the side effects of drugs

D. Nursing management

1. Medications

   a. Monoamine oxidase (MAO) inhibitors

   b. Dopaminergics: levodopa (L-dopa), carbidopa–levodopa (Sinemet), amantadine (Symmetrel)

   c. Dopamine agonists: bromocriptine (Parlodel), pergolide (Permax)

   d. Anticholinergics

2. Monitor for symptom control and adverse reactions to medications such as anemia, dystonia (prolonged muscle contraction that may cause twisting and repetitive movements or abnormal posture), nausea, darkened urine and sweat, orthostatic hypotension, changes in mentation and vision, tachycardia, urinary retention, dry mouth, constipation, and impaired glucose tolerance

NCLEX!

3. Encourage mobility with daily exercise directed by physical therapy; use of assistive devices as needed

   a. Spring-loaded chair/straight-backed chair with arms and slight elevation of back legs

   b. Elevated toilet seat

   c. Slip-on shoes or Velcro-fastened shoes

   d. Velcro fasteners on clothes

   e. Canes, splints, braces as needed

   f. Rope tied to foot of bed to assist getting to sitting position

   g. Instruct client who "freezes" to think about stepping over something

   h. Instruct client to lift legs and take big steps when walking

   i. Instruct client to hold an object to decrease resting tremors

NCLEX!

4. Provide a safe environment

   a. Remove throw rugs and excess furniture

   b. Provide grab bar in bathroom, handrails on both sides of stairs

   c. Ensure adequate lighting in the home

5. Promote a well-balanced diet

   a. Assess client's nutritional status, ability to feed self and swallow

   b. Consult with dietician, speech and occupational therapists to develop individual interventions

   c. Provide food of proper consistency to prevent aspiration as determined by client's swallowing function

   d. Provide stabilized dishes and utensils, flexible straw for drinking

   e. Offer small frequent meals and snacks

   f. Encourage high fiber and 3,000 mL of water intake a day

6. Promote adequate rest

   a. Assess client's perception of adequacy of rest, sleep pattern and existing conditions, medications that might impact sleep

   b. Avoid exercise or napping close to bedtime

   c. Limit caffeine and alcohol intake; drink milk before bedtime

   d. Provide a firm mattress with a small pillow, sheepskin or air mattress

   e. Darken the bedroom and decrease noise

7. Allow client to participate in own care; the client should be treated respectfully and not made to feel left out

8. Maintain an unhurried environment to allow sufficient time for the client to attempt his or her own ADLs

XII. Multiple Sclerosis (MS)

A. Overview

1. Defined as a chronic disorder of the CNS where the myelin and nerve axons in the brain and spinal cord are destroyed

2. Most prominent in women and European-Americans

3. Four forms based on the rate of progression: benign, relapsing-remitting, primary progressive, and secondary progressive

4. Four syndromes based on which nerve tract is originally affected: corticospinal syndrome, brainstem syndrome, cerebellar syndrome, and cerebral syndrome; symptoms will usually be suggestive of one of these areas

5. Exacerbations of the illness can be precipitated by stress, pregnancy, illness, fever, fatigue

6. Causes: unknown etiology, possibly an autoimmune or genetic basis; also suggested is childhood viral infections

B. Pathophysiology

1. The destruction of myelin and nerve axons causes a temporary, repetitive, or sustained interruption in the conduction of nerve impulses which causes the symptoms of MS

2. Plaque formation occurs throughout the white matter of the CNS which also affects the nerve impulses; affects the optic nerves, cervical spinal cord, thoracic and lumbar spine

3. Inflammation occurs around the plaques as well as normal tissue; astrocytes (gliosis) appear in the lesions and scar tissue forms, replacing the axons and leading to permanent disability; the term "gliosis" leads to the term sclerosis, which means scarring

4. The immune response

   a. Helper T-cells are elevated in CSF at the onset

   b. T-suppressor cells are decreased in serum before and during an exacerbation of the illness

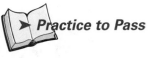

Practice to Pass

A client with Parkinson's disease has dysphagia (difficulty swallowing). What mealtime interventions should the nurse consider to prevent aspiration and ease swallowing?

NCLEX!

      c. Immunocompetent cells are present within the plaques

      d. Antibody production is evident intrathecally

    5. Types (based on rate of progression of the disease)

      a. *Benign*—nervous system dysfunction will occur in different episodes, full recovery follows

      b. *Relapsing-remitting* (most common)—neurological exacerbations occur but improvement can be seen with either complete or partial recovery

      c. *Primary progressive*—sudden loss of neurological function occurs, which may not resolve; leaves severe functional impairments; these may actually worsen over time; no remission follows

      d. *Secondary progressive*—starts similar to relapsing-remitting; changes to a primary progressive form; no remission follows

    6. Signs and symptoms include visual disturbances or blindness (retrobulbar neuritis), sudden, progressive weakness of one or more limbs, spasticity of muscles, nystagmus, tremors, gait instability, fatigue, bladder dysfunction (UTIs, incontinence), depression

C. Nursing assessment

    1. Assessment includes symptoms analysis of complaints, neurovascular assessment, movement, mental assessment, and eye exam

    2. Diagnostic tests: lumbar puncture for CSF (clonal IgG bands present), MRI, CT scans, muscle testing

D. Nursing management

    1. Medications include immunosuppressant therapy, antiviral drugs, corticosteroids, antibiotics for UTIs, interferon-alpha, and glatiramer, anticholinergic drugs, and antispasmodics

    2. No cure is available, supportive care should be maintained

    3. Maximum support to the client and family is usually needed

    4. Client education should include medications, symptoms, bladder training, self-intermittent catheterization, sexual functioning, avoiding complications, and possible triggers

    5. Safety should be assessed in the home and work environment

XIII. Amyotropic Lateral Sclerosis (ALS)

A. Overview

    1. Defined as a degenerative disease of the upper and lower motor neurons of the cerebral cortex, brain stem, and spinal cord that results in total paralysis (except for cranial nerves III, IV, and VI); also known as Lou Gehrig's disease

    2. Occurs in the fourth or fifth decade of life; more common in men; usually fatal in 3 to 5 years

    3. Causes include unknown etiology, viral infections, metabolic disorders, and trauma; familial patterns and autoimmune responses have been indicated

B. Pathophysiology

1. Motor neurons in the cortex, brain stem, and spinal cord are lost; the disease is noninflammatory; axon degeneration causes demyelination

2. The effect on UMN function leads to spastic, weak muscles and increased deep-tendon reflexes

3. The effect on LMN function causes muscle atrophy and flaccid paralysis

4. Only one muscle group may be affected initially; clinical symptoms will vary according to the muscle groups involved; loss of muscle innervation ➔ muscle atrophy ➔ decrease in muscle mass ➔ increasing fatigue

5. The difficulty of ALS is that mentality, cognitive ability, vision, hearing, and sensation are not lost; the client loses control of function without losing control of mental awareness

6. Signs and symptoms

    a. Musculoskeletal: weakness, fatigue, loss of fine motor control, spasticity, paresis, hyperreflexia, atrophy, paralysis; fasciculations of tongue, slurred speech and facial muscles

    b. Respiratory: dyspnea, ineffective airway clearance, upper respiratory infection (URI), respiratory failure

    c. Nutritional: dysphagia, inability to chew, malnutrition

    d. Other: depression, impotence, loss of bowel and bladder control

C. Nursing assessment

1. Assessment includes coordination, muscle stiffness and wasting, gait, signs of atrophy, dysarthria, dysphagia, dyspnea, reflexes, respiratory function, VS, weight, mental status, bowel function

2. Diagnostic tests: creatinine phosphokinase (CPK) (elevated), CSF (elevated protein), myelography, CT scan, muscle biopsy, electromyelogram, nerve conduction studies

D. Nursing management

1. Medications: anticholinesterase agents, steroids, antibiotics, muscle relaxants

2. Administer oxygen and ventilatory support as needed; suction as needed

3. Monitor cardiac status, vital signs

4. Monitor fluids status and offer nutritional support

5. Initiate physical therapy

6. Auscultate breath sounds

7. Encourage client to administer own ADLs as long as possible

8. Monitor bowel and bladder function, avoid constipation

9. Turn every two hours as needed; encourage ambulation; avoid strenuous exercise and plan rest periods

10. Encourage client and family to ventilate feelings

11. Involve client in support group

12. Client education should include avoiding complications, importance of outpatient care, needs of physical mobility, use of assistive devices

XIV. Pain

A. Overview

1. Pain is a subjective feeling, an individual response to noxious stimuli on the sensory nerve endings

2. Components of pain are affective (emotional), behavioral (behavioral responses), cognitive (beliefs, attitudes), sensory (perceptual), and physiologic

3. Unrelieved pain has harmful effects that slow healing; stimulation of the stress response causes increased muscle tension, local vasoconstriction, increased myocardial activity and oxygen consumption

   a. Pain tolerance is the degree of pain an individual can withstand; differences in affect, behavioral response, and cognitive factors vary from one person to the next

   b. Pain threshold is the point of pain recognition; it varies somewhat from person to person also

4. Pain can be classified according to source, speed, duration, and as "referred pain"

   a. Sources of pain

      1) Cutaneous: from skin and subcutaneous tissue

      2) Deep somatic: from muscles, tendons, joints

      3) Visceral/splanchnic: from abdominal organs; contractions, distention, colic

      4) Psychogenic/functional: pain of unknown physical cause

   b. Speed

      1) Fast: carried by A-delta fibers that are myelinated and carry sharp, bright, well-localized pain

      2) Slow: carried by C-fibers, which are unmyelinated and carry dull, burning, aching diffuse sensations

   c. Duration is considered either acute or chronic with different times and physiological and/or psychological responses

      1) Acute pain: defined as pain for six months or less, usually of sudden onset with localization in the affected area; physiological response (often see in autonomic sympathetic "flight or fight" response), psychological response (heightened emotional response with anxiety, fear)

      2) Chronic pain: defined as pain for six months or greater, persists over an indefinite period, is poorly localized, often diffuse; physiological response (may be none or may be a fatigued autonomic response with depressed vital signs); psychological response (characterized by attention to pain as all-consuming and signs of depression such as a sleeping disorder, anorexia or overeating, crying, flat or sad affect, and withdrawal)

   d. Referred pain is pain that is perceived at a site different from its origin

5. **Phantom pain** (pain that exists in a removed part) occurs in an amputated body part or limb, possibly caused by spontaneous firing of spinal cord neurons that have lost their normal sensory input

6. Intractable pain or malignant pain is chronic progressive pain that is unrelenting and severely debilitating

7. Causes include surgery, injury, trauma, chronic diseases (cancer, arthritis, AIDS, etc.), strenuous work, hormone shifts (migraines, menstruation), pregnancy, earache, toothaches, and infections

B. **Pathophysiology**

1. Nociception is the process of how pain is recognized consciously and can be considered conceptually in four steps: transduction, transmission, perception, and modulation

    a. Transduction: conversion of a stimulus to an action potential at the site of tissue injury

        1) Chemicals are released with cellular damage from such things as burns, radiation, pressure, tears, and cuts

        2) These chemicals sensitize the primary afferent nociceptors (PANs), fibers that carry painful stimuli; PANs are: A-delta (fast pain); C-fibers (slow pain)

        3) Analgesics that work to block transduction by interfering in the production of the chemicals that sensitize the PANs to begin the action potential and send the signal to the spinal cord include: corticosteroids, which block the formation of arachidonic acid; NSAIDS (nonsteroidal anti-inflammatory drugs), which block the formation of prostaglandins

    b. Transmission: the neuronal action potential is transmitted to and through the CNS so that it can be perceived

        1) The impulse is projected to the spinal cord

        2) It is processed in dorsal horn

        3) It is then transmitted to the brain

        4) Analgesics that work at the level of transmission stabilize membranes by inactivating sodium channels, thus inhibiting the action potential

        5) Referred pain occurs when nerve fibers from visceral areas and somatic areas that converge in the same area in the dorsal horn are processed in such a way that they are perceived as originating in the area of the somatic sensory A-delta fiber rather than the visceral C-fiber (e.g., myocardial ischemia is perceived as pain in the left arm)

        6) The gate control theory of pain offers an explanation for why such interventions as the TENS (trans electrical nerve stimulator), heat and cold, and massage are effective

            a) There are theoretical gates in the dorsal horn

            b) Small-diameter nerve fibers carry pain impulses through a gate, but large-diameter sensory nerve fibers going through the same gate can close the gate and inhibit transmission

c. Pain perception, the experience of pain, occurs in the cortex; may occur at a basic level in the thalamus

d. Modulation, inhibition of nociception

1) Efferent fibers descending from the brain stem modulate or alter pain; mechanisms include:

a) Endogenous opioids (naturally occurring, morphine-like chemicals) made in the CNS inhibit transmission of pain by binding to opioid receptors in the CNS to block transmission of nociceptive signals (e.g., endorphin, norepinephrine, enkephalin)

b) The endogenous analgesia center in the midbrain produces profound analgesia when stimulated

2) Many analgesics modulate pain by mimicking endogenous neuromodulators; examples include tricyclic antidepressants block serotonin reuptake (work well for neuropathic pain that is dull, aching, burning); synthetic opioids [e.g., morphine sulfate, meperidine (Demerol), hydromorphone (Dilaudid)]; the variability of individual endorphin levels may explain the fact that pain thresholds to the same stimulus are different from person to person

3) Surgical treatment of intractable pain (chronic, progressive pain that is unrelenting and severely debilitating) interrupts the pain pathways; types include: nerve block (destroys nerve roots chemically with phenol or alcohol); rhizotomy (destroys sensory nerve roots at the level of entry into the spinal cord); and cordotomy (transects the spinal pain pathway before the impulses ascend the spinothalamic tracts)

2. Signs and symptoms include elevated BP, increased HR, increased RR, grimacing, crying, sweating, posturing, depression, dilated pupils, anxiety and/or agitation, hypermotility

C. Nursing assessment

1. Assessment

a. Sensory components of pain (location, character or quality, pattern, duration, quantity or severity)

1) Location: Where is the pain? Is the pain on the surface or deep? Can you put your finger on it? Does it radiate or spread?

2) Character or quality: Describe how it feels (aching, burning, shooting, stinging, constant, intermittent, sharp, dull)

3) Pattern: How often does it come? Is it different at different times? Does anything make it start, make it worse or better?

4) Duration: How long have you had the pain?

5) Quantity or severity: How long have you had the pain? Can you rank the pain on a scale of 0 to 10, with 0 as no pain and 10 as the worst possible?

      b. Affective, behavioral, and cognitive components of pain; emotion will influence pain; expression of pain and beliefs about pain will vary from culture to culture; questions to ask include:

         1) What does the pain mean to you? Does it interfere or hinder you in any way?

         2) What do you think is causing the pain?

         3) What do you think will make it better?

         4) What home remedies have you tried or are you using?

         5) What prescription or over-the-counter (OTC) medications have you tried or are you using to treat the pain?

2. Diagnostic tests: not recommended generally; rating scale 1 to 10 and symptom analysis of the complaints are used; specific diagnostic tests to determine the cause of the pain are used according to the complaints voiced and location of pain

D. Nursing management

1. Medications include OTC analgesics such as acetaminophen (Tylenol), NSAIDs such as ibuprofen (Motrin), opioid analgesics such as morphine or meperidine (Demerol), anticonvulsants for chronic pain, and antiemetics

2. General principles in nursing management of pain

      a. Establish a trusting nurse-client relationship

      b. Always listen; believe and respect the client

      c. Clarify responsibilities, collaborate with the client to promote control and participation: discuss the client's role in reporting pain, the client's acceptable level of pain and the nurse's commitment when the client reports pain

      d. Be with the client during pain; offer support, concern, empathy and reassurance

      e. Explain all interventions for pain and how they work

3. Intervene to relieve pain

      a. Administer pain medications as ordered early in the pain episode to reach the client's acceptable pain level

      b. Consider round-the-clock administration of pain medication if pain is present most of the day

      c. If client has patient-controlled analgesia (PCA) (intravenous delivery of opioid by pump that allows the client to deliver analgesia on demand with preset dose and frequency limits and the option of preset continuous dosage):

         1) Instruct in concept and demonstrate

         2) Emphasize that client controls the device, not the family

      d. If client has an epidural catheter, assess for orthostatic hypotension and inspect insertion site for infection

NCLEX!

    e. Assess pain with the use of an analgesic scale each time vital signs are taken, after each administration of medication and with peak effect

    f. Assess for side effects of pain medications and symptoms that aggravate pain: sedation, nausea, constipation, respiratory depression, urinary retention, and hypotension.

    g. Include pain management in discharge teaching

NCLEX!

  4. Promote rest and relaxation; implement nondrug pain treatments (alternative or complementary therapies) as appropriate; these include:

    a. Cognitive strategies, such as distraction (music, TV, reading, humor), guided imagery, and positive suggestion; suggest the desired effect will be obtained when administering medications and alternative therapies; use words like "episode" and "experience" instead of "attack," "comfort" instead of "pain"

    b. Behavioral approaches such as rhythmic, slow breathing

    c. Therapeutic touch

    d. Cutaneous stimulation such as pressure, acupressure, heat and cold therapy, and massage

    e. Lower lights and reduce noise

    f. Reposition, support body parts, encourage mild activity such as gentle ROM

    g. Plan care and schedule visitors to provide uninterrupted rest periods

  5. Chronic pain requires a comprehensive approach to manage it effectively; how the pain affects the client's ability to perform ADLs should be assessed and included in the plan of care

NCLEX!

  6. Monitor constraints to effective pain management including the following misconceptions:

    a. Use of opioids (formerly narcotics) for management of acute pain will lead to addiction (compulsive drug-seeking): research indicates that only 0.1 percent of persons using opioids for acute pain management in the postoperative period will become addicted; addiction should *not* be confused with:

      1) Physical dependence: experience of physiological withdrawal symptoms with rapid discontinuance of opioids

      2) Tolerance: the need for increasing amounts of opioids to achieve the same level of pain relief

    b. It is better to wait until pain peaks to take analgesics: less analgesic is needed and better relief is obtained when the analgesic is given at the onset of pain

    c. Oral analgesics do not work as well as intravenous or intramuscular routes: if an **equianalgesic chart** (same pain relief obtained with different drugs, doses, and routes) is used, the oral route is equally effective; amount of drug needed is increased because of the first-pass effect of the liver

7. Intervene to alter the affective and cognitive components of pain

    a. Encourage the client to discuss factors that may impact and contribute to the experience of pain such as sociocultural influences, economic stress, and past experiences with pain

    b. Assist the client to identify previously effective coping strategies

    c. Refer to appropriate healthcare resources for counseling and therapy such as the psychologist, occupational therapist, physical therapist, or social worker as needed

XV. Alzheimer's Disease

A. Overview

1. Defined as a chronic, progressive form of dementia (cognitive impairment from organic syndrome) with cerebral degeneration

2. Occurs most often after age 65 (senile dementia); but can occur between 40 to 60 years of age (presenile dementia)

3. Causes include unknown etiology but has been linked to genetic tendency

B. Pathophysiology

1. Plaques, pathological changes, and neuronal tangles occur in the brain; within these plaques are dying nerve terminals, aluminum deposits, and abnormal protein fragments

2. Theories as to the cause

    a. An abnormal processing of a protein known as the amyloid precursor protein (APP) allows part of the protein to kill cells

    b. Inheritance of a gene coding for apolipoprotein E (APO-E4), which causes neuronal cell death

3. The number of functioning neurons is decreased, which accounts for the decline in cognition, memory and thought

NCLEX!

4. Signs and symptoms include forgetfulness, decreased judgment, personality changes, behavioral changes, loss of short-term memory, speech and language problems; in the terminal stages, loss of the ability to perform ADLs, seizures, delusions, paranoia, depression, inability to recognize loved ones; death usually results from the complications of immobility

C. Nursing assessment

1. Assessment includes: mental status, memory (short- and long-term), ability to make decisions or plans, ability to calculate, speech, energy level, mood, sleep patterns, initiative and motivation, VS, indications or gastrointestinal (GI) or urinary problems (anorexia, dysphagia, urinary or fecal incontinence); emotional status; skin assessment for trauma

2. Diagnostic tests: no specific tests are available for diagnosing the disease; MRI, positron emission tomography (PET), and single photon emission computed tomography (SPECT) scans support the diagnosis

D. Nursing management

1. Medications include tacrine (Cognex)

2. Client education should include memory aids, diet, and safety

3. Plans should be made with the family present for support measures and safety issues

4. Assist with reality orientation: repeat caregivers' names on a regular basis, use written instructions and directions, large-face clocks, orient the client as needed, use familiar objects and memory aids

5. Be consistent, use simple instructions, avoid rushing

6. Allow the client to perform ADLs as long as possible, assisting as necessary

7. Monitor fluid and nutritional status

Case Study

F. J. is an elderly man with newly diagnosed Parkinson's disease who has just been admitted to an extended-living facility. He is admitted, reluctantly, by his family who cannot care for him at home where he lives alone. F. J. does not feel he needs to be admitted and wants his family to leave him alone.

❶ What signs and symptoms should the nurse anticipate?

❷ What nursing diagnosis will be the highest priority?

❸ When will be the best time to schedule his physical therapy session?

❹ When it takes him a long time to get dressed in the morning, the nurse offers assistance. He becomes very upset. How should the nurse handle this?

❺ What are some specific instructions the nurse should give him to assist with his mobility problems?

For suggested responses, see pages 565–566.

Posttest

1. A young female with a diagnosis of multiple sclerosis (MS) has just discovered she is also pregnant. She and her husband have been trying to conceive for several years and are very excited. What client education should be given to the client concerning her disease and pregnancy?

(1) Immediately report weakness that progresses upward in the extremities.

(2) Report a change in level of consciousness, severe headache, or slow pulse.

(3) Recognize that a sore/stiff neck and pain when the neck is flexed are critical signs to report.

(4) Immediately report spasticity, weakness, or visual changes.

2 A client has seizure activity that is continuous in nature. When the nurse leaves to obtain an oxygen set-up, the seizures resume. The client's coloring is getting worse. The nurse decides to enact standing orders to treat:

(1) Anticonvulsant syndrome.
(2) Status epilepticus.
(3) Brain herniation.
(4) Syphilitic posturing.

3 Which of the following assessment findings should concern the nurse in a 35-year-old client with an intracranial hematoma?

(1) Hamstring pain when the hip and knee are flexed and then extended
(2) Curling of the toes when stroking the bottom of the foot upward
(3) Muscle aches and cramping, especially at night
(4) Cogwheel and lead pipe rigidity

4 After a magnetic resonance imaging (MRI) to rule out an expanding brain lesion, the nurse prepare the client for a lumbar puncture. Information for the client would include:

(1) The risk of paralysis because the needle is inserted through the spinal cord.
(2) Maintaining a full bladder for better visualization.
(3) Keeping his head flat to avoid a headache.
(4) Directions to straighten the legs slowly.

5 The nurse at the community clinic assesses a client with complaints of a pounding headache. The client is known to have a T4 level spinal cord injury that occurred some time ago. The nurse should first assess for:

(1) Sinus infection.
(2) Spinal shock.
(3) Upper motor neuron deficit.
(4) Autonomic dysreflexia.

6 Corneal abrasion in the client with myasthenia gravis can be prevented by which of the following?

(1) Saline soaks applied every shift
(2) Instilling artificial tears in the eyes every 1 to 2 hours
(3) Ensuring the client's contact lenses are on while awake
(4) Providing sunglasses when client is outside

7 To reduce risks for meningitis, the nurse's best advice to an elderly client is:

(1) Stay mentally active and engaged.
(2) Get pneumococcal pneumonia and influenza vaccinations.
(3) Drink at least 3,000 mL fluids per day.
(4) Exercise 15 to 30 minutes most days of the week.

8 The nurse is providing care for a client with Guillain-Barré syndrome who has plasmapheresis. Which other neurological condition is sometimes treated with plasmapheresis?

(1) Meningitis
(2) Parkinson's disease
(3) Myasthenia gravis
(4) Amyotrophic lateral sclerosis

9 The client with newly-diagnosed Parkinson's disease states, "I just don't think I can handle having Parkinson's disease." The nurse's best first response is:

(1) "You are really feeling overwhelmed, aren't you?"
(2) "I am sure you can. A lot of other people do!"
(3) "What do you think will be the hardest thing to handle?"
(4) "The entire healthcare team will help you manage the disease."

10 The client's postoperative pain seems to be getting worse instead of better. When the nurse asks the client, "Why do you think it's getting worse?" the client replies, "My wife died last month. It's all I can think about." The nurse must now consider:

(1) Calling the physician for an increased dosage of pain medication.
(2) Calling the physician for a sedative.
(3) Referring the client for a psychiatric consult.
(4) Developing interventions for grief and loss.

See pages 164–165 for Answers and Rationales.

Answers and Rationales

Pretest

1 Answer: 3 *Rationale:* Although a ventilator is not required for injury below C3, the innervation of intercostal muscles is affected. Hemorrhage and cord swelling extends the level of injury making it likely that this client will need a ventilator.
Cognitive Level: Application
Nursing Process: Planning; *Test Plan:* PHYS

2 Answer: 2 *Rationale:* Keeping the head of the bed elevated to 30 degrees promotes venous drainage, which is important in decreasing ICP. Alignment of the head prevents obstruction of the jugular veins. Obstruction would impede venous drainage.
Cognitive Level: Application
Nursing Process: Implementation; *Test Plan:* PHYS

3 Answer: 1 *Rationale:* Momentary loss of consciousness followed by a lucid period and rapid deterioration is a classic picture resulting from a torn cerebral artery, producing an epidural bleed.
Cognitive Level: Application
Nursing Process: Assessment; *Test Plan:* PHYS

4 Answer: 4 *Rationale:* The period after the clonic phase of a seizure is the postictal period. Typically, the client slowly regains consciousness, moving from a relaxed, quiet state to confusion or disorientation on awakening.
Cognitive Level: Application
Nursing Process: Implementation; *Test Plan:* SECE

5 Answer: 1 *Rationale:* Protective pads/diapers should be used only after all other treatment modes have been tried. Early dependency on incontinence products may decrease motivation to seek evaluation and treatment.
Cognitive Level: Application
Nursing Process: Evaluation; *Test Plan:* HPM

6 Answer: 3 *Rationale:* Clients with meningitis will be less able to protect themselves from both internal and external injury. Providing cognitive stimulation and increasing cardiac output are contraindicated with meningitis. Enhancing coping skills may be a focus if the client has residual effects from meningitis but is not a major focus.
Cognitive Level: Application
Nursing Process: Planning; *Test Plan:* SECE

7 Answer: 1 *Rationale:* Presyndrome to Guillain-Barré syndrome is often a viral infection or immunization. Lower extremity weakness or paralysis that progresses upward is classic in Guillain-Barré. Fatigue is not usually seen, nor are tremors or seizures.
Cognitive Level: Analysis
Nursing Process: Assessment; *Test Plan:* PHYS

8 Answer: 3 *Rationale:* The client should know the signs of crisis and should report them immediately. There is often more fatigue and weakness later in the day than in the morning, so the client should plan important activities for early in the day. It may be easier to eat three small meals with snacks because chewing may cause fatigue.
Cognitive Level: Application
Nursing Process: Implementation; *Test Plan:* HPM

9 Answer: 3 *Rationale:* The resting or nonintentional tremor may be controlled with purposeful movement, such as holding an object. Deep-breathing, a warm bath, and diazepam will promote relaxation but are not specific interventions for the tremor.
Cognitive Level: Application
Nursing Process: Implementation; *Test Plan:* PHYS

10 Answer: 2 *Rationale:* Always believe the client's report and ranking of pain. The client tolerated the last full dose of medication so he should be given a full dose now. The nurse would reassess the client's pain level within 30 minutes of administering pain medication depending on peak action time of the drug. The nurse would not need to take vital signs unless indicated.
Cognitive Level: Analysis
Nursing Process: Implementation; *Test Plan:* SECE

Posttest

1 Answer: 4 *Rationale:* Stresses such as pregnancy can increase the chance of an exacerbation of MS. Signs of an exacerbation are spasticity, weakness, or visual changes. Option 1 indicates Guillain-Barré syndrome; option 2 indicates increased intracranial pressure or hematoma; option 3 indicates meningitis.
Cognitive Level: Analysis
Nursing Process: Analysis; *Test Plan:* PHYS

2 Answer: 2 *Rationale:* When seizure activity becomes continuous and repetitive, respirations are affected and the progression of status epilepticus is life-threatening. Nursing interventions address prevention of hypoxia, acidosis, hypoglycemia, hyperthermia, and exhaustion.
Cognitive Level: Analysis
Nursing Process: Analysis; *Test Plan:* PHYS

3 **Answer: 1** *Rationale:* A positive Kernig's sign, which is described in option 1, is common in intracranial hematomas. Option 2 is a negative Babinski; with a hematoma the nurse should expect a positive Babinski (fanning of the toes in an adult). Option 3 is common in many illnesses; option 4 is specific to Parkinson's disease.
Cognitive Level: Application
Nursing Process: Assessment; *Test Plan:* PHYS

4 **Answer: 3** *Rationale:* The spinal needle is inserted into the area below the spinal cord eliminating the likelihood of paralysis. A misdirected needle may puncture a distended bladder. The client must maintain the knees to chest position until completion of the lumbar puncture. Because cerebrospinal fluid (CSF) has been removed during the lumbar puncture, time must be allowed for production and replacement of the CSF.
Cognitive Level: Application
Nursing Process: Analysis; *Test Plan:* PHYS

5 **Answer: 4** *Rationale:* Spinal cord injury at or above the level of T6 can experience an exaggerated sympathetic response, seen only after recovery from spinal shock. If untreated, autonomic dysreflexia is potentially fatal as bradycardia and severe hypertension progress.
Cognitive Level: Analysis
Nursing Process: Analysis; *Test Plan:* SECE

6 **Answer: 2** *Rationale:* Corneal abrasion in the client with myasthenia gravis is caused by dryness of the cornea from inability to close the eyelids and blink. It can be prevented by application of artificial tears every 1 to 2 hours.
Cognitive Level: Application
Nursing Process: Implementation; *Test Plan:* PHYS

7 **Answer: 2** *Rationale:* Meningitis bacteria or viruses often gain entry into the cerebrospinal fluid secondary to an upper respiratory tract infection. Options 1, 3, and 4 are generally healthy practices for the elderly client but not specific health promotion for prevention of meningitis.
Cognitive Level: Application
Nursing Process: Implementation; *Test Plan:* HPM

8 **Answer: 3** *Rationale:* Plasmapheresis is performed to remove autoantibodies that attack the myelin sheaths of motor and sensory nerves in Guillain-Barré and attack the acetylcholine receptors at the neuromuscular junction in myasthenia gravis. The other diseases have not been identified with autoimmune disorder.
Cognitive Level: Knowledge
Nursing Process: Implementation; *Test Plan:* PHYS

9 **Answer: 1** *Rationale:* The nurse should first encourage the client experiencing a loss to express his feelings. Option 1 acknowledges the client's feelings, is open-ended, and promotes further discussion.
Cognitive Level: Analysis
Nursing Process: Implementation; *Test Plan:* PSYC

10 **Answer: 4** *Rationale:* The client's pain is affective as well as sensory. Grieving his wife's death is a normal response that does not necessarily require psychiatric consult. Options 1 and 2 address the sensory, not affective, component of his pain.
Cognitive Level: Application
Nursing Process: Implementation; *Test Plan:* PSYC

References

Ball, J., & Binder, R. (1999). *Pediatric nursing: Caring for children* (2nd ed.). Upper Saddle River, NJ: Prentice Hall.

Black, J. M., Hawks, J. H., & Keene, A. M. (Eds.). (2001). *Medical-surgical nursing: Clinical management for positive outcomes*. Philadelphia: W.B. Saunders, pp. 461–503, 1944–1947, 2016–2023, 2028.

Ebersole, P. & Hess, P. (1998). *Toward healthy aging: Human needs and nursing response* (5th ed.). St. Louis, MO: Mosby, pp. 332–347, 405–409.

Corbett, J. V. (2000). *Laboratory tests and diagnostics procedures* (5th ed.). Upper Saddle River, NJ: Prentice Hall, p. 649.

Ignatavicius, D. D., Workman, M. L., & Mishler, M. (Eds.). (1999). *Medical-surgical nursing across the health care continuum* (3rd ed.). Philadelphia: W.B. Saunders, pp. 1035–1038, 1040–1043, 1085–1098.

LeMone, P. & Burke, K. M. (2000). *Medical-surgical nursing: Critical thinking in client care* (2nd ed.). Upper Saddle River, NJ: Prentice Hall, pp. 72–97, 1743–1748, 1836–1846, 1853–1860.

Lewis, S. M., Heitkemper, M. M., & Dirksen, S. R. (1999). *Medical surgical nursing: Assessment and management of clinical problems* (5th ed.). St. Louis, MO: Mosby, pp. 126–154, 1638–1641, 1694–1702, 1719–1720.

McCaffery, M. (1999). *Pain: Clinical manual* (2nd ed.). St. Louis, MO: Mosby, pp. 15–34, 36–102, 121–122.

McCance, K. L., & Huether, S. E. (Eds.). (2001). *Pathophysiology: The biologic basis for disease in adults and children* (4th ed.). St. Louis, MO: Mosby, pp. 423–432, 548–549, 554–558, 565–567.

Sullivan, E. J., & Decker, P. J. (2001). *Effective leadership and management in nursing*. Upper Saddle River, NJ: Prentice Hall, p. 224.

Venes, D., Thomas, C. L., & Taber, C. W. (Eds.). (2001). *Taber's cyclopedic medical dictionary* (19th ed.). Philadelphia: F.A. Davis.

CHAPTER 5

Musculoskeletal Health Problems

Cathy Cormier, MN, RN, C

CHAPTER OUTLINE

OBJECTIVES

▌ Define key terms associated with musculoskeletal health problems.

▌ Identify risk factors associated with the development of musculoskeletal health problems.

▌ Discuss the common etiologies of musculoskeletal health problems.

▌ Describe the pathophysiologic processes associated with specific musculoskeletal health problems.

▌ Distinguish between normal and abnormal musculoskeletal findings obtained from nursing assessment.

▌ Prioritize nursing interventions associated with specific musculoskeletal health problems.

[*Media Link*]

Use the CD-ROM enclosed with this text, or log onto the address given to access the free, interactive Companion Website created for this series. The CD-ROM and Companion Website accompanying this book offer additional practice opportunities and information—NCLEX Review, Case Studies, Glossary, In Depth with NCLEX, and more.

www.prenhall.com/hogan

REVIEW AT A GLANCE

ankylosis *joint immobility or fixation secondary to an underlying disease process*

articular cartilage *connective tissue covering the epiphysis where joint surfaces meet; it acts as a cushion between joint surfaces*

bone remodeling *formation of new bone by osteoblasts and removal of old bone by osteoclasts; this process is regulated by the actions of parathyroid hormone, calcitonin, and vitamin D*

Bouchard's node *the formation of hard nodules in the proximal interphalangeal (PIP) joints resulting in joint deformity characteristic of osteoporosis*

boutaniere deformities *joint deformity associated with rheumatoid arthritis, characterized by flexion of the PIP joint and hyperextension of the distal interphalangeal (DIP) joint*

calcinosis *abnormal deposits of calcium salts on the skin*

diaphysis *the shaft, or long portion of long bones; the inner portion of the diaphysis contains the medullary cavity which* is comprised of bone marrow, this is surrounded by cortical bone

epiphysis *proximal and distal end of long bones; it is comprised of cancellous bone surrounded by cortical bone*

fascia *fibrous connective tissue responsible for supporting and connecting structures of the musculoskeletal system*

Heberden's node *the formation of a hard nodule in the distal interphalangeal (DIP) joints resulting in joint deformity characteristic of osteoarthritis (OA)*

metaphysis *located in the area of flaring between the epiphysis and the diaphysis of long bones; it contains the growth plates that are responsible for longitudinal growth of bones during growth years*

osteolysis *softening and breakdown of bone*

osteophytes *outgrowth of bony tissue commonly referred to as spurs*

pannus *vascular granulation tissue that forms in the synovial membrane of clients with rhumatoid arthritis (RA); it is* responsible for destruction of bones and surrounding tissue in affected joints

periosteum *membrane covering bone, except in areas where articular cartilage is present, which contains nerve, lymph, and blood vessels*

rheumatoid nodules *subcutaneous masses found in 20 percent of clients with rhumatoid arthritis (RA); they are characterized as firm, nontender masses usually found on olecranon bursae or along the extensor surface of the forearm*

scleradactyly *scleroderma that is localized within fingers*

swan neck *joint deformity associated with rheumatoid arthritis (RA), characterized by hyperextension of the proximal interphalangeal joint with flexion of the distal interphalangeal joints*

telangiectasis *small, dilated blood vessels with a bright-red center point and spiderlike branches that may occur in clients with scleroderma*

ulnar drift *joint deformity characteristic of rheumatoid arthritis (RA)*

Pretest

1 The nurse has completed instructions on health maintenance for a client diagnosed with osteoarthritis. The nurse verifies that the client understood the instructions if the client states that participation in which of the following sports would be beneficial?

(1) Tennis
(2) Jogging
(3) Swimming
(4) Volleyball

2 A health history and physical assessment on a client with rheumatoid arthritis (RA) may reveal which of the following assessment data?

(1) Heberden's nodes
(2) Morning stiffness no longer than 30 minutes
(3) Asymmetric joint swelling
(4) Swan neck deformities

3 Which of the following over-the-counter (OTC) agents should the client on uricosuric drugs be instructed to avoid?

(1) Acetaminophen (Tylenol)
(2) Ibuprofen (Motrin)
(3) Aspirin (ASA)
(4) Naproxen (Naprosyn)

4 Which of the following nursing interventions is contraindicated in the care of a client with acute osteomyelitis?

(1) Apply heat compresses to the affected area
(2) Immobilize the affected area
(3) Administer narcotic analgesics for pain
(4) Administer OTC analgesics for pain

5 Which of the following lab data would be most significant in the client with Paget's disease?

(1) Elevated white blood count (WBC)
(2) Elevated erythrocyte sedimentation rate (ESR)
(3) Positive tissue biopsy for *Staphylococcus*
(4) Elevated serum alkaline phosphatase

6 Which of the following individuals is at greatest risk for developing an osteosarcoma?

(1) Male, age 42
(2) Female, age 52
(3) Female, age 20
(4) Male, age 15

7 A drug history is important in a client with systemic lupus erythematosus (SLE) because the disease may be associated with use of which of the following drugs?

(1) Procainamide (Procan SR)
(2) Acetylsalicylic acid (aspirin)
(3) Diazepam (Valium)
(4) Azathioprine (Imuran)

8 To prevent occurrences of Raynaud's phenomenon, what should the client diagnosed with systemic scleroderma be instructed to do?

(1) Wear gloves
(2) Perform range-of-motion exercises daily
(3) Limit sodium intake
(4) Avoid warm temperature

9 Which of the following occurs during the remodeling phase of bone healing?

(1) Callus formation occurs.
(2) Callus is replaced with mature bone.
(3) Osteoclasts resorb excess callus to return the bone to its original shape.
(4) Proliferation of osteoblast and fibroblasts occurs within the hematoma at the fracture site.

10 Which of the following statements applies to compartment syndrome?

(1) Increased pressure within the tissues results from excessive edema at the fracture site.
(2) Capillary pressures over 15 mm Hg can result in permanent muscle and nerve damage.
(3) The presence of a peripheral pulse will rule out compartment syndrome.
(4) Pain associated with compartment syndrome will be relieved with use of analgesics.

See pages 198–199 for Answers and Rationales.

I. Risk Factors Associated with Musculoskeletal Health Problems

A. Osteoarthritis (OA): obesity, age, gender (affects genders equally up to age 55, incidence increases in women after this time), heredity

B. Rheumatoid arthritis (RA): gender (occurs 2 to 3 times more frequently in females); age (onset usually occurs during middle-age, however it can occur at any time); possible genetic link

NCLEX!

C. Gouty arthritis: gender (increased frequency in men, may occur postmenopausal or in women with a genetic link), obesity, heavy alcohol intake, familial trait, disease states (malignancies, diabetes mellitus [DM], kidney disease, hypertension [HTN], acidosis); clients taking the following medications may experience drug-induced gout—thiazide diuretics, cytotoxic drugs, low-dose acetylsalicylic acid (aspirin), and ethambutol (Myambutol)

D. Osteomyelitis

NCLEX!

1. Hematogenous: children under 10 with recent history of throat, ear or skin infections; debilitated clients with recurrent upper respiratory infection (URIs), urinary tract infections (UTIs), and skin infections; and intravenous (IV) drug-abusers

2. Direct entry: recent history of puncture wound, gunshot wound, fracture, surgery

E. **Paget's disease:** adults over 40 years of age, more common in males

F. **Muscular dystrophy (MD):** male children with family history

G. **Fibromyalgia:** more common in women; stress

H. **Bone tumors:** genetic link, exposure to chemotherapy or radiation (osteosarcomas), Paget's disease

I. **Systemic lupus erythematosus (SLE):** women of childbearing years, family history, ethnicity (African Americans, Asians, and Hispanics)

J. **Scleroderma:** women of childbearing years; African-American women; coal miners; occupational exposure to polyvinyl chloride, epoxy resins, and aromatic hydrocarbons; genetic link probable

K. **Fractures:** trauma, active participation in sports, elderly clients at risk for falls, clients with bone disease

L. **Compartment syndrome:** more frequent in crushing injuries and fractures of the forearm or lower leg

M. **Osteoporosis:** postmenopausal women; ethnicity (Caucasian and Asians); clients with the following endocrine disorders: hyperparathyroidism, hyperthyroidism, Cushing's syndrome, diabetes mellitus; use of the following substances: glucocorticoids, caffeine, nicotine, tetracycline, and aluminum-containing antacids; sedentary lifestyle; both genders over 80 years of age

II. Osteoarthritis (OA)

A. Overview

1. Defined as a form of arthritis with progressive destruction of the cartilage in both the synovial joints and vertebrae

2. Characteristics

   a. Most common form of arthritis, also referred to as *degenerative arthritis*

   b. Chronic, progressive, nonsystemic disease

   c. Characterized by degeneration of the **articular cartilage** (connective tissue covering the **epiphysis** [proximal and distal end of long bones] where joint surfaces meet) in the hands: proximal interphalangeal (PIP) and distal interphalangeal (DIP) joints, feet (metatarsophalangeal [MTP] joints), shoulder, lumbar and cervical spine, hips, and knees

3. Classifications and causes

   a. *Primary idiopathic:* unknown etiology, however, risk factors usually present

   b. *Secondary disorder:* OA resulting from conditions that predispose a client to degenerative changes in the joints; for example: rheumatoid arthritis, diabetes mellitus, congenital deformities, joint trauma, or repetitive movement of a joint related to participation in sports or work activities

B. Pathophysiology

1. Primary idiopathic OA: articular cartilage decreases friction during joint movement and displaces the force of the workload onto the subchondral bone, thereby decreasing stress within the joint itself

   a. Type II collagen, normally present in healthy articular cartilage, contains proteoglycans; proteoglycans are macromolecules that provide elasticity and stiffness to articular cartilage allowing it to resist compression

   b. It is thought that clients with primary idiopathic OA have some type of malfunction in the production of proteoglycans; the body attempts to compensate by producing more proteoglycans and collagen; however, these substances are destroyed faster than they can be synthesized

   c. Type II collagen is eventually replaced with Type I collagen (normally present in skin and tendons); as Type I collagen continues to replace Type II collagen with disease progression, the composition of the articular cartilage is altered, and it is unable to perform its original function

   d. In response to changes in the articular cartilage, synovitis (inflammation of a synovial joint) often occurs within the joint and the subchondral bone responds to cartilage damage by producing **osteophytes** (outgrowth of bony tissue commonly referred to as spurs)

2. Secondary OA

   a. Repetitive movements that apply excessive workloads to joints will result in breakdown of the cartilage and changes in the subchondral bone

   b. The ability of cartilage to lubricate the joint is depleted and friction between joint surfaces increases during joint motion

   c. The outcome is similar to that of primary idiopathic OA; joint narrowing occurs with cartilage breakdown, and synovitis and formation of osteophytes occurs with disease progression

3. Signs and symptoms

   NCLEX!

   a. Dull, aching pain in the affected joint relieved with rest

   b. Numbness or tingling at night, associated with disease progression secondary to nerve damage

   c. Crepitus with joint movement

   d. Edema and stiffness in the affected joint

   e. Decreased range of motion (ROM) and ability to participate in activities of daily living (ADLs)

   NCLEX!

   f. Joint deformities: **Heberden's nodes** (formation of hard nodules in the DIP joints, resulting in joint deformity) and **Bouchard's nodes** (formation of hard nodules in the PIP joints resulting in joint deformity)

   g. Symptoms vary in severity and may range from mild intermittent discomfort to complete disability

C. Nursing assessment

1. Assessment includes baseline ROM, participation in ADLs and work/leisure activities, pain assessment, safety with ambulation, baseline weight and dietary habits, presence of Heberden's nodes and Bouchard's nodes

2. Diagnostic tests

   a. X-ray: loss of joint cartilage, narrowing of space between adjacent bones, and formation of osteophytes in progressive disease states

   b. Eosinophil sedimentation rate (ESR): normal, slight increase with synovitis, used to differentiate other forms of arthritis

D. Nursing management

1. Medications include acetaminophen (Tylenol) preferred or acetylsalicylic acid (aspirin), corticosteroids (intra-articular injection or other forms), nonsteroidal antiinflammatory drugs (NSAIDs)

2. Instruct on weight reduction

3. Collaborate with physical therapy (PT) regarding an aerobic exercise program to reduce and eliminate strain on joints: swimming, biking, walking, water aerobics

4. Collaborate with occupational therapy (OT) regarding assistive devices for ADLs

5. Implement and assess effectiveness of pain relief measures

   a. Teach action and side effects of medications used for pain control

   b. Application of heat before exercising and application of cold after exercising

   c. Splints designed to immobilize the joint

   d. Cotton gloves at night

   e. Paraffin dips

   f. Warm water soaks

   g. Neck collar and lumbar corsets for OA of vertebrae

   h. Firm mattress for sleeping

6. Preoperative teaching as required for the following surgeries:

   a. Arthroscopy (use of an arthroscope to examine the interior of a joint)

   b. Total joint replacements for OA of hip and knee

   c. Joint fusions for OA of cervical spine

7. Instruct on safety in home (see Box 5-1)

III. Rheumatoid Arthritis (RA)

A. Overview

1. Defined as a chronic, progressive, systemic, autoimmune disease with inflammation of the joints and deformity

- Eliminate throw rugs in home.
- Use good body mechanics when performing ADLs and work/leisure activities.
- Use a shower chair and hand rails when bathing.
- Use cane and walker as directed to decrease workload on hips and knees.
- Use well-fitting, supportive shoes when ambulating.

2. Characteristics

   a. Onset is insidious and characterized by periods of remissions and exacerbations

   NCLEX!

   b. Characterized by chronic inflammation of bilateral joints and surrounding structures; multiple joints are usually involved

3. Unknown etiology; however, evidence supports that disease progression is related to autoimmune processes in middle age

4. Systemic complications

   a. Extrasynovial rheumatoid nodules on the heart, lungs, eyes, or spleen

   b. Vasculitis

   c. Anemia

B. Pathophysiology

1. Exposure to a viral pathogen may initiate the inflammatory response; immunoglobulin G (IgG) is formed in response to the antigen, but for some unknown reason the body begins to produce autoantibodies (called rheumatoid factors) against IgG

   a. The rheumatoid factors combine with IgG to form immune complexes

   b. The continued presence of the immune complexes within the joint cavity results in chronic inflammation and destruction of the articular cartilage as well as surrounding joint structures

   NCLEX!

2. The synovial membrane (located within the joint capsule and responsible for producing synovial fluid to lubricate joint structures) hypertrophies and thickens secondary to chronic inflammation

   a. Blood supply to the area is occluded and cellular necrosis occurs

   b. These events lead to the formation of **pannus** (vascular grannulation tissue that forms in the synovial membrane of clients with RA)

   c. Pannus gradually extends from the synovial membrane and surface of the articular cartilage into the joint capsule and subchondral bone causing destruction of the bone

3. Fibrous adhesions and bony **ankylosis** (joint immobility or fixation secondary to an underlying disease process) occurs as the involved bone is destroyed; the inflammatory process extends to the support structures of the bone, tendons and ligaments, and joint instability and deformities occur

4. Signs and symptoms

    a. Initially may present with vague systemic symptoms such as anorexia, weight loss, fever, and loss of energy

NCLEX!

    b. Early disease states will present with inflammation, swelling, and decreased movement of the joints in the hand (PIP and MCP), feet (MTP), wrists, and elbows; as RA progresses, joints of the knees, hips, and cervical spine may also be involved

    c. The American Rheumatism Association has developed diagnostic criteria for rheumatoid arthritis; evidence of four out of seven criteria must be present to confirm the diagnosis (see Box 5-2)

C. Nursing assessment

NCLEX!

    1. Assessment includes low-grade temperature; decreased ROM; signs and symptoms of inflammation (tenderness, swelling, redness) involving multiple joints bilaterally; morning stiffness lasting greater than one hour; change in energy level and ability to participation in ADLs as well as work/leisure activities; pain assessment; neurological assessment (complaints of headache, numbness, or tingling with involvement of cervical vertebrae); baseline weight and history of recent weight loss; presence of:

    a. Joint deformities

        1) **Swan neck** (hyperextension of the PIP joints with flexion of the DIP joints)

        2) **Ulnar drift** (joint deformity characteristic of RA)

        3) **Boutonnière deformities** (flexion of the PIP joint and hyperextension of DIP joint)

NCLEX!

    b. Rheumatoid nodules (firm, nontender subcutaneous masses found on olecranon bursae or extension surface of forearm) over pressure areas

    2. Diagnostic tests

    a. X-ray: may show minimal changes early in the disease; however, as disease progression occurs, narrowing of joint space, bone erosion, and bone deformities are evident bilaterally

    b. Serum rheumatoid factor: not exclusive for RA but positive in the majority of clients

    c. Evidence of anemia with complete blood count (CBC)

Box 5-2	
Diagnostic Criteria for Rheumatoid Arthritis	• Morning stiffness lasting for at least 1 hour and persisting over at least 6 weeks
	• Arthritis with swelling or effusion of three or more joints persisting for at least 6 weeks
	• Arthritis of wrist, MCP, or PIP joints persisting for at least 6 weeks
	• Symmetric arthritis with simultaneous involvement of corresponding joints on both sides of the body
	• Rheumatoid nodules
	• Positive serum rheumatoid factor
	• Characteristic radiologic changes of rheumatoid arthritis noted in hands and wrists

d. Elevated ESR

e. Synovial fluid analysis: increased white blood cells (WBCs), increased turbidity, decreased viscosity

D. Nursing management

1. Medications

   a. NSAIDs, used early in the disease

   b. Systemic corticosteroids: long-term use is associated with severe side effects; they are usually utilized when NSAIDs are no longer effective

   c. Disease-modifying drugs (DMARDs): once the last drug of choice for treatment, these drugs are now being used earlier in the treatment regime because evidence suggests that they may play a role in arresting disease progression

      1) Most drugs in this category are contraindicated in clients with a history of kidney and liver disease

      2) Drugs included in this category are auranofin, (Ridaura), azathioprine (Imuran), hydroxychloroquine, (Plaquenil), and cyslosporine (Neoral)

2. Instruct on disease process and treatment regimen

3. Refer to support groups including Arthritis Foundation

4. Emphasize rest to decrease joint stress

   a. Pace activities

   b. Perform activities while sitting when possible

   c. Splints for hands and wrists

   d. Relaxation techniques

   e. Guided imagery

5. Collaborate with physical therapist (PT) regarding therapeutic exercise program, isotonic exercises, passive range of motion (PROM), and active range of motion (AROM) to maintain muscle strength and ROM

6. Collaborate with occupational therapist (OT) regarding assistive devices for ADLs, tips for joint protection and work simplification

7. Teach action and side effects of medications used for pain control

8. Implement and assess effectiveness of pain relief measures

   a. Medications

   b. Application of heat or cold, depending on what works for client

   c. Paraffin dips

   d. Firm mattress for sleeping and proper positioning in bed for comfort

9. Pre-operative teaching as required for the following surgeries:

   a. Synovectomy (removal of the synovial membrane)

   b. Total joint replacements for OA of hip and knee

   c. Joint fusions for RA of cervical spine

► *Practice to Pass*

When providing health maintenance teaching to the client with rheumatoid arthritis (RA), what information should the nurse include regarding the best methods to increase joint mobility and maintain joint function?

NCLEX!

10. Instruct on home safety (refer back to Box 5-1)

11. Instruct on hazards of immobility if bedridden and teach prevention

IV. Gouty Arthritis

A. Overview

1. Defined as a metabolic disease marked by increased serum uric acid levels (hyperuricemia) and joint inflammation

2. Characteristics

NCLEX!

NCLEX!

   a. Not all clients with hyperuricemia will develop gouty arthritis

   b. Acute, painful episodes of monoarticular joint inflammation lasting about 10 to 14 days

   c. Acute episodes vary in frequency and are often precipitated by some stress: surgery, joint trauma, and emotional stress; it is self-limiting with treatment

3. Classifications and causes

   a. *Primary:* genetic alteration in purine (end product of nucleoprotein digestion, breaks down from uric acid) metabolism resulting in an increased production of uric acid or a decrease in the excretion of uric acid

   b. *Secondary:* hyperuricemia secondary to disease state or medications

B. Pathophysiology

NCLEX!

1. Increased levels of serum uric acid precipitate within the joint and initiate the inflammatory response; sodium urates are deposited, around or within the joints

2. Phagocytosis of urate crystals occurs, leading to cell death and release of lysosomal enzymes

3. If untreated, chronic inflammation will lead to involvement of multiple joints, destruction of cartilage, bone, and formation of tophi

4. Signs and symptoms

NCLEX!

   a. Sudden onset of severe pain in one joint; the great toe is most commonly affected; however, it may occur in the instep, wrist, tarsal joints, knees, elbows, and ankles

   b. Joint appears red or dusky, swollen, edematous, and is extremely tender to touch

NCLEX!

   c. Tophi: hard, movable, nodules with irregular surfaces occur in synovium, helix of ear, olecranon bursa, and Achilles' tendon (most common locations); associated with chronic untreated gout; can resolve with treatment

C. Nursing assessment

1. Assessment includes: complete health history, determination of risk factors; pain assessment; inspection of affected joint for signs and symptoms of inflammation; and mobility and safety with ADLs

2. Diagnostic tests

   a. Serum uric acid level greater than 7.5 mg/dL (normal: male 2.1 to 8.5 mg/dL; female 2.0 to 6.6 mg/dL)

   b. Increased WBC and ESR during acute episodes

c. 24-hour urine to evaluate uric acid excretion

1) Levels will correlate with increased serum uric acid levels if there is an overproduction of uric acid

2) In cases where the excretion of uric acid is a problem, serum uric acid will be increased; however, 24-hour urine levels will be decreased

d. Synovial fluid analysis (positive for urate crystals)

D. Nursing management

1. Medication

a. Colchicine (Novocolchine): effective in the treatment of acute attacks if treatment is initiated as soon as symptoms occur; IV administration will increase response and decrease nausea and vomiting associated with oral administration; instruct client to stop taking orally if diarrhea occurs

b. Narcotic analgesics and NSAIDs effectively relieve pain associated with acute attacks; acetylsalicylic acid (aspirin) is contraindicated because it decreases the excretion of uric acid and interferes with the action of uricosuric drugs

c. Uricosuric agents: used in the prophylactic treatment of gouty arthritis and chronic gouty arthritis; allopurinol (Zyloprim) and probenecid (Benemid)

2. Instruct client on disease process and treatment plan; emphasis that the disease prognosis is good with treatment compliance

3. Administer medications as ordered and instruct client on medication regime; instruct clients to increase fluid intake to 3 L/day to decrease incidence of kidney stones associated with use of uricosuric agents

4. Instruct on strict bedrest for first 24 hours of acute attack, activity may aggravate and prolong acute symptoms; provide a bedcradle to relieve pressure from linens at affected area

5. Assist with weight reduction

6. Instruct on limiting intake of alcohol to a moderate level

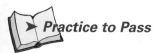

Practice to Pass

Explain how the results of a 24-hour urine for uric acid assists the healthcare provider in determining the etiology of gout.

V. Osteomyelitis

A. Overview

1. Defined as an acute or chronic infection of the bone

2. Characteristics

a. Early diagnosis critical to prevent disease progression

b. Most common causative agent: *Staphylococcus aureus*

3. Classifications and causes: osteomyelitis is classified by the mode of entry as well as course of the disease

a. Entry

1) Hematogenous: bloodborne infection localized in bone

2) Direct entry: contamination through an open wound; most common form in adults

    b. Course

       1) Acute: less than 6 weeks

       2) Chronic: more than 6 to 8 weeks, can last years

B. Pathophysiology

  1. Entry of pathogen occurs; organism lodges in bone, multiplies, and initiates the inflammatory response

  2. As pus accumulates, pressure within the bone cavity increases, and blood supply to the area diminishes

  3. If the infection enters the chronic stage, infection spreads through the bone

  4. Bone cells become necrotic and break off into segments called sequestra

  5. Sequestra remain surrounded by pus and become a great medium for the spread of bacteria to surrounding bone tissue

  6. New bone formation, called involucrum, develops around the necrotic bone cells and sinus tract formation often occurs

  7. Signs and symptoms

    a. Hematogenous

       1) Acute onset of fever, chills, pain, and limited ROM at site of infection

       2) Involvement of **metaphysis** (growth plates located in the area of flaring between epiphysis [proximal and distal end of long bones] and **diaphysis** [shaft or long portion of long bones]) of tibia, humerus, or femur in children

       3) Involvement of vertebrae in adults

    b. Direct entry

       1) Afebrile or low-grade temperature

       2) Erythema, pain, tenderness at site of infection

C. Nursing assessment

  1. Health history

    a. Recent episode of *Staphylococcus* infection in children less than 10 years

    b. Illicit IV drug use

    c. Recent trauma, surgery, or puncture wound in adults

  2. Assessment includes determining drug allergies; pain assessment (abrupt onset of pain, guarding of affected site); vital signs (VS); discomfort; decreased ROM at affected site; wound drainage; and decreased activity level

  3. Diagnostic tests

    a. X-ray: no changes in early stages, elevation of **periosteum** (membrane covering the bone that contains nerve, lymph and blood vessels) and increased osteoclastic (bone cells responsible for the resorption of bony tissue) activity with disease progression

    b. Bone scan (positive for active infection)

    c. Computed tomography (CT) scan or magnetic resonance imaging (MRI) (positive for sinus tracts, abscesses, and may assist in determining boundaries of infection)

    d. ESR and WBC (elevated)

    e. Blood and tissue cultures (positive)

D. Nursing management

    1. Medications include: antibiotics as ordered, over-the-counter (OTC) analgesics or narcotic analgesics for pain relief

    2. Administer medications as ordered, assess therapeutic/nontherapeutic effects

    3. Implement and assess effectiveness of pain relief measures; immobilize the affected area

    4. Prevent the spread of infection

        a. Implement aseptic technique

        b. Instruct on the importance of proper handwashing

        c. Instruct on strict bedrest, mobility may mobilize bacteria

        d. Application of heat during acute infection is contraindicated; bacteria may spread as a result of vasodilatation

    5. Splint foot to prevent foot drop

    6. Pre-operative teaching as required for incision and drainage (I & D) of wound

    7. Instruct on nutritious diet for optimal wound healing

    8. Instruct on safety measures with use of assistive devices; crutches, walkers, wheelchair

VI. Paget's Disease (Osteitis Deformans)

A. Overview

    1. Defined as a chronic bone disease with inflammation of the bone; hypertrophy of long bones; and deformity of flat bones

    2. Characteristics

        a. Early diagnosis is important to arrest disease progression

        b. Occurs most commonly in spine, cranium, hip, pelvis, thighs, and lower extremities

    3. Cause is unknown, may be viral

    4. Long-term complications

        a. Heart failure secondary to increased demand for blood to achieve **bone remodeling** (formation of new bone by osteoblasts and removal of old bone by osteoclasts)

        b. Lung disease if ribs are involved

        c. Neurological deficits secondary to pressure on brain from enlarged cranium

        d. Increased incidence of sarcoma

NCLEX!

NCLEX!

NCLEX!

        e. Arthritis

        f. Renal calculi secondary to hypercalcemia

B. Pathophysiology

NCLEX!

    1. Osteolytic phase: characterized by rapid growth of abnormal osteoclasts; formation of new bone cannot occur at the same rate that bone resorption (destruction of bone) is taking place, and healthy bone is replaced with vascular, fibrous connective tissue

NCLEX!

    2. Osteoblastic sclerotic phase: bone deformities occur as bone eventually become enlarged, rough, thicker, and weaker; the bone assumes a mosaic pattern called cement lines

    3. Signs and symptoms

        a. May remain asymptomatic for years

        b. Bone pain is the most common symptom

NCLEX!

        c. Headache and hearing loss occur with involvement of the cranium

        d. Increased head size

NCLEX!

        e. Bowing of legs

        f. Fatigue

C. Nursing assessment

    1. Assessment

        a. Pain assessment: increasing pain with weight bearing may indicate long bone involvement; headaches may indicate cranial bone involvement

        b. Waddling gait

        c. Bone deformities: kyphosis, enlarged skull, and bowing of legs

        d. Decrease in height

        e. Cardiac assessment: hypertension (HTN) and arteriosclerosis

        f. Hearing or vision loss secondary to pressure on cranial nerves

        g. Pathological fractures

        h. Complaints of fatigue

    2. Diagnostic tests

        a. Serum alkaline phosphatase (elevated)

        b. Urine for hydroxyproline (elevated), an amino acid present in urine of clients with Paget's disease

        c. X-rays (reveal bone deformities, bone enlargement, widening of bone cortex)

        d. Bone scans (reveal active bone remodeling)

D. Nursing management

    1. Medications include NSAIDs; bone metabolism regulators: calcitonin (Calcimar); antineoplastic: plicamycin (Mithramycin)

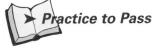

Practice to Pass

A client diagnosed with Paget's disease wants to know why physical therapy is needed. Relate the bone deformities common in clients with Paget's disease to the disease's pathophysiology.

2. Implement and assess effectiveness of pain relief measures

 a. Medications

 b. Collaborate with PT or OT regarding proper fitting for a brace or corset

 c. Heat and massage therapy

3. Assess therapeutic/nontherapeutic effects of medication therapy

4. Encourage client to remain active

5. Assess for signs and symptoms of hypercalcemia caused by increased osteoclast activity (fatigue, depression, mental confusion, nausea, vomiting, increased urination, and electrocardiogram [EKG] changes)

6. Instruct on safety to prevent pathological fractures

7. Instruct client to increase fluid intake 2L to 3L/day to prevent renal calculi unless contraindicated because of other conditions

8. Assist with adaptation to hearing or vision loss

VII. Muscular Dystrophy (MD)

A. Overview

1. Defined as a genetically transmitted disease that is progressive and involves specific muscles

2. Characteristics

 a. Condition includes several disease states characterized by progressive muscle wasting

 b. Has an insidious onset associated with progressive muscle weakness

3. Genetically transmitted by recessive gene on X-chromosome (mother to son) or spontaneous mutation form may occur in females

4. Classifications: there are several forms of the disease; characterized by age of onset, clinical manifestations, and disease progression

 a. Rapidly progressing: Duchenne's muscular dystrophy (DMD)

 1) X-linked recessive, onset usually by age 5

 2) Most common form

 b. Slower-progressing forms

 1) Becker's: onset 5 to 15 years of age; X-linked recessive

 2) Fascioscapulohumeral: onset 10 to 30 years; autosomal dominant

 3) Limb-girdle: onset 10 to 30 years; cause varies

B. Pathophysiology

1. Defect in gene that produces the protein dystrophin, which affects the contraction of muscles and is normally found next to the sarcolemma membrane

2. Muscle cells die, are phagocytized, and eventually replaced with fatty tissue

3. Muscle size increases causing pseudohypertrophy (false appearance of being enlarged), muscles become progressively weakened because of the fatty deposits and connective tissue that enters the muscle fibers

4. Signs and symptoms

   a. Duchenne's MD

      1) Symptoms present around 2 to 3 years of age with frequent falls

      2) Waddling gait and toe walking

      3) Pseudohypertrophy of muscles in lower extremities

      4) Kyphosis

      5) Progressive immobility, confined to wheelchair by teen years

      6) Death in early adulthood secondary to respiratory or cardiac failure

      7) Cardiac involvement in later stage of illness

   b. Becker's MD: generalized muscle involvement; normal life span

   c. Facioscapulo-humeral MD: face, neck, and shoulder muscles involved with muscle inflammation

   d. Limb-girdle MD: shoulder and pelvic muscle involvement; upper- and lower-extremity weakness in proximal muscles

C. Nursing assessment

1. Assessment includes: family history; gait and walking in toddlers; kyphosis in pre-teen years; muscle strength; history of recurrent URIs with aging

2. Diagnostic tests

   a. Serum creatinine phosphokinase (CPK), lactic dehydrogenase (LDH), glutamic transaminase, and glucose phosphate elevated

   b. Electromyograms (reveals decreased electrical signals within muscles)

   c. Muscle biopsy (muscle cell necrosis and scar tissue present)

   d. Prenatal testing for dystrophin gene for prevention

D. Nursing management

1. No medications are recommended

2. Access available resources and refer client and family to support groups

3. Prevent upper respiratory infections

4. Goal is to maintain mobility and prevent contractures

   a. Collaborate with PT regarding therapeutic exercise program

   b. Collaborate with OT regarding use of splints to prevent contractures

5. Instruct on safe use of wheelchair

6. Incorporate growth and developmental activities appropriate for age

VIII. Fibromyalgia

A. Overview

1. Defined as a condition of the muscles and joints resulting in chronic pain without evidence of arthritis

2. Characteristics

   a. Condition may be precipitated or aggravated by stress or exertion

   b. Onset is usually gradual, but it can occur suddenly

3. Cause: unknown etiology, may be associated with endocrine disorders, affective disorders and disturbances in sleep; may be acute or chronic

B. Pathophysiology

1. Unclear; inappropriate levels of neurotransmitters have been investigated

2. Lacks the characteristics of arthritis such as inflammation or structural changes in muscles or joints

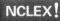

3. Signs and symptoms

   a. Muscle pain: local or generalized over entire body

   b. Most commonly occurs in the neck, shoulders, lower back, and hips

   c. Fatigue

   d. Headache

   e. Sleep disturbances, particularly lack of non-REM sleep (stage 4)

   f. Irritable bowel syndrome

   g. Muscle spasms

C. Nursing assessment

1. Assessment includes: pain, mobility, sleep patterns, sources of stress, bowel patterns, and psychosocial assessment

2. Diagnostic tests: physical exam and the presence of 11 consistent tender points; tests to rule out other disorders such as OA or RA may be performed

D. Nursing management

1. Medications include: NSAIDs for pain; tricyclic antidepressants for sleep such as amitriptyline (Elavil)

2. Encourage activity and assist with exercise program

3. Refer to support groups

4. Instruct on importance of rest

5. Stress management

6. Nutritious diet

IX. Bone Tumors

A. Overview

1. Defined as a tumor or neoplasm involving the skeletal tissue

2. Characteristics

   a. *Primary bone tumors:* originate in the bone; account for 1 percent of cancer in adults and 15 percent in children

      1) Commonly referred to as sarcomas

      2) Pathology may be malignant or benign

   b. *Metastatic bone tumors:* originate from a tumor somewhere else in the body

      1) Occurs more commonly than primary bone tumors

      2) Associated with primary cancer of the breast, lung, prostate, and kidney

      3) Usually located in the spine, pelvis, femur, humerus, or ribs

3. Osteosarcoma

   a. Primary malignant bone tumor characterized by rapid growth, etiology unknown

   b. Occur more frequently in males between the ages of 10 and 25 years, with the greatest incidence during teenage years

   c. Tissue of origin: metaphysis of long bones

   d. Common sites: distal femur, proximal tibia, and proximal humerus

   e. Frequently discovered following an injury

4. Chondrosarcoma

   a. Primary malignant bone tumor characterized by slow growth, etiology unknown

   b. Occurs more frequently in adult males

   c. Tissue origin: cartilage

   d. Common sites: pelvis, femur, and humerus

5. Ewing's sarcoma

   a. Primary malignant bone tumor characterized by rapid metastasis to lung tissue, etiology unknown

   b. Occurs between the ages of 10 and 25, with the greatest incidence in the teen years

   c. Tissue origin: nerve tissue within bone marrow

   d. Common sites: pelvis, humerus, femur, and ribs

B. Pathophysiology

1. Growth of neoplastic cells in tissue of origin causes **osteolysis** (softening and breakdown of bone)

2. Alteration in bone remodeling occurs, resulting in destruction of normal bone tissue

3. Enlargement of bony surfaces occurs with tumor growth; bones become weak, leaving the client at risk for pathological fractures

4. Structures surrounding bone tissue are invaded as neoplastic cells continue to multiply

5. Signs and symptoms vary based on the size and location of the tumor and include:

   a. Pain and swelling at site of tumor

   b. Decreased ROM

   c. Neuralgia secondary to nerve compression

   d. Palpable mass

   e. Pathological fractures

   f. Temperature

C. Nursing assessment

1. Assessment includes symptom analysis of pain or swelling at affected site, activity level, complaints of weakness; conduct health history to determine risk factors; palpate for masses; and assess vital signs

2. Diagnostic tests

   a. X-rays

      1) Benign tumors: well-defined tumor margins

      2) Malignant tumors: undefined tumor borders, extension of tumor beyond bone structure

   b. CT scan and MRI: can detect soft tissue sarcomas not detected on X-ray; they also identify the location of the tumor, extent of tumor growth, as well as metastases

   c. Bone scans

   d. Bone biopsy

   e. Serum calcium and serum alkaline phosphatase: elevated

   f. Red blood count (RBC): elevated

NCLEX!

D. Nursing management

1. Medications include nonopioid and opioid analgesics (codeine products); and chemotherapy prior to surgery

2. Implement and assess effectiveness of pain relief measures

   a. Proper positioning

   b. Use of assistive devices for ambulation

NCLEX!

3. Instruct on safety in home

4. Provide rest periods between activities

5. Instruct on chemotherapy and radiation therapies as treatment options

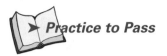

Practice to Pass

Identify the characteristics that differentiate osteosarcomas, chondrosarcomas, and Ewing's sarcomas.

6. Pre-operative teaching as required for the following surgeries: limb-salvage surgery (surgical removal of a bone tumor that prevents limb amputation) and limb amputation

7. Incorporate growth and developmental stage in nursing interventions

8. Collaborate with PT and/or OT regarding therapeutic exercise regime following surgery

9. Assist client and family in developing coping strategies in dealing with diagnosis and treatment plans and refer to cancer support groups

X. Systemic Lupus Erythematosus (SLE)

A. Overview

1. Defined as a chronic inflammatory, rheumatic, autoimmune disease, characterized by remissions and exacerbations

2. Characteristics

   a. Prognosis improves with early diagnosis and treatment

   b. May affect connective tissue of any body organ, disease progression varies from mild to severe depending on organ involvement

3. Classifications

   a. *Drug-induced lupus:* associated with use of procainamide (Procan SR), hydralazine (Apresoline), isoniazid (INH), and some antiepileptic drugs; symptoms usually subside after the drugs are discontinued

   b. *Discoid lupus:* limited to involvement of the skin

   c. *Systemic lupus:* involvement of one or more of the following systems: musculoskeletal, lungs, kidneys, CNS, cardiovascular, hematological

4. Causes

   a. Infections from leukemia and renal failure are major causes of mortality

   b. Etiology is unknown but may be attributed to: exposure to ultra-violet rays, genetic defect, or hormonal imbalance (which may explain increased incidence during pregnancy)

B. Pathophysiology

1. The body produces autoantibodies, specifically against DNA, secondary to hyperactivity of B-cells

2. These autoantibodies combine with antigens to form immune complexes; accumulation of immune complexes within connective tissue triggers the inflammatory response

3. Chronic inflammation destroys connective tissue; tissue damage varies with organ involvement

4. Signs and symptoms

   a. May be unpredictable and vary with organs involved

   b. General presenting symptoms include; fever, malaise, fatigue, weakness, and weight loss

    c. Musculoskeletal: polyarthralgia, symmetrical arthritis

    d. Integumentary: alopecia, butterfly rash, sclerosis of skin on fingers, discoid lesions

    e. Painless lesions in oral mucosa

    f. Cardiac: pericarditis

    g. Lungs: pleural effusions, pleuritis

    h. Kidney: glomerulonephritis, renal failure

    i. CNS: seizures, psychosis, cerebral vascular accident (CVA), senile dementias

    j. Hematological: anemia, leukopenia, and thrombocytopenia

    k. Infections

C. Nursing assessment

    1. Assessment includes conducting a health history to identify risk factors; complete drug history; nutrition (baseline weight and history of recent weight loss); skin assessment (rashes, hair loss, photosensitivity, ecchymosis and petechiae may indicate hematologic involvement); respiratory assessment (pleural effusion and pleuritis); renal assessment: obtain intake and output (I & O); neurological assessment (seizure activity, changes in affect and/or cognitive abilities); cardiovascular assessment (vital signs, signs and symptoms of pericarditis); musculoskeletal assessment (symmetrical joint pain, assess ability to participate in ADLs, history of weakness)

    2. Diagnostic tests

        a. X-ray of affected joints (will not show degenerative changes or bone deformities characteristic of arthritis)

        b. Serum syphilis (false positive)

        c. Serum antinuclear antibody (ANA) (positive), but this is not exclusive to SLE

        d. Anti-DNA antibody (positive), which is definitive for SLE

        e. Serum complement levels (decreased)

        f. CBC (positive for anemia, leukocytopenia, and/or thrombocytopenia)

        g. Urinalysis (UA): positive for proteinuria and/or hematuria

        h. Blood urea nitrogen (BUN) and creatinine (Cr): elevated

        i. ESR (elevated)

D. Nursing management

    1. Medications

        a. NSAIDs: used for treatment of joint pain

        b. Antimalarials: used for treatment of joint pain and skin disorders

        c. Corticosteroids: used during acute exacerbations, may also use a low-maintenance dose during remissions

        d. Immunosuppressive drugs: toxic drugs used during acute life-threatening exacerbations only

2. Instruct on disease process and treatment regimen

3. Instruct on factors that may trigger exacerbations

   a. Pregnancy: provide counseling regarding family planning and alternatives to birth control pills

   b. Exposure to UV rays: use sunscreen with sun protection factor (SPF) of 15, wear sun hats, avoid sunbathing, and use a beach umbrella

   c. Medication: avoid the use of birth control pills, sulfonamides, penicillin

4. Refer to support groups

5. Implement and assess effectiveness of joint pain relief measures

   a. Medications

   b. Application of heat

   c. Therapeutic exercise program

6. Administer medications as directed and assess therapeutic and nontherapeutic responses

   a. Educate about side effects of corticosteroids (cushingoid effects, HTN, weight gain)

   b. Advise regarding side effects of immunosuppressive drugs

   c. Blindness can occur with antimalarials; routine eye exams should be done

7. Instruct on importance of good nutrition

8. Instruct on handwashing and infection control in the home to prevent infection

9. Instruct on oral care

10. If alopecia occurs from the SLE, make referral for hair wig if appropriate to maintain positive body image

11. Assist family and client in developing coping strategies to deal with cognitive changes

12. Instruct family and client on appropriate safety interventions related to cognitive changes

XI. Scleroderma (Systemic Sclerosis)

A. Overview

1. Defined as a chronic, autoimmune, connective tissue disorder involving the skin and other organs, characterized by remissions and exacerbations

2. Classifications are systemic sclerosis, CREST syndrome, and limited

3. Unknown etiology; may include genetic, immune, or environmental factors

B. Pathophysiology

1. Unknown etiology

2. Overproduction of collagen leads to fibrosis and inflammation resulting in damage to affected area

3. Types of scleroderma

   a. *Systemic sclerosis* (SS): involvement of the skin of the fingers, hands, face, and trunk as well as visceral organs

      1) The most common visceral organs affected are esophagus, intestines, lungs, heart, and kidney

      2) May progress quickly and be life-threatening depending on extent of organ involvement

   b. *CREST syndrome:* acronym representing

      1) **Calcinosis** (abnormal deposits of calcium salts on the skin)

      2) Raynaud's syndrome

      3) Esophageal dysfunctions

      4) **Sclerodactyly** (scleroderma localized within fingers)

      5) **Telangiectasia** (small, dilated blood vessels with a bright-red center point and spikerlike branches)

      6) Prognosis is good and disability is limited

   c. Limited: involvement of the skin on the fingers, hands, and face; self-limiting with good prognosis

4. Signs and symptoms

   a. Skin

      1) Shiny, thick skin on the fingers, hands progressing to arms, trunk, and face

      2) Pursed lips

      3) Nonpitting edema of affected areas

      4) Calcium deposits on skin

      5) Telangiectasis

      6) Hyperpigmentation

   b. Vascular: Raynaud's syndrome

   c. Musculoskeletal: polyarthralgia and joint stiffness

   d. Esophageal: heartburn and dysphagia

   e. Intestinal: constipation, diarrhea, malabsorption, abdominal distention

   f. Heart: ECG changes, signs and symptoms of pericarditis

   g. Lungs: shortness of breath (SOB) on exertion

   h. Kidneys: renal failure

C. **Nursing assessment**

   1. Assessment

      a. Skin assessment

      b. Baseline height and weight; recent weight loss

    c. Gastrointestinal: dietary intake, bowel patterns, abdominal assessment, complaints of heartburn and dysphagia

    d. Musculoskeletal: decreased ROM in affected areas, complaints of polyarthalgia and joint stiffness, clawlike appearance of hands

    e. Respiratory assessment

    f. Cardiac: heart rate and rhythm, hypertension

    g. Renal: I & O

2. Diagnostic tests

    a. ESR (elevated)

    b. Urinalysis (proteinuria)

    c. BUN and Cr (elevated with renal failure)

    d. ANA (elevated)

    e. Skin biopsy (results indicate dermal collagen thickening, confirms diagnosis)

    f. Pulmonary function test (abnormal)

D. Nursing management

1. Medications

    a. NSAIDs for joint pain

    b. H_2 antagonists and proton pump inhibitors for gastrointestinal (GI) symptoms

    c. Beta blockers and calcium channel blockers to promote vasodilation

    d. Corticosteroids and immunosuppressive drugs are used in advanced life-threatening disease states

2. Instruct on disease process and treatment regimen

3. Refer to support groups

4. Musculoskeletal symptoms

    a. Collaborate with PT regarding therapeutic exercises to maintain joint mobility

    b. Collaborate with OT regarding assistive devices and ADL training

5. GI symptoms

    a. Consult dietitian for nutritional support

    b. Maintain high-Fowler's position during and following meals

    c. Small frequent meals

6. Raynaud's syndrome

    a. Instruct to avoid cold temperatures

    b. Wear gloves and socks to warm hands and improve circulation

    c. Avoid smoking

7. Skin care: instruct to inspect skin daily for breakdown and utilize skin moisturizers

XII. Fractures

A. Overview

1. Defined as a break in the bone, which occurs secondary to trauma or bone disease

2. Classifications: the location of the break, angle of the break, and/or relationship with external environment

   a. Relationship to external environment

   1) Open or compound: penetration of skin, bone protrudes through

   2) Closed: no penetration of bone through the skin

   b. Type of break

   1) Complete: bone broken all the way through

   2) Incomplete: partially broken or splintered

   c. Name of fracture

   1) Comminuted: bone shatters into pieces

   2) Compression: bone is crushed

   3) Impacted: ends of broken pieces are jammed together

   4) Spiral: bone twists and causes jagged break

   5) Greenstick: incomplete break

   6) Transverse: complete break at right angle to long axis of bone

3. A client may be able to move the affected area even though a fracture exists

4. Causes include accidents, trauma, motor vehicle accidents, abuse, neglect, and disease processes such as osteoporosis

B. Pathophysiology

1. Hematoma formation: bleeding occurs immediately following the fracture secondary to ruptured blood vessels within the bone and trauma to surrounding tissue; the presence of clotting factors within the hematoma leads to the formation of a fibrin mesh around the fracture site

2. Granulation tissue: during the first 48 to 72 hours, new capillary beds form and the proliferation of osteoblasts (bone cell responsible for formation of new bone) and fibroblast occurs within the hematoma

   a. Granulation tissue replaces the hematoma

   b. Phagocytosis also occurs and removes necrotic bone tissue

3. Callus formation: within a week the granulation tissue changes and becomes callus (composed of new cartilage, calcium, phosphorus, and osteoblasts)

   a. Callus becomes interlaced among bony fragments and delicately links the distal ends of the fracture

   b. Eventually callus formation extends beyond the fracture and serves as a temporary splint

NCLEX!

    c. The process continues leading to increase strengthening of the bone

    d. X-rays will confirm this stage of bone healing and help to determine the treatment regimen

  4. Ossification: formation of mature bone replaces callus; the delicate link between distal ends of the fracture solidifies and a strong connection is restored

  5. Remodeling: osteoclasts resorb excess callus and the bone returns to pre-injury strength and shape

  6. Signs and symptoms

    a. Pain and muscle spasms

    b. Asymmetrical appearance of limb secondary to bone displacement

    c. Numbness and or tingling at affected site secondary to nerve compression

    d. Loss of function

    e. Edema secondary to tissue trauma

    f. Crepitus with movement

C. Nursing assessment

  1. Assessment includes

    a. Subjective data describing the event

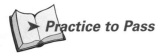

Practice to Pass

A 10-year-old client diagnosed with a fractured humerus is discharged from the Emergency Department after application of a cast. Develop a teaching plan for the child and significant other regarding cast care.

    b. Conducting a pain assessment, assess for guarding of affected site

    c. Loss of function

    d. Crepitus

    e. Edema, ecchymosis, and tenderness at affected site

    f. Presence of pulses

    g. Asymmetrical appearance

  2. Diagnostic test: X-ray will confirm fracture

D. Nursing management

  1. Medications include analgesics to control pain, antibiotics for open fracture

  2. Emergency nursing care: immobilize the fracture, control bleeding, and clean the wound

  3. Assess five Ps (see Figure 5-1)

  4. Teach action and side effects of medications; obtain consent for operation prior to medicating, if surgery is pending

  5. Pre-operative teaching as required for the following surgeries

    a. Closed reduction

    b. Open reduction

  6. Instruct on safety and use of assistive devices

  7. Elevate the extremity and apply an ice pack to relieve edema

Figure 5-1

5 Ps in assessing circulation.

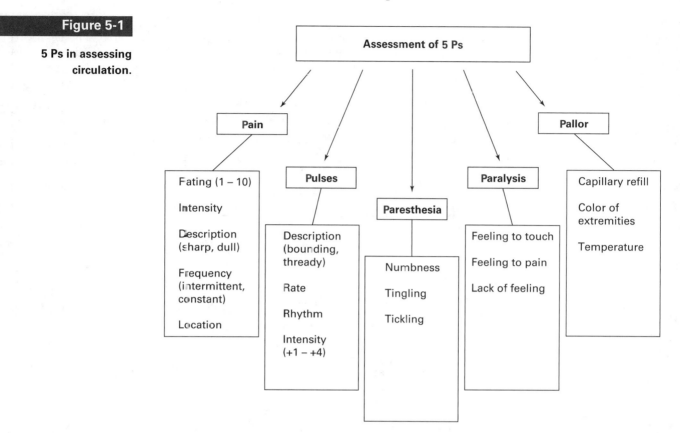

Figure 5-1

5 Ps in assessing circulation.

8. Assess and provide client teaching on prevention of hazards of immobility

9. Recognize and treat early complications

    a. Hypovolemic shock

    b. Fat emboli (petechial rash, tacycardia, tachcepnia)

    c. Deep vein thrombosis

    d. Compartment syndrome (see below)

10. Instruct on cast care if applicable (see Box 5-3)

11. Provide traction care if applicable (see Box 5-4)

12. Maintain nutritional status

XIII. Compartment Syndrome

    A. Overview

        1. Defined as muscle and nerve damage related to excessive swelling in the area of a fracture

Box 5-3

Teaching Tips for Clients with Casts

- During the first 24 hours after application of the cast, apply ice directly over the fracture, elevate the extremity, and promote drying of the cast by leaving it exposed to air and supporting it on pillows.
- Report any of the following symptoms to your healthcare provider: increased pain, change in color, coolness of extremity, lack of movement, or numbness and tingling.
- Do not place any item in the cast; use a blowdryer on the cool setting to relieve itching.
- Keep plaster casts dry at all times; cover with plastic during bathing.
- Fiberglass casts may get wet; be sure to dry them completely with a blowdryer on cool setting.
- Report drainage or cast odor to your healthcare provider.

   2. Classifications

      a. *Acute:* occurs following a crushing injury or bone fracture, when a cast has been applied

      b. *Chronic:* occurs most frequently in young adults who participate in activities that require repetitive motion, causing excessive strain on the lower extremities; for example, long-distance running

   B. Pathophysiology

      1. Two factors leading to compartment syndrome

      a. Hemorrhage and edema occur following a fracture, causing a reduction in the ability of the **fascia** (fibrous connective tissue responsible for supporting and connecting structures of the musculoskeletal system) to accommodate excessive edema

      b. A closed compartment may be created with application of a tightly fitting external dressing, splint, or cast, which causes increased pressure on the limb

      2. As pressure within the compartment increases, both venous and arterial circulation become obstructed and tissue perfusion is diminished

      3. Consequently, tissue ischemia, loss of function, and nerve damage occur; pressures of 30 mmHg or more can result in permanent muscle and nerve damage

NCLEX!

Box 5-4

Nursing Implications for Clients Receiving Traction

- Maintain correct alignment at all times.
- All weights should clear the floor at all times.
- Inspect the skin at pressure points for skin breakdown.
- Implement skin care measures that prevent skin breakdown.
- Implement nursing interventions that prevent hazards of immobility.
- Inspect pin sites for signs and symptoms of infection.
- Provide pin care according to agency policy.

4. Signs and symptoms

    a. Severe pain unrelieved by analgesics

    b. Paresthesis

    c. Loss of function and decreased reflexes

    d. Pallor, extremity cool to touch

    e. Pulse may or may not be present

C. Nursing assessment

    1. Assessment

        a. Symptom analysis of pain

        b. Neurovascular checks following fractures; pulses may be present during early stages of compartment syndrome

        c. Assess external dressings, splint, or cast for tightness

        d. Excessive edema at fracture site

    2. Diagnostic tests: no tests are recommended

D. Nursing management

    1. Medications include analgesics for pain

    2. Notify physician

    3. Elevate extremity and apply ice immediately to increase venous return and decrease edema

    4. Remove or loosen constrictive dressings and or splint, assist with bivalving the cast if directed

    5. Conduct pre-operative teaching as indicated for a fasciotomy (surgical procedure to cut and divide a fascia)

XIV. Osteoporosis

    A. Overview

        1. Defined as a musculoskeletal disorder characterized by loss of bone mass

        2. Disease process predisposes clients to fractures

        3. Classifications

            a. *Type I:* associated with early postmenopausal estrogen deficiency

            b. *Type II:* senile osteoporosis associated with calcium deficiency

        4. Cause related to endocrine disorder, malignancy, or the aging process

    B. Pathophysiology

        1. The disease process is characterized by an increase in the activity of osteoclasts and a decrease in the activity of osteoblasts; this leads to bone resorption that exceeds bone formation

        2. The outer cortex (outer surface of the bone composed of hard, cortical bone) of the diaphysis and metaphysis becomes thinner secondary to enlargement of bone

3. Advanced disease process leads to loss of trabeculae (spongy bone containing red bone marrow located in the area of the metaphysis of long bones) from cancellous (spongy bone located towards the interior of the bone containing red or yellow bone marrow) bone and thinning of the cortex; these changes in bone structure increase the risk of a client experiencing a bone fracture

4. Signs and symptoms: loss of height, kyphosis, low back pain, fractures of the forearm, spine, and hip

C. Nursing assessment

1. Assessment includes analysis of possible risk factors; height (pattern of decrease); pain assessment; and any recent fractures

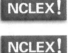

2. Diagnostic test: bone density studies; X-rays (will not show changes in bone mass until a loss greater than 30 percent exists)

D. Nursing management

1. Medications include calcium supplements; estrogen therapy replacement in postmenopausal women

2. Instruct clients at risk and those diagnosed on the following:

   a. Implement an exercise regimen that incorporates weight bearing exercises; jogging, walking, rowing, and weight lifting

   b. Instruct on adequate calcium intake through diet or supplements

      1) Premenopausal women 1,000 mg/day

      2) Postmenopausal women 1,500 mg/day

   c. Instruct elderly clients at risk on safety with ambulation in home (see Box 5-1)

Case Study

A 45-year-old client sustains fractures of the right leg and arm because of a motor vehicle accident. The client is treated in the Emergency Department and then admitted to an orthopedic unit for observation.

❶ What are the priorities of care at the scene of the accident?

❷ Outline the nursing care of the client after casts are placed on the right arm and leg.

❸ What discharge instructions should the nurse give to the client?

❹ Forty-eight hours after the accident, the client complains of excruciating pain in his right arm unrelieved by analgesics. What complication should the nurse suspect?

❺ What are the priorities of care?

For suggested responses, see page 566.

Posttest

1. To determine if a client is experiencing compartment syndrome, which of the following is a priority area for nursing assessment?

   (1) Assessing for edema at the fracture site
   (2) Palpating pulse at the fracture site
   (3) Performing a pain assessment
   (4) Assessing for the presence of drainage on the cast

2. Beta blockers are given to clients with scleroderma to treat which of the following symptoms?

   (1) Telangiectasis
   (2) Pericarditis
   (3) Bradycardia
   (4) Raynaud's phenomenon

3. Which of the following lab values is most significant when assessing complications associated with Paget's disease?

   (1) Calcium level of 15 mg/dL
   (2) Positive RF factor
   (3) Blood urea nitrogen (BUN) of 140 mg/dL
   (4) Eosinophil sedimentation rate (ESR) of 30 mm/hr

4. Which of the following statements applies to Ewing's sarcoma?

   (1) Occurs most frequently in men between the ages of 20 and 40 years of age
   (2) Is a primary bone tumor characterized by rapid growth and lung metatastisis
   (3) Is a metatastic bone tumor that occurs secondary to colon cancer
   (4) Usually originates in bone cartilage

5. The pathophysiology underlying gouty arthritis may be attributed to:

   (1) Increased immune complexes within the joint cavity.
   (2) An alteration in purine metabolism resulting in hyperuricemia.
   (3) Excessive bone remodeling secondary to increased levels of phosphorus.
   (4) The presence of fibrous adhesions within bony cartilage.

6. A client is diagnosed with osteomyelitis involving the foot. The highest priority during the implementation of nursing care is:

   (1) Maintaining adequate pain control.
   (2) Implementing aseptic technique.
   (3) Promoting adequate nutrition.
   (4) Splinting the foot to prevent foot drop.

7. When counseling the parents of a child diagnosed with muscular dystrophy, which of the following statements most accurately describes the disease progression?

   (1) "Prognosis is favorable with early detection."
   (2) "With aggressive physical therapy and the use of a walker, your child will remain ambulatory through adulthood."
   (3) "The muscles and the lungs may also become involved, and this can shorten your child's lifespan."
   (4) "Muscle weakness is progressive and rapid, and your child will most likely be confined to a wheelchair by the age of 5."

8. Which of the following statements best describes the underlying pathology of osteoarthritis (OA)?

   (1) Changes in the composition of the articular cartilage contribute to increased friction during joint movement.
   (2) Joint inflammation occurs secondary to the presence of immune complexes within the joint cavity.
   (3) Excessive bone necrosis within the joint occurs secondary to increased osteoclastic activity.
   (4) Bone damage occurs secondary to osteolysis and excessive bone remodeling.

9 In the early treatment of rhumatoid arthritis (RA), which of the following drugs would the nurse expect to be included in the client's drug regime?

(1) Non-steroidal antiinflammatory drugs (NSAIDs)
(2) Systemic corticosteroids
(3) Disease modifying anti-rheumatoidal drugs (DMARDs)
(4) NSAIDs and DMARDs

10 Which of the following statements best describes the pathophysiology underlying osteoporosis? The disease process is related to:

(1) Increased amounts of estrogen in postmenopausal women.
(2) A decrease in osteoblasts and an increase in osteoclasts.
(3) A decrease in blood supply to the bone resulting in bony necrosis.
(4) Invasion of a pathogen leading to osteolysis of bone.

See pages 199–200 for Answers and Rationales.

Answers and Rationales

Pretest

1 **Answer: 3** *Rationale:* Aerobic exercises such as swimming help the client to maintain maximum range of motion (ROM) and mobility while minimizing strain on joints. Isotonic exercises such as tennis, jogging, and volleyball place excessive strain on diseased joints.
Cognitive Level: Application
Nursing Process: Evaluation; Test Plan: HPM

2 **Answer: 4** *Rationale:* Swan neck deformities of the hand are classic deformities associated with rheumatoid arthritis secondary to the presence of fibrous connective tissue within the joint space. Clients with RA do experience morning stiffness, but it can last from 30 minutes up to several hours. RA is characterized by symmetrical joint involvement, and Heberden's nodes are characteristic of osteoarthritis.
Cognitive Level: Application
Nursing Process: Assessment; *Test Plan:* PHYS

3 **Answer: 3** *Rationale:* Aspirin interferes with the action of uricosuric drugs. Acetaminophen, naproxen, or ibuprofen may be used effectively as an analgesic in the treatment of pain associated with acute gout, and they do not interfere with the action of uricosuric drugs.
Cognitive Level: Application
Nursing Process: Implementation; *Test Plan:* SECE

4 **Answer: 1** *Rationale:* Options 2, 3, and 4 are appropriate nursing interventions when caring for a client diagnosed with osteomyelitis. The application of heat can increase edema and pain in the affected area and spread bacteria through vasodilatation.
Cognitive Level: Application
Nursing Process: Implementation; *Test Plan:* SECE

5 **Answer: 4** *Rationale:* Serum alkaline phosphatase is elevated because of increased activity of bone cells. Inflammation is in the bone and usually doesn't reveal an elevated serum WBC, ESR, or the presence of *Staphylococcus*.
Cognitive Level: Application
Nursing Process: Assessment; *Test Plan:* PHYS

6 **Answer: 4** *Rationale:* Osteosarcomas are most commonly seen in males during optimal growth years. Middle-aged males (option 1), females age 50 to 60 (option 2), and females of childbearing age (option 3) are less likely to develop osterosarcoma.
Cognitive Level: Application
Nursing Process: Assessment; *Test Plan:* HPM

7 **Answer: 1** *Rationale:* Although the etiology of SLE is unknown, certain environmental factors have been associated with the onset of symptoms. The administration of procainamide (Procan SR) and hydralazine (Apresoline) have been associated with SLE symptoms, which usually subside after the drug is discontinued.
Cognitive Level: Application
Nursing Process: Analysis; *Test Plan:* PHYS

8 **Answer: 1** *Rationale:* Raynaud's disease is characterized by spasms of the blood vessels within the fingers of the hands resulting in diminished circulation. Gloves protect the hands from cold temperatures and provide warmth, which promotes blood flow to the affected areas. Raynaud's syndrome is in the CREST syndrome, a type of scleroderma.
Cognitive Level: Application
Nursing Process: Implementation; *Test Plan:* PHYS

9 **Answer: 3** *Rationale:* During earlier stages of bone healing, overproduction of callus enlarges the bone and acts as a splint. Callus is eventually replaced with mature bone during the ossification phase of bone healing, and then the excess callus is resorbed during the remodeling phase to return the bone to its original shape.
Cognitive Level: Comprehension
Nursing Process: Analysis; *Test Plan:* PHYS

10 **Answer: 1** *Rationale:* Edema is expected immediately following a fracture, but because the fascia is non-elastic, excessive swelling will lead to increased capillary pressure within the area resulting in nerve and muscle damage if left untreated. Damage is irreversible if the capillary pressure reaches 30 mmHg. A pulse may still be present during early stages of compartment syndrome. One factor that can differentiate pain associated with trauma from the fracture, and that from compartment syndrome, is the ineffectiveness of analgesics when compartment syndrome occurs.
Cognitive Level: Comprehension
Nursing Process: Analysis; *Test Plan:* PHYS

Posttest

1 **Answer: 3** *Rationale:* Although assessing for edema, pulses, and the presence of drainage is important in the care of a client with a fracture, pain unrelieved by analgesics is the symptom most indicative of compartment syndrome.
Cognitive Level: Analysis
Nursing Process: Assessment; *Test Plan:* SECE

2 **Answer: 4** *Rationale:* When clients with scleroderma develop Raynaud's phenomenon, which is characterized by vasospasms of the arteries and veins of the hands, beta blockers are the treatment of choice. Bradycardia is not specific to scleroderma. Clients may experience pericarditis, but this is not treated with beta blockers.
Cognitive Level: Application
Nursing Process: Implementation; *Test Plan:* PHYS

3 **Answer: 1** *Rationale:* Hypercalcemia (option 1) can occur as a complication of Paget's disease secondary to increased osteoclast activity. The other tests are not specific to Paget's disease, although they are all abnormal values.
Cognitive Level: Application
Nursing Process: Assessment; *Test Plan:* PHYS

4 **Answer: 2** *Rationale:* Ewing's sarcoma is a primary bone tumor associated with rapid metastasis to the lung. It occurs most frequently in males during optimal growth periods.
Cognitive Level: Application
Nursing Process: Analysis; *Test Plan:* PHYS

5 **Answer: 2** *Rationale:* The pathophysiology of gouty arthritis is related to overproduction or decreased excretion of uric acid in the primary form. The other options are incorrect.
Cognitive Level: Application
Nursing Process: Analysis; *Test Plan:* PHYS

6 **Answer: 2** *Rationale:* Although all the items listed are important in the plan of care for the client diagnosed with osteomyelits, maintaining aseptic technique and preventing the spread of infection is crucial to resolving the disease process. Maslow's hierarchy may identify option 1 as highest priority, but infection is the cause of the pain. Think of what causes the problem and deal with that first in a question like this one.
Cognitive Level: Analysis
Nursing Process: Implementation; *Test Plan:* PHYS

7 **Answer: 3** *Rationale:* Symptoms of muscular dystrophy usually manifest themselves in the toddler years. The child has a waddling gait and experiences frequent falls. There is no cure for the disease, and as muscles become progressively weak. Most children are confined to a wheelchair by the teen years. As the disease progresses, heart and lung muscle are affected, resulting in cardiac and pulmonary failure. These complications frequently occur by the age of 20.
Cognitive Level: Application
Nursing Process: Analysis; *Test Plan:* PHYS

8 **Answer: 1** *Rationale:* Articular cartilage is responsible for decreasing friction during joint movement and displacing the force of the workload onto the subchondral bone. In OA, the composition of the articular cartilage is changed because of a malfunction in the production in proteoglycans. Consequently, the articular cartilage can no longer perform its original function.
Cognitive Level: Comprehension
Nursing Process: Analysis; *Test Plan:* PHYS

9 Answer: 4 *Rationale:* DMARDs are now being used earlier in the treatment regime for RA because evidence suggests that they may play a role in arresting the disease process. NSAIDs are used in combination with this drug classification for pain management. Systemic corticosteroids are not used until NSAIDs are no longer effective because of the severe side effects associated with their use.
Cognitive Level: Application
Nursing Process: Implementation; *Test Plan:* PHYS

10 Answer: 2 *Rationale:* Osteoporosis is characterized by excessive bone resorption that exceeds the body's ability to produce new bone. It is more prevalent in postmenopausal women with low levels of estrogen. A decrease in the number and activity of osteoblasts and an increase in the number and activity of osteoclasts occurs.
Cognitive Level: Application
Nursing Process: Analysis; *Test Plan:* PHYS

References

Arthritis Foundation (2001). DMARDs. Retrieved on June 24, 2001: http://www.arthritis.org/answers/drugguide/dmars.asp

Bancroft, D. & Piggs, J. (1998). Alterations in skeletal function: rheumatic disorders. In C. Porth (Ed.), *Pathophysiology: Concepts of altered health states* (5th ed.). Philadelphia: Lippincott, pp. 1121–1144.

Bush, M. (2000). Nursing management of arthritis and connective tissue diseases. In S. Lewis, M. Heitkemper, & S. Dirkson (Eds.), *Medical-surgical nursing: Assessment and management of clinical problems* (5th ed.). St. Louis, MO: Mosby.

Corwin, E. (2000). *Handbook of pathophysiology* (2nd ed.). Baltimore: Lippincott Williams & Wilkins, pp. 319–321.

Gunta, K. (2002). Alterations in skeletal function: Congenital disorders, metabolic bone disease, and neoplasms. In C. Porth (Ed.), *Pathophysiology: Concepts of altered health states* (6th ed.). Philadelphia: Lippincott, pp. 1109–1111.

Gunta, K. (2002). Alterations in skeletal function: Trauma and infection. In C. Porth (Ed.), *Pathophysiology: Concepts of altered health states* (6th ed.). Philadelphia: Lippincott, pp. 1079–1094.

Jenkins, D. (1998). Organ and organ systems. *Hollinshead's functional anatomy of the limbs and back* (7th ed.), Philadelphia: W.B. Saunders, pp.17–23.

LeMone, P. & Burke, K. (2000). *Medical surgical nursing: Critical thinking in client care* (2nd ed.). Upper Saddle River, NJ: Prentice Hall, pp. 1511–1526, 1572–1616.

Ruda, S. (2002). Nursing assessment: Musculoskeletal system. In S. Lewis, M. Heitkemper, & S. Dirkson (Eds.), *Medical-surgical nursing: Assessment and management of clinical problems* (5th ed.). St. Louis, MO: Mosby, pp. 1762–1818.

Thomas, C. L. (Ed.). (2000). *Taber's cyclopedic medical dictionary* (19th ed.). Philadelphia: F. A. Davis.

Wilson, B. A., Shannon, M. T., & Stang, C. L. (2001). *Nursing drug guide: 2001.* Upper Saddle River, NJ: Prentice Hall.

CHAPTER 6

Eye, Ear, Nose, and Throat Health Problems

Diane Smith, MSN, RN

CHAPTER OUTLINE

OBJECTIVES

▌ Define key terms associated with eye, ear, nose, and throat health problems.

▌ Identify risk factors associated with the development of eye, ear, nose, and throat health problems.

▌ Discuss the common etiologies of eye, ear, nose, and throat health problems.

▌ Describe the pathophysiologic processes associated with specific eye, ear, nose, and throat health problems.

▌ Distinguish between normal and abnormal eye, ear, nose, and throat findings obtained from nursing assessment.

▌ Prioritize nursing interventions associated with specific eye, ear, nose, and throat health problems.

[Media Link]

Use the CD-ROM enclosed with this text, or log onto the address given to access the free, interactive Companion Website created for this series. The CD-ROM and Companion Website accompanying this book offer additional practice opportunities and information—NCLEX Review, Case Studies, Glossary, In Depth with NCLEX, and more.

www.prenhall.com/hogan

REVIEW AT A GLANCE

audiometry *test used to evaluate the ability to hear pure tones of varying intensity*

Caldwell-Luc procedure *procedure used to treat epistaxis and chronic sinusitis involving entry into the maxillary sinus through an incision under the upper lip; when used for epistaxis, involves ligating the artery responsible for bleeding; when used for sinusitis, allows for creation of a window to increase aeration of the sinus and promote drainage*

cholesteatoma *an inflamed cyst or mass filled with epithelial cells and debris that remains infected, enlarges, and may destroy the ossicles, causing permanent hearing loss; results from chronic otitis media*

endolymph *pale, transparent fluid within the membranous labyrinth*

gonioscopy *test used to measure the depth of the anterior chamber of the eye; used to differentiate open-angle from narrow (angle-closure) glaucoma*

intraocular pressure (IOP) *pressure of the aqueous humor within the eye; normally ranges from 12 to 20 mmHg*

labyrinth *term used to describe the inner ear; composed of two parts: the bony labyrinth, a system of open channels that houses the second part, the membranous labyrinth; the bony labyrinth contains the vestibule, semicircular canals, and the cochlea*

laryngectomy *removal of all or part of the larynx; partial laryngectomy is used for tumors confined to a specific portion of the larynx; supraglottic laryngectomy is used for tumors located above the glottis (true vocal cords); total laryngectomy involves removal of the entire larynx and surrounding structures and is used for tumors extending beyond the vocal cords; permanent tracheostomy is always required following total laryngectomy*

miotic *pharmacological agents that cause pupil constriction*

mydriatic *pharmacological agents that cause pupil dilation*

myringotomy *incision into the tympanic membrane to relieve pressure; also known as tympanocentesis*

nystagmus *involuntary, rapid movements of the eye*

otosclerosis *familial condition of the stapes (ossicles of the middle ear) characterized by resorption of bone followed by overgrowth of new, hard sclerotic bone; sclerotic changes impact the stapes and oval window and impair sound transmission into the inner ear*

presbycusis *age-related loss of ability to hear high-frequency sounds; may impair the ability to hear normal speech*

Rinne test *test done by alternately placing a tuning fork on the mastoid bone and in front of the ear canal to compare air and bone conduction; with conductive hearing loss, bone conduction is greater than air conduction; with sensorineural loss, the opposite results are noted*

stapedectomy *surgical removal and replacement of diseased stapes to restore hearing*

tonometry *indirect measure of intraocular pressure using contact or noncontact methods*

tympanocentesis *aspiration of fluid/pus from the middle ear using a needle*

tympanometry *also known as impedance audiometry; an indirect measurement of the compliance of the middle ear to sound transmission; an audiometer with a sealed probe tip is used to deliver a continuous tone to the tympanic membrane; an instrument records the energy reflected from the surface of the membrane; compliance is reduced in the presence of effusions in the middle ear*

tympanoplasty *surgical reconstruction of the ossicles and tympanic membrane of the middle ear to help restore hearing*

Weber test *diagnostic test using a tuning fork held against the midline of the top of the head to differentiate conductive hearing loss from sensorineural hearing loss*

Pretest

1 A client has just been diagnosed with closed-angle (narrow-angle or acute angle-closure) glaucoma. The nurse assesses the client for which of the following most common presenting symptoms of this disorder?

(1) Halo vision
(2) Dull eye pain
(3) Severe eye and face pain
(4) Impaired night vision

2 The nurse notes a cloudy appearance to the lens of an 80-year-old client's eye. Which of the following additional assessment findings would help confirm the diagnosis of cataracts?

(1) Sense of a curtain falling over the visual field
(2) Persistent, dull eye pain
(3) Loss of red reflex
(4) Double vision

3 The priority nursing measure for the client with a penetrating eye injury from a visible foreign body is to:

(1) Patch both eyes.
(2) Immobilize the foreign body and cover the eye.
(3) Irrigate the eye with copious amounts of water.
(4) Administer carbonic anhydrase inhibitors as prescribed.

4 A client is diagnosed with conductive hearing loss and asks how this occurred. The nurse should respond by stating that conductive hearing loss:

(1) Has an unknown etiology.
(2) Occurs as a result of damage to the hair cells of the inner ear.
(3) Usually results from chronic exposure to loud noise.
(4) Occurs as a result of damage to the ear structures.

5 A client with sensorineural hearing loss should be assessed using which of the following?

(1) Tympanocentesis
(2) Transillumination of the sinuses
(3) Electronystagmography
(4) Weber and Rinne tests

6 The teaching plan for the parents of an infant with acute otitis media should include which of the following?

(1) Antibiotics can be discontinued when the infant is afebrile.
(2) When bottle-feeding, the infant should be maintained in an upright position.
(3) Orange juice and other fruit juices should be eliminated from the diet.
(4) Cigarette smoke in the home is not a significant risk factor in acute otitis media.

7 The nurse developing a teaching plan for a client with atrophic macular degeneration should include information concerning:

(1) Surgical treatment options.
(2) The availability of aids to enhance vision and promote safety.
(3) The risks associated with the loss of peripheral vision.
(4) Antibiotic therapy.

8 Which of the following ophthalmic medications would be indicated for the client with open-angle glaucoma?

(1) Pilocarpine (Pilocar)
(2) Scopolamine hydrobromide (Hyoscine)
(3) Atropine sulfate (Isopto Atropine)
(4) Epinephrine (Epitrate)

9 A 60-year-old male presents to the clinic complaining of hoarseness and a cough. His spouse states his voice has changed in the last few months. The nurse interprets that the client's symptoms are consistent with which of the following disorders?

(1) Gastroesophageal reflux disease (GERD)
(2) Coronary artery disease (CAD)
(3) Laryngeal cancer
(4) Chronic sinusitis

10 The priority postoperative nursing action following nasal packing for epistaxis is:

(1) Providing frequent oral care.
(2) Ensuring adequate intake of oral fluids.
(3) Monitoring respiratory function and oxygen saturation.
(4) Administering analgesics as prescribed.

See pages 228–229 for Answers and Rationales.

I. Risk Factors Associated with Eye, Ear, Nose, and Throat Health Problems

A. Glaucoma: advancing age, ethnicity, diabetes, and family history

B. Cataracts: advancing age, tobacco smoking associated with alcohol consumption, exposure to ultraviolet light, ocular trauma, and family history

C. **Eye injury:** environmental and workplace hazards, motor vehicle accidents, sports injuries, and physical assault

D. **Macular degeneration:** advancing age, family history, and nutritional factors have been implicated

E. **Retinal detachment:** advancing age and trauma (i.e., sudden blows to the head)

F. **Sensorineural hearing impairment:** advancing age, ototoxic medications, and persistent exposure to loud noise

G. **Conductive hearing impairment:** otosclerosis, infections of the external or middle ear, trauma to the tympanic membrane and middle ear

H. **Otitis media:** age (i.e., common in infants and children), upper respiratory infections, and allergies

I. **Meniere's disease:** age (i.e., increased incidence in middle-age) and family history

J. **Epistaxis:** nasal trauma (i.e., blunt trauma or mild irritation from manipulation), nasal allergies, substance abuse (i.e., cocaine) sinusitis, upper respiratory infections (URI), nasal allergies, tobacco smoking, use of oxygen, certain climates or altitudes, prescription medications, and anatomic variations (i.e., deviated nasal septum, nasal polyps)

K. **Laryngeal cancer:** tobacco smoking, alcohol consumption associated with tobacco smoking, occupational exposure to chemicals and toxins, and family history

II. Glaucoma

A. Overview

1. Defined as a group of conditions characterized by increased **intraocular pressure (IOP);** if untreated, it results in ischemia and degeneration of the retina and optic nerve, loss of vision, and complete blindness

2. Normal intraocular pressure ranges from 12 to 20 mmHg

3. Caused by alterations in the circulation and resorption of aqueous humor

4. Classified as *open-angle* (wide-angle) or *closed-angle* (narrow-angle or acute-angle closure)

5. Manifests as a *primary* or *secondary* disorder and may be congenital or acquired

   a. Primary glaucoma occurs without evidence of preexisting eye or systemic disease

   b. Secondary glaucoma results from inflammatory processes, tumors, long-term steroid use, or ocular trauma

B. Pathophysiology

1. Aqueous humor serves to maintain IOP and support metabolism of the lens and posterior cornea

2. The formation/secretion of aqueous humor is an active process that begins at the ciliary body (ciliary epithelium) in the posterior chamber; aqueous humor flows through the pupil into the anterior chamber; resorption into the venous system occurs through the trabecular meshwork of the anterior chamber into the Canal of Schlemm (Figure 6-1)

Figure 6-1

Internal structures of the eye.

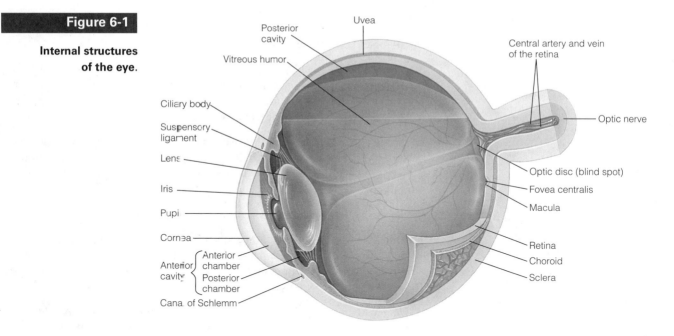

Posterior cavity

Uvea

Central artery and vein of the retina

Vitreous humor

Ciliary body

Suspensory ligament

Lens

Iris

Pupil

Cornea

Anterior cavity { Anterior chamber / Posterior chamber }

Canal of Schlemm

Optic nerve

Optic disc (blind spot)

Fovea centralis

Macula

Retina

Choroid

Sclera

3. Open-angle (wide-angle) glaucoma

   a. Etiology is unclear; there is no obstruction between the trabecular meshwork and the anterior chamber

   b. May occur because of an abnormality of the trabecular meshwork (network) that impairs flow of aqueous humor into the Canal of Schlemm; the resulting increased pressure in the anterior chamber causes increased pressure in the posterior chamber

   c. Usually affects both eyes, has a genetic component, and is frequently seen in adults over 60 years of age

   d. Onset is insidious with no symptoms in the early stages

   e. Signs and symptoms include tunnel vision (an initial symptom), pain (persistent, dull eye pain, lasting over 20 minutes), halo and/or blurred vision, inability to detect colors

4. Closed-angle (narrow-angle or acute-angle closure) glaucoma

   a. An *acute medical emergency* resulting in narrowing of the angle between the pupil and lateral cornea resulting in impaired outflow of aqueous humor

   b. Symptoms relate to sudden, intermittent increases in IOP and may occur following prolonged sitting in a darkened room, during emotional upset or stress, or any condition causing prolonged pupil dilation

   c. Often unilateral; other eye may be affected at a later time and accounts for only 5 to 10 percent of the cases

   d. Signs and symptoms include sudden, severe eye pain, severe headache accompanied by nausea and vomiting (may be confused with migraine), blurred vision and/or complaints of halos around lights, redness of the eye, haziness (steaminess) of the cornea, and dilated pupil that is nonreactive to light

C. Nursing assessment

1. Open-angle (wide-angle) glaucoma

   a. Assessment includes eye examination for loss of peripheral vision, tunnel vision or complaints of seeing halos around lights; ability to focus on near objects or differentiate colors, symptom analysis of headaches and eye pain, and family history of glaucoma

   b. Diagnostic tests: intraocular pressure measurement (**tonometry**), examination of the optic disk, visual field testing, **gonioscopy** (visualization and measurement of the angle of the anterior chamber) to differentiate open-angle from closed-angle glaucoma

2. Closed-angle (narrow-angle or acute-angle closure) glaucoma

   a. Assessment includes symptom analysis of acute onset of severe eye pain, headaches associated with nausea and vomiting, assess the eye for color and clarity as well as pupil response, and obtain recent history of prolonged exposure to darkened room, high stress or emotional distress

   b. Diagnostic tests: same as those used for open-angle glaucoma; blindness can occur if increased intraocular pressure persists for 24 to 48 hours

D. Nursing management

1. Medications

   a. Beta-adrenergic blocking eyedrops such as timolol maleate (Timoptic) are used to decrease production of aqueous humor; watch for systemic effects

   b. **Miotics** (drugs that constrict the pupil); constriction of pupil stimulates the ciliary muscle to pull on the trabecular meshwork surrounding the Canal of Schlemm, which facilitates the flow of aqueous humor; pilocarpine hydrochloride (Pilocar) is a typical drug

   c. Carbonic anhydrase inhibitors (CAIs) such as acetazolamide (Diamox) and dichlorphenamide (Daranide) are used in closed-angle glaucoma to reduce the secretion/formation of aqueous humor by the ciliary body

2. For closed-angle glaucoma, surgical procedures to facilitate drainage of aqueous humor can include trabeculectomy, laser trabeculoplasty, iridectomy, or laser iridotomy

3. Teach the importance of early detection; urge clients to begin regular eye examinations at age 40 and continue annually

4. Avoid **mydriatrics** (drugs that dilate the pupils) such as atropine sulfate (Isopto Atropine); memory trick: "d" is in both mydriatic and dilate

5. Obtain Medic-alert card or bracelet

6. Use safety precautions (i.e., lights, handrails) to compensate for reduced vision

7. Client teaching

   a. Importance of daily compliance with medication; stress that noncompliance may lead to permanent loss of vision

   b. Actions and side effects of specific medications (i.e., systemic effects of ophthalmic beta blockers)

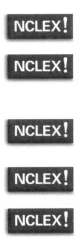

▶ Practice to Pass

A client who has just been diagnosed with open-angle glaucoma states that her mother "went blind" from glaucoma and that she fears the same will happen to her. How should the nurse respond?

    c. Procedures for correct and safe self-administration of eye drops

    d. Postoperative home care

NCLEX!

    e. Importance of reading over-the-counter (OTC) labels since many of these drugs can increase IOP

II. Cataracts

A. Overview

1. Defined as a progressive clouding or opacity of the lens of the eye that interferes with the transmission of light to the retina, leading to painless loss of vision

2. Found in 50 percent of clients between 65 to 74 years and 70 percent of clients over 75 years (Curtis & Carroll, 1998)

3. Cataracts due aging (senile cataracts) are the most common; other cause are foreign body ocular trauma causing lens swelling and rupture, congenital factors (i.e., Down's syndrome, intrauterine rubella infection, and fetal exposure to radiation), metabolic disorders (i.e., diabetes mellitus, hypoparathryoidism), certain medications such as systemic corticosteroids, chlorpromazine (Thorazine) and busulfan (Myleran), exposure to ultraviolet light (UV-B)

B. Pathophysiology

1. As a result of aging or injury, cells in the lens degenerate beginning at the periphery and moving to the center; with progression, the entire lens becomes involved

2. Cellular debris from the deteriorating lens escapes through the degenerating lens capsule into the aqueous humor and may contribute to obstruction of outflow of aqueous humor resulting in increased IOP

3. Partial opacity is termed "immature cataract"; opacity of entire lens is termed "mature cataract"

4. Age-related (senile) cataracts are usually bilateral but may be asymmetrical in development

NCLEX!

5. Signs and symptoms include blurred vision, visual distortion, decreased night vision, glare and/or abnormal presence of light in visual field, decline in near and distant vision, white or gray opacity filling the pupil opening (aperture); as cataract matures, retina becomes impossible to visualize; loss of red reflex occurs

C. Nursing assessment

1. Assessment includes an eye examination, determining client's understanding of the cause, symptoms, and treatment options related to cataracts, and assess client's fears of blindness and/or permanent disability related to cataracts and proposed cataract surgery

2. Diagnostic tests: direct examination of the eye using an ophthalmoscope or slit-lamp (lens opacity and absence of red reflex) and Snellen vision testing to assess loss of visual acuity

D. Nursing management

1. Medications include postoperative management with analgesics, anti-inflammatories, and antibiotics to decrease discomfort and prevent infection; no effective medicine is available to remove a cataract

2. Surgical interventions: lens extraction and intraocular lens implantation or use of convex corrective lens; methods utilized include:

   a. Extracapsular extraction: involves removal of lens nucleus and cortex; posterior lens capsule remains intact to help support the lens implant; currently the most popular method

   b. Phacoemulsification (use of sound waves to break up the lens) has enhanced the success of extracapsular extraction

   c. Cryoextraction involves the use of forceps or a supercooled probe to extract the lens through a small incision in the cornea

   d. Intracapsular extraction involves the removal of the entire lens and surrounding capsule

   e. Newest technology involves laser removal of lens opacities

3. Surgical procedures are done on outpatient basis using local anesthesia; usually they are performed on one eye at a time with the second procedure completed within several weeks or months

4. Identify safety concerns in the environment related to the loss of visual acuity and propose adaptive measures; if a lens implant is not performed, safety measures must be reinforced related to the loss of accommodation

5. Caution clients to avoid night driving prior to surgical correction

6. Client teaching related to surgery (see Box 6-1)

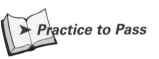

Practice to Pass

Following cataract surgery with lens implantation, the client asks the nurse to explain at-home activity restrictions. What specific instructions should be given to the client?

NCLEX!

NCLEX!

NCLEX!

Box 6-1	The following should be included when teaching clients undergoing cataract surgery:
Teaching Clients Undergoing Cataract Surgery	• Anticipated pre- and postoperative procedures

The following should be included when teaching clients undergoing cataract surgery:

- Anticipated pre- and postoperative procedures
- Importance of leaving eye patch in place until changed or removed by surgeon at postoperative visit, usually within 24 to 48 hours
- Importance and procedure for administering eye drops and/or ointments during the postoperative period
- Need for eye protection such as sunglasses during the day and eye shields at night
- Need to avoid sleeping on operative side and bending over
- Insertion and care of postoperative contact lenses if prescribed
- If convex corrective lens are prescribed, explain the loss of peripheral visual fields and need for *turning* the head from side to side to prevent accidents; measures to compensate for loss of depth perception should be emphasized

IV. Eye Injury

   A. Overview

      1. Defined as any injury to a part of the eye; since even minor injuries can threaten vision, all should be considered emergencies and immediate evaluation and care should be obtained

      2. Major causes of eye injury include corneal abrasion, blunt trauma, penetrating trauma, and burns

   B. Pathophysiology

      1. *Corneal abrasion*

        a. Characterized by a disruption of the superficial epithelium of the cornea

        b. Common causative agents include contact lenses, foreign bodies (i.e., dust, dirt, fingernails, eyelashes), and chemical irritants

        c. Drying of the surface of the eye contributes to corneal abrasion

        d. Superficial cornea abrasions are extremely painful but generally heal without scarring; deeper abrasions may lead to infection and scar formation

        e. Signs and symptoms include pain, tearing, photophobia, and visual impairment (usually temporary)

NCLEX!

      2. *Blunt trauma*

        a. Common causes include sports injuries from baseballs, tennis rackets, handballs as well as from contact sports such as basketball, football, boxing, and wrestling; motor vehicle accidents, physical assault, and falls

        b. Signs and symptoms include lid ecchymosis (black eye), subconjunctival hemorrhage, hyphema, and orbital blowout fracture

NCLEX!

          1) Subconjunctival hemorrhage is caused by blood vessel rupture under the conjunctiva, the membrane that lines the inner surface of the eye; manifests as a well-defined, red, painless area; usually requires no treatment; blood reabsorbs within 2 to 3 weeks

          2) Hyphema is characterized by bleeding into the anterior chamber of the eye; symptoms include pain, decrease visual acuity and reddish tint in the visual field; blood is visible to the examiner

          3) Orbital blowout fracture is caused by fracture of any part of the orbit; the ethmoid bone on the orbital floor is most common site; with fracture, the orbital contents including the fat, muscles and eye can herniate into the maxillary sinus; symptoms include diplopia, pain, decreased sensation on the affected cheek, limited movement of the eye, and enophthalmos (sunken appearance to the eye)

      3. *Penetrating trauma*

        a. Common causes of penetrating eye injuries include shards of glass pieces of metal produced from high-speed drilling, gunshot wounds (including BBs), arrows, and knives

        b. In penetrating injuries, layers of the eye reapproximate immediately after the injury, and injury may not be readily apparent

      c. In perforating injuries, layers of the eye do not reapproximate and rupture of the globe and loss of ocular contents may occur

      d. Symptoms include pain, loss of vision, bleeding, and possible loss of eye contents

  4. *Burns*

      a. Chemical burns are the most common; other causes include heat, radiation, and explosions

      b. Sources of chemical burns include both acid substances (i.e., acid from car batteries) and alkaline substances (i.e., ammonia, lye from oven cleaners)

      c. Alkaline burns are generally more serious because of progressive damage from particles of the offending agent remaining in contact with the conjunctival sac; acid burns are generally less serious

      d. Symptoms include eye pain, decreased vision, swollen eyelids, conjunctival reddening and edema and cloudiness of the cornea; ulcerations of the cornea and sloughing of conjunctival tissue may be present with chemical burns

C. Nursing assessment

  1. Assessment includes presence of other injuries (i.e., nasal fractures, skin abrasions, facial and scalp lacerations/burns), eye movement, and visual acuity

  2. Diagnostic tests: examination of the eye under magnification using topical anesthetics to facilitate examination, fluorescein staining to identify abrasions, and facial x-rays or computed tomography (CT) scanning to identify orbital fractures and/or to evaluate foreign bodies

D. Nursing management

  1. Corneal abrasions

      a. Medications include application of ophthalmic antibiotics and eye pad to reduce pain and photophobia

      b. If foreign body present, removal with sterile applicator and/or irrigate with sterile solution

      c. Client education to prevent reinjury

  2. Blunt trauma

      a. Medications include carbonic anhydrase inhibitors to reduce IOP as ordered

      b. Place client on bedrest in semi-Fowler's position

      c. Patch affected eye; unaffected eye may also be patched to decrease eye movement

      d. Client education about the importance of protective eyewear during sports activities

3. Penetrating trauma

   a. Medications include narcotic analgesics, sedatives and/or antiemetics for vomiting, topical and/or intravenous antibiotics as ordered to prevent infection

   b. Do not attempt to remove embedded foreign body

   c. Immobilize foreign body and cover eye to protect from further injury with metal eye shields; paper cups may be substituted for metal shield if the foreign body is too large

   d. Patching the unaffected eye decreases movement of affected eye

   e. Institute bed rest to prevent further injury

   f. Client education to avoid future injuries

4. Burns

   a. Medications include topical anesthetics to decrease pain during irrigation; following irrigation, apply topical antibiotics as ordered

   b. For chemical burns, immediately flush with copious amounts of normal saline or water

   c. Following irrigation, evaluate vision with and without any corrective eyeglasses

   d. During irrigation, evert the eyelid to ensure thorough irrigation of conjunctival sac

   e. Client education on importance of protective eyewear

V. Macular Degeneration

A. Overview

1. Defined as degeneration of the macular area of the retina in the eye; the most common type is termed age-related macular degeneration (ARMD)

2. The macula is in the center of the retina, it receives light from the center of the visual field, and has the greatest visual acuity

3. Causes of age-related macular degeneration are unknown; injury, inflammation, nutritional and hereditary factors have been implicated; males and females are affected equally

B. Pathophysiology

1. In ARMD, gradual failure of the outer layer of the retina, the pigmented epithelium occurs; the pigmented epithelium attaches the retina to the choroid layer and functions to remove cellular wastes; as the outer layer fails, photoreceptor cells are lost, waste products and toxins accumulate in the subretinal space, and cell death occurs

2. Types

   a. Atrophic ("dry") form: characterized by gradual, progressive bilateral loss of vision caused by atrophy and degeneration of the outer pigmented layer of the retina that is attached to the choroid

   b. Exudative ("wet") form: characterized by more rapid, severe loss of vision because of accumulation of serous or hemorrhagic fluid into the subretinal space; the accumulated fluid leads to separation of the retina from the choroids; scar formation leads to death of retinal cells and loss of vision

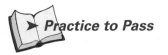

The client asks the nurse to explain the term "macular degeneration." How should the nurse respond?

3. Signs and symptoms include loss of central vision (peripheral vision remains intact), pale yellow spots called "drusen" appear on the macula, visual distortion of images (i.e., straight lines may appear wavy), and difficulty with activities requiring close central vision (i.e., reading and sewing)

C. Nursing assessment

1. Assessment includes eye examination and symptom analysis of appearance of wavy lines and changes in ability to perform close-up work

2. Diagnostic tests: ophthalmologic examination, visual acuity, visual field and color vision tests, and electroretinography (ERG) to measure retinal responses to light

D. Nursing management

1. No medications are required for macular degeneration; treatment modalities include:

   a. Laser photocoagulation for exudative macular degeneration

   b. No current therapy for atrophic macular degeneration

2. Early referral for ophthalmologic examination and early intervention may preserve vision and slow progression of disease

3. Reassurance that loss of central vision does not progress to loss of peripheral vision

4. Assessment of the home environment to prevent injuries related to loss of vision

5. Client education

   a. Availability of aids to enhance vision and promote safety (i.e., magnification devices, enhanced lighting)

   b. Availability of large-print books and newspapers as well as audio books

   c. Importance of home safety evaluation to minimize risk of injuries and falls

VI. Retinal Detachment

A. Overview

1. Defined as the separation of the sensory layer of the retina from the choroid

2. Usually occurs spontaneously but may result from trauma such as sudden blows to the head

3. Spontaneous retinal detachment occurs most frequently in clients older than 50 years

4. Causes include eye tumors, inflammatory disorders, myopia, and cataract extraction

B. Pathophysiology

1. The retina may tear and fold back onto itself or remain intact and be pulled away from the choroid as the vitreous humor shrinks because of aging

2. Breaks in the retina allow fluid from the vitreous cavity to seep into the defect; additionally, fluids from choroid vessels, the pull of gravity, and traction imposed by the vitreous enhance separation

3. Separation of the retina from the choroid causes ischemia, death of retinal neurons, and permanent loss of vision

4. Retinal damage can progress slowly or can enlarge quickly resulting in complete detachment

5. It is considered a medical emergency requiring immediate intervention

6. Signs and symptoms include sudden appearance of floaters, irregular lines and/or flashes of light in the visual field, sensation of having a curtain drawn across the field of vision, progressive deterioration of vision, blurred vision, weeping of eye (when trauma occurs), loss of central vision if macula is involved, hemorrhage into the vitreous, and ophthalmic examination may reveal gray opaque appearance of retina and/or evidence of tears, holes, or folds in retina; detachment is usually not accompanied by any pain

C. Nursing assessment

1. Assessment includes symptom analysis of visual changes such as floating spots and/or flashing lights, loss of visual acuity, blurred vision, and/or sense of curtain or veil coming down into visual field, any history of trauma to the eye, and physical examination for weeping and visual redness

2. Diagnosis based on ophthalmoscope examination

D. Nursing management

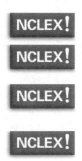

➤ Practice to Pass

A client is admitted to the outpatient surgery unit for scleral buckling of a detached retina. How should the nurse explain retinal detachment and respond to the client's fears about permanent loss of vision?

1. Medications include antibiotics, anti-inflammatories, and analgesics as ordered

2. Treatment modalities include the following surgical interventions:

   a. Scleral buckling utilizes laser photocoagulation or cryothermy to produce adhesions which seal the retinal layers; silicone is used to indent or "buckle" the sclera to enhance contact between layers

   b. Pneumatic retinopexy involves injecting air/gas into the vitreous to force the detached retina into contact with the choroid

   c. Laser photocoagulation or cryothermy can also be used without scleral buckling to create areas of inflammation and adhesions, which fuse separated layers together

   d. Surgical instrumentation is used to manipulate the detached retina into place

3. Provide for emergency care with an ophthalmologist

4. Ensure that client's head is positioned with detached area in a dependent position to assist gravity to pull retina back closer to the choroid

5. Instruct client to avoid bending forward or making sudden head movements

6. Cover both eyes with patches to limit ocular movement

7. Protect client from injury (i.e., bed in low position, side rails up, call bell within reach)

8. Provide pre- and postoperative instructions

9. Offer psychological support to alleviate anxiety related to sudden loss of vision and fear of permanent blindness

VII. Sensorineural Hearing Impairment

A. Overview

1. Defined as abnormalities of the cochlear apparatus or auditory nerve decreasing and/or distorting the transfer of sounds to the brain, resulting in loss of hearing; sound transmission to the inner ear is normal

2. Occurs with disorders affecting the inner ear, auditory nerve, or auditory pathways to the brain

3. Characterized by loss of perception of high-frequency tones, making speech recognition difficult in noisy environments

4. Causes of sensorineural hearing loss include persistent exposure to loud noise, trauma to the head or inner ear, vascular lesions, ototoxicity from medications (i.e., aminoglycosides, salicylates, diuretics, vancomycin, antineoplastic agents); infections (i.e., bacterial meningitis), Meniere's disease, **presbycusis** (degenerative changes resulting from aging), endocrine disorders (i.e., diabetes mellitus, hypothyroidism), intrauterine infections (i.e., maternal rubella), developmental malformations, and tumors (i.e., acoustic neuroma, meningioma, metastatic brain tumors)

5. In presbycusis, degenerative changes may begin in early adulthood but not be clinically significant until later in life; men are affected earlier and experience greater hearing loss than women

6. Hearing loss is usually permanent

7. May occur along with conductive hearing loss; termed mixed hearing loss

B. Pathophysiology

1. The inner ear (**labyrinth**) contains the vestibule, semicircular canals, and the cochlea; the cochlea houses the organ of Corti (see Figure 6-2)

2. Exposure to high levels of noise on an intermittent or constant basis damages the hair cells of the organ of Corti

3. With presbycusis, hair cells of the organ of Corti degenerate; gradual, progressive hearing loss results in difficulty hearing high-pitched tones and conversational speech; eventually, the ability to hear middle and lower tones is lost

4. Signs and symptoms of sensorineural hearing loss include deafness (usually bilateral), inability to hear low, middle and/or high-pitched sounds, tinnitus (ringing in ear), dizziness, and pain

C. Nursing assessment

1. Nursing assessment includes signs of hearing loss (i.e., increased voice volume, requests for information to be repeated, inappropriate responses to questions, lack of response, and turning head to the direction of a speaker)

2. Diagnostic tests: **audiometry** to assess hearing, **Weber** and **Rinne** tests (tuning fork tests) to differentiate sensorineural hearing loss from conductive hearing loss, brainstem auditory evoked response (BAER), and brain imaging studies to rule out intracranial lesions

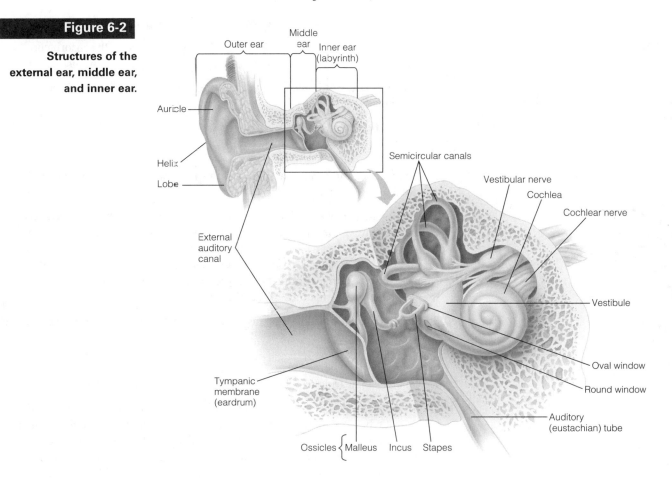

Figure 6-2

Structures of the external ear, middle ear, and inner ear.

D. **Nursing management**

1. Medications are not recommended; treatment modalities are limited but include:

   a. Cochlear implants: provide clients with perception of sound but not normal hearing; allow clients to recognize warning sounds of telephones, sirens, and automobiles; alert clients to incoming communication; and provide some help for clients even if no auditory nerve function exists

   b. Hearing aids not generally helpful; serve only to intensify the distorted sounds

   c. Use of devices that provide "white noise" to mask the unpleasant or distressing sounds associated with tinnitus

2. Avoid shouting; address clients in normal, low-pitched voice

3. Provide adequate visual contact and lighting when communicating with clients to foster lip reading; face client directly

4. Provide alternative means of communication (i.e., use sign language, provide written instructions)

5. Reduce background noises when communicating with clients

6. Use short sentences and gestures (i.e., pointing) when appropriate

7. Educate the family about the social isolation associated with sensorineural hearing loss including apparent inattention, withdrawal, and/or disinterest

NCLEX!

8. Evaluate safety of home environment (i.e., ability to hear smoke detectors, telephones)

VIII. Conductive Hearing Impairment

A. Overview

1. Defined as an interruption in sound transmission from the external auditory canal to the inner ear

2. Causes include obstruction of the external auditory canal by impacted cerumen; edema of the canal lining, foreign objects, and neoplasms; rupture or scarring of the tympanic membrane; disruption or fixation of the bones in the middle ear secondary to trauma or **otosclerosis** (a familial disorder of hearing loss); otitis externa or otitis media, presence of fluid in the middle ear; and congenital malformations of the external or middle ear

3. Termed mixed hearing loss if occurs in conjunction with sensorineural hearing loss

B. Pathophysiology

1. Changes in hearing may be sudden or gradual depending upon cause

2. With otosclerosis, bone resorption is followed by overgrowth of new, hard sclerotic bone; the stapes (ossicle in middle ear) becomes immobilized against the oval window thus decreasing the transmission of sound to the inner ear; pressure of otosclerotic bone on inner ear structures or the 8th cranial nerve may also result in sensorineural hearing loss

3. Often unilateral; may be bilateral if caused by otosclerosis

NCLEX!

4. Signs and symptoms include loss of sound at all frequencies and tinnitus with otosclerosis

C. Nursing assessment

1. Assessment includes presence of foreign bodies, infection and/or cerumen in external auditory canal, integrity of tympanic membrane and presence of otitis media

2. Diagnostic tests: Weber and Rinne tests, audiometry, **tympanometry** (an indirect measurement of compliance of the middle ear to sound transmission), and otoscopic examination

D. Nursing management

1. No medications are recommended; treatment modalities include:

   a. Hearing aids to amplify sound

   b. Assistive listening devices ("pocket talker")

   c. Reconstructive procedures to restore hearing: **stapedectomy** (making an incision in stapes to improve hearing) for otosclerosis and **tympanoplasty** (surgical procedures to restore the function of the middle ear to transmit sound more efficiently)

2. Client teaching related to conductive hearing loss (see Box 6-2)

3. Utilize techniques appropriate for the hearing impaired as noted in the section on nursing management of sensorineural hearing loss

4. Provide appropriate pre- and postoperative care

IX. Otitis Media

A. Overview

1. Defined as inflammation and/or infection of the middle ear

2. Primarily affects infants and young children; may occur in adults

3. Major cause of conductive hearing loss

4. Two common forms of otitis media include *serous otitis media* and *acute otitis media*

5. Causes

   a. Serous otitis media: upper respiratory infections, allergies, and narrow or edematous Eustachian tubes

   b. Acute otitis media: *Streptococcus pneumoniae, Haemophilus influenzae,* and *Streptococcus pyogenes*

B. Pathophysiology

1. The tympanic membrane protects the middle ear from the external auditory canal; the Eustachian tube (auditory tube) connects the middle ear with the nasopharynx and serves to equalize pressure in the middle ear with atmospheric pressure

2. *Serous otitis media*

   a. Occurs when the Eustachian tube is obstructed for a prolonged period of time, causing impaired equalization of air pressure within the middle ear

   b. Air in the middle ear is absorbed; continued obstruction of the Eustachian tube prevents more air from entering, and negative pressure

---

Box 6-2

Teaching Clients with Conductive Hearing Loss

The following points should be included in a teaching plan for clients with conductive hearing loss:

- Technique for proper insertion and cleaning of hearing aids
- Proper insertion of hearing aid batteries; need for extra batteries
- Availability of assistive listening devices (i.e., "pocket talkers")
- Postoperative and home care following stapedectomy or tympanoplasty
- Methods to protect ears from injury; use of ear plugs while swimming and diving
- Care of ears and ear canal, including cleaning and removal of cerumen
- Signs of middle ear infection and the importance of early and complete treatment

in the middle ear results; serous fluid moves into the middle ear forming a sterile effusion

    c. Signs and symptoms of serous otitis media include: decreased hearing in affected ear, complaints of "snapping" or "popping," decreased mobility of the tympanic membrane, retracted or bulging of the tympanic membrane indicating the presence of fluid or air bubbles, pain, bleeding and/or rupture of the tympanic membrane, rupture of the round window with sensory hearing loss, and vertigo

  3. *Acute otitis media*

    a. Results from the entry of pathogens from the oronasopharynx via the Eustachian tube into the normally sterile environment of the middle ear

    b. Typically follows upper respiratory infections

    c. Common in infants and children because of short, straight Eustachian tubes; higher incidence noted in bottle-fed infants/toddlers who maintain a more horizontal position during feeding and in those living with smokers

    d. Invasion and colonization by bacteria along with white blood cell invasion leads to pus formation; pus increases middle ear pressure and may lead to rupture of the tympanic membrane

    e. Signs and symptoms of acute otitis media include: pain, often severe, in affected ear; infants and young children may pull at affected ear; fever; impaired hearing; dizziness and vertigo; red, inflamed or dull, bulging tympanic membrane; decreased movement of membrane; tenderness over mastoid area indicating the development of mastoiditis

  4. Chronic, recurring otitis media may result in permanent perforation of the tympanic membrane, permanent hearing loss, and/or the formation of a benign epithelial-cell tumor, called **cholesteatoma**

  5. Complications of untreated acute otitis media include meningitis, osteomyelitis of the skull, and facial paralysis

C. Nursing assessment

  1. Assessment includes visualization of tympanic membrane using otoscope, pain (quality, severity, and location); note that pain associated with otitis media, unlike that of external otitis, is not aggravated by ear movement; history for recurrent otitis media

  2. Diagnostic tests: visualization of the tympanic membrane with pneumatic otoscope, tympanometry, complete blood count (CBC) to assess for an elevated white blood cell count, and culture of middle ear effusion if membrane has ruptured or **myringotomy** (incision into the tympanic membrane) has been done

D. Nursing management

  1. Serous otitis media

    a. Medications include systemic or intranasal decongestants to reduce edema of the Eustachian tube and maintain patency; analgesics, and antipyretics

    b. Treatment includes autoinflation of the middle ear by forcefully exhaling against closed nostrils

    c. Avoidance of air travel and underwater diving

NCLEX!

Practice to Pass

A young mother brings her 12-month-old child in with recurrent acute otitis media. What should the nurse suggest to help prevent recurrence of these middle ear infections?

2. Acute otitis media

    a. Medications include antibiotic therapy with or without decongestants; therapy often continued for 10 to 12 days; analgesics, and antipyretics

    b. Tympanocentesis: aspiration of fluid from the middle ear

    c. Myringotomy with or without the insertion of tympanostomy tubes (ventilation tubes)

3. Stress importance of completing full course of antibiotic therapy

4. Stress importance of increasing fluid intake and consuming nutritious diet to enhance immune system and hasten resolution of the infection

5. Alert clients or parents of possibility of superinfections due to antibiotic therapy

6. If tympanostomy tubes are present, caution clients to avoid swimming, diving, or allowing water to enter the ear

7. Provide appropriate pre- and postoperative care for myringotomy and/or insertion of tympanostomy tubes

X. External Otitis

A. Overview

1. Defined as an inflammation of the outer ear canal; known as swimmer's ear

2. Caused by excess moisture in ear canal, fungi or bacteria, trauma, or local hypersensitivity; common organisms include *Pseudomonas aerugenosa*

B. Pathophysiology

1. Removal of the cerumen, which has water-repellant and antimicrobial properties, leaves the ear canal susceptible to infection; excess moisture, vigorous cleaning, or excess drying of the ear canal can assist in removing the cerumen

2. Signs and symptoms include severe pain, fullness in the ear, and decreased hearing; pain with application of pressure on the tragus is a hallmark sign; visual examination shows clusters of white particles on the side of the canals and edema; the tympanic membrane may be difficult to see but will appear normal and pearly gray

C. Nursing assessment

1. Assessment includes a symptom analysis of when the pain began (frequency, description), occupation or frequency in swimming, physical palpation of tragus

2. Diagnostic tests: ear examination with otoscope

D. Nursing management

1. Medications include topical antibiotics, topical corticosteroids such as polymixin B-neomycin hydrocortisone (Cortisporin otic), tolnaftate solution (Tinactin) for fungal infection, pain medication as needed, and Dome Burrow solution to irrigate the ear

2. Instruct client to use topical antibiotic for prescribed time in order to completely eliminate the organism and avoid swimming for 7 to 10 days

3. Educate the client to use drying agents before and after swimming such as Swimmer's Ear™ or a 2 percent acetic acid solution with alcohol; earplugs should be used for clients with ear tubes

XI. Meniere's Disease

A. Overview

1. Defined as a chronic disorder of the inner ear characterized by a triad of symptoms including vertigo, tinnitus, and sensorineural hearing loss, known as *endolymphatic hydrops*

2. Usually unilateral, affecting men and women equally; high-risk group includes adults between the ages of 35 and 60

3. Causes include trauma, infection, allergies, adrenal-pituitary insufficiency, hypothyroidism, immune system dysfunction, increased sodium intake, stress, and premenstrual fluid retention; a genetic predisposition may exist

B. Pathophysiology

1. Most common form is idiopathic

2. An overaccumulation of fluid (**endolymph**) in the membranous labyrinth of the inner ear results in dilation of the lymphatic channels and labyrinth dysfunction; autonomic nervous system control of the labyrinthine circulation may be impaired also contributing to labyrinth dysfunction

3. The excess fluid is thought to be caused by an impaired absorption of endolymph

4. Onset of symptoms may be gradual or sudden

NCLEX!

5. Signs and symptoms include severe rotary vertigo (lasting from minutes to hours, may be associated with nausea and vomiting and may cause immobility), tinnitus, sensorineural hearing loss, sense of fullness in ears, hypotension, diaphoresis, and **nystagmus** (irregular eye movements) during acute attacks

C. Nursing assessment

1. Assessment includes subjective complaints of dizziness, nausea, vomiting, sweating, tinnitus, blurred vision, sensitivity to light, and roaring sensation to ears; objective assessment should include heart rate (HR) (bradycardia), incapacitating vertigo, gastrointestinal (GI) tract symptom (diarrhea), and disequilibrium; history often includes past otitis media, allergies, and arteriosclerosis

2. Diagnostic tests

   a. Electronystagmography (ENG): a series of tests used to evaluate the vestibular-ocular reflexes by identifying nystagmus as a response to specific stimuli; caloric ice water test is one part of ENG

   b. Caloric ice water testing involves the instillation of ice water into the external auditory canal; in clients with impaired inner ear function, the normal nystagmus response is blunted or absent

   c. X-rays and CT scans are used to evaluate anatomic changes of the central portion of the inner ear known as the vestibule

   d. Rinne and Weber tests utilize a tuning fork to test hearing

   e. Auditory dehydration test involves the administration of fast-acting diuretics or hyperosmolar substances (i.e., glycerin) to decrease fluid pressure in the inner ear; acute, temporary improvement is considered diagnostic

   f. Audiometry testing

D. Nursing management

1. Medications for *acute attacks*

   a. Anticholinergics: atropine sulfate (Isopto Atropine) and scopolamine (Isopto Hyoscine)

   b. Central nervous system (CNS) depressants: diazepam (Valium), lorazepam (Ativan)

   c. Antiemetics: prochlorperazine (Compazine), meclizine (Antivert)

   d. Sedatives/antiemetics: droperidol (Inapsine)

   e. Antihistamines: diphenhydramine (Benadryl)

   f. Antibiotics for bacterial labyrinthitis

2. Medications *between attacks* include oral diuretics to decrease pressure in the labyrinth and vasodilators

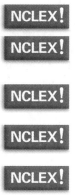

3. Ensure client safety *during attacks* (i.e., assist with ambulation, side rails up, bed in low position, call bell within reach), limit movement, and replace fluid and electrolytes

4. Medical treatment options *between* acute attacks focus on prevention and include sodium-restricted diet and avoidance of substances causing vasoconstriction (i.e., tobacco, alcohol, and caffeine)

5. Surgical interventions

   a. Endolymphatic sac decompression and shunting, which releases pressure in the labyrinth and shunts endolymph from membranous labyrinth to subarachnoid space

   b. Vestibular nerve resection: removal of part of 8th cranial nerve

   c. Labyrinthectomy: complete removal of the labyrinth

6. When administering diuretics, monitor for electrolyte imbalance

7. Ensure adequate hydration and nutrition if attacks are frequent

8. Client teaching

   a. Signs of impending attack (i.e., feeling of ear fullness, increasing tinnitus, vertigo, nausea and vomiting)

   b. Avoidance of attack triggers (i.e., stress, fatigue, blinking lights, loud noises, quick or jerky body movements)

   c. Safety measures if attack occurs while driving (i.e., pull off to the side of the road, need for car phone and "HELP POLICE" sign)

   d. Need for adequate rest and sleep

   e. Relaxation techniques

   f. Availability of organizations offering information and support (i.e., Vestibular Disorders Association and Meniere's Network)

   g. Need for Medic-alert bracelet, card, or necklace

XII. Epistaxis

A. Overview

1. Defined as a nosebleed; the nose is highly vascular, receiving blood from major arterial vessels originating from both the internal and external carotid arteries

2. Men are affected by nosebleeds more often than women

3. Bleeding may originate in the anterior or posterior nose

4. Identified by the area where the bleeding originates: *anterior epistaxis* or *posterior epistaxis*

5. Causes include medications, particularly antiplatelets or anticoagulants, and the following:

    a. Anterior epistaxis: drying, infection, blunt trauma or trauma from manipulation, cocaine use, and local infection

    b. Posterior epistaxis: blood dyscrasias, hypertension, diabetes, and trauma

B. Pathophysiology

1. Ninety percent of all nosebleeds arise from Kiesselbach's area, a rich vascular plexus in the anterior nasal spectum or from rupture of vessels caused by trauma

2. Posterior epistaxis tends to be more severe; occurs more often in older adults

C. Nursing assessment

NCLEX!

1. Assessment includes identifying the amount of blood lost and source of bleeding by examining both nares and back of throat to rule out posterior bleeding, client's health history, medication history including use of herbal products, and vital signs

2. There are no diagnostic tests; a CBC may be obtained if severe blood loss has been experienced

D. Nursing management

1. Medications include topical application of vasoconstrictors such as phenylephrine (Neo-Synephrine), oxymetazoline hydrochloride (Afrin), or adrenaline; chemical cauterization using silver nitrate or Gelfoam, topical antibacterial ointment to inner nares, and analgesics (particularly if packing has been placed)

2. Treatment options

NCLEX!

    a. First aid measures

    1) Assess for respiratory distress; administer supplemental oxygen as indicated

    2) Instruct client to sit upright with head tilted forward

    3) Apply pressure, by pinching nose toward the septum, for 5 to 10 minutes

    4) Apply ice packs to the nose and/or forehead to promote vasoconstriction

    5) Encourage client to expectorate blood to prevent nausea and vomiting resulting from swallowed blood

      6) Estimate blood loss when possible

      7) Maintain an attitude of calm reassurance

    b. Nasal packing

    c. Surgery including cauterization and ligation of the vessels (i.e., **Caldwell-Luc procedure**)

3. Following nasal packing

    a. Monitor respiratory function and oxygen saturation

    b. Assess packing for odor, color, and amount of drainage

    c. Administer analgesics as needed

    d. Monitor vital signs to assess for cardiovascular complications and infection

    e. Monitor position of catheter (i.e., rubber or inflatable type) if used to provide hemostasis

    f. Provide frequent oral care; use bedside humidifier to reduce drying of oral mucous membranes

4. Provide pre- and postoperative teaching and care as indicated

XIII. Sinusitis

A. Overview

1. Defined as inflammation with resulting infection of the mucous membranes of one or more of the paranasal sinuses

2. Commonly follows upper respiratory tract infections or viral rhinitis

3. Classified as *acute*, *subacute*, or *chronic*

    a. Acute sinusitis lasts from 1 day to 3 weeks

    b. Subacute sinusitis persists from 3 weeks to 3 months

    c. Chronic sinusitis lasts longer than 3 months.

4. Immunocompromised clients may be at greater risk for sinusitis and may be more difficult to treat

5. Causes include: upper respiratory infections, viral rhinitis, nasal polyps, deviated nasal septum, tooth abscess, prolonged nasotracheal or nasogastric intubation in the hospitalized client, abuse of nasal decongestants, swimming and diving, exposure to frequent changes in barometric pressure (i.e., pilots, flight attendants), smoking, nasal packing (epistaxis), and allergies

B. Pathophysiology

1. The paranasal sinuses are air cells that connect with the nasal cavity and are named for the bone in which they are located (i.e., frontal, sphenoid, ethmoid, and maxillary)

2. Sinuses are lined with cilia; cilia facilitate movement of fluids and microorganisms into the nasal cavity for exit from the body

3. Viral illness produces inflammation of the sinus mucosa causing obstruction of the normal ciliary action; creating an ideal environment for bacterial growth

4. Following invasion of microorganisms into the sinuses, the inflammatory response increases swelling and congestion, further compromising normal ciliary action; bacterial growth continues

5. Common organisms associated with sinusitis include *Streptococcus pyogenes*, *Staphylococcus aureus*, *Streptococcus pneumoniae*, and *Haemophilus influenzae*; gram-negative species and fungi may also be causative

NCLEX!

6. Signs and symptoms

   a. Acute sinusitis: constant, often severe pain and tenderness over infected sinuses, pain in the teeth may indicate maxillary sinusitis, headache, fever, malaise, and fatigue, nasal congestion, purulent nasal discharge, halitosis, sore, and inflamed throat because of swallowed secretions

   b. Subacute or chronic sinusitis: dull, intermittent or constant pain, purulent nasal discharge, chronic cough, and loss of sense of smell

7. Local and intracranial complications of sinusitis

   a. Periorbital abscesses and/or cellulitis

   b. Osteomyelitis of the facial bones

   c. Cavernous sinus thrombosis

   d. Meningitis

   e. Brain abscess

   f. Sepsis

C. Nursing assessment

1. Assessment includes frequency of sinusitis, precipitating factors, pain, and need for analgesics

2. Diagnostic tests: physical examination including inspection of the nose and throat, cultures of nasal discharge, transillumination of the sinuses, x-rays and CT scans to detect opacity of sinuses, and nasal endoscopy to visualize the anterior nasal cavity and sinus openings

D. Nursing management

1. Medications include antibiotic therapy, oral or intranasal decongestants, intranasal corticosteroids, expectorants such as guaifenesin (Robitussin) to liquefy secretions, saline nasal sprays and/or steam inhalation, saline irrigation of the maxillary sinus (i.e., antral irrigation) using needle access to the sinus, and analgesics

2. Surgical interventions

   a. Endoscopic sinus surgery

   b. Caldwell-Luc procedure

   c. External sphenoethmoidectomy: removal of diseased tissue from the sphenoid or ethmoid sinuses via a surgical incision along the side of the nose

   d. Administer analgesics as necessary; institute comfort measures (i.e., application of ice packs, elevate head of bed)

e. Provide teaching

1) Importance of completing full course of antibiotic therapy

2) Uses and hazards of nasal decongestants

3) Signs and symptoms of recurrent infection

4) Importance of adequate hydration

5) Postoperative management including avoidance of strenuous activity and blowing the nose

XIV. Laryngeal Cancer

A. Overview

1. Defined as cancer of the glottis (true vocal cords), supraglottis, or subglottis

NCLEX!

2. Causes are prolonged use of tobacco and alcohol, chronic laryngitis, occupational exposure to chemicals and toxins, exposure to selected types of human papilloma virus, and genetic predisposition

3. Squamous cell carcinoma is the most common type of laryngeal malignancy

4. With early diagnosis and treatment, 80 to 90 percent of small lesions can be cured; without treatment, 90 percent of clients die within 3 years (LeMone & Burke, 2000)

B. Pathophysiology

1. Exposure to irritants (i.e., tobacco smoke, chemicals, toxins) result in changes to the laryngeal mucosa

2. Precancerous leukoplakia (white, patchy lesions) and erythroplakia (red, velvet-like patches) appear on the laryngeal mucosa

3. Lesions may occur in any of three areas of the larynx (i.e., the glottis, the supraglottis, or the subglottis); lesions along the edges of the glottis (the true vocal cords) are the most common (see Figure 6-3)

4. Lesions of the glottis are usually well-differentiated and slow-growing

Figure 6-3

Visualization of lesion along edge of glottis.

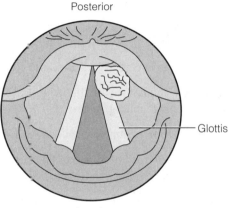

Posterior

Glottis

Anterior

5. Structures in the supraglottis include the epiglottis, arytenoid muscles and cartilage, and the false vocal cords; the subglottis is located below the vocal cords and terminates at the tracheal ring; tumors of the supraglottis are often large before symptoms are noted and very rare

6. Laryngeal tumors initially metastasize to the regional lymph nodes; metastasis to the lungs may follow

NCLEX!

7. Signs and symptoms include hoarseness, change in voice, dyspnea, pain and burning in throat when drinking hot liquids or citrus juices, dysphagia, foul-smelling breath, pain radiating to the ear, persistent cough, and palpable lump in the neck

C. Nursing assessment

1. Assessment includes early recognition of signs and symptoms, signs of respiratory distress, nutritional status, and psychosocial needs; prompt assessment and early referral of clients presenting with symptoms of laryngeal cancer; early diagnosis is critical to survival

2. Diagnostic tests

NCLEX!

a. Laryngoscopy with biopsy of leukoplakia (precancerous lesions) and erythroplakia (precancerous patches)

b. X-ray studies of head, neck, and chest; CT or MRI scans

c. Barium swallow to evaluate swallowing and/or presence of tumor in esophagus

D. Nursing management

1. Medications include adjunctive chemotherapy

2. Treatment options

a. Surgical interventions: partial, supraglottic, or total **laryngectomy** (removal of part or all of the larynx) depending upon tumor location; radical neck dissection with cervical lymph node involvement

b. External beam radiation or implants for early tumors

NCLEX!

3. Monitor respiratory status

4. Provide supplemental nutrition

5. Assess emotional status and possible grieving, encourage client to ventilate feelings and concerns

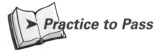
▶ Practice to Pass

6. Provide postoperative care as indicated and client teaching as follows:

a. Postoperative and home care following partial or total laryngectomy (i.e., tracheotomy care, enteral nutrition)

The client asks the nurse about the methods available to restore speech following total laryngectomy. How should the nurse respond?

b. Need for radiation treatments and/or chemotherapy

c. Options available for restoration of speech (i.e., esophageal speech, battery-operated speech generator)

d. Availability of support services (i.e., American Cancer Society, support groups, pastoral care)

Case Study

R. M., a 48-year-old female client, has been admitted to the Emergency Department with severe vertigo accompanied by nausea and vomiting. She also complains of tinnitus and a sense of fullness in the left ear. She is diagnosed with acute Meniere's disease.

❶ What other assessment findings can be expected?

❷ What medical interventions can be anticipated during the acute phase of this illness?

❸ What diagnostic tests can be anticipated for this client?

❹ How should the nurse explain Meniere's disease to the client?

❺ What discharge instructions should be given to the client?

For suggested responses, see pages 566–567.

Posttest

1. A client reports sudden onset of continuous eye pain and impaired vision. Pupil dilation is noted. The nurse concludes that this assessment data is consistent with which of the following disorders?

(1) Closed-angle (narrow-angle) glaucoma
(2) Open-angle glaucoma
(3) Cataracts
(4) Retinal detachment

2. A client with Meniere's disease would probably complain of which of the following?

(1) Bilateral hearing impairment
(2) Vertigo and nausea
(3) Pain when the tragus is touched
(4) Tenderness over the mastoid area

3. A male client has just had a cataract operation without a lens implant. In discharge teaching, the nurse will instruct the client's wife to:

(1) Prepare only soft foods for several days to prevent facial movement.
(2) Keep the eye dressing on for 10 days.
(3) Have her husband remain in bed for 3 days.
(4) Allow him to walk upstairs only with assistance.

4. An adult client presents to the Emergency Department after having a rock hit his eye while weeding along a ditch near a busy highway. The event occurred several hours earlier. The nurse assesses the eye and finds redness and weeping, but the client denies any pain. Which of the following early symptoms would help confirm retinal detachment?

(1) Pain
(2) Floaters
(3) Subconjunctival hemorrhage
(4) Halo vision

5 A client is diagnosed with a cholesteatoma and asks the nurse to explain what this is. The best explanation by the nurse would be, "Cholesteatoma is an:

(1) Overaccummulation of fluid in the membranous labyrinth of the inner ear."
(2) Inflamed cyst or mass filled with epithelial cell debris resulting from chronic middle ear infection."
(3) Irritation to part of the uvea; the middle coat of the eyeball."
(4) Inflammation of the center of the retina."

6 Which of the following clients is at highest risk for macular degeneration?

(1) A biochemist exposed to various toxins
(2) An elderly client
(3) A youth hit in the eye with a baseball
(4) A young adult with multiple allergies

7 A client presents to the clinic with complaints of sinusitis. The nurse anticipates that the most useful technique for diagnosis would be:

(1) The Weber test.
(2) Fluorescein staining.
(3) Transillumination.
(4) Caloric ice water testing.

8 Which of the following is a priority nursing diagnosis for a client with epistaxis?

(1) Anxiety with risk for aspiration
(2) Risk for infection
(3) Pain
(4) Impaired verbal communication

9 Which of the following clients is at highest risk for laryngeal cancer? A client who:

(1) Has an injury to the larynx.
(2) Is 85 years old.
(3) Has chewed tobacco for 20 years.
(4) Suffers from chronic sinusitis.

10 Nursing interventions for a client with sensorineural hearing loss include:

(1) Providing information about the availability of hearing aids to amplify sound.
(2) Educating family members about social isolation and depression.
(3) Administering antibiotics as prescribed.
(4) Preparing the client for tympanoplasty.

See pages 229–230 for Answers and Rationales.

Answers and Rationales

Pretest

1 Answer: 3 *Rationale:* Narrow-angle glaucoma develops abruptly and manifests with acute face and eye pain and is a medical emergency. Halo vision, dull eye pain, and impaired night vision are symptoms commonly associated with open-angle glaucoma.
Cognitive Level: Application
Nursing Process: Assessment; *Test Plan:* PHYS

2 Answer: 3 *Rationale:* A cloudy-appearing lens is symptomatic of cataract development. As the cataract matures, the red reflex is lost. A sense of a curtain falling over the visual field is associated with de-

tached retina. Eye pain and double vision are not associated with cataracts.
Cognitive Level: Application
Nursing Process: Assessment; *Test Plan:* PHYS

3 Answer: 2 *Rationale:* The foreign body should not be removed or manipulated. It should be immobilized if possible and the eye covered to protect from further injury. A paper cup can be used in place of an eye patch. Patching both eyes is an appropriate intervention to prevent ocular movement but follows immobilization of the foreign body. Irrigation with water is an intervention for chemical burns to the eyes. Car-

bonic anhydrase inhibitors are used to decrease intraocular pressure following blunt trauma.
Cognitive Level: Analysis
Nursing Process: Implementation; *Test Plan:* SECE

4 **Answer: 4** *Rationale:* Conductive hearing loss results from changes that occur in the external or middle ear. Hearing aids, assistive listening devices (i.e., "pocket talkers"), and reconstructive surgeries can improve or correct hearing loss. Exposure to high levels of noise on an intermittent or constant basis damages the hair cells of the Organ of Corti, resulting in sensorineural hearing loss.
Cognitive Level: Application
Nursing Process: Implementation *Test Plan:* PHYS

5 **Answer: 4** *Rationale:* Weber and Rinne tests are used to differentiate conductive hearing loss from sensorineural. Tympanocentesis is the aspiration of fluid/pus from the middle ear to identify the causative organism of acute otitis media. Transillumination of the sinuses is a diagnostic tool used to assess for sinusitis. The diagnosis of Meniere's disease is confirmed by electronystagmography, a series of tests to evaluate vestibular-ocular reflexes.
Cognitive Level: Application
Nursing Process: Assessment; *Test Plan:* PHYS

6 **Answer: 2** *Rationale:* A higher incidence of acute otitis media is noted in infants who are bottle-fed in a horizontal position and who live in homes with smokers. The full 10- to 12-day course of antibiotic therapy must be administered. There is no relationship between the ingestion of fruit juices and acute otitis media.
Cognitive Level: Application
Nursing Process: Planning; *Test Plan:* HPM

7 **Answer: 2** *Rationale:* Atrophic macular degeneration causes loss of central vision. Magnification devices and enhanced lighting help to promote safety. Peripheral vision remains intact. Although laser photocoagulation is effective for exudative macular degeneration, there is no treatment for the atrophic form. Since macular degeneration is not an infectious process, antibiotic therapy is not indicated.
Cognitive Level: Application
Nursing Process: Planning; *Test Plan:* PHYS

8 **Answer: 1** *Rationale:* Pilocarpine (Pilocar) is a miotic and the most commonly prescribed drug for glaucoma. Scopolamine (Hycoscine) and atropine are anticholinergics; epinephrine is an adrenergic agonist.

All three are mydriatrics. The pupil dilation caused by mydriatrics is contraindicated in glaucoma.
Cognitive Level: Application
Nursing Process: Analysis; *Test Plan:* SECE

9 **Answer: 3** *Rationale:* These symptoms, along with dysphagia, foul-smelling breath, and pain when drinking hot or acidic fluids, are common signs of laryngeal cancer. Chronic sinusitis can produce foul breath and pain or burning in the throat. GERD and CAD may produce epigastric and/or chest pain, but hoarseness and change of voice do not occur.
Cognitive Level: Application
Nursing Process: Assessment; *Test Plan:* PHYS

10 **Answer: 3** *Rationale:* All of the nursing actions listed are appropriate for the client following nasal packing for epistaxis; however, the risk of aspiration is high, and monitoring respiratory function essential. Notice the question asks for the *priority* intervention.
Cognitive Level: Application
Nursing Process: Implementation; *Test Plan:* SECE

Posttest

1 **Answer: 1** *Rationale:* Closed or narrow-angle glaucoma has an abrupt onset and is characterized by severe pain of sudden onset. The pain usually lasts longer than 20 minutes with closed-angle glaucoma. Eye pain that comes and goes quickly can be indicative of allergies. Open-angle glaucoma occurs gradually with no initial manifestations. Pain is not associated with cataracts or retinal detachment.
Cognitive Level: Application
Nursing Process: Analysis; *Test Plan:* PHYS

2 **Answer: 2** *Rationale:* Meniere's disease is associated with vertigo that may last for hours as well as fluctuating hearing loss, nausea, and vomiting. The disorder is unilateral, but because hearing is bilateral, the client often does not realize the extent of the hearing loss. Option 3 is indicative of swimmer's ear, and option 4 is indicative of acute otitis media.
Cognitive Level: Application
Nursing Process: Analysis: *Test Plan:* PHYS

3 **Answer: 4** *Rationale:* Without a lens, the eye cannot accommodate. Since it is difficult to judge distance and climb stairs when the eyes cannot accommodate, for safety reasons the client should have assistance when climbing stairs.
Cognitive Level: Analysis
Nursing Process: Implementation; *Test Plan:* SECE

4 **Answer: 2** *Rationale:* Retinal detachment is painless, but eventually floaters and visual loss will be manifested, especially if hemorrhage has occurred. Subconjunctival hemorrhage is a manifestation of blunt trauma to the eye. Halo vision is characteristic of glaucoma.
Cognitive Level: Analysis
Nursing Process: Assessment; *Test Plan:* PHYS

5 **Answer: 2** *Rationale:* Cholesteatomas are benign, slow-growing tumors of the middle ear that are filled with epithelial cell debris. Untreated cholesteatomas may enlarge to fill the middle ear, destroy the ossicles, and cause profound hearing loss. Option 1 (endolymph) is indicative of Meniere's disease. Options 3 and 4 are distracters.
Cognitive Level: Analysis
Nursing Process: Implementation; *Test Plan:* PHYS

6 **Answer: 2** *Rationale:* Age-related macular degeneration is the leading cause of loss of vision in clients over 50 years of age. Blunt trauma, exposure to toxins, and allergies are not known causes of macular degeneration.
Cognitive Level: Application
Nursing Process: Analysis; *Test Plan:* HPM

7 **Answer: 3** *Rationale:* Transillumination of the sinuses in a non-invasive technique used to detect fluid in the maxillary and frontal sinuses. The Weber test differentiates conductive hearing loss from sensorineural hearing loss. Fluorescein staining helps identify corneal abrasions and caloric testing is used to evaluate nystagmus in Meniere's disease.
Cognitive Level: Application
Nursing Process: Planning; *Test Plan:* PHYS

8 **Answer: 1** *Rationale:* Since the amount of blood lost in a nosebleed can be frightening to clients, anxiety is a priority nursing diagnosis. Blood draining into the nasopharynx poses a risk of aspiration. Risk for infection and pain are appropriate nursing diagnoses related to nasal packing but are not the priorities. Impaired verbal communication is unlikely.
Cognitive Level: Analysis
Nursing Process: Analysis; *Test Plan:* PHYS

9 **Answer: 3** *Rationale:* The two major risk factors for laryngeal cancer are prolonged smoking along with concomitant use of alcohol. Although the majority of cases occur in men ages 50 to 75, advancing age does not significantly increase risk. Injury to the larynx and chronic sinusitis are not risk factors.
Cognitive Level: Application
Nursing Process: Analysis; *Test Plan:* HPM

10 **Answer: 2** *Rationale:* The client with sensorineural hearing loss experiences social isolation and depression and may appear withdrawn. Amplification devices such as hearing aids are helpful for clients with conductive hearing loss but only amplify noxious sounds for the client with sensorineural hearing loss. Antibiotics are not helpful for sensorineural hearing loss, and tympanoplasty is used to correct damage to structures in the middle ear.
Cognitive Level: Application
Nursing Process: Implementation; *Test Plan:* PSYC

References

Brashers, V. & Davey, S. (2002). Alterations in pulmonary function. In K. McCance & S. Heuther (Eds.), *Pathophysiology: The biologic basis for disease in adults and children* (4th ed.). St. Louis, MO: Mosby, pp. 1190–1191.

Curtis, S. & Carroll, E. (2002). Alterations in vision. In C. Porth (Ed.), *Pathophysiology: Concepts of altered health states* (6th ed.). Philadelphia: Lippincott, pp. 1025–1053.

Henze, R. (2000). Normal and altered function of the special senses. In B. Bullock & R. Henze (Eds.), *Focus on pathophysiology*. Philadelphia: Lippincott, p. 1040.

Lemone, P. & Burke, K. (2000). *Medical surgical nursing: Critical thinking in client care* (2nd ed.). Upper Saddle River, NJ: Prentice Hall, pp. 1348–1352, 1357–1360, 1368–1389, 1876–1882, 1898–1948.

Mackin, L. & Bullock, B. (2000). Altered pulmonary function. In B. Bullock & R. Henze (Eds.), *Focus on pathophysiology*. Philadelphia: Lippincott, p. 578.

Nelsen-Marsh, J. (2000). Alterations in special sensory function. In L. E. Copstead & J. Banasik (Eds.), *Pathophysiology: Biological and behavioral perspectives* (2nd ed.). Philadelphia: W. B. Saunders, pp. 1060–1078.

Porth, C. (2002). Alterations in respiratory function: Respiratory tract infections, neoplasms, and childhood disorders. In C. Porth (Ed.), *Pathophysiology: Concepts of altered health states* (6th ed.). Philadelphia: Lippincott, pp. 503–504.

Porth, C. & Curtis, R. (2002). Alterations in hearing and vestibular function. In C. Porth (Ed.), *Pathophysiology: Concepts of altered health states* (6th ed.). Philadelphia: Lippincott, pp. 1053–1066.

Schlosser, S., Bullock, B., Kaudewitz, L., & McDaniel, G. (2000). Developmental stages and health alterations. In B. Bullock & R. Henze (Eds.), *Focus on pathophysiology*. Philadelphia: Lippincott, p. 113.

Tupper, S. (1999). When the inner ear is out of balance. *RN* 62 (11): 36–40.

CHAPTER 7

Gastrointestinal Health Problems

Eugenia H. Tickle, RN, MSN, EdD

CHAPTER OUTLINE

OBJECTIVES

▌ Define key terms associated with gastrointestinal health problems.

▌ Identify risk factors associated with the development of gastrointestinal health problems.

▌ Discuss the common etiologies of gastrointestinal health problems.

▌ Describe the pathophysiologic processes associated with specific gastrointestinal health problems.

▌ Distinguish between normal and abnormal gastrointestinal findings obtained from the nursing assessment.

▌ Prioritize nursing interventions associated with specific gastrointestinal health problems.

[*Media Link*]

Use the CD-ROM enclosed with this text, or log onto the address given to access the free, interactive Companion Website created for this series. The CD-ROM and Companion Website accompanying this book offer additional practice opportunities and information—NCLEX Review, Case Studies, Glossary, In Depth with NCLEX, and more.

www.prenhall.com/hogan

REVIEW AT A GLANCE

borborygmus *rumbling sounds in the gastrointestinal (GI) tract*

Crohn's disease *an inflammatory condition of the bowel in which there are patchy areas of inflammation anywhere along the entire GI tract; also known as regional enteritis*

dumping syndrome *rapid emptying of stomach contents into the small intestine, causing sweating and weakness after a meal; usually occurs after a gastric resection*

dyspepsia *burning, epigastric pain*

erythroplakia *red patches in the mouth*

fecalith *a hard piece of stool that is stone-like and may cause bleeding*

gastroparesis *delayed gastric emptying time*

hematemesis *vomiting up blood*

Helicobacter pylori *Gram-negative bacteria that plays a role in the development of peptic ulcers*

intussusception *the intrusion of a part of the intestine into another part that is distal to it*

leukoplakia *white patches on the mouth*

McBurney's point *the point halfway between umbilicus and the right iliac crest*

melena *black, tarry feces caused by the presence of blood*

peptic ulcer disease (PUD) *an ulcer that may be located in the lower end of the esophagus, the stomach, or the duodenum*

peritonitis *infection of the membrane that lines the peritoneum or abdominal cavity*

pyrosis *severe epigastric pain or heartburn*

rebound tenderness *severe pain over an area of tenderness when pressure is applied to that area by the examiner and quickly released*

volvulus obstruction *a twisting of the bowel resulting in a large bowel obstruction*

Zollinger-Ellison syndrome *a condition in which a pancreatic tumor causes secretion of excess amounts of gastrin, which stimulates the secretion of hydrochloric acid and pepsin; these events can lead to the formation of a peptic ulcer*

Pretest

1 A client is being admitted to a hospital unit complaining of severe pain in the lower abdomen and is lying on the bed with his knees flexed. Admission vital signs reveal an oral temperature of 101.2°F. Which of the following would confirm a diagnosis of appendicitis?

(1) The pain is localized at a position halfway between the umbilicus and the right iliac crest.
(2) The client describes the pain as occurring 2 hours after eating.
(3) The pain subsides after eating.
(4) The pain is in the left lower quadrant.

2 An elderly client presents with fever, leukocytosis, lower left quadrant pain, and diarrhea alternating with constipation. The nurse concludes that these are frequently seen in clients with:

(1) Appendicitis.
(2) Diverticulitis.
(3) Peptic ulcer disease.
(4) Irritable bowel syndrome.

3 A client says to the nurse, "My doctor told me my ulcer may have been caused by bacteria. I thought ulcers were caused by diet and too much stress." Which of the following responses by the nurse is the best?

(1) "If it was caused by bacteria, you would have a fever as a result of the inflammatory process."
(2) "We know that ulcers are communicable. They can be spread easily. Be careful you don't spread it to your children."
(3) "Diet and stress have nothing to do with developing an ulcer."
(4) "Even though the bacteria *Heliobacter pylori* causes inflammation, other factors may cause increased acid in the stomach."

4 In caring for a client with a hiatal hernia, which of the following should be included in a teaching plan regarding causes?

(1) To avoid heavy lifting
(2) A dietary plan based on soft foods
(3) Its prevalence in young adults
(4) Its prevalence in fair-skinned individuals

5 An elderly male client is worried about bright red blood in his stool along with feeling tired and worn out. The nurse determines that these symptoms are characteristic of:

(1) Ascending (right-sided) colon cancer.
(2) Descending (left-sided) colon cancer.
(3) Gallbladder disease.
(4) Gastric ulcers.

6 A client states, "My doctor told me to quit taking aspirin since I've developed this ulcer. I have to take aspirin to keep my arthritis from hurting. I don't know what to do." Which response on the part of the nurse is best?

(1) "Let's worry about treating your ulcer—your arthritis will have to wait."
(2) "Aspirin is one of the medications that makes an ulcer worse; another medicine can be ordered by the doctor for your arthritis."
(3) "Go ahead and take the aspirin if it helps, but watch closely for bleeding."
(4) "The doctor knows what is best for you, and you should follow those instructions."

7 The nurse is caring for a female client during recuperation following development of a duodenal ulcer. The client suddenly experiences severe abdominal pain, increased heart rate, increased respiratory rate, and diaphoresis. On palpation, the abdomen is rigid; bowel sounds are faint and diminished. Which of the following nursing actions is appropriate?

(1) Immediately place her in high Fowler's position to facilitate breathing.
(2) Help her walk to the bathroom to get rid of any flatus.
(3) Check to see if she has food allergies and see if she ate anything to which she might be allergic.
(4) Establish IV access and call the doctor to report the assessment data.

8 A female client complains of a burning, cramping pain in the top part of the abdomen that becomes worse in the middle of the afternoon and sometimes awakens her at night. She reports that eating something usually helps the pain go away but that the pain is now becoming more intense. Which of the following is the best conclusion for the nurse to draw?

(1) These symptoms are consistent with an ulcer.
(2) The client is probably developing cholelithiasis.
(3) The client probably has indigestion and needs to watch what she eats.
(4) A snack before bed should be recommended.

9 Which of the following clients would be most at risk for an intestinal obstruction?

(1) A Jewish client who smokes and consumes large amounts of caffeine
(2) An elderly client who is on bedrest because of postoperative abdominal surgery
(3) An individual eating a low-fiber, high-fat diet
(4) An adult diagnosed with cirrhosis of the liver

10 A client is complaining of dyspepsia, frequent belching, and increased salivation. The nurse suspects which of the following?

(1) Peptic ulcer disease (PUD)
(2) Ulcerative colitis
(3) Rolling hiatal hernia
(4) Gastroesophageal reflux disease (GERD)

See pages 252–253 for Answers and Rationales.

I. **Risk Factors Associated with Gastrointestinal Health Problems**

A. *Gastroesophageal reflux disease:* prolonged gastric intubation, infections, systemic diseases, systemic lupus erythematosus (SLE), ingestion of corrosive substances, acidic foods, obesity, smoking, and alcohol intake

B. *Peptic ulcer disease (PUD):* chronic diseases such as COPD, rheumatoid arthritis, or cirrhosis; stress; smoking; continued or excessive use of nonsteroidal antiinflammatory drugs (NSAIDs) or aspirin products; *H. pylori* infection; duodenal ulcers are more prominent with type O blood and may be genetically transmitted

C. **Hiatal hernia:** aging, trauma, surgery, hereditary, obesity

D. *Crohn's disease*: Genetic and familial predisposition, race (Jewish highest), stress

E. **Ulcerative colitis:** race, genetic predisposition, stress, autoimmune disease

F. **Diverticular disease:** diseases such as ulcerative colitis and Crohn's disease; obesity; poor dietary habits (high intake of refined foods), especially in the elderly

G. **Intestinal obstruction:** clients having abdominal surgeries; elderly; trauma

H. **Appendicitis:** fecal impactions, kinking of the bowel, parasites, infections

I. *Peritonitis*: diseases such as Laennec's cirrhosis, tuberculosis, PUD, inflammatory conditions, trauma or perforation of the abdominal viscus, surgery

J. **Neoplasms of the gastrointestinal (GI) tract:** tobacco use (oral cancer); excessive alcohol and tobacco consumption; diet lacking fruits and vegetables; esophageal disorders (esophageal cancer); genetic predisposition; diet high in gastric irritants; conditions such as chronic gastritis or achlorhydria (stomach cancer); low-fiber, high-fat diet and diseases such as Crohn's disease, polyps, ulcerative colitis (intestinal cancer)

II. **Gastroesophageal Reflux Disease (GERD)**

A. **Overview**

1. Defined as the backflow of gastric contents into the esophagus; also known as heartburn or esophagitis

2. Etiologies include high-fat diet; hiatal hernia; pregnancy, obesity; conditions that reduce lower esophageal sphincter tone (such as excess caffeine intake); congenital defects; **gastroparesis** (delayed gastric emptying time); activities such as vomiting, coughing, lifting, or bending

B. **Pathophysiology**

1. Gastric contents that are regurgitated into the esophagus are acidic and irritate the lining of the esophagus; the lower esophageal sphincter (LES) should completely close when food is consumed into the stomach; when the LES is weakened or incompetent, higher pressure within the stomach forces the contents into the esophagus where the pressure is less; this same concept of a higher pressure area emptying into a lower pressure area accounts for incidence of gastroesphageal reflux disease (GERD) in conditions such as pregnancy, obesity, and overindulgence of food

2. The esophagus has mucus-producing cells to protect the lining, but in less quantity than the stomach, where a high acid environment is normal

3. Severe GERD can cause epithelial cell damage and erosion of the muscularis

4. Complications include strictures, bleeding, reflux-induced asthma, laryngitis

5. Signs and symptoms include **dyspepsia** (burning, epigastric pain); frequent belching with a sour taste; pain after eating, when lying down, and after straining or lifting; increased salivation; flatulence; history of high stress level

C. Nursing assessment

1. Assessment includes symptom analysis of pain (1–2 hours after eating), nutritional assessment, analysis of any other symptoms, and evidence of complications

2. Diagnostic tests: pH probe test is used to determine the number and length of declines in the pH of stomach contents (less than 4.0); barium swallow; otherwise history determines the diagnosis

D. Nursing management

1. Medications include antacids, H_2-receptor antagonists, proton pump inhibitors, antihistamines; separate all antacids from meals by 1 hour and from other medications by 1 to 2 hours

2. Teach client about possible surgery (fundoplication)

3. Offer several small meals rather than three large ones; suggest weight loss if necessary; limit or eliminate caffeine, heavy spices, and smoking

4. Elevate the head of the bed while sleeping

5. Instruct the client to avoid eating in a supine position and to drink extra fluids unless contraindicated

6. Instruct the client to keep a diary of the foods that seem to increase the symptoms and avoid these when determined

7. Discuss stress reduction methods and resources

III. Peptic Ulcer Disease (PUD)

A. Overview

1. Defined as an ulcer, which may be located in the lower end of the esophagus, the stomach, or the duodenum

2. Occurs equally between males and females; mortality increases with age over 75

3. Causes include: excessive stress, **Helicobacter pylori** infection (a gram-negative bacteria), excessive use of NSAIDs and aspirin products; any situation where there is damage to the mucosa; and **Zollinger-Ellison syndrome** (a pancreatic tumor that causes excess amounts of gastrin to be excreted)

4. Three main types are gastric, duodenal, and stress; may be acute or chronic

   a. Gastric ulcers: etiologies include ingestion of medications, tobacco, caffeine, alcohol; *H. pylori* infection; chronic bile reflux and increased serum gastrin

   b. Duodenal ulcers: etiologies include hypersecretion of pepsinogen, autosomal dominant trait, *H. pylori* infection (95–100% of cases)

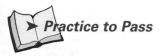

Practice to Pass

A 42-year-old male client is diagnosed with GERD after being admitted with severe pains in his chest, frequent indigestion, and pain after meals. Since he thought he was having a heart attack, how should the nurse explain the difference in the symptoms between the two diagnoses?

B. Pathophysiology

1. Ulcers may be contributed to by three main factors

   a. *Excess acid* can lead to a break or ulceration in the mucosa of the stomach or duodenum; the break allows the mucosa to be subjected to an acid or alkaline environment and thus autodigestion occurs

   b. *Decreased mucus production* can leave the mucosal cells unprotected from the acid environment; hypoxia, shock, severe burns, etc., can lead to the injury of the mucus-producing cells

   c. *Increased delivery of acid* can cause the protective mucus layer to be irritated because of the rapid movement of stomach contents, such as in **dumping syndrome** (rapid emptying of stomach contents into the small intestine causing sweating, weakness, etc., after a meal)

2. Ulcers can be superficial or deep

   a. Superficial ulcers are also called erosions

   b. Deep lesions extend through the musculature and penetrate blood vessels causing hemorrhage; can also cause perforation of the wall of the stomach or the intestines

3. Infection with the bacteria *H. pylori* is a major factor in gastric and duodenal ulcers, causing death of mucosal epithelial cells; it also releases toxins and enzymes that produce inflammation and ulcer development; increased levels of gastrin and/or pepsinogen have been attributed to presence of the bacteria

Figure 7-1

The pathophysiology of dumping syndrome.

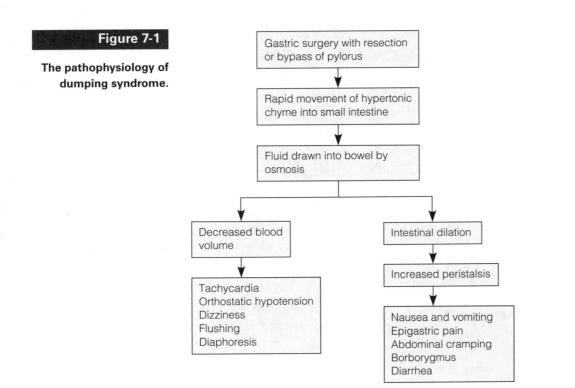

4. Rapid gastric emptying (such as in dumping syndrome) may cause increased acid in the duodenum and aid ulcer development (Figure 7-1)

5. Stress, caffeine, cigarette smoking, and alcohol consumption increase acid production; aspirin and NSAID medications inhibit prostaglandin, which helps protect the lining of the stomach

6. Gastric ulcers are usually small and singular, located at the lesser curvature of the stomach; duodenal ulcers are usually deep and occur in the beginning area of the duodenum next to the pyloric sphincter

7. A Curling's ulcer is an acute stress ulcer that usually follows a severe illness (especially burns, trauma, surgery, shock, renal failure); is a form of stress ulcer; tends to be multiple, superficial, and tends to erode several areas of the gastric mucosa

8. Signs and symptoms

   a. Gastric ulcers: severe **pyrosis** (epigastric pain or heartburn); may radiate to back or flank; usually occurs immediately after or during a meal; food usually does not relieve the pain

   b. Duodenal ulcers: right epigastric pain; radiates to back or thorax; often occurs when stomach is empty; food and antacids relieve the pain

   c. Other: fullness after eating, nausea, vomiting, bloating, anorexia, gnawing type of pain; weight loss or weight gain (with duodenal ulcers because eating relieves the pain); pain may come and go; **hematemesis** (vomiting up blood) and **melena** (black, tarry feces because of the presence of blood)

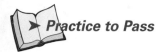

Practice to Pass

A client asks the nurse, "How can I prevent development of an ulcer? My father had lots of trouble with them." How should the nurse answer the client?

C. **Nursing assessment**

1. Assessment includes symptom analysis of pain; relationship of pain to food intake; any hematemesis or melena; use of NSAID medications, list of all medications taken at home; intake of alcohol or use of cigarettes; history of stress level

2. Diagnostic tests: blood serum for presence of *H. pylori* antibodies; endoscopy, barium studies and upper GI (ulcer craters present); CBC (decreased RBC, hemoglobin, hematocrit); stool specimen (positive for occult blood), electrolytes

D. **Nursing management**

1. Medications include an H₂ antagonist such as cimetidine (Tagamet), ranitidine (Zantac), or famotidine (Pepcid); proton pump inhibitor such as omeprazole (Prilosec); mucosal barrier drug such as sucralfate (Carafate); antacids to neutralize gastric acid (with the exception of bicarbonate of soda); cytoprotective agent such as synthetic *E. prostaglandin* (Cytotec) to promote mucus production for healing; and antibiotics to destroy *H. pylori*

   a. Frequently this can be done by giving two antibiotics such as tetracycline hydrochloride (Achromycin) and metronidazole (Flagyl)

   b. Often recommended to give bismuth compound (Pepto-Bismol) with the antibiotics (but may make stools appear as melena)

2. Individualize the diet by determining which foods cause pain and eliminating them; suggest six small meals daily rather than three large ones; limit food intake, caffeine, and alcohol late at night

3. Limit milk to one glass per meal

4. Avoid caffeine, cigarettes, and alcohol

5. Encourage rest and stress reduction

6. Monitor for indications of perforation such as severe abdominal pain, rigidity in the abdomen, distention, absent bowel sounds, and signs of shock

7. Monitor weight periodically

8. Avoid use of NSAIDs and acetylsalicylic acid (aspirin) products; instruct the client that many pain medications and most arthritis medications contain these agents and should be avoided

IV. Hiatal Hernia

A. Overview

1. Defined as the protruding of the stomach into the mediastinal cavity by way of the diaphragm (see Figure 7-2)

2. Types

   a. *Sliding esophageal hernia* (most common, 90%): the herniated section of stomach slides back and forth through the hiatus with position changes and increased peristalsis

   b. *Rolling esophageal hernia:* the fundus and greater curvature of the stomach roll into the thorax next to the esophagus; can have serious complications

3. Causes include weakening of the esophageal muscles due to aging, trauma, surgery or an anatomic defect; heavy straining or lifting

B. Pathophysiology

1. In a sliding esophageal hernia, there is gastroesophageal reflux caused by the weakened esophageal hiatus muscles; this accounts for the symptoms experienced

2. In a rolling or paraesophageal hernia, increased intrathoracic pressure occurs because of the protrusion of the thoracic contents by the hernia

3. It may by asymptomatic, or signs and symptoms may vary according to the type of hernia

   a. Sliding: dysphagia, pyrosis, regurgitation, bloating, and heartburn

   b. Rolling: shortness of breath, chest pain (similar to anginal pain), and tachycardia

C. Nursing assessment

1. Assessment includes symptom analysis of pain, vital signs (VS), complaints of shortness of breath, analysis of symptoms that would suggest angina versus GI pain (description of the pain)

2. Diagnostic tests: upper GI, arterial blood gases (ABGs) if shortness of breath is experienced, CXR shows stomach in thorax

D. Nursing management

1. Medications include antacids, H_2-receptor antagonists, analgesics

2. Monitor and educate about proper diet and taking six small meals rather than three large ones; begin on weight reduction program if necessary

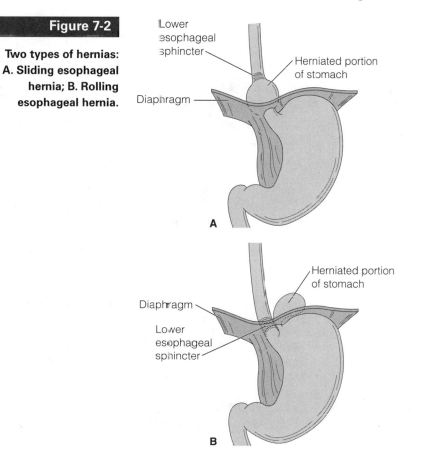

Figure 7-2

Two types of hernias: A. Sliding esophageal hernia; B. Rolling esophageal hernia.

Lower esophageal sphincter

Herniated portion of stomach

Diaphragm

A

Herniated portion of stomach

Diaphragm

Lower esophageal sphincter

B

NCLEX!

3. Educate the client about head elevation for sleep and eating

4. Explain surgery if indicated

NCLEX!

5. Discourage intake of alcohol, high amounts of caffeine, and cigarettes

V. Crohn's Disease (Regional Enteritis)

A. Overview

1. Defined as a chronic inflammatory condition of the bowel in which there are patchy areas of inflammation anywhere in the entire GI tract; most common in the ileum or colon; referred to as inflammatory bowel disease (IBD) and grouped with ulcerative colitis because symptoms are similar

2. Incidence is higher among young adults and teenagers; occurs equally in both genders; more often seen in clients of Jewish and Caucasian race

NCLEX!

3. Develops slowly, with remissions and exacerbations; emotional factors related to family matters or work aggravate the illness

4. Cause is unknown but thought to be multifactoral, probably involving an infectious process (bacteria, viruses, mycobacteria), allergy or immune disorder, psychosomatic, dietary, hormonal, and environmental factors

B. Pathophysiology

1. Inflammatory lesions may occur anywhere from the mouth to the anus; more often lesions occur in the ascending colon, distal ileum, and anorectal areas

2. The lesions are local and involve all layers of the intestinal wall; the wall contains shallow long ulcers with long or short areas of stricture

3. The lesions involve some areas of the bowel but not all areas (called skip lesions)

4. Because of the involvement of the submucosal layers, the mucosa has a granuloma (tumor-like growth) that gives the tissue a cobblestone appearance

5. The bowel wall becomes congested, thickened, and may develop abscesses; fistulas may develop between the infected area and the bladder or other areas of intestine, resulting in malabsorption of nutrients (see Figure 7-3)

6. Scar tissue may interfere with movement of chyme and perforation or obstruction may occur

7. Complications caused by excessive diarrhea include fluid and electrolyte imbalance as well as dehydration; deficiency in absorption of folic acid, calcium, and vitamin D; anal fissures, perianal abscesses, and fistula

8. Signs and symptoms include nausea, vomiting, flatulence, malaise, weight loss cause by anorexia, three to five semisolid foul-smelling stools/day; intermittent, localized pain in the right lower quadrant (worsening as the disease progresses); mucus in stools with possible pus (blood may also be present); urgency in the night to defecate; fluid and electrolyte imbalance, dehydration, fever, elevated WBC, iron-deficiency anemia, perianal abscesses and fistulas, and hypoalbuminemia

Figure 7-3

Pathophysiology leading to the symptons of Crohn's disease.

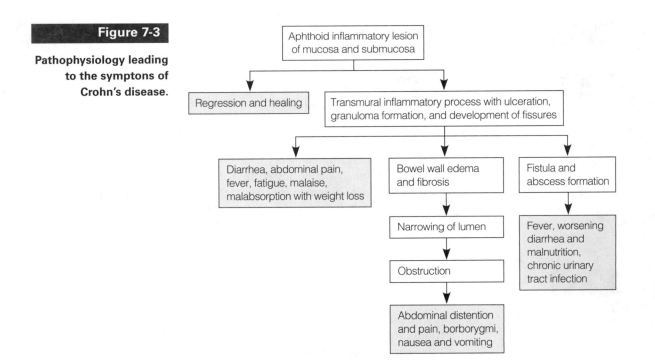

C. Nursing assessment

1. Assessment includes nutritional and fluid status, symptom analysis of symptoms and pain, bowel pattern assessment, daily weight, activity tolerance, visual examination of stool, history of risk factors/stress level and emotional factors, vital signs, skin/nail color changes secondary to anemia

2. Diagnostic tests: CBC (elevated WBC, low RBC, Hgb, and Hct), barium enema (reveals characteristic "string sign," or skip lesions), albumin level (low), high erythrocyte sedimentation rate (ESR), electrolytes (hypocalcemia)

D. Nursing management

1. Medications include sulfasalazine (Azulfidine) to control infection; corticosteroids to decrease inflammation; analgesics to control abdominal pain; anticholinergics to control diarrhea; vitamin and mineral replacements; electrolyte replacements as needed; antipyretics if fever occurs; many of the electrolytes (especially potassium and calcium) should be given with food to decrease GI irritation

2. Attempt to control the diarrhea since the distended intestinal wall may lead to perforation; monitor temperature

3. Fluid replacement may be given to correct dehydration; monitor for symptoms of dehydration; TPN may be added if necessary to provide for nutritional needs while allowing GI tract to rest

4. Give low-residue, low-fat, high-protein, high-calorie diet

5. Instruct about lifestyle management to reduce stress

VI. Ulcerative Colitis

A. Overview

1. Defined as an inflammatory disease affecting the mucous membranes of the colon; affects part of or all of the colon and rectum

2. Occurs between ages of 10 to 40; more common in Caucasian and Jewish race

3. Considered under the general heading of inflammatory bowel disease along with Crohn's disease; disease has stages of exacerbations and remissions

4. The disease is labeled as mild, moderate, or fulminating

5. The disease is of unknown etiology; suggested causes include a genetic basis, viruses, bacteria, autoimmunity, and stress

B. Pathophysiology

1. Ulcerated lesions form small erosions in the mucosal layer; there are no skip lesions as in Crohn's disease

2. These cavities may feature small hemorrhages and abscesses

3. The wall of the bowel thickens and the ulcerations are fibrotic in the later stages of the illness

4. Complications can include intestinal obstruction, dehydration, fluid and electrolyte imbalances, malabsorption, iron-deficiency anemia

5. Signs and symptoms include chronic, bloody diarrhea mixed with mucus (worsens as the disease increases in severity); fever; weight loss; abdominal cramping and pain; nausea and vomiting; urge to defecate

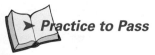

Practice to Pass

How should the nurse determine whether a client with Crohn's disease is becoming dehydrated?

NCLEX!

NCLEX!

NCLEX!

NCLEX!

C. Nursing assessment

1. Assessment includes bowel habits, visual inspection of stool, vital signs, weight, nutritional status, symptom analysis of pain, activity tolerance, bowel sounds, and nutritional status

2. Diagnostic tests: CBC (low RBC, Hgb, Hct), electrolytes (low potassium), sigmoidoscopy, stool for occult blood

D. Nursing management

1. Medications include antipyretics; anti-inflammatory drugs such as sulfasalazine (Azulfidine); antibiotics; corticosteroids; antimicrobial agents, metronidazole (Flagyl); antidiarrheals; antispasmodics

2. Offer bulk-free diet and nutritional supplements as necessary; weigh client weekly

3. Offer psychological support and counseling

4. Monitor bowel sounds and bowel movements

5. Assess for signs of dehydration; monitor intake and output; administer IV fluids as ordered

VII. Diverticular Disease

A. Overview

1. Defined as *diverticula* or *diverticulum*: an outpouching of the walls of the colon; *diverticulitis:* inflammation of a diverticulum within the intestinal tract; *diverticulosis:* the condition of having diverticula within the colon without any inflammation or symptoms

2. More common in clients over 60 years of age eating a low-residue diet

3. May be *acute* (similar to appendicitis) or *chronic* (characterized by severe constipation and pain, distention, and flatulence)

4. Causes include severe constipation, obesity, lack of dietary fiber or roughage

B. Pathophysiology

1. An increase in intraluminal pressure causes the outpouching of the colon wall; there is usually a weakness in the intestinal wall from effects of diet

2. Bacteria from food that becomes trapped in the pouches then causes diverticulitis

3. A lack of adequate blood supply or nutrients from the diet may also contribute to the development of this disease

4. Chronic diverticulitis may cause thickening of the intestinal walls and possibly obstruction

5. Complications include rupture of the intestinal wall leading to peritonitis; obstruction, and abscesses (rare)

6. Signs and symptoms include constipation, lower left-sided abdominal pain, signs of peritonitis (fever, guarding, abdominal rigidity); occasional rectal bleeding; diarrhea (not as common as constipation); elevated WBC; may be asymptomatic

C. Nursing assessment

1. Assessment includes: symptom analysis of complaints and any pain, vital signs, palpation of abdomen, auscultation of bowel sounds, bowel habits, any posturing

2. Diagnostic tests: ultrasound, sigmoidoscopy, guaiac stool, barium enema, CTscan

D. Nursing management

1. Medications include antidiarrheals and antispasmodics (occasionally), laxatives (bulk-forming), stool softeners, analgesics, antipyretics if fever occurs

2. Monitor vital signs and treat fever as necessary

3. Encourage 2 to 3 liters of fluid per day unless contraindicated

4. Assess stools for color, consistency, frequency, presence of blood

5. Encourage rest periods and discourage lifting, straining, or bending

6. Offer high dietary roughage (fruit, vegetables, fiber)

7. Educate the client about the symptoms of the disease and a lifestyle that can decrease these symptoms

8. Encourage the cessation of smoking and alcohol use for general GI health

VIII. Intestinal Obstruction

A. Overview

1. Defined as the inability of the intestinal contents to progress through the bowel in a normal manner; sites of blockage may be in the small intestine (high blockage) or in the colon (low blockage)

2. Classified as mechanical or paralytic obstructions

   a. *Mechanical* is caused by any condition that hinders the patency of the lumen of the bowel (tumors, adhesions); most common type overall

   1) A **volvulus obstruction** refers to a twisting of the bowel and results in a large bowel obstruction; most common in elderly clients

   2) **Intussusception** is the intrusion of a part of the intestine into another part that lies distal to it; most common in infants 10–15 months

   b. *Functional* or *paralytic* is caused by neurogenic or muscular impairment that hinders peristalsis (postsurgery, prolonged bedrest)

3. Children most commonly have mechanical obstructions (especially younger than 2 years) rather than paralysis obstructions

4. Causes include intestinal adhesions, hernias, tumors, severe constipation, surgery, debilitated state with prolonged bedrest

B. Pathophysiology

1. Blockage of the intestine (regardless of cause) leads to intestinal distention by gas and air, pooling of gastric and biliary secretions, and loss of fluids, electrolytes, and proteins

2. Distention caused by pooling of the secretions leads to decreased absorption of water and electrolytes through the bowel wall; vomiting and pooling lead to hypovolemia, dehydration, and ultimately hypovolemic shock

NCLEX!

NCLEX!

NCLEX!

3. The impaired blood supply leads to increased peristalsis initially, ischemia and acidosis, bacterial invasion, and possibly subsequent necrosis and peritonitis

4. Cellular disruption and tissue hypoxia, along with stasis of the secretions, provide an excellent medium for bacteria growth

5. Complications include fluid and electrolyte imbalances, gangrene of the bowel, strangulation of a bowel segment, and perforation

6. Signs and symptoms include colicky pain, distention of bowel; bowel sounds may be **borborygmus** (rumbling sounds) initially, then change to hypoactive or absent; nausea and vomiting (bilious, feculent); anorexia; diarrhea or lack of bowel movement; abdominal tenderness, rigidity, fever; restlessness; electrolyte abnormalities; hypovolemic or septic shock may occur

C. Nursing assessment

1. Assessment includes bowel habits and patterns, symptom analysis of pain, bowel sounds, palpation of the abdomen, visual inspection of stool, intake and output, nutritional status, vital signs and oxygen saturation, abdominal girth

2. Diagnostic tests: CBC, electrolytes, abdominal x-ray, amylase level, barium enema, CT scan, ultrasound of abdomen

D. Nursing management

1. Medications include laxatives (oral or suppository), enemas, electrolyte replacements as needed

2. Monitor bowel sounds and bowel movements; check for a fecal impaction and remove if possible

3. Measure intake and output (I & O); weight, and amount of food consumed each meal

4. Provide privacy to have a bowel movement; offer air freshener

5. Decompression of the bowel through a nasogastric tube or surgical intervention may be needed

6. Postsurgery, encourage early ambulation and increased fluid intake

7. Monitor vital signs; provide IV fluids as ordered

8. Client education should be given regarding the need to prevent constipation (use of natural laxatives, stool softeners, increased fluid intake, and increased activity)

9. Monitor the use and frequency of opioid analgesics that decrease motility

IX. Appendicitis

A. Overview

1. Defined as an inflammation of the vermiform appendix

2. Occurs often in children and young adults ages 10 to 30 years; males are affected more often than females

3. May be acute (sudden, severe), chronic (follows an acute attack), or gangrenous (extreme inflammation); an appendix may rupture

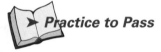

Practice to Pass

An elderly female client presents with a distended abdomen, hypoactive bowel sounds, tenderness and pain upon palpation and states her last bowel movement was 7 days ago. What changes could occur within the next few hours that would warrant immediate attention if the obstruction is not treated?

4. Symptoms in females must be differentiated from ovarian cysts, ectopic pregnancy, and pelvic inflammatory disease

5. Causes include unknown etiology, obstruction of appendix from stool, or necrosis of organ

B. Pathophysiology

1. The appendix is attached to the cecum just below the ileocecal valve and in normal individuals is small, serving no known purpose

2. Obstruction of the lumen can occur due to stool (**fecalith**—a hard piece of stool which is stone-like), tumors, or foreign bodies

3. Due to the obstruction, inflammation and bacterial invasion can occur

4. Occlusion of capillaries and venules causes increased intraluminal pressure, leading to decreased blood flow to the mucosa and hypoxic tissue

5. Gangrene can develop from thrombosis of the luminal blood vessels, which may lead to perforation and possibly resultant **peritonitis** (infection of the membrane that lines the peritoneum or abdominal cavity)

6. Signs and symptoms include pain in the right lower quadrant of the abdomen that may localize at **McBurney's point** (halfway between umbilicus and right iliac crest); GI disturbances (anorexia, nausea, vomiting, diarrhea, or sometimes constipation); **rebound tenderness** (severe pain over the area of tenderness when pressure is applied to the appendix area by the examiner and quickly released); posturing by lying on side or back with knees flexed; fever, elevated BP and/or heart rate caused by pain and fever; malaise

7. If a confirmed diagnosis of appendicitis is made and the pain suddenly stops without any intervention, the appendix may have ruptured; the pain is lessened because the appendix is no longer distended; surgery is still needed

C. Nursing assessment

1. Assessment includes vital signs, symptom analysis of pain, palpation of abdomen (rebound tenderness) until diagnosis is made, history of bowel movements, history of menses in women, and activity tolerance

2. Diagnostic tests: CBC (elevated WBC with rupture), ultrasound, CT scan

D. Nursing management

1. Medications include IV antibiotics, analgesics for pain, and antipyretics for fever

2. Comfort measures until a diagnosis is confirmed; surgery is the recommended treatment

3. Administer IV fluids in preparation for surgery if diagnosis is confirmed; in the absence of rebound tenderness, IV fluids are given to confirm a possible GI virus (pain improves after fluids are given with a virus)

4. Avoid enemas, cathartics, heating pads, or abdominal palpation with a confirmed diagnosis to prevent a rupture

5. Monitor vital signs, especially temperature

6 Administer standard postoperative care: turn, cough, deep-breathing; early ambulation, assess bowel sounds, monitor urinary output, and provide wound care

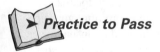

Practice to Pass

A 15-year-old is brought to the Emergency Department complaining of right lower quadrant pain and diarrhea. There are no other signs and symptoms present. What assessment and nursing intervention would help to rule out appendicitis?

NCLEX!

X. Peritonitis

A. Overview

1. Defined as local or generalized inflammation of the peritoneum (lining that covers the abdominal viscera)

2. May be primary (bacterial infection), secondary (trauma, surgical injury, chemical irritation), or as a complication of GI accessory organ disease

3. Caused by a ruptured appendix or peptic ulcer, diverticulitis, bowel obstruction, ruptured urinary bladder, infection from the reproductive tract, or as a postoperative complication resulting in leakage from an intestinal anastomosis

B. Pathophysiology

1. The peritoneum is a semipermeable membrane; as an attempt to maintain homeostasis, fluid shifts may occur with third-spacing into the peritoneal cavity; dehydration, decreased urinary output, hypovolemia, electrolyte imbalance, and even shock may occur

2. If the secretions or chemical irritants leaking into the peritoneum are sterile, the irritation is primarily chemical; if they are infected, an intense inflammatory response is generated

3. Generalized peritonitis progresses to septicemia, which leads to septic shock and multiple organ failure; symptoms may be overlooked in the elderly client until the condition is severe

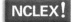

4. Signs and symptoms include abdominal pain that is intense, often localized at site of involvement; chills and fever; anorexia, nausea, and vomiting; guarding and rigidity of the abdomen; abdominal distention; diminished or absent bowel sounds; sweating, tachycardia, tachypnea; oliguria; restlessness, disorientation; elevated WBC; pallor; reduce urine output from dehydration

C. Nursing assessment

1. Assessment includes symptom analysis of pain and other complaints, vital signs, auscultation of bowel sounds, palpation of abdomen, urinary output, mental status, skin color, and nutritional assessment

2. Diagnostic tests: CBC, electrolytes, abdominal ultrasound, BUN, creatinine, peritoneal aspiration with cultures

D. Nursing management

1. Medications include antibiotic therapy (after cultures are obtained); analgesics for pain control; potassium replacement if kidney function is adequate

2. Replacement of fluid and electrolytes

3. Monitor urinary output and venous pressure

4. Mechanical ventilation or monitoring of pulmonary artery pressure by a Swan-Ganz catheter may be necessary for severely ill clients

5. TPN may be used for nutritional needs

6. NG tube is often necessary for abdominal distention and reduced peristalsis; postoperative feeding may be done by jejunostomy tube if client is unable to take an oral diet

7. Emotional support for both the client and family is important

8. Routine postoperative care, discharge planning and referrals are essential

XI. Neoplasms of the Gastrointestinal Tract

A. Overview

1. Defined as oral cancer (lips, pharynx, tongue, soft palate, and uvula); esophageal, stomach, or colon and rectum (colorectal) cancer

2. **Leukoplakia** (white patches on the mouth) and **erythroplakia** (red patches in the mouth) are pre-cancerous lesions that should be reported; ulcers on lips or in the mouth that don't heal, as well as enlarged lymph nodes, should be investigated as possible harmful lesions

3. Early diagnosis is essential in both oral and colorectal cancer for higher survival rates to be achieved

4. Causes include tobacco and alcohol use; diet low in fiber, high in fat, and low in fruits and vegetables; genetic disposition

B. Pathophysiology

1. Squamous cells in the mouth are susceptible to developing squamous cell carcinoma; oral cancer spreads very rapidly because of the rich vascular supply in the mouth

2. Esophageal tumors encircle the esophagus and invade the lymphatic system

3. Stomach cancer includes adenocarcinoma occurring within the pyloric region of the stomach; spreads through the lymphatic system and into other organs

4. Most colorectal cancers are moderately differentiated adenocarcinomas; colorectal cancers tend to grow slowly; start in the mucosa and most extend over a considerable amount of tissue before reaching the lymph channel and metastasizing

5. Signs and symptoms

   a. Oral: difficulty or pain in chewing, swallowing, or speaking; presence of a precancerous lesion or an ulcer in the tissue

   b. Esophageal: dysphagia, pulmonary complications, regurgitation, aspiration, or fistula formation

   c. Stomach: loss of appetite, weight loss, gastric discomfort, weakness, pain

   d. Colorectal

      1) Right-sided (ascending): mild bleeding; weakness, fatigue, lack of energy; anorexia and weight loss

      2) Left-sided (descending): change in bowel habits such as going from diarrhea to constipation; small or pencil-shaped stools, gas or bloating, dark blood in the stool or rectal bleeding; another complaint is the feeling of not completely emptying on defecation

   e. Anorexia, weakness, and weight loss are indications of any tumor growth; in advanced stages the tumor mass would be palpable

C. Nursing assessment

1. Assessment includes changes in bowel habits, nutritional status, weight loss or gain, palpation of the abdomen, activity tolerance, symptom analysis of any pain, visual inspection of any oral lesions; (oral lesions frequently can be palpated with a gloved finger before they are visible, any firm, asymmetric enlargement should be suspect and reported); visual inspection of stool specimen

2. Diagnostic tests: guaiac test for occult blood, biopsy, colonoscopy or sigmoidoscopy, barium enema, CBC, liver function tests, CT scan/MRI, bronchoscopy, endoscopy, carcinoembryonic antigen (CEA), upper and lower GI series, coagulation panel

D. Nursing management

1. Medications and treatment

   NCLEX!

   a. Radiation and/or surgery is often the treatment recommended

   b. Chemotherapy may be given alone or in combination with radiation therapy and surgery

   c. Other: analgesics, antiemetics, stool softeners, antibiotic therapy if indicated

   NCLEX!

2. Client teaching is important regarding detection of any of the GI cancers, use of sunscreens, necessity for annual physical examinations, and avoidance of potential risk factors such as smoking

   NCLEX!

3. Over the age of 40, a colonoscopy is recommended, especially if a family history exists or a client has rectal polyps or diverticulosis; an annual guaiac test is recommended for clients over the age of 50

4. If surgery is performed, provide standard postoperative care

5. Provide pain management

6. Maintain patent airway after oral surgery

7. Monitor nutritional status; provide good oral care; hydrate well after an endoscopy of GI series

8. Provide emotional support and referral as needed for the client and family

9. After surgery for colorectal cancer, monitor bowel patterns closely for frequency, volume, and consistency of bowel movements

Case Study	A 34-year-old female is admitted complaining of abdominal pain and diarrhea. She is very pale and emaciated. Her admitting diagnosis is rule out Crohn's disease.

❶ What specific questions should the nurse ask her as part of the admission history?

❷ What objective data should the nurse collect?

❸ What information will be helpful regarding the client's social history? Why?

❹ What nursing measures are important to prevent the complication of dehydration?

❺ What other nursing interventions should the nurse anticipate providing?

For suggested responses, see page 567.

Posttest

1 A client presents to the clinic with "bad pain" in the middle of the abdomen, vomiting, and "not knowing what is wrong." Palpation reveals rebound tenderness with increased pain halfway between the umbilicus and the top of the pelvis. The client seems to have less pain when lying on the left side and flexing the knees. What is the best conclusion for the nurse to draw?

(1) To make sure the client does not have an impaction, an enema should be given.
(2) Since the client is vomiting, the problem is probably gastroenteritis.
(3) The client should be checked for possible appendicitis.
(4) Since the client has been vomiting, nourishment may help.

2 A client with Zollinger-Ellison syndrome thinks she has a rare form of cancer. The nurse explains that this syndrome is characterized by which of the following?

(1) A destruction of the mucus-protecting cells of the stomach that could lead to an ulcer
(2) A condition that causes increased secretion of pepsin and hydrochloric acid
(3) A twisting of the bowel that leads to intestinal obstruction
(4) Crohn's disease, which is an inflammatory bowel disorder

3 A client who is exhibiting borborygmi, cramping pain, vomiting, and diarrhea has a diagnosis of peptic ulcer disease (PUD) with recent surgical treatment. The client is probably experiencing which of the following?

(1) Dumping syndrome
(2) Complications of the PUD
(3) Perforation of the stomach
(4) Peritonitis

4 A client diagnosed with peptic ulcer disease wants to know why he is being given antibiotics. The nurse's best answer would be:

(1) "Antibiotics help calm the stomach and decrease the symptoms."
(2) "Antibiotics decrease dumping syndrome, which can lead to PUD."
(3) "*H. pylori* is a bacterial cause for PUD and antibiotics will treat the cause."
(4) "The excess acid can be decreased when the stomach is sterile."

5 Which of the following foods should be avoided in a client with peptic ulcer disease?

(1) Vegetables
(2) Meats
(3) Fruits
(4) Chocolate

6 The nurse explains to a family that a main physiologic reason for weight loss in a client with Crohn's disease is which of the following?

(1) The symptoms of anorexia prevent the client from eating.
(2) The inflammation of the disease decreases the appetite.
(3) The thickening and congestion of the bowel wall results in malabsorption.
(4) The "skip lesions" interfere with food passage through the bowel.

7 The nurse explains to a certified nursing assistant (CNA) who is also a nursing student that the reason elderly clients are more prone to diverticulitis is because of:

(1) Poor, deficient diet.
(2) Chronic diarrhea.
(3) Frequent laxative use.
(4) Sedentary lifestyle.

8 A client who has Crohn's disease and is noncompliant should be cautioned about the risk for which of the following?

(1) Perforation of the bowel
(2) Colorectal cancer
(3) Peptic ulcer disease (PUD)
(4) Ulcerative colitis

9 Prior to giving an analgesic for pain to a postoperative client who has a history of peptic ulcer disease (PUD), the nurse should check to see that the agent does not contain which of the following?

(1) An opioid product
(2) Acetaminophen (Tylenol)
(3) Acetylsalicylic acid (aspirin)
(4) Hydrocodone

10 A client is admitted to the unit with a large, distended bowel, acute tenderness upon palpation of the abdomen, fever, rigidity, and absent bowel sounds. After being on the unit, the client's level of consciousness decreases, and he begins to have feculent vomit. The priority therapeutic intervention would be to:

(1) Reduce the fever through antipyretics.
(2) Insert an NG tube to wall suction and monitor the output.
(3) Administer pain medications to relax the client.
(4) Listen to bowel sounds.

See pages 253–254 for Answers and Rationales.

Answers and Rationales

Pretest

1 **Answer: 1** *Rationale:* Pain over McBurney's point, the point halfway between the umbilicus and the iliac crest, is diagnostic for appendicitis. Assessment for rebound tenderness would also assist in the diagnosis. Options 2 and 3 are common with ulcers; option 4 may suggest ulcerative colitis or diverticulitis.
Cognitive Level: Application
Nursing Process: Assessment; *Test Plan:* PHYS

2 **Answer: 2** *Rationale:* Fever indicates an infection, ruling out options 3 and 4. Appendicitis typically causes pain in the umbilical area or right lower quadrant and is not usually accompanied by diarrhea. Fever and diarrhea accompany diverticulitis.
Cognitive Level: Application
Nursing Process: Assessment; *Test Plan:* PHYS

3 **Answer: 4** *Rationale:* *H. pylori* causes release of toxins and enzymes that promote inflammation and ulceration. It is not spread from one person to another. Contributing factors are those that increase secretion of acid and pepsin.
Cognitive Level: Application
Nursing Process: Analysis; *Test Plan:* PHYS

4 **Answer: 1** *Rationale:* Heavy lifting is one factor that leads to development of a hiatal hernia. Dietary factors involve limiting fat intake or spicy foods, not restricting the client to soft foods. It is more prevalent in individuals who are middle-aged or older. Fair-skinned individuals are not prone to this condition.
Cognitive Level: Application
Nursing Process: Assessment; *Test Plan:* HPM

5 **Answer: 2** *Rationale:* Red blood in the stool is more characteristic of left-sided cancer of the colon. If blood occurs in the stool at all in right-sided cancer of the colon or gastric ulcers, it will be black or tarry. There is no blood in the stool of a client with gallbladder disease. Remember, bright red blood can also occur with hemorrhoids, but this choice was not available.
Cognitive Level: Application
Nursing Process: Assessment; *Test Plan:* HPM

6 **Answer: 2** *Rationale:* Aspirin is one of the nonsteroidal anti-inflammatory drugs (NSAIDs). These drugs are predisposing or contributing factors in the development of an ulcer, because of the effect on prostaglandins. Many of the medications used for arthritis may also irritate an ulcer; therefore, a physician should be consulted.
Cognitive Level: Application
Nursing Process: Implementation; *Test Plan:* PHYS

7 **Answer: 4** *Rationale:* These are all signs of perforation. If the client is going into shock, it is important to establish IV access before the veins collapse. The doctor will probably schedule emergency surgery. If a client has a possible perforation, she should be in low Fowler's position (option 1) to contain the secretions in the abdomen. Walking (option 2) is not recommended, and food allergies (option 3) are not as likely to be the problem.
Cognitive Level: Analysis
Nursing Process: Analysis; *Test Plan:* PHYS

8 **Answer: 1** *Rationale:* This description of pain is consistent with ulcer pain. The pain is epigastric and is worse when the stomach is empty and is relieved by food. These symptoms are not common with

cholelithiasis. Ordinary indigestion does not present with this clinical scenario.
Cognitive Level: Application
Nursing Process: Assessment; *Test Plan:* PHYS

9 **Answer: 2** *Rationale:* One form of intestinal obstruction is paralysis, caused by decreased movement of the intestinal contents by normal peristalsis. The client in option 1 is at high risk for Crohn's disease and ulcerative colitis. Option 3 enhances the risk of cancer of the colon and diverticular disease; option 4 is consistent with peritonitis.
Cognitive Level: Application
Nursing Process: Assessment; *Test Plan:* PHYS

10 **Answer: 4** *Rationale:* Gastroesophageal reflux disease causes epigastric pain that is usually described as burning; it is accompanied by belching with a sour taste, pain after eating, increased salivation, and flatulence. The symptoms of a sliding hiatal hernia are similar to GERD, but not those of a rolling hernia. Symptoms of PUD are more pronounced and reflective of a full or empty stomach. Ulcerative colitis symptoms are related to pain and bowel movements.
Cognitive Level: Application
Nursing Process: Assessment; *Test Plan:* PHYS

Posttest

1 **Answer: 3** *Rationale:* Lying on the side with legs flexed, pain over McBurney's point, and rebound tenderness are characteristic symptoms of appendicitis. Vomiting frequently accompanies the pain. The client definitely should *not* have an enema if appendicitis is suspected. If surgery is needed for appendicitis, the client needs to be NPO.
Cognitive Level: Analysis
Nursing Process: Assessment; *Test Plan:* PHYS

2 **Answer: 2** *Rationale:* Zollinger-Ellison syndrome is a condition usually caused by a gastrin-secreting tumor of the pancreas, stomach, or intestines that leads to the increased secretion of pepsin and hydrochloric acid. This often leads to peptic ulcer disease. Option 1 explains one of the pathologic reasons for peptic ulcer disease; option 3 explains a volvulus obstruction, and another name for Crohn's disease is regional enteritis.
Cognitive Level: Application
Nursing Process: Analysis; *Test Plan:* PHYS

3 **Answer: 1** *Rationale:* Dumping syndrome is the rapid influx of stomach contents into the duodenum or jejunum causing increased peristalsis and dilation

of the intestines. Although this occurs primarily after a gastrectomy, the condition can cause an ulcer.
Cognitive Level: Application
Nursing Process: Analysis; *Test Plan:* PHYS

4 **Answer: 3** *Rationale:* The bacteria *H. pylori* has been discovered to be the leading cause of many ulcers and can be treated with success by antibiotics. Options 1, 2, and 4 are unrealistic answers for the action of antibiotics.
Cognitive Level: Application
Nursing Process: Implementation; *Test Plan:* PHYS

5 **Answer: 4** *Rationale:* Caffeine stimulates the acid secretion and can interfere with the function of the lower esophageal sphincter. Chocolate contains caffeine and should be limited along with other drinks and foods with caffeine. Spicy or hot foods, smoking, and alcohol should also be avoided.
Cognitive Level: Application
Nursing Process: Implementation; *Test Plan:* PHYS

6 **Answer: 3** *Rationale:* The bowel wall becomes congested, thickens, and sometimes develops fistulas, which can become infected. This leads to malabsorption and deficiency in absorption of folic acid, calcium, and vitamin D. The anorexia can play a role in weight loss, but most clients eat and cannot explain why they have weight loss.
Cognitive Level: Application
Nursing Process: Analysis; *Test Plan:* PHYS

7 **Answer: 1** *Rationale:* Elderly clients often eat less food with less roughage and fiber and therefore do not obtain the proper nutrients from their diet, which

can aid in the development of the disease. Most often chronic constipation, not diarrhea, is a cause.
Cognitive Level: Application
Nursing Process: Assessment; *Test Plan:* PHYS

8 **Answer: 2** *Rationale:* Clients with Crohn's disease are at risk of developing cancer of the GI tract. A noncompliant client increases that risk and should be educated that Crohn's can be successfully kept under control.
Cognitive Level: Application
Nursing Process: Analysis; *Test Plan:* HPM

9 **Answer: 3** *Rationale:* A client with any GI disorder, especially a peptic ulcer, should never receive any aspirin product. Many pain medications contain aspirin and are combinations of an opioid analgesic and a non-opioid analgesic such as aspirin. The nurse administering the pain medication should know what ingredients are in it. Hydrocodone is a schedule III opioid analgesic in agents such as Lortab.
Cognitive Level: Analysis
Nursing Process: Implementation; *Test Plan:* SECE

10 **Answer: 2** *Rationale:* Inserting an NG tube will decompress the bowel, which will relieve the vomiting and pain and hopefully prevent the client from going into shock. This may be a measure to institute only until surgery can be performed. All of the interventions are appropriate, but vomiting fecal matter can be dangerous (as well as unpleasant) because of the possibility of aspiration, especially with a decreasing level of consciousness.
Cognitive Level: Analysis
Nursing Process: Implementation; *Test Plan:* SECE

References

Corwin, E. J. (2000). *Handbook of pathophysiology* (2nd ed.). Philadelphia: Lippincott, pp. 551–554.

Bullock, B. A. & Henze, R. L. (2000). *Focus on pathophysiology*. Philadelphia: Lippincott, pp. 721–741.

Hansen, M. (1998). *Pathophysiology: Foundations of disease and clinical intervention*. Philadelphia: W. B. Saunders, pp. 692–762.

Ignatavicius, D., Workman, M., & Mishler, M. (1999). *Medical surgical nursing across the health care continuum* (3rd ed.). Philadelphia: W. B. Saunders, pp. 1355–1377, 1379–1403, 1405–1431.

LeMone, P. & Burke, K. (2000). *Medical surgical nursing: Critical thinking in client care* (2nd ed.). Upper Saddle River, NJ: Prentice Hall, pp. 422–509, 769–875.

McCance, K. & Huether, S. (2002). *Pathophysiology: The biologic basis for disease in adults and children* (4th ed.). St. Louis, MO: Mosby, pp. 1335, 1344, 1367.

Porth, C. M. (2002). *Pathophysiology: Concepts of altered health states* (6th ed.). Philadelphia: Lippincott, pp. 719–742.

Sands, J. (1999). Management of persons with problems of the stomach and duodenum. In W. Phipps, J. Sands, & J. Marek. (Eds.), *Medical-surgical nursing: Concepts and clinical practice* (6th ed.). St. Louis: Mosby, pp. 1277–1371.

Thomas, C. L. (Ed.). (2001). *Taber's cyclopedic medical dictionary*. Philadelphia: F. A. Davis.

Wilson, B. A., Shannon, M. T., & Stang, C. L. (2001). *Nursing drug guide: 2001*. Upper Saddle River, NJ: Prentice Hall.

CHAPTER 8

Hepatobiliary Health Problems

Carol D. Clark, MS, RN, ANP, GNPC

CHAPTER OUTLINE

OBJECTIVES

▌ Define key terms associated with hepatobiliary health problems.

▌ Identify risk factors associated with the development of hepatobiliary health problems.

▌ Discuss the common etiologies of hepatobiliary health problems.

▌ Describe the pathophysiologic processes associated with specific hepatobiliary health problems.

▌ Distinguish between normal and abnormal hepatobiliary findings obtained from nursing assessment.

▌ Prioritize nursing interventions associated with specific hepatobiliary health problems.

[*Media Link*]

Use the CD-ROM enclosed with this text, or log onto the address given to access the free, interactive Companion Website created for this series. The CD-ROM and Companion Website accompanying this book offer additional practice opportunities and information—NCLEX Review, Case Studies, Glossary, In Depth with NCLEX, and more.

www.prenhall.com/hogan

REVIEW AT A GLANCE

ascites *increased amount of fluid in the abdominal cavity*

bile *a thick, yellow-green fluid secreted from the biliary tract and duodenum; responsible for digestion of food, absorption of fats and fat-soluble vitamins, and stimulation of peristalsis*

biliary cirrhosis *cirrhosis characterized by a prolonged state of jaundice because of retention of bile and bile duct inflammation*

cholecystitis *inflammation of the gallbladder*

cholelithiasis *condition in which there are stones present in the gallbladder*

cirrhosis *scarring of liver tissue, which interferes with normal liver function and results in structural changes within the liver*

fulminant hepatitis *necrosis and shrinking of the liver, possibly resulting in liver failure; a complication of viral hepatitis*

hemochromatosis *a genetically transmitted disease where iron is excessively absorbed and accumulated*

hepatic encephalopathy *damage to brain tissue, which occurs as a complication of cirrhosis of the liver caused by ammonia in brain tissue*

hepatitis *an inflammation of the liver*

jaundice *yellow-tinged color of the skin, body organs, or body fluids caused by abnormally high accumulation of bile pigment (bilirubin) in the blood*

Laënnec's cirrhosis *development of cirrhosis associated with chronic alcoholism*

melena *black tarry-colored feces as a result of secretions from intestines on free blood*

pancreatitis *inflammation of the pancreas*

portal hypertension *increase in pressure in the portal vein caused by obstruction or congestion; a complication of cirrhosis of the liver*

splenomegaly *an enlarged spleen*

steatorrhea *excessive elimination of fat; fatty stools*

thrombocytopenia *a decrease in the number of platelets*

varices *dilation of a vein that is usually tortuous*

Wilson's disease *an autosomal recessive disorder where ceruloplasmin is decreased, which leads to increased copper in several organs (liver, brain, kidney, and cornea)*

Pretest

1 Hepatic fat accumulation in a 55-year-old male is usually a result of which type of cirrhosis?

(1) Biliary
(2) Metabolic
(3) Postnecrotic
(4) Laënnec's

2 A concerned mother doesn't understand how her child acquired hepatitis A, when he was perfectly healthy up to a week ago. One characteristic of hepatitis A that may help her to understand is that hepatitis A has:

(1) An incubation period of 60 to 180 days.
(2) A fecal-oral mode of transmission.
(3) A positive carrier state.
(4) A sexual mode of transmission.

3 The physical assessment findings of spider angiomas, palmar erythema, peripheral edema, ascites, and change in mental status are consistent with which of the following disorders?

(1) Cholelithiasis
(2) Cholecystitis
(3) Cirrhosis
(4) Pancreatitis

4 A 45-year-old female hospitalized with acute pancreatitis has orders for meperidine (Demerol) 50 mg IM every 4 hours as needed for pain. Demerol has been ordered rather than morphine for this client because it:

(1) Has a faster onset of action than morphine.
(2) Is less addictive than morphine.
(3) Causes fewer spasms of the sphincter of Oddi.
(4) Has fewer cognitive side effects.

5 A 65-year-old female with a history of hepatic encephalopathy is hospitalized for pneumonia and dehydration. When she complains to the nurse about the small portions of meat ordered by the dietitian, the best response would be:

(1) "Ask your doctor about it in the morning."
(2) "I will call and order larger portions for you."
(3) "The amount of meat on your tray is dictated by certain blood test results."
(4) "Your protein is being limited, but you can have more food from another group."

6 The physical assessment of a 55-year-old female with end-stage cirrhosis reveals a protuberant abdomen with bulging flanks and dullness to the dependent side while lying on the right. The appropriate terminology for documentation of this assessment is:

(1) Fluid overload.
(2) Malnutrition.
(3) Ascites.
(4) Distention.

7 Which of the following statements is true regarding cancer of the pancreas?

(1) Clients with pancreatic cancer have often had a long history of painful sitting.
(2) Clients with pancreatic cancer will describe recent onset of black tarry stools.
(3) Clients with pancreatic cancer will describe a slow onset of anorexia and weight loss.
(4) Clients with pancreatic cancer will have no symptoms to report.

8 When providing discharge teaching to the client with chronic cirrhosis, his wife asks the nurse to explain why there is so much emphasis on bleeding precautions. Which of the following provides the most appropriate response?

(1) "The liver affected by cirrhosis is unable to produce clotting factors."
(2) "The low protein diet will result in reduced clotting factors."
(3) "The increased production of bile decreases clotting factors."
(4) "The required medications reduce clotting factors."

9 Which of the following statements is true regarding viral hepatitis infection?

(1) Hepatitis B is transmitted by the fecal-oral route.
(2) Hepatitis A is a sexually transmitted disease.
(3) The posticteric phase follows jaundice and lasts several weeks.
(4) Hepatitis D has a slow onset.

10 When explaining the rationale for the use of lactulose (Chronulac) syrup to the client with chronic cirrhosis, the nurse would use which of the following statements?

(1) "Chronulac syrup reduces constipation, which is a frequent complaint with cirrhosis."
(2) "Chronulac syrup suppresses the metabolism of ammonia and aids in its elimination through feces."
(3) "Chronulac syrup helps to reverse cirrhosis of the liver."
(4) "Chronulac syrup can be taken intermittently to reduce side effects."

See pages 276–277 for Answers and Rationales.

I. Risk Factors Associated with Hepatobiliary Health Problems

A. *Cirrhosis:* alcoholism (primary); viral hepatitis, toxic reactions to drugs and chemicals, biliary obstruction, cardiac disease; **hemochromatosis** (a genetically transmitted disease where iron is excessively absorbed and accumulated); **Wilson's disease** (an autosomal recessive disorder where ceruloplasmin is decreased which leads to increased copper in several organs [liver, brain, kidney, and cornea])

B. *Hepatitis*

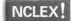

1. Hepatitis A: drinking contaminated milk or water and consumption of shellfish from contaminated waters; children in daycare centers and institutionalized adults are at increased risk

2. Hepatitis B: contact with blood or serum and oral or sexual contact

3. Hepatitis C: intravenous drug abusers, persons receiving blood transfusions, healthcare workers, persons on hemodialysis, those with high-risk sexual behavior and organ transplant recipients

4. Hepatitis D: intravenous drug users and those receiving clotting factor concentrates

5. Hepatitis E: pregnant women in developing countries

C. **Cancer of the liver:** persons with chronic hepatitis B infection, hepatitis C, or cirrhosis, and consumption of the hepatocarcinogens in food such as aflatoxin in moldy peanuts

D. *Cholecystitis:* diet high in fat content, cholelithiasis

E. *Cholelithiasis:* aging process, family history, cirrhosis, Crohn's disease, sickle-cell anemia, hyperlipidemia, congenital malformation of biliary ducts, obesity and rapid weight loss, diabetes mellitus, drugs that reduce cholesterol, and hyperalimentation; other risk factors include: Native American, Caucasian or Mexican-American ethnicity and female gender (pregnancy or use of oral contraceptives)

F. *Pancreatitis:* alcohol in men, gallstones in women, hyperlipidemia, hyperparathyroidism, viral infections, and abdominal trauma

G. **Cancer of the pancreas:** smoking (major risk); industrial chemicals, environmental toxin exposure, high-fat diet, pancreatitis, age, and diabetes mellitus

II. **Cirrhosis**

A. **Overview**

1. Cirrhosis is defined as scarring of liver tissue, which interferes with normal liver function and results in structural changes within codes of the liver

2. Characterized by structural and functional disorganization as a result of diffuse fibrosis and nodules of regenerated tissue

3. Two types

a. Laënnec's cirrhosis

b. Biliary cirrhosis

4. Causes

a. Laënnec's cirrhosis: consumption of a pint or more of alcohol per day

b. Biliary cirrhosis: hepatotoxins, any obstruction of common bile duct, severe congestive heart failure (CHF)

B. **Pathophysiology**

1. **Laënnec's cirrhosis:** development of cirrhosis associated with chronic alcoholism

a. Alcohol is transformed to acetaldehyde, which begins to alter hepatocyte function

b. The presence of acetaldehyde inhibits the removal of proteins from the liver and alters metabolism of vitamins and minerals

c. As large amounts of alcohol are consumed, fat accumulates in the liver, known as "fatty liver"

2. **Biliary cirrhosis** is cirrhosis characterized by a prolonged state of bile duct inflammation and jaundice (late manifestation) because of retention of **bile** (a thick yellow-green fluid secreted from the biliary tract to duodenum; responsible for digestion of food, absorption of fat and fat-soluble vitamins, and stimulation of peristalsis)

   a. *Primary:* inflammation, destruction, fibrosis, and obstruction of the intrahepatic bile ducts results in nodular regeneration and cirrhosis; women are more commonly affected than men are and this type of cirrhosis does not usually begin before the age of 30

   b. *Secondary:* inflammation and scarring of bile ducts occurs proximal to an obstruction caused by neoplasms, strictures or gallstones

3. Postnecrotic cirrhosis: fibrous, nodular scar tissue replaces necrotic tissue because of viral hepatitis B or C, drugs, toxins, or autoimmune disease

4. Metabolic cirrhosis: inflammation and scarring, which is a result of defects or storage diseases; examples are antitrypsin deficiency, glycogen storage disease, Wilson disease, and galactosemia

5. Progression of disease

   a. Fatty infiltration results in inflammation, which in turn results in necrosis and fibrosis of the liver, followed by regeneration and scarring

   b. Damage is increased if the client has a poor nutritional state

   c. Normal structure of liver is lost and replaced by disorganized arrangement of scars and nodules

   d. Widespread scarring puts pressure on and obstructs blood vessels and biliary ducts

   e. Increased capillary pressure causes increased fluid in abdomen and development of **portal hypertension** (increase in pressure in the portal vein caused by obstruction or congestion; a complication of cirrhosis of the liver)

   f. Decreased production of albumin results in decreased colloidal osmotic pressure, fluid leaves blood vessels and enters abdomen (third spacing)

   g. Decreased metabolism of aldosterone results in sodium retention and increased fluid retention

   h. Portal hypertension causes collateral circulation to develop in stomach, rectum, and esophagus; these vessels become distended and cause **varices** (tortous dilation of a vein); in the esophagus the varices are irritated by alcohol and food causing rupture and excessive bleeding, **melena** (black tarry-colored feces as a result of secretions of free blood from intestines), hematemesis; this is also aggravated by coughing, vomiting, lifting, or straining

   i. Portal hypertension causes back up of blood in spleen, which results in **splenomegaly** (enlarged spleen) and increased breakdown of white blood cells (WBCs), red blood cells (RBCs), platelets resulting in anemia, bleeding, **thrombocytopenia** (decreased platelet count) and decreased defense against infection

j. Decreased liver function results in inability to inactivate adrenocortical hormones, estrogen, testosterone, and aldesterone

k. Normally, ammonia is produced by bacteria and enzymes, which break down amino acids

1) The ammonia goes to the liver to be converted to urea and eliminated

2) If the liver is not functioning, the ammonia is not broken down; it accumulates in the blood stream, crosses the blood-brain barrier and goes in to the brain tissue, and leads to **hepatic encephalopathy** (damage to brain tissue, which occurs as a complication of cirrhosis of the liver due to ammonia in brain tissue); precipitated by any major hemodynamic insult to the body such as bleeding, shock, toxins to the body, hypovolemia, or anything that can increase the metabolic needs on the liver

6. Signs and symptoms of cirrhosis include weakness, fatigue, fever, anorexia, weight loss, nausea, vomiting, indigestion, increased flatulence, change in memory or level of consciousness, sexual dysfunction (loss of libido, change in menstrual pattern), edema, ascites, change in secondary sex characteristics (gynecomastia), bruising or hematoma, spider angiomas (a telangiectasis with a red, elevated center and small radiating blood vessels), palmar erythema (redness of the palm), jaundice, dark urine, light-colored feces, enlarged liver and spleen, muscle wasting, decreased strength, insomnia

7. Signs and symptoms of hepatic encephalopathy include restlessness, change in level of consciousness, inability to concentrate, altered sleep, forgetfulness, confusion, asterixis (flapping tremor of the hands when extending the arms), muscle twitching, and coma

C. Nursing assessment

1. Assessment includes hyponatremia (thirst, confusion, lethargy, and apprehension), vital signs (VS), bowel sounds, abdominal girth, dilation of abdominal wall veins, pulse quality, **ascites** (increased amount of fluid in the abdominal cavity), peripheral edema, color, mental status, reproductive history, urine and stool color, palpate abdominal muscle strength, weight, gastrointestinal (GI) complaints

2. Diagnostic tests: electrocardiogram (ECG), potassium, sodium, blood urea nitrogen (BUN), creatinine (CR), stool for occult blood, ultrasound (US) of abdomen, complete blood count (CBC), clotting studies, prothrombin time (PT), partial thromboplastin time (PTT), urine specific gravity, arterial blood gases (ABGs), liver function tests: alanine aminotransferase (ALT), aspartate aminotransferase (AST), alkaline phosphatase, gamma-glutamyl transpeptidase (GGT), bilirubin levels, liver biopsy (to verify cirrhosis), protein, albumin, ammonia levels

D. Nursing management

1. Medications

a. Diuretics for ascites

b. Lactulose (Chronulac) and neomycin (Mycifradin) to reduce high ammonia levels by the metabolism of lactulose to organic acids by intestinal bacteria and decreasing the pH of the colon; a more acid pH converts ammonia to a nonabsorbable food so that it is expelled in the feces

NCLEX!

    c. Vitamin K (Aquamephyton) for clotting

    d. Antacids if gastritis is present

  2. Avoid medications highly metabolized by the liver such as barbiturates, sedatives, acetaminophen (Tylenol), and alcohol-containing products

  3. Monitor daily weight, abdominal girth, and peripheral edema daily

NCLEX!

  4. Administer low-sodium, low-protein diet of 500 to 2,000 mg of sodium with restricted fluids; protein is controlled to eliminate the ammonia; sodium is controlled to limit fluid accumulation

  5. Inspect skin integrity every 8 hours

  6. Be cautious about the amount and frequency of medications administered

  7. Monitor neurologic functioning for early signs of encephalopathy

  8. Check VS each 8 hours

NCLEX!

  9. Institute bleeding precautions

    a. Avoid manipulation of rectum, including prevention of constipation

    b. Avoid injections

    c. Assess and report echymosis and purpura

    d. Apply extra pressure for areas that begin to bleed

    e. Use a soft toothbrush and assess gums for bleeding

    f. Avoid harsh blowing of the nose

    g. Try to coordinate timing of lab work to prevent excess venipunctures

 10. Position in high Fowler's with feet elevated, avoid supine position

 11. Monitor respiratory status and administer oxygen as indicated

 12. Use warm—not hot—water for bathing to reduce pruritus

 13. Institute skin protocols to prevent breakdown

 14. Be cautious in administering antihistamines for itching due to the liver disease and impaired metabolism

 15. Priority nursing diagnoses are Fluid volume excess; Altered tissue perfusion; Risk for injury: bleeding; Risk for impaired gas exchange; Impaired skin integrity

E. Complications

  1. Portal hypertension

    a. Overview

      1) Defined as an abnormally high blood pressure in the portal venous system

      2) Occurs when blood flow through the portal system is obstructed or impeded due to thrombosis, inflammation, or fibrous changes in the hepatic sinuses with cirrhosis or hepatitis; parasitic diseases and right-sided congestive heart failure can also cause portal hypertension

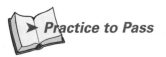

➤ Practice to Pass

How should the nurse determine if a client is developing ascites? What lab data are important?

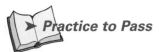

➤ Practice to Pass

A known client with alcoholism is admitted with a BP of 210/110, strong ammonia odor, tenderness in the abdomen, anorexic look, and reports eating only one meal per day containing less than nutritional foods. The client develops a GI hemorrhage and is treated for a GI bleed. Relate the signs and symptoms to Laënnec's cirrhosis.

b. Pathophysiology

1) Portal veins carry blood from the gastrointestinal tract, pancreas and spleen to the liver

2) Blood then flows through the liver, empties into the inferior vena cava, and is delivered to the right atrium

3) Normal pressure in this system is 3 mmHg; with portal hypertension, pressure reaches 10 mmHg

4) Obstruction causes blood to back up into the portal circulation and increase pressure; high pressure in the portal veins causes collateral circulation to develop between the portal veins and the systemic veins

5) Decreased protein synthesis results in a decrease in albumin, which leads to edema and ascites

6) Long-term portal hypertension causes distended, twisted collateral veins; gradually these become transformed to varicosities

7) The major complication is hemorrhage

c. Nursing assessment

1) Assess the abdomen for distention of collateral veins radiating over the abdomen; hematemesis, melena; signs of shock (cool, pale skin, drop in blood pressure [BP], increase in heart rate [HR] and respirations) review the history for jaundice, hepatitis, or alcoholism

2) Diagnostic tests: CBC, clotting factors

d. Nursing management

1) There is no effective medical treatment for portal hypertension, and nursing care is the same as treatment of cirrhosis

2) Nursing diagnoses are: Risk for injury: bleeding; Risk for impaired gas exchange; Risk for impaired skin integrity; and Altered nutrition

2. Esophageal varices

a. Overview

1) Defined as distended, tortuous collateral veins that occur from prolonged elevation of pressure

2) Most commonly located in the stomach and lower esophagus but may also be found in the rectum

3) Mortality from ruptured esophageal varices ranges from 30 to 60 percent, and many individuals die within 1 year

b. Pathophysiology

1) Increased pressure in the portal veins causes the development of collateral vessels to develop between the portal veins and the systemic veins where blood pressure is lower

2) Blood then bypasses the obstructed portal vessels and is carried via the collateral veins in the esophagus, anterior abdominal wall, and rectum

    3) The first sign of esophageal varices is usually the vomiting of copious amounts of dark-colored blood; ruptured varices do not cause pain and the rupture is usually precipitated by increased venous pressure and gastric acid

  c. Nursing assessment

    1) Assessment includes: hematemesis and melena

    2) Diagnostic tests: CBC, clotting studies, type and cross-match

  d. Nursing management

    1) Medications include: vasopressin (Pitressin) to lower portal blood pressure; beta blockers to lower blood pressure; antacids; lactulose (Chronulac) or neomycin (Mycifradin) for decreasing production of ammonia if caused by cirrhosis; vitamin K (Aquamephyton) for clotting

    2) Ruptured esophageal varices are a medical emergency, and management includes compression with the insertion of a Sengstaken-Blakemore tube; varices may be managed by injection of a sclerosing agent (sclerotherapy) or surgical construction of a portacaval shunt

    3) Replace blood loss with administration of blood and intravenous (IV) fluids

    4) Maintain patent airway

    5) Monitor VS every 30 minutes

    6) Use gastric lavage with cool saline to control bleeding

    7) Monitor for signs of shock

III. Hepatitis

A. Overview

1. **Hepatitis** is defined as an inflammation of the liver, usually viral in nature

2. The known hepatitis viruses are (see Table 8-1)

  a. Hepatitis A (HAV)

  b. Hepatitis B (HBV): causes high amount of liver damage

  c. Hepatitis B–associated delta virus (HDV)

  d. Hepatitis C virus (HCV): causes high amount of liver damage

  e. Hepatitis E (HEV)

  f. Hepatitis F

  g. Hepatitis G

3. Each virus differs in mode of transmission, incubation period, degree of liver damage, and ability to create a carrier state

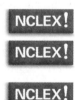

  a. HAV and HEV are both spread by fecal-oral contamination; inadequate handwashing, infected food handlers, contaminated food or water, and improper cleaning of utensils are major sources of infection

  b. HBV, HCV, and HDV are all spread by bloodborne organisms; control of contaminated needles, universal precautions for healthcare workers, and control of blood administration are primary means to control infection

Table 8-1	Classification and Characteristics of Viral Hepatitis				
	Hepatitis A HAV	**Hepatitis B HBV**	**Hepatitis C HCV**	**Hepatitis D HDV**	**Hepatitis E HEV**
Onset	Abrupt	Insidious	Insidious	Insidious	Abrupt
Transmission	Fecal-oral	Blood and body fluids	Blood and body fluids	Blood and body fluids	Fecal-oral
Incubation Period	2–6 weeks	6 weeks to 4 months	2–12 weeks	1–6 months	3 weeks to 2 months
Antibody- Antigens	Anti-HAV*	Anti-HBs HBsAg+	Anti-HCV (indicates infection, no confir- mation of immunity +HCV RNA	Anti-HDV* HDVAg+	Anti-HEV*
Carrier State	No	Yes	Yes	Yes	No
Post-Exposure Treatment	Gamma globulin	Hepatitis B immune globulin	None available	Immune globulin	Gamma globulin does not offer protection
Vaccination	Immune globulin HAV vaccine	HBV vaccine	None	HBV vaccine	None

*Demonstrates immunity
+Presence of this antigen signifies acute infection or carrier state

    c. Hepatitis F and G, little is known yet of transmission and mechanism of hepatic injury; hepatitis F is an enteric virus isolated from human stool and hepatitis G is associated with acute and chronic non-ABCDE hepatitis; hepatitis G is transmitted parenterally

    d. Depending upon the cause, hepatitis can exist in either an acute or chronic form; the chronic form results in cirrhosis

    e. Causes other than viruses include hepatobiliary obstruction from gallstones or from the toxic effects of alcohol, drugs, toxins, or infectious agents

B. Pathophysiology

    1. Viral infections of the liver create the same pathologic lesions as viral infections in other parts of the body; hepatic cell necrosis, scarring, Kupffer cell hyperplasia, and infiltration by mononuclear phagocytes occur in varying amounts and severity

    2. The cytotoxic T-cells and natural killer cells activated by the immune response promote cellular injury; the hepatic cells begin to regenerate within 48 hours of injury

    3. Distortion of the normal structure of the liver interferes with the flow of blood and bile

    4. Obstruction of portal and hepatic blood flow increases portal pressure causing engorgement, hepatomegaly, and splenomegaly

    5. Cholestasis and obstructive **jaundice** (yellow-tinged color of the skin body organs, or body fluids caused by abnormally high accumulation of bile [bilirubin] in the blood) are a result of the inflammatory effect on the bile canaliculi

NCLEX!

NCLEX!

6. Signs and symptoms are specific to the stages

   a. Preicteric stage (before jaundice occurs): malaise, fatigue, nausea, vomiting, diarrhea, anorexia (and aversion to food, especially protein and fat), enlarged liver and lymph nodes, electrolyte imbalances; conjunctivitis; skin rash; pain (headache, muscle aches, painful joints, fever, and sore throat)

   b. Icteric stage (onset of jaundice): jaundice, pruritus, light-colored stools, brown urine, malaise, preicteric symptoms improve or subside

   c. Posticteric stage (convalescent phase): decrease in fatigue, appetite returns to normal, laboratory work improves, and pain subsides

7. A complication of hepatitis is **fulminant hepatitis** (necrosis and shrinking of the liver, possibly resulting in liver failure): develops 6 to 8 weeks after initial symptoms, anorexia, and vomiting, abdominal pain, progressive jaundice followed by ascites, GI bleeding, lethargy, disorientation, and coma develop; mortality rate is high

C. **Nursing assessment**

1. Assessment

   a. Preicteric: assess for energy level; nutritional status; GI complaints; genitourinary (GU) patterns; presence of any pain; palpate liver and lymph nodes; VS

   b. Icteric phase: assess skin for color and integrity; stools and urine characteristics; VS; GI symptoms; nutritional status

   c. Posticteric: assess for improvement in all laboratory results and symptoms

2. Diagnostic tests

   a. Preicteric stage

      1) Electrolytes: abnormal

      2) Liver function tests (AST, ALT, alkaline phosphatase): elevated

      3) Virus and antibodies present in serum

   b. Icteric stage

      1) Total, conjugated, and unconjugated serum bilirubin: elevated

      2) Urinalysis: bilirubinuria

   c. Posticteric stage

      1) Serum bilirubin and enzymes: normal or returning to normal

      2) Serum antibodies: elevated

   d. Other diagnostic tests

      1) Hepatitis A: anti-HAV (antibody to HAV demonstrates immunity); IgM anti-HAV (antibody to HAV in recent infections to 6 months)

      2) Hepatitis B: HBsAG (Hepatitis B surface-antigen indicating active disease); HBeAg (antigen in chronic carriers of hepatitis B); Anti-HBs (immunity following hepatitis B vaccine); anti-HBc-IgM (indicates core infection in hepatitis B)

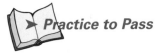

Practice to Pass

A client asks, "How can I keep from developing hepatitis B?" What should the nurse tell him?

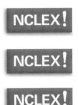

3) Hepatitis C: anti-HCV (antibody found in hepatitis C clients that indicates an infection but not necessarily immunity)

4) Hepatitis D: HDAg (antigen in acute infection); anti-HDV (antibody found in hepatitis D)

D. Nursing management

1. Medications include antiemetics to control nausea; use of antihistamines such as diphenhydramine (Benadryl), dimenhydrinate (Dramamine) or trimethobenzamide hydrochloride (Tigan) are best; emollient creams and lotions on skin

2. Avoid acetaminophen (Tylenol), prochlorperazine (Compazine), or other drugs detoxified in the liver

3. Eliminate the risk for infection (transmission): standard precautions and meticulous handwashing are essential to prevent the transmission of hepatitis A and E

4. Diet should consist of 16 carbohydrate kcalories per kilogram of ideal body weight; calories should be consumed in the morning hours since most clients are nauseated by afternoon and evening; decrease fat content as fat is generally not appetizing

5. Monitor fluid and electrolytes

6. Prevent skin breakdown and avoid the use of hot water for bathing

7. In fulminant hepatitis, protein is restricted

8. Supportive care with rest and gradual return to normal activities

9. Prevention for healthcare workers

   a. Use of Standard (Universal) Precautions

   b. Good handwashing

   c. Hepatitis A and B vaccines

IV. Cancer of the Liver

A. Overview

1. Defined as metastatic carcinoma or primary neoplasm of the liver

2. Cancer of the liver as a primary site is not common in the United States, but frequently metastasis occurs from pulmonary, breast, and gastrointestinal primary sites

3. Primary cancers arise from the bile duct in 10 percent of cases; alcohol-induced cirrhosis and hepatitis A or B account for most of the primary cancer of the liver in the United States

4. Causes include chronic cirrhosis, vinyl chloride exposure, inorganic arsenic, mycotoxin aflatoxin, nitrosamines, pesticides, prolonged androgen therapy, and contraceptive steroids

B. Pathophysiology

1. Major types

   a. Hepatocellular carcinoma, arising from the liver cells

   b. Cholangiocarcinoma, primary cancer of the cells of the bile duct

2. Hepatocellular carcinoma is classified as nodular, massive, or diffuse

3. Metastasis to the heart, lung, brain, kidney, and spleen is rapid because of the invasion of the hepatic and portal veins

4. Benign tumors of the liver are adenomas often affecting women and related to oral contraceptives

5. Manifestations are usually related to the effects of the tumor or the functional changes in the liver

   a. Bile products are secreted because of the secretion of substances by the tumors

   b. The tumor secretes hormones that lead to polycythemia, hypoglycemia, and hypercalcemia

   c. Obstruction of the biliary system leads to jaundice, portal hypertension, ascites

   d. The impairment of hepatocytes results in metabolic disturbances

   e. Invasion of the tumor into the liver, which is often inoperable, causes hepatomegaly, hemorrhage and liver failure

   f. Other signs and symptoms

      1) GI: nausea, vomiting, fullness, pressure, and dull ache in the right upper abdomen

      2) Pain, as a result of enlargement of the tumor

      3) Debilitation, weight loss, cachexia

      4) Symptoms of cirrhosis

C. Nursing assessment

1. Assessment includes presence of GI symptoms, pain, weight, nutritional status, fluid status (I & O), measure abdominal girth, and presence of bleeding

2. Diagnostic tests: magnetic resonance imagery (MRI), computed tomography (CT) scans, ultrasound, and alpha-fetoprotein serum markers (specific to detecting hepatocellular carcinoma)

D. Nursing management

1. Medications include narcotics and analgesics for pain; chemotherapeutic agents [5-fluorouracil (5-FU), methrotrexate (MRX), doxorubicin (Adriamycin)]

2. There is no cure; palliative care is the goal

3. Monitor for and prevent infection

4. Inspect skin and prevent breakdown

5. Manage pain and instruct client to ask for pain medication prior to onset of severe pain

6. Offer support for client and family for grief and coping

V. Cholelithiasis

A. Overview

1. **Cholelithiasis** is defined as the formation of stones in the biliary duct system or the gallbladder

2. Approximately 10 to 20 percent of men and 20 to 40 percent of women are affected

3. Causes include obesity, oral contraceptives and estrogen therapy, family history, diseases (cirrhosis, Crohn's disease, hyperlipidemia, diabetes mellitus), hyperalimentation

B. Pathophysiology

1. Gallstones form when cholesterol and calcium precipitate as solid crystals within the mucous lining of the gall bladder

2. This process is enhanced by delayed emptying of the gallbladder

3. If the gallstone obstructs the cystic duct, acute cholecystitis occurs

4. Manifestations are a result of the presence and location of the stone (see Figure 8-1)

   NCLEX!

   a. Stones lodged in the cystic duct cause distention of the gallbladder, colicky pain (severe, cramplike)

   NCLEX!

   b. Pain may radiate to the subscapular area

   c. The obstruction of the common bile duct causes reflux of bile into the liver and jaundice

   NCLEX!

   d. Other signs and symptoms include nausea, vomiting, epigastric pain, heartburn, and intolerance to fat-containing foods

C. Nursing assessment

   NCLEX!

1. Assessment includes pain, color, stool characteristic, nutritional status, GI symptoms (epigastric pain, heartburn, nausea, vomiting, right upper abdominal pain)

2. Diagnostics tests: serum bilirubin (direct bilirubin elevated if biliary ducts involved, indirect bilirubin elevated if liver damage occurs), alkaline phosphatase (elevated), cholangiography or radioactive scan, ultrasound of the gallbladder, HIDA (gallbladder) scans

Figure 8-1

Common location of gallstones.

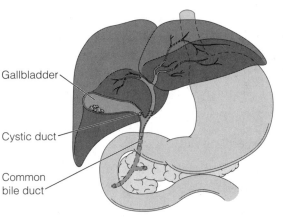

Gallbladder

Cystic duct

Common bile duct

D. Nursing management

1. Medications include: oral bile acids or dissolvers: ursodeoxycholic acid (UDCA), chenodeoxycholic acid (Chenodiol); analgesics such as meperidine (Demerol); cholestyramine (Questran) for pruritis

2. Clients should be taught to avoid high-fat foods because these stimulate gall-bladder contractions: avoid whole-milk products, fried foods, nuts, gravies, cooking oils, hot dogs, chocolate, and cheese

3. Obese clients should be instructed in weight loss

4. The goal is to reduce the inflammation and the blockage

VI. Cholecystitis

A. Overview

1. **Cholecystitis** is defined as an inflammation of the cystic duct caused by the lodging of a gallstone in the duct

2. May be acute or chronic

3. Causes

   a. Cholelithiasis

   b. Without cholelithiasis: trauma, fasting, hyperalimentation, surgery

B. Pathophysiology

1. A lodged gallstone in the cystic duct exerts pressure against the wall of the gallbladder, decreasing blood flow

2. Ischemia follows with the possibility of necrosis and perforation of the gallbladder

3. Chemical irritation from the obstruction or the presence of a bacterial infection prevents the outflow of the bile from the gallbladder

4. Signs and symptoms include pain that suddenly or gradually develops (classically in the back or the right shoulder), fever, nausea, vomiting, jaundice, clay-colored stools, intolerance to fat-containing foods, epigastric pain, heartburn

C. Nursing assessment

1. Assessment includes rebound tenderness, VS, abdominal muscle guarding, GI distress (epigastric pain, heartburn, nausea, vomiting, right upper abdominal pain), skin color, stool characteristics, and nutritional status

2. Diagnostics tests: serum bilirubin (direct bilirubin elevated if biliary ducts involved, indirect bilirubin elevated if liver damage), alkaline phosphatase (elevated), serum amylase (normal unless pancreas involved), complete blood count (elevated WBC), electrolytes, cholangiography or radioactive scan, ultrasound of the gallbladder, HIDA (gallbladder) scans

D. Nursing management

1. Medications include: oral bile acids or dissolvers: ursodeoxycholic acid (UDCA), chenodeoxycholic acid (Chenodiol); antibiotics, antipyretics; analgesics such as meperidine (Demerol); cholestyramine (Questran) for pruritis

2. Clients should be taught to avoid whole-milk products, fried foods, nuts, gravies, cooking oils, hot dogs, chocolate, and cheese

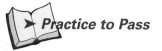

Practice to Pass

A client with cholelithiasis is admitted to the medical-surgical unit. What nursing diagnoses are appropriate for the plan of care and what specific interventions would be necessary to institute?

NCLEX!

NCLEX!

NCLEX!

3. Obese clients should be instructed in weight loss

4. For surgical interventions, the nurse's focus in on Knowledge deficit, both pre- and postoperatively; other nursing diagnoses include: Pain, Risk for impaired gas exchange, and Risk for infection

5. Teaching for home care

   a. The focus for nonsurgical interventions is diet management and instructions for the stone dissolving medications; include information about the function of the gallbladder and purpose of bile

   b. Teaching for the postoperative client is focused upon pain control, monitoring for infection, eating low-fat foods; and managing a T-tube by:

      1) Ensuring patency of the tube

      2) Monitoring the amount of drainage: as much as 500 mL within first 24 hours, 200 mL the next 2 to 3 days, and minimal after that

      3) Maintaining a Fowler's position to promote drainage

      4) Assessing the skin around the tube for integrity

      5) Assisting and teaching the client to ambulate with the tube

      6) Monitoring for signs of infection

VII. Pancreatitis

A. Overview

1. **Pancreatitis** is defined as an inflammation of the pancreas

2. Classification

   a. Acute: necrosis, suppuration (abscesses), gangrene, and hemorrhage occurs

   b. Chronic: formation of scar tissue that interferes with the function of the organ

3. Causes

   a. Alcoholism (excessive intake of liquor or wine for 6 years or more)

   b. Biliary (obstruction of the pancreatic duct by a gallstone)

   c. Other: high triglyceride levels, hypercalcemia, or infections

B. Pathophysiology

1. *Acute*

   a. When the pancreas is injured and/or the function is disrupted, pancreatic enzymes (phosopholipase A, lipase, and elastase) leak into the pancreatic tissue and initiate autodigestion

   b. Trypsin and elastase are activated proteolases and along with lipases, break down tissue and cell membranes, resulting in edema, vascular damage, hemorrhage and necrosis

   c. Replacement of pancreatic tissue by fibrous changes causes exocrine and endocrine changes with loss of function of the islets of Langerhans, which secrete insulin, resulting in diabetes mellitus

      d. Multiple-organ failure and mortality occurs when toxic enzymes are released into the bloodstream and distributed by vessels into major organs

         1) Activation of kinin occurs, resulting in vasodilation

         2) Increased stickiness of leukocytes occurs, causing emboli

         3) Coagulopathy occurs, which causes disseminated intravascular coagulation

         4) Increased permeability causes movement of fluid and circulatory insufficiency

         5) Myocardial depressant factor is released, which decreases cardiac function

         6) Activation of the renin-angiotensin processes decreases kidney function as a result of decreased renal perfusion

      e. Types

         1) Acute interstitial: the pancreas and the surrounding tissue are engorged with interstitial fluid; this form may progress to hemorrhagic

         2) Acute hemorrhagic: bleeding into the gland and other structures occurs

  2. *Chronic:* a structural or functional impairment of the pancreas, most commonly associated with chronic alcohol abuse

      a. The chronic form of pancreatitis is irreversible and leaves connective tissue in place of pancreatic tissue

      b. Pancreatic cysts are common lesions found in chronic pancreatitis, which are walled-off pockets of pancreatic juice, necrotic debris, or blood

      c. Types

         1) Chronic calcifying pancreatitis is the form associated with alcoholism; the alcohol causes a spasm of the sphincter of Oddi resulting in a blockage of the passage of secretions out of the pancreas and the enzymes pass into the tissue, resulting in autodigestion of pancreatic tissue

         2) Chronic obstructive pancreatitis is the form associated with gallstones in women

  3. Signs and symptoms

      a. Acute pancreatitis

         1) Sudden onset of severe epigastric and abdominal tenderness and pain that radiates to the back; may be relieved by sitting up and leaning forward, flexing the left leg or by walking

         2) GI: nausea, vomiting, and distention

         3) Cardiac: tachycardia, hypotension

         4) Other: fever, decreased bowel sounds, and cold, clammy skin; mild jaundice may occur within 24 hours of acute symptoms, retroperitoneal bleeding after 3 to 6 days, weakness, anxiety, pallor

b. Chronic pancreatitis

    1) Left upper abdominal pain radiating to the back

    2) GI: nausea, vomiting, weight loss, flatulence, constipation, **steatorrhea** (excessive elimination of fat, fatty stools), malabsorption

C. Nursing Assessment

1. Assessment includes symptom analysis of pain, GI complaints, nutritional status, energy level, stool characteristics, VS, skin color, bleeding—positive Turner's sign (flank bruising) or Cullen's sign (umbilical bruising)

2. Diagnostic tests

    a. Acute

        1) Serum amylase: elevated

        2) Serum lipase: elevated

        3) Serum calcium: decreased

        4) ABGs

    b. Chronic

        1) Serum and urinary amylase levels: elevated

        2) Serum bilirubin: elevated

D. Nursing management

1. Medications

    a. Opioid narcotic analgesics such as meperidine hydrochloride (Demerol); avoid morphine because it causes spasms of the sphincter of Oddi and doesn't allow the pancreas to rest

    b. Antibiotics

    c. Antacids

    d. H$_2$-blockers such as cimetidine (Tagamet) or rantidine (Zantac)

    e. Proton pump inhibitors such as omeprazole (Prilosec)

    f. Carbonic anhydrase inhibitors: acetazolamide (Diamox)

    g. Antispasmodics: dicyclomine (Bentyl)

    h. Antiemetics

    i. Antipyretics

2. Assess and reassess at regular intervals for the location, radiation, duration, character and intensity of the pain

3. Maintain nothing by mouth (NPO) status (3 to 7 days) in order to reduce gastric secretions and the aggravation of pancreatic pain; gastric suction may be ordered to minimize secretions

4. Decrease physical movement and mental stimulation to minimize gastric secretions and pain

5. Provide moisture to dry mucous membranes, which are a result of NPO status

6. Prevent visualization of food since gastric secretions are stimulated by the sight of food

7. Encourage a position of comfort, which is elevation of the head at 45 degrees, side lying with knees flexed

8. Daily weight

9. Assess bowel sounds

10. Assess cardiovascular status at regular intervals, monitor VS

11. Assess respiratory function at regular intervals because abdominal pain causes shallow respirations; pleural effusion is also a complication of pancreatitis

12. IV fluid replacement with electrolytes and possibly total parenteral nutrition (TPN)

13. IV albumin may be needed to combat third-spacing

14. Monitor O_2 saturation

VIII. Cancer of the Pancreas

A. Overview

1. Defined as tumors of the pancreas that are ductal adenocarcinomas; nearly all cases are fatal

2. Seventy percent of tumors are located in the pancreatic head, 20 percent in the body of the pancreas, and 10 percent in the tail

3. Causes include longstanding diabetes, chronic pancreatitis, and smoking; it is not associated with coffee drinking, alcoholism, and cholelithiasis

B. Pathophysiology

1. Pancreatic cancer has a slow onset and is usually not detected until the tumor has spread

2. Cancer of the head of the pancreas obstructs bile flow while tumors in the body of the pancreas press on the celiac ganglion

3. Cancer cells often invade the stomach, duodenum, bile duct, colon, spleen, kidney, and major blood vessels

4. Signs and symptoms

   a. Common symptoms: weight loss, anorexia, nausea, vomiting, flatulence, epigastric pain, malaise, diarrhea and constipation, palpable abdominal mass, hematemesis, melena

   b. Cancer of the head of the pancreas specifically causes jaundice (from biliary obstruction), clay-colored stools, dark urine, and pruritus

   c. Cancer in the tail of the pancreas may cause no symptoms until metastasis has occurred

   d. Tumors in the body of the pancreas may cause pain and nausea during eating or when lying supine

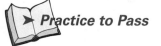

Practice to Pass

In trying to determine the etiology of a client's abdominal pain, various laboratory tests are ordered. What specific symptoms and lab work would differentiate cholecystitis, pancreatitis, and cirrhosis?

C. Nursing assessment

1. Assessment includes weight, GI symptoms, symptom analysis of pain, stool and urine characteristics, skin color, fluid and electrolyte status, nutritional status, energy level

2. Diagnostic tests: carcinoembryonic antigen (elevated), bilirubin levels (increased), urine urobilinogen (decreased), alkaline phosphatase (elevated), ultrasonography

D. Nursing management

1. Medications

   a. Opioid narcotic analgesics such as meperidine hydrochloride (Demerol)

   b. Antiemetics

2. The client with pancreatic cancer may be a candidate for resection called a Whipple's procedure (removal of the head of the pancreas, entire duodenum, one-third of stomach, part of the jejunum, and lower-half of the common bile duct with restructuring of the pancreas, stomach and common bile duct); postoperative care is consistent with that of any abdominal surgery and demands special attention to:

   a. Pain management

   b. Respiratory expansion

   c. Monitoring of complications related to oxygenation

   d. Renal function

   e. Level of consciousness

   f. Blood chemistries

3. Avoid the use of morphine that causes spasms of the pancreatic duct smooth muscle, which can complicate the flow of pancreatic juices

4. Have dietitian evaluate clients needs, especially during NPO status

5. Palliative care as with any cancer client

Case Study

M. S. is a 55-year-old female presenting as a hospital admission for surgery in the morning. She is a divorced mother of three adult children and has smoked one pack of cigarettes daily for 30 years. In the past month, she has lost 20 pounds, cannot sleep lying on her back, and is unable to tolerate solid foods. The client became jaundiced in the past 48 hours and computed tomography (CT) scan confirmed a mass in the pancreas.

❶ What are the primary risk factors present for pancreatic cancer?

❷ Where is the likely location of the tumor based upon the client's symptoms?

❸ What are the primary preoperative nursing interventions?

❹ What are the primary postoperative nursing interventions?

❺ What is the likely prognosis for this client?

For suggested responses, see page 567.

Posttest

1 Which of the following clients is more likely to develop pancreatitis?

(1) A 59-year-old male with a history of occasional alcohol use
(2) A client with renal problems and hypocalcemia
(3) A client recovering from myocardial infarction with hypercholesterolemia
(4) A client with a stone lodged in the pancreatic duct

2 Which of the following actions of pancreatic enzymes can cause pancreatic damage?

(1) Utilization by the intestine
(2) Autodigestion of the pancreas
(3) Reflux into the pancreas
(4) Clogging of the pancreatic duct

3 Which of the following laboratory tests indicates a diagnosis of pancreatitis?

(1) Lipase 230 IU/L
(2) Calcium 6.0 mEq/L
(3) Blood glucose 65 mg/dL
(4) White blood cell count 5,000/mm^3

4 The client with pancreatitis may exhibit Cullen's sign on physical examination. Which of the following data best describes Cullen's sign?

(1) Jaundiced sclera
(2) Pain that occurs with movement
(3) Bluish discoloration of the left flank area
(4) Bluish discoloration of the periumbilical area

5 Which of the following findings would strongly indicate the possibility of cirrhosis?

(1) Dry skin
(2) Hepatomegaly
(3) Peripheral edema
(4) Pruritus

6 A client with cirrhosis may have alterations in which of the following laboratory values?

(1) Carbon dioxide level
(2) pH
(3) Prothrombin time (PT)
(4) White blood cell count (WBC)

7 Which of the following clients is most likely to acquire hepatitis?

(1) A child with a bacterial infection
(2) A client with dysfunction of the biliary system
(3) A client with metastasis of liver cancer
(4) An adult with varicella zoster

8 In reviewing the possible causes of hepatitis A in a 22-year-old male, which of the following would be the most likely factor?

(1) Contact with blood in his profession as a policeman
(2) Receiving a blood transfusion during surgery
(3) Eating shrimp at the local pub
(4) Admitting to being sexually active

9 A client is admitted to the unit with complaints of malaise, nausea, vomiting, anorexia, and headaches. The lab work shows abnormal electrolytes and elevated aspartate aminotransferase (AST), alanine aminotransferase (ALT), and alkaline phosphatase (ALP); hepatitis B surface antigen (HBsAG) is present. The nurse would assume the client has:

(1) Hepatitis A.
(2) Hepatitis B.
(3) Cirrhosis.
(4) Pancreatitis.

10 A client is admitted with possible liver cancer. Which of the tests below would be the most confirming of this diagnosis?

(1) Abdominal ultrasound
(2) Abdominal flat plate X-ray
(3) Alpha-fetoprotein markers
(4) Computed tomography (CT) scan

See pages 277–278 for Answers and Rationales.

Answers and Rationales

Pretest

1 **Answer: 4** *Rationale:* A fatty liver is one of the main effects of alcohol consumption, known as Laënnec's cirrhosis. Other factors such as dietary intake of fat, body stores of fat, and hormonal status can also contribute to fatty liver.
Cognitive Level: Application
Nursing Process: Analysis; *Test Plan:* PHYS

2 **Answer: 2** *Rationale:* Hepatitis A has an acute onset, and accounts for about 25 percent of hepatitis cases in the United States. The usual incubation period is 15 to 40 days. The disease is spread where there is fecal contamination of water supplies and from oral contamination (such as in daycare).
Cognitive Level: Application
Nursing Process: Analysis; *Test Plan:* PHYS

3 **Answer: 3** *Rationale:* Portal hypertension and liver cell failure contribute to the late manifestations of cirrhosis. Cholelithiasis and cholecystitis will be accompanied by pain, food intolerances, and/or vomiting. Pancreatitis presents with pain radiating to the back, mild cardiovascular changes, and hypocalcemia.
Cognitive Level: Comprehension
Nursing Process: Assessment; *Test Plan:* PHYS

4 **Answer: 3** *Rationale:* The onset of action for meperidine is 10 to 15 minutes and the onset for morphine is 20 to 60 minutes. Both drugs are equal in the potential for addiction. Demerol is less sedating than morphine. The most important difference is that the meperidine causes fewer spasms of the sphincter of Oddi, which contributes to the goal of giving the pancreas a rest.
Cognitive Level: Application
Nursing Process: Analysis; *Test Plan:* PHYS

5 **Answer: 4** *Rationale:* The client is at increased risk for a return of the encephalopathy because of the diagnosis of pneumonia and dehydration. She has volume depletion and the potential for electrolyte imbalance, both of which can contribute to the development of encephalopathy. Dietary protein intake must be controlled (or eliminated) in order to minimize the ammonia levels in the blood stream.
Cognitive Level: Analysis
Nursing Process: Implementation; *Test Plan:* PHYS

6 **Answer: 3** *Rationale:* In the cirrhotic liver, fibrous tissue develops among the parenchymal cells preventing the production of adequate plasma proteins. The consequence of low plasma proteins leads to a decrease in colloid osmotic pressure and generalized edema. When combined with high portal capillary pressures, large amounts of fluid and protein form in the abdominal cavity, which is called ascites. Gravity causes the fluid to sink and gas-filled loops of the bowel rise creating the shifting dullness and tympany during assessment.
Cognitive Level: Analysis
Nursing Process: Assessment; *Test Plan:* PHYS

7 **Answer: 3** *Rationale:* The cancer cells alter enzyme secretion and flow to the duodenum in addition to causing fat and protein malabsorption. These changes result in weight loss and nausea, which are common signs and symptoms of cancer of the pancreas regardless of location.
Cognitive Level: Knowledge
Nursing Process: Analysis; *Test Plan:* PHYS

8 **Answer: 1** *Rationale:* When bile production is reduced, the body has reduced ability to absorb fat-soluble vitamins. Without adequate vitamin K absorption, clotting factors II, VII, IX, and X are not produced in sufficient amounts.
Cognitive Level: Application
Nursing Process: Implementation; *Test Plan:* PHYS

9 **Answer: 3** *Rationale:* The posticteric phase follows jaundice. Symptoms decrease and the serum enzymes begin to return to normal. Hepatitis B is transmitted by parenteral, sexual, or perinatal routes. Hepatitis A is transmitted by the fecal-oral route. Hepatitis D has a rapid onset.
Cognitive Level: Knowledge
Nursing Process: Analysis; *Test Plan:* PHYS

10 **Answer: 2** *Rationale:* Chronulac is a synthetic nonabsorbable disaccharide metabolized to organic acids by enteric bacteria and causes osmotic catharsis while reducing the growth of ammonia-forming bacteria. Chronulac also lowers the pH of the colon, which converts ammonia to a nonabsorbable form allowing expulsion through the laxative action of the drug. The dose required is 15 to 30 mL orally every 4 to 6 hours and may be titrated to a lower dose if diarrhea occurs.
Cognitive Level: Analysis
Nursing Process: Implementation; *Test Plan:* PHYS

Posttest

1 **Answer: 4** *Rationale:* Causes of pancreatitis include alcohol abuse of excessive intake of liquor or wine for 6 years or more, high triglyceride levels, and hypercalcemia. Stones lodged in the pancreatic duct can cause obstruction and lead to inflammation of the pancreas. Options 1, 2, 3 are worded incorrectly.
Cognitive Level: Analysis
Nursing Process: Analysis; *Test Plan:* PHYS

2 **Answer: 2** *Rationale:* When the pancreas is injured and/or has an impaired or disrupted function, the pancreatic enzymes (phosopholipase A, lipase, and elastase) leak into the pancreatic tissue and initiate autodigestion. Options 3 and 4 can be causes of pancreatitis. Option 1 is incorrect to this situation.
Cognitive Level: Comprehension
Nursing Process: Analysis; *Test Plan:* PHYS

3 **Answer: 1** *Rationale:* In pancreatitis, the lipase, amylase, glucose and white blood count (WBC) are all elevated. The calcium is low for 7 to 10 days and is a sign of severe pancreatitis. This question draws on your knowledge of laboratory results and what is normal and abnormal. If this question was problematic, review your normal lab values for each of these tests and as you study.
Cognitive Level: Analysis
Nursing Process: Assessment; *Test Plan:* PHYS

4 **Answer: 4** *Rationale:* Bleeding is a complication of pancreatitis and is usually identified through a positive Turner's sign (flank bruising) or Cullen's sign (umbilical bruising). Options 1 and 3 are correct in pancreatitis, but do not answer the question. Read the stem carefully when taking the test. Option 2 is incorrect; remember the pain may be relieved by flexing the left leg or by walking.
Cognitive Level: Comprehension
Nursing Process: Assessment; *Test Plan:* PHYS

5 **Answer: 2** *Rationale:* Although option 4 is correct, it is not a *strong* indicator of cirrhosis. Pruritus can occur for many reasons. Options 1 and 3 are incorrect, fluid accumulation is usually in the form of ascites in the abdomen. Hepatomegaly is an enlarged liver, which is correct. The spleen may also be enlarged.
Cognitive Level: Application
Nursing Process: Assessment; *Test Plan:* PHYS

6 **Answer: 3** *Rationale:* Clients with cirrhosis have used their clotting factors, and the liver is unable to provide enough clotting factors. A prothrombin time

is an indication of the time needed for blood to clot. If clotting factors aren't present, bleeding is more likely.
Cognitive Level: Application
Nursing Process: Assessment; *Test Plan:* PHYS

7 **Answer: 4** *Rationale:* Although hepatitis is associated with cholestasis (option 2), the most likely candidate would be someone with a viral infection. A classic example is someone with varicella zoster. Options 1 and 3 are not related to hepatitis. Other causes include alcohol, toxins, and severe hepatocellular damage.
Cognitive Level: Analysis
Nursing Process: Assessment; *Test Plan:* PHYS

8 **Answer: 3** *Rationale:* Hepatitis A is transmitted by fecal-oral route. The virus is excreted in oropharyngeal secretions (nose and throat) and transmitted by direct contact of person to person, or by fecal contamination of food or water. A worker at the pub could have hepatitis A and transfer it to the food that is

being prepared. Options 1, 2, and 4 are classic of hepatitis B, C, and D.
Cognitive Level: Application
Nursing Process: Analysis; *Test Plan:* PHYS

9 **Answer: 2** *Rationale:* The symptoms in preicteric hepatitis are vague and more flu-like as described above. The physician usually needs laboratory work to verify a diagnosis. In this case, the presence of the antigen HBsAG concludes that the client has an active form of the disease since hepatitis B surface antigen is present.
Cognitive Level: Analysis
Nursing Process: Assessment; *Test Plan:* PHYS

10 **Answer: 3** *Rationale:* Although an abdominal ultrasound, x-ray, and CT scan are useful in the diagnosis of cancer of the liver, the alpha-fetoprotein serum markers are specific to detecting primary hepatocellular carcinoma.
Cognitive Level: Application
Nursing Process: Assessment; *Test Plan:* PHYS

References

Bickley, L. (1998). *Bates' guide to physical examination and history taking* (7th ed.). Philadelphia: Lippincott, pp. 374–375.

Goroll, A. & Mulley, A. (2000). *Primary care medicine.* Philadelphia: Lippincott Williams & Wilkins, p. 467.

Guyton, A. & Hall, J. (2000). *Textbook of medical physiology* (10th ed.). Philadelphia: W.B. Saunders.

Johnson, A. (1999). Disorder of the liver. In D. Ignatavicius, M. Workman, & M. Mishler. *Medical-surgical nursing across the health care continuum.* Philadelphia: W. B. Saunders, p. 1477.

Karch, A. (2000). *Focus on nursing pharmacology.* Philadelphia: Lippincott, p. 292.

LeMone, P. & Burke, K. (2000). *Medical-surgical nursing: Critical thinking in client care* (2nd ed.). Upper Saddle River, NJ: Prentice Hall, pp. 511–552.

McCance, K. & Huether, S. (2002). *Pathophysiology: The biologic basis for disease in adults and children* (4th ed.). St. Louis, MO: Mosby, pp. 1358, 1363, 1371.

Porth, C. (Ed.). (2002). *Pathophysiology: Concepts of altered health status* (6th ed.). Philadelphia: Lippincott, pp. 745–772.

Sands, J. (1999). Management of persons with problems of the stomach and duodenum. In W. Phipps, J. Sands, & J. Marek (Eds.), *Medical-surgical nursing: Concepts and clinical practice* (6th ed.). St. Louis: Mosby, p. 1374.

Stobo, J., Hellman, D., Ladenson, P., Petty, B., & Thomas, T., (1999). *The principles and practice of medicine* (24th ed.). Stamford, CT: Appleton & Lange, pp. 517, 538.

Vaughn, G. (1999). *Understanding and evaluating common laboratory tests.* Stanford, CT: Appleton & Lange, p. 185.

CHAPTER 9

Endocrine and Metabolic Health Problems

Joseann Helmes DeWitt, MSN, RN, C, CLNC

CHAPTER OUTLINE

OBJECTIVES

▮ Define key terms associated with endocrine and metabolic health problems.

▮ Identify risk factors associated with the development of endocrine and metabolic health problems.

▮ Discuss the common etiologies of endocrine and metabolic health problems.

▮ Describe the pathophysiologic processes associated with specific endocrine and metabolic health problems.

▮ Distinguish between normal and abnormal endocrine and metabolic findings obtained from nursing assessment.

▮ Prioritize nursing interventions associated with specific endocrine and metabolic health problems.

[Media Link]

Use the CD-ROM enclosed with this text, or log onto the address given to access the free, interactive Companion Website created for this series. The CD-ROM and Companion Website accompanying this book offer additional practice opportunities and information—NCLEX Review, Case Studies, Glossary, In Depth with NCLEX, and more.

www.prenhall.com/hogan

REVIEW AT A GLANCE

Addison's disease *chronic adrenocortical insufficiency as a result of destruction of adrenal glands*

Addisonian crisis *acute adrenocortical insufficiency precipitated by stress or abrupt withdrawal of glucocorticoids; signs and symptoms include hypotension and shock*

antidiuretic hormone (ADH) *hormone secreted by the posterior pituitary gland; purpose is to control serum osmolality*

Conn's syndrome (hyperaldosteronism) *primary hyperaldosteronism; hypersecretion of aldosterone in which hypertension is a major complication*

Cushing's syndrome *symptoms produced by excess cortisol from adrenal cortex; classic signs and symptoms are moon face, truncal obesity, purple striae on abdomen*

diabetes insipidus *disorder caused by antidiuretic hormone (ADH) insufficiency, results in excess fluid excretion*

diabetes mellitus *most common disorder of the endocrine system; lack of secretion or inadequate secretion of insulin, or insulin resistance, resulting in hyperglycemia, and leading to multisystem effects*

diabetic ketoacidosis (DKA) *life-threatening state of hyperglycemia and metabolic acidosis*

exophthalmos *abnormal protrusion of eyeballs; seen in hyperthyroidism, and may affect one or both eyes*

goiter *enlargement of the thyroid gland, most often seen in hyperthyroidism, but also may occur in hypothyroidism or euthyroidism*

Graves' disease *hyperthyroidism leading to a hypermetabolic state*

hyperparathyroidism *increase in the secretion of parathyroid hormone (PTH)*

hyperthyroidism *increase in the secretion of thyroid hormone (TH)*

hypoparathyroidism *decrease in the secretion of parathyroid hormone (PTH)*

hypothyroidism *decrease in the secretion of thyroid hormone (TH)*

insulin *hormone produced by the pancreas, responsible for controlling level of glucose*

myxedema *form of hypothyroidism characterized by non-pitting edema that is generally found in the periorbital and pretibial areas*

myxedema coma *life-threatening state of hypothyroidism*

pheochromocytoma *tumor (usually benign) of the adrenal medulla resulting in excessive secretion of catecholamines which leads to severe hypertension*

syndrome of inappropriate antidiuretic hormone (SIADH) *excessive secretion of antidiuretic hormone (ADH) from the pituitary gland; results in excessive water retention*

thyroid storm *life-threatening form of hyperthyroidism, characterized by extreme state of hypermetabolism*

Pretest

1 The nurse is obtaining a health history on a 36-year-old female who reports an increase in appetite, weight loss, intolerance to heat, and nervousness. On physical assessment, the client is noted to have thin hair and moist skin. Based on this information, the nurse would suspect which of the following?

(1) Hypothyroidism
(2) Hyperthyroidism
(3) Hypoparathyroidism
(4) Hyperparathyroidism

2 A client is returning from a subtotal thyroidectomy for the treatment of hyperthyroidism. The immediate priority in assessing this client would include which of the following?

(1) Assess for respiratory distress
(2) Assess fluid volume status
(3) Assess neurological status
(4) Assess for pain

3 A client with hypothyroidism is taking levothyroxine sodium (Synthroid), a thyroid replacement hormone. Which of the following statements made by the client would indicate additional teaching is required?

(1) "I know I will be on this medication for the rest of my life."
(2) "I don't eat excessive amounts of cabbage or spinach."
(3) "I take my Synthroid with food."
(4) "I take my Synthroid in the mornings."

4 In providing care for a client being admitted for hyperparathyroidism, the nurse anticipates implementing which of the following actions?

(1) Administering intravenous calcium gluconate
(2) Administering large amounts of intravenous saline
(3) Maintaining strict fluid restriction
(4) Monitoring for tetany

5 The nurse evaluating a client receiving supplemental calcium treatment for hypoparathyroidism knows that the client has achieved therapeutic effects of the calcium supplement when which of the following serum calcium levels is obtained?

(1) 5.6 mg/dL
(2) 12.0 mg/dL
(3) 9.0 mg/dL
(4) 7.0 mg/dL

6 A client with Cushing's syndrome is admitted with the symptoms of hypertension, fatigue, and edema. The priority nursing diagnosis for this client would be which of the following?

(1) Fluid volume deficit
(2) Fluid volume excess
(3) Anxiety related to lack of knowledge
(4) Knowledge deficit

7 A client with Conn's syndrome (hyperaldosteronism) who will not be treated surgically is receiving spironnolactone (Aldactone). The nurse explains the purpose of this drug to the client as being which of the following?

(1) To reverse the hyperaldosteronism
(2) To decrease the serum potassium level
(3) To promote fluid retention
(4) To treat hypertension and hypokalemia

8 A client with Addison's disease is being discharged home and will be taking hydrocortisone (Cortisol). The client requires further instructions about this medication when which of the following statements is made?

(1) "I will monitor closely for any signs of infection."
(2) "I will wear a Medic-Alert bracelet indicating disease and treatment."
(3) "I will report any rapid weight gain or fluid in my legs if it persists for over 1 week."
(4) "I will take safety measures at home to prevent injuries."

9 The nurse is establishing a plan of care for a client newly admitted with syndrome of inappropriate antidiuretic hormone secretion (SIADH). The priority diagnosis for this client would be which of the following?

(1) Fluid volume deficit
(2) Anxiety related to disease process
(3) Fluid volume excess
(4) Risk for injury

10 The nurse is discussing the treatment regimen for a client newly diagnosed with Type I diabetes mellitus. During the discussion of insulin administration, the client asks the nurse, "Why can't I just take a pill like my friend does?" Which of the following statements indicates the client understands the nurse's explanation?

(1) "My body does not produce insulin, therefore I must receive the injections."
(2) "I will be on insulin for a short while, then I can take the pills."
(3) "The pills are not as effective as the insulin injections."
(4) "When my body starts making insulin again, I can stop taking the injections."

See page 311–312 for Answers and Rationales.

I. Risk Factors Associated with Endocrine and Metabolic Health Problems

A. Thyroid hyperfunction disorders

1. Graves' disease: immunological factors, genetic predisposition, infection, stress, excessive intake of thyroid medications; occurs 8 times more frequently in females

2. Goiter: inadequate intake of iodine, increase in thyroid hormone demand

3. Thyroid storm: stress, injury, infection, surgery

B. **Thyroid hypofunction disorders**

1. Hypothyroidism: congenital defect, immunological factors, elderly, infection, iodine deficiency, antithyroid drugs

2. Myxedema: undiagnosed or untreated hypothyroidism

C. **Parathyroid disorders**

1. Hyperparathyroidism: elderly, female, thyroid adenoma

2. Hypoparathyroidism: accidental removal or damage to parathyroid during thyroidectomy

D. **Adrenal cortex hyperfunction disorders**

1. Cushing's syndrome: tumor of pituitary gland, excess administration of corticosteroids or ACTH (although exogenous hormone may also suppress endogenous function)

2. Conn's disease: tumors of adrenal gland

E. **Adrenal cortex hypofunction disorders (Addison's disease):** immunological factors, surgical removal of adrenal glands, infection of adrenal glands, tumor of adrenal gland, head trauma (affects pituitary gland), withdrawal of exogenous glucocorticoids or ACTH

F. **Adrenal medulla hyperfunction disorder (pheochromocytoma):** genetic predisposition, middle-age

G. **Anterior pituitary disorders**

1. Gigantism: pituitary adenoma (hyperfunction)

2. Acromegaly: pituitary adenoma (hyperfunction)

3. Dwarfism: pituitary adenoma, congenital, inheritance, trauma, and radiation (hypofunction)

H. **Posterior pituitary disorders**

1. Diabetes insipidus (hypofunction of ADH secretion): head trauma, brain tumor, removal of pituitary gland, irradiation of pituitary gland, genetic predisposition, renal disease

2. Syndrome of inappropriate antidiuretic hormone (SIADH; hyperfunction of ADH): head trauma, brain tumor, infection, brain surgery, some pharmacologic agents

I. **Diabetes mellitus**

1. Type I diabetes mellitus: genetic predisposition, immunological factors, environmental factors, age > 45, increased in African Americans and Native Americans; hypertension, and elevated cholesterol are common associated conditions

2. Type II diabetes mellitus: age > 30 years, obesity, genetic predisposition

3. Diabetic ketoacidosis: increased insulin requirements, insufficient exogenous insulin

4. Hyperosmolar hyperglycemic non-ketotic coma (HHNC): stressors such as infection, trauma, surgery coupled with underlying (and perhaps unknown) hyperglycemia

II. Thyroid Hyperfunction Disorders

A. Overview

1. The thyroid gland is located in the lower neck anterior to the trachea; its primary function is to produce, store, and secrete hormones:

   a. Thyroxine (T_4)—responsible for cellular metabolism

   b. Triiodothyronine (T_3)—responsible for regulating cellular metabolism

   c. Thyrocalcitonin (calcitonin)—role is calcium regulation

   d. T_3 and T_4 are known collectively as thyroid hormone

2. Iodine is necessary for the thyroid gland to synthesize and secrete hormones

3. Thyroid hormone (T_3 and T_4) stimulates body growth, increases metabolic rate, heart rate, and glucose; overall role is to maintain metabolism and regulate growth and development

4. Calcitonin acts on kidneys and bones to decrease serum calcium levels

5. Causes of thyroid hyperfunction disorders include autoimmune responses, neoplasms, excessive intake of thyroid medications, and excess secretion of thyroid-stimulating hormone (TSH) from the anterior pituitary gland

B. Pathophysiology

1. The production of thyroid hormone (TH) is dependent on adequate secretion of thyroid stimulating hormone (TSH) from the anterior pituitary; the hypothalamus regulates pituitary secretion of TSH by negative feedback

2. **Hyperthyroidism** (hyperfunction of the thyroid gland) leads to an excess of thyroid hormone (TH) in the body

   a. The presence of excess TH leads to a hypermetabolic state, which causes an increase in metabolic function, oxygen consumption by tissues, and heat production

   b. Thyroid hyperfunction disorders

      1) Graves' disease

      2) Toxic goiter

      3) Thyroid storm: leads to increased protein, lipid, carbohydrate, and vitamin metabolism

3. **Graves' disease,** the most common cause of hyperthyroidism, is seen most often in women under age 40

   a. Though the exact cause is unknown, it is considered an autoimmune disorder in response to stimulation of the thyroid gland from a long-acting thyroid stimulator (LATS)

   b. The result is an excess production of TH, which leads to a *hypermetabolic state*

4. **Goiter** describes the enlargement or hypertrophy of the thyroid gland in an attempt to compensate for inadequate TH, and may be present in hyperthyroidism or hypothyroidism

   a. Goiter may be the result of response to excess TSH stimulation, excess growth-stimulating immunoglobulins, or the presence of substances that inhibit thyroid hormone synthesis

   b. The goiter may become so large that respiratory complications arise as a result of compression to the neck and chest

5. *Toxic multinodular goiter* exists when small, independently functioning nodules in the thyroid gland tissue are present and secrete TH

   a. The nodules may be benign or malignant

   b. The manifestations develop more slowly than Grave's disease

   c. Toxic goiter is most often seen in women age 60 or older, who have had goiter for several years

6. **Thyroid storm** (also known as thyroid crisis or thyrotoxicosis) is a *life-threatening condition,* which describes an extreme state of hyperthyroidism

   a. The presence of excessive thyroid hormone causes a rapid increase in metabolic rate

   b. Immediate treatment is necessary to avoid death

7. Signs and symptoms

   a. Hyperthyroidism (see Figure 9-1): note all the symptoms are elevated or high except weight loss, sex drive, and fluid volume

   b. Symptoms caused by excessive stimulation of:

      1) Sympathetic (adrenergic) branch of central nervous system (CNS): cardiac activity, reflexes

      2) Thyroxine: increased metabolism, weight loss, and psychological symptoms

   c. Thyroid storm: leads to extreme hyperthermia (102°F to 106°F), tachycardia, agitation, seizures

   d. Classic symptoms are weight loss, nervousness, **exophthalmos** (protrusion of eyeballs), increased appetite, palpitations, and heat intolerance

C. **Nursing assessment**

1. Assessment for hyperthyroidism includes assessment of eyes, vital signs (VS), cardiac monitor for rhythm changes, signs of congestive heart failure (CHF), nutritional assessment, complaints of GI distress, muscle strength and appearance, presence of goiter, reproductive history, integument assessment, weight, fluid status

2. Assessment findings for thyroid storm include elevated temperature, symptom analysis of pain, bowel/GI complaints, neurological, development of seizures, changes in VS, respiratory status

3. Diagnostic tests

   a. Serum thyroid antibodies (Serum TA): elevated

   b. Thyroid-stimulating hormone (TSH): decreased

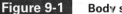 **Figure 9-1**   **Body system effects of hyperthyroidism.**

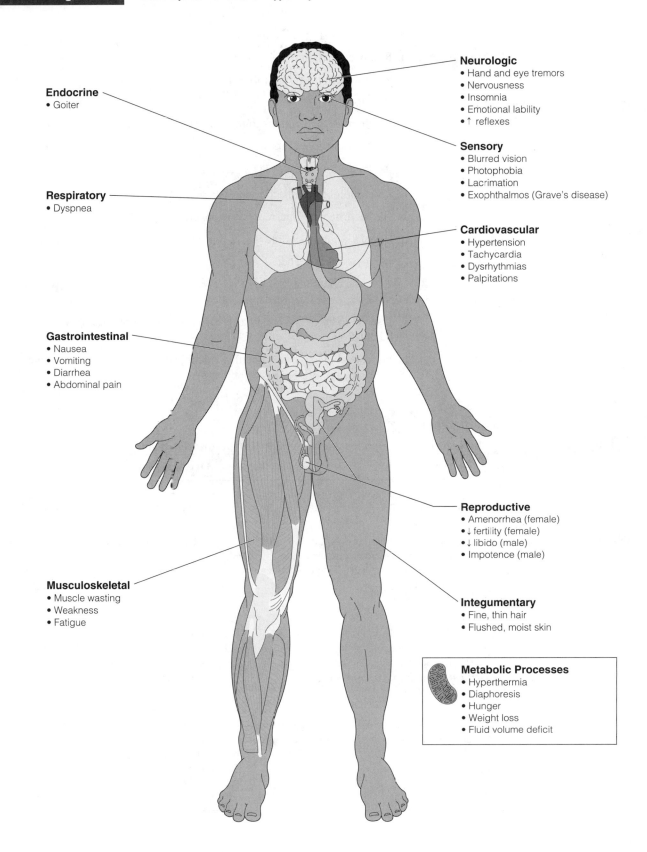

Endocrine
• Goiter

Respiratory
• Dyspnea

Gastrointestinal
• Nausea
• Vomiting
• Diarrhea
• Abdominal pain

Musculoskeletal
• Muscle wasting
• Weakness
• Fatigue

Neurologic
• Hand and eye tremors
• Nervousness
• Insomnia
• Emotional lability
• ↑ reflexes

Sensory
• Blurred vision
• Photophobia
• Lacrimation
• Exophthalmos (Grave's disease)

Cardiovascular
• Hypertension
• Tachycardia
• Dysrhythmias
• Palpitations

Reproductive
• Amenorrhea (female)
• ↓ fertility (female)
• ↓ libido (male)
• Impotence (male)

Integumentary
• Fine, thin hair
• Flushed, moist skin

Metabolic Processes
• Hyperthermia
• Diaphoresis
• Hunger
• Weight loss
• Fluid volume deficit

       c. Serum thyroxine (T_4): increased; decreased in primary hyperthyroidism

       d. Serum triiodothyronine (T_3): increased

       e. T_3 uptake test (T_3RU): increased

       f. Radioactive iodine (RAI) uptake with thyroid suppression test: increased

D. Nursing management (see Table 9-1)

NCLEX!

  1. Medications

    a. Antithyroid medications to reduce TH production

      1) Methimazole (Tapazole)

      2) Propylthiouracil (PTU, Propyl-Thracil)

    b. Propranolol (Inderal) to treat dysrhythmias

    c. Glucocorticoids: interfere with conversion of T_4 to T_3

    d. Lugol's solution (iodine) to decrease vascularity and size of thyroid

    e. Antipyretics if needed

  2. Educate the client that it may take several weeks before the therapeutic effects of antithyroid medications are noticed

    a. Instruct to take medication as prescribed and to not abruptly discontinue medication

    b. Educate about signs of hypothyroidism, which may occur if too much medicine is taken or dose needs adjusting

---

Table 9-1	Comparison of Symptoms and Treatment of Hyperthyroidism and Hypothyroidism	
	Hyperthyroidism	**Hypothyroidism**
Etiology	Autoimmune responses, excess secretion of thyroid-stimulating hormone (TSH), neoplasms, excessive intake of thyroid medications	Congenital defects, antithyroid medications, iodine deficiency, damage to thyroid from surgery or radiation
Clinical Manifestations	Emotional liability, agitation, exophthalmos, increased reflexes, tachycardia, diarrhea, muscle weakness, fatigue, flushed skin, goiter, hyperthermia, weight loss, heat intolerance, diaphoresis *Hint:* Everything is elevated except weight	Memory impairment, confusion, decreased reflexes, periorbital edema, hypotension, bradycardia, constipation, muscle weakness, goiter, edema, weight gain, hypothermia, cold intolerance *Hint:* Everything is decreased except weight
Laboratory Values	• Elevated serum thyroid antibodies (Serum TA), • Decreased thyroid-stimulating hormone (TSH) in primary hyperthyroidism • Increased serum triiodothyronine (T_3) • Increased T_3 uptake	• Increased thyroid-stimulating hormone (TSH) in primary hyperthyroidism • Decreased serum thyroxine (T_4) • Decreased serum triiodothyronine (T_3) • Decreased T_3 uptake • Hyponatremia
Treatment	Pharmacologic agents: methimazole (Tapazole), propylthiouracil (PTU), propranolol (Inderal), glucocorticoids Lugol's Solution Radioactive therapy Thyroidectomy	Pharmacologic agents Levothyroxine sodium (Levothroid) liotrix (Euthroid) Vasopressor agents

3. Monitor for cardiac dysrhythmias, tachycardia

4. Implement antipyretic measures

5. Elevate head of bed to decrease eye pressure

6. Teach eye care and monitor for vision changes if exophthalmos occurs, since it will not change even after medications have been started

7. Monitor dietary intake: client may require up to 4,000 to 5,000 calories a day during hypermetabolic state

8. Monitor intake and output

9. Monitor weight

10. Keep environment cool and quiet because of symptoms

11. Radioactive therapy may be recommended to destroy thyroid cells in order to reduce production of TH

    a. Give radioactive iodine orally; results are expected in 6 to 8 weeks

    b. Does not require hospitalization or radiation precautions

    c. Contraindicated in pregnant women

    d. Monitor for signs of *hypothyroidism*

12. Preoperative and postoperative care for surgical intervention to remove all or part of the thyroid (thyroidectomy)

    a. Subtotal thyroidectomy leaves part of the thyroid gland intact in order to produce adequate amounts of TH

    b. If a total thyroidectomy is performed (usually for treatment of cancer), *lifelong* thyroid hormone replacement is necessary; educate client about importance of compliance with medication regime

    c. Preoperative care includes administering antithyroid medications to promote an euthyroid state, and iodine preparations to decrease vascularity of the gland; teach client how to support neck with both hands while sitting up, moving, or coughing following surgery to reduce strain on suture line

    d. Postoperative care includes monitoring for complications such as hemorrhage, respiratory distress, laryngeal nerve damage, and tetany

13. Priority nursing diagnoses for thyroid hyperfunction disorders: Activity intolerance; Altered nutrition; Hyperthermia; Risk for injury

III. Thyroid Hypofunction Disorders

A. Overview

1. Hypofunction of the thyroid leads to an insufficient amount of thyroid hormone (TH), a condition known as **hypothyroidism**

2. Decreased TH results in a *hypometabolic state* manifested by a decrease in metabolic function, a decrease in oxygen consumption by tissue, and a decrease in heat production

    3. Thyroid hypofunction disorders

        a. Hypothyroidism

        b. Myxedema

        c. Myxedema coma

    4. Classified as primary or secondary

    5. Causes of primary and secondary hypothyroidism

        a. Causes of primary hypothyroidism include congenital defects, loss of thyroid tissue from surgery or radiation, antithyroid medications, endemic iodine deficiency, or thyroiditis

        b. Causes of secondary hypothyroidism include peripheral resistance to thyroid hormones or pituitary TSH deficiency

B. Pathophysiology

    1. *Hypothyroidism* describes an insufficient amount of thyroid hormone (TH), which leads to a decrease in metabolic rate; manifestations develop slowly over months to years

    2. Myxedema describes a generalized hypometabolic state occurring with untreated hypothyroidism

        a. Accumulation of proteins in the interstitial spaces results in an increase in interstitial fluids, causing mucinous edema (myxedema)

        b. This non-pitting edema is most commonly found in the pretibial and facial areas

    3. Myxedema coma (also known as *hypothyroid crisis*) is the result of extreme or prolonged hypothyroidism; though rare, it is a life-threatening condition

        a. Characterized by a severe metabolic state: lactic acidosis, hypoglycemia, hyponatremia, hypotension, bradycardia, cardiovascular collapse, hypothermia, hypoventilation, and coma

        b. Precipitated by inadequate thyroid replacement, infection, trauma, exposure to cold temperatures, central nervous system depressants

    4. *Iodine deficiency:* iodine is necessary for TH synthesis and secretion

        a. Iodine deficiency occurs as a result of antithyroid drugs and lithium or iodine intake

        b. In the United States, thyroid deficiency because of inadequate iodine intake is rare with the use of iodized salt

    5. *Hashimoto's thyroiditis* is an autoimmune disorder generally affecting women age 30 to 50, in which antibodies develop and destroy thyroid tissue

        a. TH levels decrease as a result of fibrous tissue replacing functional thyroid tissue

        b. Goiter develops as the thyroid enlarges to compensate for the decreasing levels of TH

6. Signs and symptoms

    a. Hypothyroidism (see Figure 9-2): notice that most symptoms are decreased except weight and fluid volume

    b. Myxedema coma: hypothermia, cardiovascular collapse, coma, hyponatremia, hypoglycemia, lactic acidosis

C. Nursing assessment

1. Assessment of hypothyroidism includes neurological assessment, presence of periorbital edema, VS, cardiac rhythm, bowel habits, muscle strength, integument assessment, presence of goiter, reproductive history, fluid status, weight, activity tolerance, respiratory status

2. Assessment in myxedema coma includes VS, cardiac assessment, neurological assessment, and other assessments performed for hypothyroidism

3. Diagnostic tests

    a. Serum thyroid antibodies (serum TA): normal; elevated in Hashimoto's thyroiditis

    b. Thyroid stimulating hormone (TSH) in primary hypothyroidism: increased

    c. Serum thyroxine (T_4): decreased (normal 5 to 12 ng/dL)

    d. Serum triiodothyronine (T_3): decreased (normal 80 to 200 ng/dL)

    e. T_3 uptake test (T_3RU): decreased

    f. Radioactive iodine (RAI) uptake test (thyroid scan) with thyroid suppression test: no change or decreased

    g. Hyponatremia (dilutional)

    h. Increased cholesterol and triglyceride levels

    i. Myxedema coma: glucose decreased, ABGs show metabolic acidosis

D. Nursing management (see Table 9-1)

1. Medications

    a. Thyroid replacement medications

        1) Levothyroxine sodium (T_4), Levoid, Levothroid, Synthroid, Synthrox

        2) Liotrix (Euthroid, Thyrolar)

    b. Vasopressor agents to maintain adequate perfusion

2. Intravenous glucose

3. Monitor for signs of digitalis toxicity if receiving digoxin (Lanoxin)

4. Monitor for hyperthyroidism; teach signs and symptoms of both hyper- and hypothyroidism

5. Monitor for hyperglycemia and also for hypoglycemia (since myxedema can lead to this)

6. Monitor vital signs, daily weight

Figure 9-2   **Body system effects of hypothyroidism.**

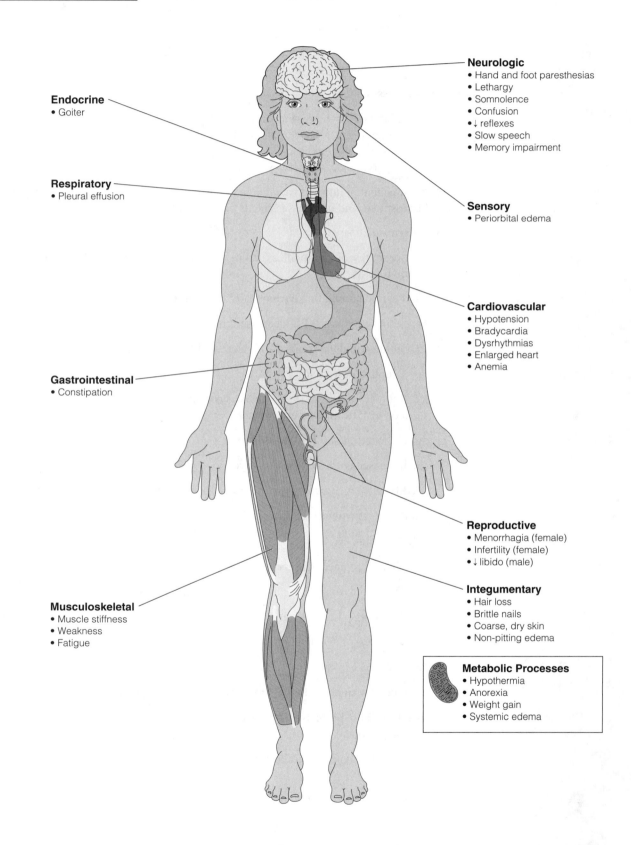

Endocrine
• Goiter

Respiratory
• Pleural effusion

Gastrointestinal
• Constipation

Musculoskeletal
• Muscle stiffness
• Weakness
• Fatigue

Neurologic
• Hand and foot paresthesias
• Lethargy
• Somnolence
• Confusion
• ↓ reflexes
• Slow speech
• Memory impairment

Sensory
• Periorbital edema

Cardiovascular
• Hypotension
• Bradycardia
• Dysrhythmias
• Enlarged heart
• Anemia

Reproductive
• Menorrhagia (female)
• Infertility (female)
• ↓ libido (male)

Integumentary
• Hair loss
• Brittle nails
• Coarse, dry skin
• Non-pitting edema

Metabolic Processes
• Hypothermia
• Anorexia
• Weight gain
• Systemic edema

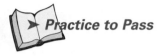

Practice to Pass

The nurse is providing teaching to a client newly diagnosed with hypothyroidism. Her family is also included in the teaching process. What instructions should the nurse provide to the client and the client's family?

7. Client education

a. Educate the client to take medications 1 hour before or 2 hours after meals for optimal absorption and to take medication in morning

b. Medication replacement is *lifelong*

c. Do not substitute drug brands or use generic equivalents without prior approval from healthcare provider as dosing may be different

d. Avoid excessive intake of foods such as cabbage, carrots, spinach, turnips, and peaches, which inhibit TH utilization

e. Report nervousness, insomnia, palpitations, excess weight loss or leg cramps to primary healthcare provider

8. Priority nursing diagnoses for thyroid hypofunction disorders: Activity intolerance; Altered nutrition; Decreased cardiac output; Hypothermia; Risk for impaired skin integrity; Risk for injury

IV. Parathyroid Disorders

A. Overview

1. The parathyroid glands are located posterior to the thyroid glands

a. Their major function is to maintain normal serum calcium levels by secreting parathyroid hormone (PTH), which increases bone resorption of calcium

b. PTH responds to decreased calcium levels by increasing calcium absorption from the bone, kidneys, and intestines

2. **Hyperparathyroidism** is an *increase* in PTH, which leads to hypercalcemia, hypophosphatemia, bone damage, and renal damage

3. **Hypoparathyroidism** is a *decrease* in PTH, which leads to hypocalcemia, hyperphosphatemia, hyperreflexia, and an altered sensorium

4. Causes of hyperparathyroidism

a. *Primary hyperparathyroidism* results from an adenoma or hyperplasia of one of the parathyroid glands

b. *Secondary hyperparathyroidism* results as a response of the parathyroid glands to chronic hypocalcemia (usually caused by renal failure)

c. *Tertiary hyperparathyroidism* results from hyperplasia of the parathyroid glands and a resulting loss of response to serum calcium levels

5. The most common cause of hypoparathyroidism is damage to or removal of the parathyroid glands during thyroidectomy

B. Pathophysiology

1. Hyperparathyroidism

a. Increased PTH causes an increased resorption of calcium by the kidneys, leading to *hypercalcemia,* and an increased excretion of phosphate by the kidneys, leading to hypophosphatemia

b. Increased PTH causes an increased release of phosphorus and calcium by the bones, leading to bone decalcification and the formation of renal calculi

c. Increased PTH causes an increased bicarbonate excretion and decreased acid excretion, leading to hypokalemia and metabolic acidosis

2. Hypoparathyroidism

a. Decreased PTH causes a decrease in bone and renal resorption of calcium, leading to *hypocalcemia,* and a decrease in renal excretion of phosphate, elevating serum phosphate levels (hyperphosphatemia)

b. Calcifications may form on eyes, causing cataracts, and on the basal ganglia, causing brain calcifications

c. Decreased serum calcium levels cause muscular excitability, tetany, and laryngeal spasms

3. Signs and symptoms

NCLEX!

a. Hyperparathyroidism

1) Neurological: depression, psychosis, paresthesias, decreased neuromuscular irritability, impaired vision, altered level of consciousness

2) Cardiovascular: hypertension, dysrhythmias

3) Gastrointestinal: nausea, abdominal pain, constipation, peptic ulcers, gastric bleeding, thirst, anorexia, pancreatitis

4) Renal: renal calculi, hypercalciuria, hyperphosphaturia

5) Musculoskeletal: muscle atrophy and weakness, bone pain, pathologic fractures, back pain, osteoporosis, demineralization of bone

6) Metabolic: metabolic acidosis, weight loss, polyuria, polydipsia, dehydration

NCLEX!

b. Hypoparathyroidism

1) Neurological: hyperactive reflexes, increased intracranial pressure, irritability, anxiety, depression, paresthesias of lips, hands, and feet, laryngeal spasms, seizure activity

2) Cardiovascular: dysrythmias

3) Gastrointestinal: malabsorption syndromes, abdominal cramps

4) Musculoskeletal: carpopedal spasms, facial grimacing, muscle spasms, tetany, seizures, positive Chvostek's sign, and positive Trousseau's sign, hyperactive deep tendon reflexes, calcification of bones

5) Renal: renal colic

6) Integumentary: dry and scaly skin, hair loss, brittle nails

C. Nursing assessment

1. Assessment of hyperparathyroidism includes neurological assessment including LOC, VS, heart rhythm, GI assessment, complaints of pain, muscle strength, weight, I & O

2. Diagnostic tests for hyperparathyroidism

a. Serum calcium level: hypercalcemia: normal 8.8 to 10 mg/dL

b. Serum phosphorus level: hypophosphatemia; normal 2.5 to 4.5 mg/dL

c. ABGs: metabolic acidosis

    d. Serum potassium level: hypokalemia

    e. Urine calcium (leads to stones): increased

    f. Urine phosphates: increased

    g. Parathyroid hormone (PTH): increased

    h. Alkaline phosphate: increased

    i. Radiological examinations reveal deposits of calcium in soft tissues and renal structures, osteoporotic changes, demineralization of bone

3. Nursing assessment of hypoparathyroidism includes reflexes and other neurological assessments, VS, cardiac rhythm, GI complaints, Chvostek's sign, Trousseau's sign, signs of tetany, any integumentary or renal complaints

4. Diagnostic tests for hypoparathyroidism

    a. Serum calcium levels (hypocalcemia)

    b. Serum phosphate levels (hyperphosphatemia)

    c. Parathyroid hormone (PTH): decreased

    d. Urine calcium: decreased

    e. Radiologic examination reveals calcification of skull

D. Nursing management

  1. Hyperparathyroidism

    a. Medications

      1) Furosemide (Lasix) (oral or intravenous) to promote diuresis

      2) Phosphates (oral or intravenous) for replacement

      3) Calcitonin (Calcimar): intravenous to decrease release of calcium by bones

      4) Plicamycin (Mithracin) to inhibit bone resorption of calcium

      5) Gallium nitrate (Gallium) to inhibit bone resorption of calcium

      6) Glucocorticoids to decrease gastrointestinal absorption of calcium

    b. Educate the client to consume diet low in calcium and vitamin D, and increase oral intake of fluids as prescribed

    c. Intravenous saline fluids to increase excretion of calcium

    d. Preoperative and postoperative care for surgical removal of the parathyroid gland (parathyroidectomy) for primary hyperparathyroidism

    e. Strain urine for stones, monitor I & O

    f. Monitor EKG rhythm, VS

  2. Hypoparathyroidism

    a. Medications

      1) Intravenous calcium gluconate (Kalcinate) initially, then supplemental oral calcium replacement

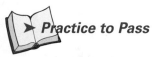

Practice to Pass

The nurse is providing care to a client who has recently had a thyroidectomy. What clinical manifestations and abnormal laboratory values should the nurse expect to observe if the client was experiencing symptoms related to damage of the parathyroid gland?

NCLEX!

NCLEX!

2) Oral vitamin D

3) Administer parathyroid hormone (PTH)

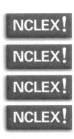

b. Educate the client to consume a diet high in calcium and low in phosphate

c. Monitor for seizure activity and laryngeal spasms; provide protective environment if seizures occur

d. Perform Chvostek's sign and Trousseau's sign for hypocalcemia

e. Tracheostomy set at bedside for respiratory emergencies caused by laryngeal spasm

f. Monitor neuromuscular function

3. Priority nursing diagnoses for parathyroid disorders: Impaired physical mobility; Risk for injury; Pain; Altered urinary elimination; Altered nutrition

V. Adrenal Cortex Hyperfunction Disorders

A. Overview

1. The adrenal glands are located superior to each kidney and composed of the adrenal medulla (the inner layer of adrenal gland) and the adrenal cortex (the outer layer of the adrenal gland)

   a. The adrenal medulla secretes the catecholamines: epinephrine, norepinephrine, and dopamine

   b. The adrenal cortex secretes mineralcorticoids (aldosterone), glucocorticoids (cortisol, androgens and estrogens [sex hormones])

2. The functions of epinephrine and norepinephrine (catecholamines) include increasing metabolic rate, increasing alertness, increasing insulin levels, and the "fight-or-flight" response

3. The functions of glucocorticoids (cortisol) include assisting the body's response to stress, suppression of inflammation, increasing serum glucose by acting as insulin antagonist, regulating metabolism of carbohydrates, fat, and protein, enhancing protein synthesis, and increasing breakdown of protein and fatty acids

4. The function of adrenocorticotropic hormone (ACTH) is in growth and development

5. The function of mineralcorticoids (aldosterone) includes sodium (Na^+) and water retention, and potassium (K^+) excretion

6. Androgens and estrogens contribute to growth and development

7. Adrenal cortex hyperfunction disorders result in excess production of

   a. Cortisol: **Cushing's syndrome**—or hypercortisolism

   b. Aldosterone: **Conn's syndrome**—hyperaldosteronism

8. Causes of hypercortisolism include adrenal tumors, adrenal hyperplasia, or exogenous glucocorticoids

9. Causes of hyperaldosteronism include an adrenal lesion or any condition that stimulates overproduction of aldosterone: heart failure, cirrhosis of liver, dehydration, renal disease

B. Pathophysiology

1. Cushing's syndrome (also known as hypercortisolism)

   a. The functions of glucocorticoids (cortisol, ACTH) include promoting gluconeogenesis, maintaining serum glucose levels, adaptation to stress, and augmenting release of catecholamines to increase blood pressure

   b. *Primary Cushing's syndrome* is caused by a benign or malignant adrenal tumor, which stimulates an increased production of cortisol

   c. *Secondary Cushing's syndrome* results from disorders of the pituitary or hypothalamus, which causes an increased release of ACTH, or from an ectopic disorder that produces ACTH

   d. *Iatrogenic Cushing's syndrome,* the most common cause of Cushing's syndrome, results from the use of long-term glucocorticoid therapy, which results in excess cortisol levels

   e. Signs and symptoms of hypersecretion of cortisol include

      1) Neurological: psychosis, emotional liability, loss of memory, depression, poor concentration

      2) Cardiovascular: hypertension, arrhythmias

      3) Gastrointestinal: peptic ulcers

      4) Musculoskeletal: muscle weakness, muscle wasting, osteoporosis, "buffalo" hump, truncal obesity

      5) Integumentary: ecchymosis, hirsutism, purple striae on abdomen, poor wound healing, skin infections, thin skin, acne

      6) Renal: glycosuria, polyuria, polydipsia, renal calculi

      7) Reproductive: decreased libido, impotence, amenorrhea, masculine characteristics in females

      8) Metabolic: hypokalemia, hypernatremia, edema, "moon face," weight gain

      9) Classic symptoms of Cushing's syndrome: moon face, buffalo hump, purple striae, truncal obesity

2. Conn's syndrome (primary hyperaldosteronism)

   a. Role of aldosterone (a mineralocorticoid) is sodium and water retention

   b. Aldosterone affects tubular resorption of sodium (Na+) and water (H_2O); also has role in excretion of potassium (K+) and hydrogen ions (H+)

   c. In *primary hyperaldosteronism* the effects of excessive secretion of aldosterone cause an increase in sodium (Na+) retention, an increase in water (H_2O) retention, and an increase in potassium (K+) excretion

      1) As blood pressure increases, renin production is suppressed

      2) Blood pressure continues to rise to dangerous levels, potentially leading to renal damage and cerebral infarcts

      3) Despite the water and sodium retention, edema is *rarely* a complication because the water is generally excreted with the potassium ions in the urine

d. In *secondary hyperaldosteronism* hypertension is uncommon

e. Signs and symptoms include visual disturbances, paresthesia, HTN, dysrhythmias, fluid retention, renal damage or failure, polyuria, muscle weakness, tetany, electrolyte and acid–base imbalance

C. Nursing assessment

1. Assessment of Cushing's syndrome includes VS; cardiac rhythm; neurological assessment; history of GI, renal, and reproductive problems; muscle strength; integument assessment; weight; presence of edema; I & O

2. Diagnostic tests for Cushing's syndrome

    a. Serum cortisol levels: increased

    b. Serum sodium levels: increased (hypernatremia)

    c. Serum potassium levels: decreased (hypokalemia)

    d. Serum glucose levels: increased (hyperglycemia)

    e. Serum ACTH levels in secondary Cushing's syndrome: increased

    f. Serum ACTH levels in primary Cushing's syndrome: decreased

    g. Urine 17-ketosteroids and 17-hydroxycorticosteroids: increased

    h. ACTH suppression test is performed in order to identify the cause

    i. White blood cell count (WBC) >10,000/mm^3

    j. Dexamethasone suppression test to determine if cause is pituitary or adrenal

    k. Radiological examinations reveal pituitary tumor or adrenal tumor

3. Assessment of Conn's syndrome includes neurological assessment, eye exam, VS, cardiac rhythm, fluid status, I & O, muscle strength, electrolytes and renal status

4. Diagnostic tests for Conn's syndrome

    a. Serum sodium levels: increased (hypernatremia)

    b. Serum potassium levels: decreased (hypokalemia)

    c. ABGs: metabolic alkalosis (elevated HCO_3^-)

    d. Serum aldosterone levels: elevated

    e. Urine aldosterone levels: elevated

    f. Serum renin levels (primary hyperaldosteronism): decreased

    g. Serum renin levels (secondary hyperaldosteronism): increased

    h. Radiological examinations reveal tumor

D. Nursing management

1. Cushing's syndrome

    a. Medications

        1) Mitotane (Lysodren): cytotoxic antihormonal agent that inhibits corticosteroid synthesis without destroying cortical cells

2) Trilostane (Modrastane) or aminoglutethimide (Cytadren): block the synthesis of glucocorticoids and adrenal steroids

3) Cyproheptadine (Periactin), somatostatin (Octreotide), or bromocriptine (Parlodel): interferes with ACTH production

4) Lifelong steroid replacement if adrenalectomy is performed

b. Preoperative and postoperative care for adrenalectomy if performed

c. Assist in monitoring effects of radiation therapy if performed

d. Monitor for *Addisonian crisis* caused by drug therapy

e. Priority nursing diagnoses for Cushing's syndrome: Fluid volume excess; Risk for infection; Risk for injury; Activity intolerance; Anxiety; Knowledge deficit; Risk for impaired skin integrity

2. Conn's syndrome

a. Medications

1) Spironolactone (Aldactone) to treat hypertension and hypokalemia for those clients who will not be treated surgically

2) Amiloride (Midamor) for those clients unable to tolerate spironolactone

3) Administer glucocorticoids preoperatively as prescribed to prevent adrenal hypofunction

b. Preoperative and postoperative care for unilateral or bilateral adrenalectomy

c. Educate client that if bilateral adrenalectomy is performed, lifetime replacement of glucocorticoids is necessary

d. Monitor blood pressure, urine output, electrolytes

e. Educate client about low-sodium diet

f. Teach side effects of medications

g. Priority nursing diagnoses for Conn's syndrome: Altered urinary elimination; Fluid volume excess; Risk for injury

VI. Adrenal Cortex Hypofunction Disorder: Addison's Disease

A. Overview

1. Addison's disease is defined as a chronic adrenocortical insufficiency as a result of destruction of the adrenal glands

2. Adrenal cortex hypofunction results in a decreased production of cortisone and aldosterone

3. Causes include destruction of the adrenal gland because of trauma, an infection, hemorrhage into the gland, or sudden stress

B. Pathophysiology

1. Also known as adrenal insufficiency

2. Gradual destruction of adrenal cortical tissue leads to hypofunction of adrenal glands

---

NCLEX!

Practice to Pass

The nurse is providing care to a client with Cushing's syndrome. What nursing interventions should be implemented for a diagnosis of Fluid volume excess?

NCLEX!

NCLEX!

3. Insufficient hormonal secretion of mineralcorticoids and glucocorticoids results in deficient aldosterone, cortisol, and androgens

4. Insufficient levels of aldosterone lead to a reduction in sodium absorption and increased sodium excretion

5. Water follows sodium, leading to increased water excretion and hypovolemia

6. Hypotension occurs as a result of hypovolemia

7. Potassium is retained (moves opposite direction of sodium), resulting in hyperkalemia

8. **Addisonian crisis** can occur, which is an acute insufficiency of adrenocortical hormone from a lack of cortisol during stress, such as surgery or pregnancy, or when exogenous corticosteroid therapy is abruptly discontinued

   a. If not treated immediately, circulatory collapse, shock, and death may occur

   b. Signs and symptoms include severe nausea and vomiting, diarrhea, dehydration, sudden pain in lower back, abdomen and legs, hypotension, tachycardia, confusion, restlessness, fatigue, shock, headache

9. Signs and symptoms of Addison's disease include

   a. Neurological: neurosis, depression

   b. Cardiovascular: hypotension, EKG changes such as tall, peaked T waves because of hyperkalemia

   c. Musculoskeletal: muscle weakness, fatigue

   d. Integumentary: skin hyperpigmentation

   e. Gastrointestinal: diarrhea, nausea, vomiting, anorexia

   f. Reproductive: decreased libido, scant pubic hair

   g. Metabolic: hyperkalemia, hyponatremia, hypoglycemia, weight loss

C. **Nursing assessment**

1. Assessment includes neurological assessment, VS, cardiac monitoring, activity tolerance, muscle strength, GI symptoms, libido, electrolyte balance, weight

2. Diagnostic tests

   a. Serum cortisol levels: low

   b. Serum ACTH levels: high

   c. Serum sodium levels: low (hyponatremia)

   d. Serum potassium levels: high (hyperkalemia)

   e. Serum aldosterone levels: decreased

   f. Urinary cortisol levels: decreased

   g. ABGs: metabolic acidosis (decreased HCO_3^-)

   h. Electrocardiogram

NCLEX!

NCLEX!

NCLEX!

▶ *Practice to Pass*

The nurse is educating a client with Addison's disease about nutritional requirements for the management of this disease. What instructions should be provided?

D. Nursing management

1. Medications include mineralocorticoid and glucocorticoid replacement

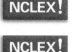

   a. Addison's disease: administer cortisone, prednisone, or fludrocortisone acetate (Florinef) as prescribed

   b. Addisonian crisis: immediate intravenous glucocorticoid replacement and fluids with sodium

2. Monitor for signs of dehydration

3. Maintain high-sodium, low-potassium diet

4. Prepare client for surgical intervention if tumor is causative factor

5. Priority nursing diagnoses for Addison's disease: Fluid volume deficit; Risk for injury

VII. Adrenal Medulla Hyperfunction Disorder: Pheochromocytoma

A. Overview

1. **Pheochromocytoma** is a catecholamine-secreting tumor (usually benign) of the adrenal medulla

2. It is a rare disorder that causes severe hypertension in addition to hyperglycemia and hypermetabolism

3. Cause is usually linked to individual with other multiple endocrine neoplasia syndromes

B. Pathophysiology

1. A tumor in the chromaffin cells of the sympathetic nervous system arises, in most cases, in the adrenal medulla

2. The tumor causes secretion of excessive amounts of the catecholamines epinephrine and norepinephrine

3. The effects of excessive amounts of epinephrine and norepinephrine can lead to a risk of cerebral hemorrhage, cardiac failure, and death if left untreated

4. Signs and symptoms

   a. Neurological: agitation, emotional outbursts, emotional instability, dilated pupils, severe headache, nervousness

   b. Cardiovascular: hypertension (may be persistent, intermittent or fluctuating; may occur rapidly and abruptly cease), tachycardia, palpitations

   c. Gastrointestinal: nausea, vomiting, diarrhea

   d. Renal: glucosuria, polyuria

   e. Musculoskeletal: tremors

   f. Metabolic: hyperglycemia, cold extremities, excessive perspiration

C. Nursing assessment

1. Nursing assessment includes VS, emotional stability, complaints of neurological symptoms or headache, GI distress, I & O, skin temperature

    2. Diagnostic tests

        a. Urine catecholamines: metanephrines and vanillylmandelic acid (VMA): positive

        b. Serum catecholamines: elevated

        c. Urine for glucose (glycosuria): elevated

        d. Serum glucose: elevated (hyperglycemia)

        e. Radiologic examinations reveal tumor

D. Nursing management

    1. Medications

        a. Phenoxybenzamine (Dibenzyline) preoperatively for hypertension control

        b. Metyrosine (Demser) to inhibit synthesis of norepinephrine

        c. Intravenous antihypertensive agents for hypertensive crisis

    2. Preoperative and postoperative care for unilateral or bilateral adrenalectomy

    3. Monitor for heart failure, cerebrovascular accident, myocardial infarction, shock, renal failure

    4. Monitor blood pressure, urinary output, neurological status

    5. Maintain seizure precautions

    6. Priority nursing diagnoses: Risk for injury; Pain

VIII. Anterior Pituitary Disorders

A. Overview

    1. The pituitary gland, referred to as the "master gland," is located at the base of the brain adjacent to the hypothalamus; it is responsible for regulating endocrine function by producing hormones that affect body systems and stimulate other endocrine glands to secrete hormones

    2. Hormones produced by the anterior pituitary gland

        a. Growth hormone (GH)

        b. Thyroid-stimulating hormone (TSH)

        c. Adrenocorticotropic hormone (ACTH)

        d. Follicle-stimulating hormone (FSH)

        e. Leutinizing hormone (LH)

        f. Prolactin (PRL)

    3. Disorders of the anterior pituitary gland result in excessive or insufficient pituitary hormones; disorders of the pituitary gland are not as common as other endocrine gland disorders

    4. *Growth hormone* (GH) is a hormone necessary for growth that regulates cell division and the synthesis of protein; exerts other metabolic effects on endocrine organs, skin, skeletal muscle, cardiac muscle, and connective tissue

5. *Hyperfunction* of the anterior pituitary (hyperpituitarism) results in excess production and secretion of one or more hormones: growth hormone (GH), prolactin (PRL), or adrenocorticotropic hormone (ACTH); leading to the manifestations such as tissue overgrowth seen in hyperpituitarism

6. The most common cause of hyperpituitarism is benign adenoma

7. *Hypofunction* of the anterior pituitary (hypopituitarism) results in a deficiency of one or more of the pituitary hormones: growth hormone (GH), follicle stimulating hormone (FSH), thyroid-stimulating hormone (TSH), leutinizing hormone (LH) and adrenocorticotropic hormone (ACTH)

8. Causes of hypopituitarism include surgical removal of the pituitary gland, pituitary tumors, pituitary infection, pituitary trauma, pituitary tumors, congenital defects, and radiation

9. Common disorders

   a. Hyperpituitarism: gigantism and acromegaly

   b. Hypopituitarism: dwarfism

B. Pathophysiology

1. Gigantism

   NCLEX!

   a. Gigantism is the result of growth hormone (GH) hypersecretion that begins *before the closure of the epiphyseal plate*

      1) This hypersecretion leads the person to become abnormally tall, often reaching 7 to 8 ft in height

      2) Body proportions are generally normal

   b. The most common cause of gigantism is tumor of the pituitary gland

   c. Early detection, diagnosis, and treatment has made this disorder rare in occurrence

   NCLEX!

   d. Signs and symptoms include excessive height and acromegaly as an adult

2. Acromegaly

   a. Acromegaly is the result of GH hypersecretion beginning *during adulthood;* bone and connective tissue continue to grow, leading to *disproportionate* enlargement of tissues

   b. The most common cause of acromegaly is a tumor of the pituitary gland

   NCLEX!

   c. Signs and symptoms include large hands and feet; protrusion of lower jaw; coarse facial features; signs of osteoporosis; change in hand, shoe, and glove size that slowly progresses; systemic symptoms: hypertension; coronary artery disease; congestive heart failure; enlarged adrenal, thyroid and parathyroid gland; amenorrhea; headache; sweating; weakness

3. Dwarfism

   a. Dwarfism results from deficient secretion of anterior pituitary hormones

   b. Inadequate secretion of these hormones leads to growth retardation and accompanying metabolic disorders

    c. Signs and symptoms include short stature, obesity, short-pitched voice, slow-maturing skeletal system, hyperlipidemia, hypercholesterolemia

C. Nursing assessment

    1. Assessment of gigantism includes growth chart for height and weight by age and visual exam

    2. Assessment of acromegaly includes VS, visual disturbances, signs and symptoms of congestive heart failure or diabetes mellitus, growth and development, symptom analysis of any pain

    3. Assessment of dwarfism includes growth chart for height and weight by age, development of sex organs

    4. Diagnostic tests: bone scan, cholesterol, lipid panel, hormone levels

D. Nursing management

    1. Medications include cortisol and thyroid replacement drugs; growth hormone for dwarfism

    2. Assist client in obtaining proper counseling to facilitate psychosocial adjustment to altered body image

    3. Monitor for diabetes insipidus since posterior pituitary gland may be affected simultaneously

    4. Priority nursing diagnoses for anterior pituitary disorders: Activity intolerance; Anxiety; Body image disturbance; Sexual dysfunction; Anticipatory grieving; Ineffective individual coping; Altered growth and development

IX. Posterior Pituitary Disorders

A. Overview

    1. The posterior pituitary gland secretes the hormones oxytocin and **antidiuretic hormone** (ADH), also known as vasopressin; the purpose of antidiuretic hormone is to control serum osmolality

    2. Disorders of the posterior pituitary gland are primarily the result of excessive or deficient ADH secretion

        a. Diabetes insipidus (DI) is the result of ADH insufficiency, resulting in excess fluid excretion

        b. Syndrome of inappropriate antidiuretic hormone secretion (SIADH) is the result of excessive excretion of ADH and excessive water retention

    3. Causes

        a. Diabetes insipidus: unknown etiology in most cases; head trauma with damage to the pituitary or a tumor

        b. SIADH: occurs most often as the result of ectopic production of ADH by malignant tumors, but may also occur as the result of pituitary surgery, head injury, or certain medications such as diuretics, anesthetics, and barbiturates

B. Pathophysiology

    1. Diabetes insipidus (DI)

a. Normally, fluid balance is maintained by actions of the hypothalamus, kidney, and pituitary gland

1) The hypothalamus detects dehydration, sends a message to the pituitary, which in turn releases ADH and sends it to the kidney

2) In the kidney it acts on the collecting and distal tubules to reabsorb water; promoting *retention* to restore fluid balance

3) When excess fluid volume occurs, the hypothalamus sends a message to the pituitary to inhibit secretion of ADH, promoting *excretion* to restore fluid balance

b. In diabetes insipidus, ADH *insufficiency* leads to the excretion of large amounts of urine (polyuria), up to 12 liters a day

c. Classifications

1) *Neurogenic diabetes insipidus* occurs when there is a decrease in the synthesis and excretion of ADH; may be idiopathic, or may result from trauma or dysfunction of the hypothalamus and pituitary gland

2) *Nephrogenic diabetes insipidus* occurs when the renal tubules are not sensitive to ADH

NCLEX!

d. If diabetes insipidus is the result of cerebral injury or other trauma, the disorder may resolve without further incident, however, if the disorder is chronic, lifelong treatment is required

NCLEX!

e. Signs and symptoms include polyuria, excess thirst, polydipsia, dehydration in the event the client is unable to replace fluid loss, weakness

2. Syndrome of inappropriate antidiuretic hormone secretion (SIADH)

a. The normal mechanisms of feedback (as previously described) from hypothalamus, pituitary gland and kidney fail despite low serum osmolality and increased fluid volume, resulting in *excessive secretion* of antidiuretic hormone (ADH), which leads to excessive water retention

b. Excessive water retention results in dilute plasma, decreased serum sodium (hyponatremia), and water intoxication

NCLEX!

c. Signs and symptoms include lethargy, confusion, and/or other changes in neurological status, cerebral edema, muscle cramps, weakness, decreased urine output, fluid retention, weight gain

C. Nursing assessment

1. Assessment of diabetes insipidus includes I & O, complaint of thirst, signs of dehydration (poor skin turgor, dry skin, sunken eyeballs, weakness, decreased urinary output, complaints of thirst, dry mucous membranes)

2. Diagnostic tests for diabetes insipidus

a. Serum sodium level (hypernatremia)

b. Urine specific gravity: low

c. Serum osmolality: high

d. Urine osmolality: decreased

e. Serum ADH levels: decreased

    f. Vasopressin test and water deprivation test: increased (hyperosmolality); diagnostic for DI

  3. Assessment of syndrome of inappropriate antidiuretic hormone includes: LOC and other neurological indicators, I & O, weight

  4. Diagnostic tests for syndrome of inappropriate antidiuretic hormone

    a. Serum sodium levels: low (hyponatremia)

    b. Serum osmolality: low

    c. Urine specific gravity: increased

D. Nursing management

  1. Diabetes Insipidus

    a. Medications include vasopressin (Pitressin, Pressyn) for treatment of neurogenic diabetes insipidus

    b. Administration of intravenous hypotonic fluids

    c. Increase oral fluid intake

    d. Treatment is lifelong for chronic diabetes insipidus

    e. Monitor intake and output

    f. Monitor daily weight

    g. Dietary instructions for low-sodium diet and to avoid caffeine, since this increases urine output

    h. Educate the client about need for Medic-Alert bracelet

  2. Syndrome of inappropriate antidiuretic hormone

    a. Medications include diuretics, demeclocycline (Declomycin)

    b. Administration of intravenous hypertonic saline fluids

    c. Oral fluid restriction

    d. Monitor intake and output

    e. Monitor daily weight

    f. Monitor for neurological changes and other signs of water intoxication

    g. Educate the client about need for Medic-Alert bracelet

  3. Priority nursing diagnoses for posterior pituitary disorders: Fluid volume excess; Fluid volume deficit; Altered urinary elimination; Risk for injury; Knowledge deficit

X. Diabetes Mellitus

  A. Overview

    1. Diabetes mellitus (DM) is defined as a lack of or inadequate secretion of insulin, or insulin resistance resulting in hyperglycemia

      a. Is the most common chronic disorder of the endocrine system

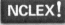

b. The pancreas (beta cells of the islets of Langerhans) fails to secrete an adequate amount of **insulin,** the hormone responsible for glucose metabolism

c. The lack of adequate insulin secretion results in inappropriate *hyperglycemia*

d. Obesity, especially when centralized in the abdomen, may lead to insulin resistance

2. Types

a. *Type 1 diabetes* (formerly insulin-dependent diabetes mellitus or IDDM) results from destruction of pancreatic beta cells, which leads to insulin dependence (no insulin is produced from beta cells of pancreas); insulin *must* be received exogenously

b. *Type 2 diabetes* (formerly non-insulin-dependent diabetes mellitus or NIDDM) results from a decrease in the beta cell weight and number or insulin resistance; may be managed with diet and exercise, and/or oral hypoglycemic agents; situations increasing stress on body (surgery, illness, trauma) may require the need for supplemental insulin temporarily

3. Causes

a. Type 1 DM: occurs as a result of genetic, environmental, or immunological factors that damage the pancreatic beta cells (the insulin secreting cells)

b. Type 2 DM: etiology is unknown; however, obesity is the single most important risk factor

B. Pathophysiology

1. Type 1 diabetes mellitus

a. Damage to the pancreatic beta cells leads to uncontrolled glucose production by the liver and subsequently results in hyperglycemia (elevated serum glucose)

b. The renal threshold for glucose is approximately 180 to 200 mg/dL, therefore glucose spills into the urine once it has surpassed the renal threshold

1) Because glucose is highly osmotic, fluids "follow" the glucose and are excreted out of the body in large amounts of urine (this force is called *osmotic diuresis*), causing an excessive loss of fluids and electrolytes; the excretion of excessive amounts of urine is known as *polyuria*

2) The loss of fluids leads to *polydipsia* (excessive thirst)

c. Because of the lack of insulin, the body is unable to utilize carbohydrates, its primary source of energy; therefore, it must use proteins and fats for energy, leading to unexplained weight loss

1) This use of fat results in *ketones,* the acid end-products of fat metabolism

2) As ketones build in the body, *acidosis* occurs

3) The breakdown of nutritional stores leads to excessive hunger, known as *polyphagia*

d. Polyuria, polydispia, and polyphagia are classic signs of diabetes and are known as the "3 Ps"

e. Failure to receive adequate amounts of insulin results in continued fat metabolism, which produces ketone bodies leading to acidosis

f. **Diabetic ketoacidosis (DKA)** results in severe metabolic, fluid, and electrolyte disturbances, and is a life-threatening condition of hyperglycemia and metabolic acidosis requiring immediate action

2. Type 2 diabetes mellitus

   a. Type 2 diabetes results from a decrease in the beta cell weight and number or from insulin resistance

   b. There is an *inadequate secretion of insulin* or an *insensitivity* (resistance) to insulin, which leads to hyperglycemia

   c. The symptoms are generally the same as in type 1 diabetes, but, type 2 has a gradual onset and may be undetected for years (later adulthood); additionally, ketones are not usually present and excess weight rather than weight loss is noted

3. Signs and symptoms

   a. Early manifestations of type 1 diabetes mellitus: polyuria, polydipsia, polyphagia, glucosuria, fatigue, weight loss, nausea, vomiting, abdominal pain

   b. Early manifestations in type 2 diabetes mellitus: polyuria, polydipsia, blurred vision, weight gain

   c. General multisystem findings (see Figure 9-3)

      1) Sensory/neurological: diabetic retinopathy, cataracts, glaucoma, paresthesias, loss of sensation, peripheral neuropathy

      2) Cardiovascular assessment: coronary artery disease, peripheral vascular disease, hypertension

      3) Gastrointestinal assessment: constipation or diarrhea

      4) Musculoskeletal assessment: contractures

      5) Integumentary assessment: atrophy, foot ulcers, poor wound healing, chronic skin infections

      6) Renal assessment: edema, chronic renal failure, albuminuria, urinary tract infections

      7) Reproductive assessment: sexual dysfunction, vaginitis

      8) Metabolic: hyperglycemia, hypokalemia, metabolic acidosis

   d. Symptoms of diabetic ketoacidosis: abdominal pain, nausea and vomiting, metabolic acidosis, fruity breath odor, Kussmaul's respirations, altered level of consciousness, coma, and death if untreated

4. Complications include diabetes ketoacidosis, hypoglycemia, atherosclerosis, CVA, PVD, diabetic retinopathy, paresthesia (especially feet), renal failure, carpal tunnel syndrome, periodontal disease, gangrene, amputation, inability to heal

Figure 9-3 Body system effects of diabetes mellitus.

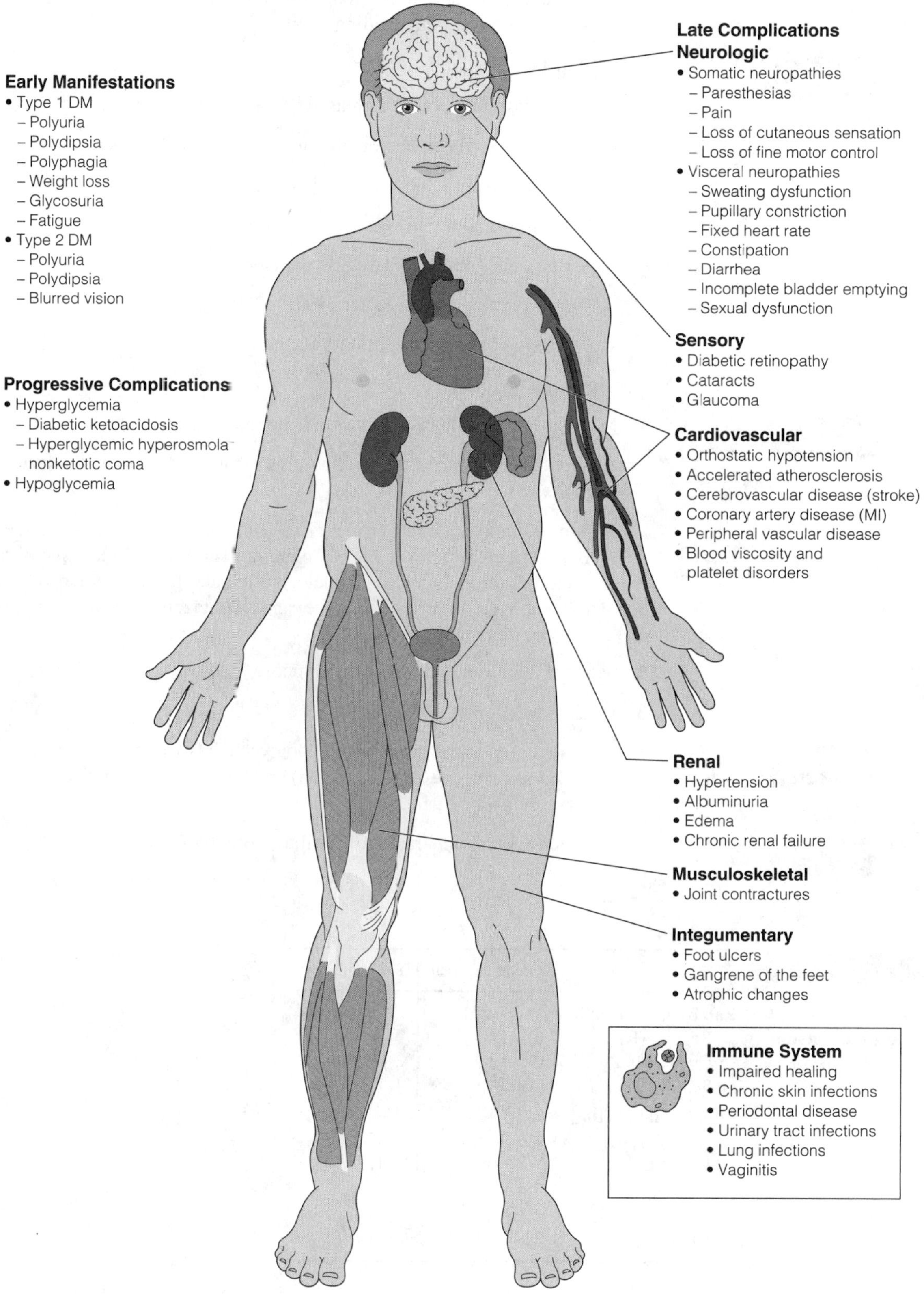

Early Manifestations
- Type 1 DM
  - Polyuria
  - Polydipsia
  - Polyphagia
  - Weight loss
  - Glycosuria
  - Fatigue
- Type 2 DM
  - Polyuria
  - Polydipsia
  - Blurred vision

Progressive Complications
- Hyperglycemia
  - Diabetic ketoacidosis
  - Hyperglycemic hyperosmolar nonketotic coma
- Hypoglycemia

Late Complications
Neurologic
- Somatic neuropathies
  - Paresthesias
  - Pain
  - Loss of cutaneous sensation
  - Loss of fine motor control
- Visceral neuropathies
  - Sweating dysfunction
  - Pupillary constriction
  - Fixed heart rate
  - Constipation
  - Diarrhea
  - Incomplete bladder emptying
  - Sexual dysfunction

Sensory
- Diabetic retinopathy
- Cataracts
- Glaucoma

Cardiovascular
- Orthostatic hypotension
- Accelerated atherosclerosis
- Cerebrovascular disease (stroke)
- Coronary artery disease (MI)
- Peripheral vascular disease
- Blood viscosity and platelet disorders

Renal
- Hypertension
- Albuminuria
- Edema
- Chronic renal failure

Musculoskeletal
- Joint contractures

Integumentary
- Foot ulcers
- Gangrene of the feet
- Atrophic changes

Immune System
- Impaired healing
- Chronic skin infections
- Periodontal disease
- Urinary tract infections
- Lung infections
- Vaginitis

C. Nursing assessment

1. Assessment includes symptom analysis, fluid status, I & O, nutritional status, weight, energy level, GI symptoms, neurological assessment, history of recent infections with difficulty healing

2. Diagnostic tests

   NCLEX!

   a. Serum fasting glucose: increased (hyperglycemia > 126 mg/dL)

   b. Serum glycosylated hemoglobin levels: increased; >7 percent

   c. Urine for glucose and ketones: positive

   d. Urine for protein: positive

   e. Serum potassium: decreased (hypokalemia)

   f. 2-hour-plasma glucose (after meal) > 200 mg/dL

   g. Cholesterol and triglyceride levels: elevated

D. Nursing management

1. Medications include insulin or oral hypoglycemic agents

   NCLEX!

   a. Type 1 diabetes: regular insulin, NPH insulin, or combination insulins such as 70/30

   b. Type 2 diabetes: oral agents such as glipizide (Glucotrol), glyburide (Dia-Beta, Micronase), tolazamide (Tolamide, Tolinase), glimepiride (Armaryl), acetohexamide (Dimelor, Dymelor), tolbutamide (Orinase), metformin (Glucophage), acarbose (Precose) and troglitazone (Rezulin), pioglitazone (Actos), rosiglitazone (Avandia)

2. Monitor intake and output, serum glucose, electrolytes

3. Client education

   NCLEX!

   a. Teach signs and symptoms of hypoglycemia (irritability, fatigue, weakness, tremors, headache. possible coma) and hyperglycemia with appropriate interventions for each

   NCLEX!

   b. Teach self administration of insulin or oral hypoglycemic agents

Table 9-2		Onset (hours)	Peak (hours)
Reaction Time of the Most Common Insulin Preparations	**Rapid-acting insulin**		
	Regular (R)	0.5–1	2–4
	Crystalline Zinc	0.5–1	2–4
	Semilente	1–1.5	4–7
	Intermediate-acting		
	NPH (N)	1–2	8–12
	Lente (L)	1–4	8–12
	Long-acting		
	Protamine Zinc	4–8	16–18
	Ultralente	4–8	16–18

    c. Teach onset and peak actions of insulin (see Table 9-2)

    d. Teach self-monitoring of glucose

    e. Teach proper dietary management of diabetes (will need nutritionist consult): include need for balanced meal plan, food groups, food exchanges and need to correlate diet with serum glucose levels

    f. Teach proper diabetic foot care and wound care

    g. Teach sick day rules: maintaining or increasing insulin when a common sickness occurs (virus, colds, etc.), along with monitoring glucose more often (every 2 to 4 hours) and maintaining fluid intake

    h. Teach proper exercise management of diabetes

4. Priority nursing diagnoses for diabetes mellitus: Altered nutrition; Risk for self-care deficit; Risk for fluid-volume deficit; Risk for impaired skin integrity; Risk for knowledge deficit

---

Case Study

A 16-year-old female, S.W., is admitted for a work-up because of symptoms of excessive weight loss, fatigue, inability to maintain her grades in school, and complaints of constant hunger. These symptoms began rather suddenly, and her mother did not recognize how severe her weight loss had become until she tried on bathing suits. Her admitting lab work was all within normal limits except: glucose 425 mg/dL and her urine tests positive for glucose and ketones. There is no family history of diabetes mellitus (DM). The doctor orders dextrostix before meals and at bedtime with regular insulin according to sliding scale along with NPH 30u SQ every morning.

❶ When the physician confirms the diagnosis of DM, how should the nurse explain the disease so she can understand?

❷ What are the most important symptoms she should be taught?

❸ The mother is frantic and doubts the diagnosis because no one in the family has DM. How should the nurse handle this situation?

❹ What should the client be taught about the possible problems associated with administration of both NPH and regular insulin?

❺ What instructions should S.W. and her mother be given about hypoglycemia and hyperglycemia and why does she need instructions on both?

For suggested responses, see pages 567–568.

Posttest

1 A client with exophthalmos as a result of Graves' disease has expressed a desire for the medications to "hurry up and work so that my eyes will go down." The nurse's response to the client will be based on which of the following?

(1) Reversal of exophthalmos occurs after a therapeutic level of the antithyroid medication is achieved.
(2) Reversal of exophthalmos occurs after treatment with ophthalmic medications.
(3) Changes in the eyes as a result of Graves' disease are not reversible, even after treatment of the disease.
(4) Exophthalmos as a result of Graves' disease is only a temporary symptom, and should resolve spontaneously.

2 The nurse is providing care to a client with myxedema coma. Priority nursing care would include which of the following?

(1) Measures to decrease body temperature
(2) Measures to decrease heart rate
(3) Measures to maintain airway, fluid and electrolyte balance, and cardiovascular status
(4) Measures to decrease blood pressure

3 A client diagnosed with primary hyperparathyroidism demonstrates that she understands the teaching plan when the client makes which of the following statements?

(1) "I know I must have surgery to remove my parathyroid gland."
(2) "I must take diuretics the rest of my life."
(3) "I must eat a diet low in potassium."
(4) "I must limit my daily fluid intake."

4 The priority nursing diagnosis for a client with hypoparathyroidism would be which of the following?

(1) Risk for fluid volume excess
(2) Risk for injury
(3) Anxiety related to lack of knowledge
(4) Knowledge deficit

5 A client with Cushing's syndrome is receiving mitotane (Lysodren), a cytotoxic antihormonal agent. When assessing the client's response to the medication, the nurse would expect therapeutic effects to be the result of which of the following?

(1) Block the utilization of glucocorticoids
(2) Suppression of adrenocorticotropic hormone (ACTH)
(3) Direct suppression of activity of the adrenal cortex
(4) Destruction of the pituitary gland

6 The health education nurse has provided preoperative teaching for a client with Conn's syndrome who is scheduled for a bilateral adrenalectomy. The client understands the teaching when which of the following statements is made?

(1) "I will need to be on lifetime replacement of glucocorticoids."
(2) "I will need to increase my salt intake."
(3) "I need to avoid salt the rest of my life."
(4) "I will need temporary replacements of glucocorticoids."

7 A client with a history of Addison's disease is admitted to the unit with Addisonian crisis manifested by severe hypotension and nonresponsiveness. Which of the following statements provided by the client's spouse would the nurse suspect precipitated the crisis?

(1) The client stopped taking the prescribed hydrocortisone several days ago.
(2) The client routinely adds salt to meals.
(3) The client is taking fludrocortisone (Florinef).
(4) The client is an insulin-dependent diabetic.

8 The nurse administering vasopressin (Pitressin) to a client with diabetes insipidus anticipates implementing which of the following actions for this medication?

(1) Maintaining fluid restriction
(2) Monitoring urine output
(3) Administering intravenous hypertonic fluids
(4) Maintaining NPO status

9 Priority nursing management of the client with pheochromocytoma would include which of the following?

(1) Monitoring blood pressure
(2) Monitoring urine output
(3) Monitoring neurological status
(4) Monitoring serum glucose levels

10 The nurse knows that a client newly diagnosed with insulin-dependent diabetes (Type I) will require further teaching when which of the following statements is made?

(1) "I will notify my healthcare provider if my glucose levels run higher or lower than target range."
(2) "I will take my insulin as prescribed, and I will not miss a dose."
(3) "I will check my glucose level 30 minutes before I eat and at bedtime."
(4) "I will not take my insulin if I am sick and cannot eat."

See page 312–313 for Answers and Rationales.

Answers and Rationales

Pretest

1 **Answer: 2** *Rationale:* Hyperthyroidism is an excess of thyroid hormone (TH), which places the body in a hypermetabolic state manifested by an increase in appetite, body temperature, and oxygen consumption. Hypothyroidism manifestations are the opposite of those seen in hyperthyroidism. The manifestations of parathyroidism are related to disturbances in calcium levels.
Cognitive Level: Analysis
Nursing Process: Assessment; *Test Plan:* PHYS

2 **Answer: 1** *Rationale:* Though fluid volume status, neurological status, and pain are all important assessments, the immediate priority for postoperative thyroidectomy is airway management. Respiratory distress may result from hemorrhage, edema, laryngeal damage, or tetany. Assessment of respiratory status should include rate, depth, rhythm, and effort.
Cognitive Level: Analysis
Nursing Process: Assessment; *Test Plan:* PHYS

3 **Answer: 3** *Rationale:* For best absorption, thyroid medications should be taken 1 hour before meals, or 2 hours after meals. Lifelong treatment of hypothyroidism is necessary. Foods that inhibit thyroid hormone (TH) synthesis, such as cabbage, spinach, and carrots, should not be consumed in excessive amounts. Thyroid medications should be taken in the morning to reduce the possibility of insomnia.
Cognitive Level: Application
Nursing Process: Evaluation; *Test Plan:* PHYS

4 **Answer: 2** *Rationale:* Hypercalcemia is the primary complication of hyperparathyroidism, and the manifestations of the disorder are directly related to the effects of hypercalcemia. Administering large amounts of intravenous saline promotes renal excretion of calcium. Calcium gluconate would increase serum calcium levels, and tetany is a symptom of hypocalcemia.
Cognitive Level: Application
Nursing Process: Implementation; *Test Plan:* PHYS

5 **Answer: 3** *Rationale:* The normal serum calcium level is 8.8 to 10 mg/dL. The therapeutic response of supplemental calcium is demonstrated by normal calcium levels.
Cognitive Level: Analysis
Nursing Process: Evaluation; *Test Plan:* PHYS

6 **Answer: 2** *Rationale:* Cushing's syndrome is manifested by sodium retention, which leads to edema and hypertension. Fluid volume excess is the appropriate diagnosis. Treatment is aimed at restoring normal body fluid balance. Anxiety and knowledge deficit should be addressed following fluid volume excess.
Cognitive Level: Application
Nursing Process: Analysis; *Test Plan:* PHYS

7 **Answer: 4** *Rationale:* Hypertension and hypokalemia are the most common signs and symptoms of hyperaldosteronism. Surgical removal of the adrenal gland(s) is the treatment of choice; however, if that is not possible, the client is treated with Aldac-

tone, a potassium-sparing diuretic, to treat the hypertension and correct the hypokalemia.
Cognitive Level: Analysis
Nursing Process: Implementation; *Test Plan:* PHYS

8 **Answer: 3** *Rationale:* Weight must be monitored *daily,* and any increase indicates fluid retention and should be reported immediately. Corticosteroids are immunosuppressants; therefore careful monitoring for infection is necessary. Additionally, an increase in the medication may be required for stressors such as infection. A Medic-Alert bracelet is recommended to inform healthcare providers of Addison's disease and cortisol treatment. Safety measures are encouraged to prevent injuries.
Cognitive Level: Analysis
Nursing Process: Evaluation; *Test Plan:* PHYS

9 **Answer: 3** *Rationale:* SIADH results in fluid retention and hyponatremia. Correction is aimed at restoring fluid and electrolyte balance. Anxiety and risk for injury should be addressed following fluid volume excess.
Cognitive Level: Analysis
Nursing Process: Planning; *Test Plan:* PHYS

10 **Answer: 1** *Rationale:* Type I, or insulin-dependent diabetes, requires lifelong replacement of insulin, as no insulin is produced from the beta cells of the pancreas. Options 2, 3, and 4 are incorrect for Type I diabetes.
Cognitive Level: Application
Nursing Process: Evaluation; *Test Plan:* PHYS

Posttest

1 **Answer: 3** *Rationale:* Exophthalmos occurs as a result of accumulation of fat deposits and by-products in the retro-orbital tissues. Even with treatment of Graves' disease, these changes are not reversible. The client should receive instructions on proper eye care.
Cognitive Level: Analysis
Nursing Process: Analysis; *Test Plan:* PHYS

2 **Answer: 3** *Rationale:* Myxedema coma is a life-threatening crisis manifested by hypothermia, hyponatremia, hypoglycemia, lactic acidosis, cardiovascular collapse, and coma. Maintaining airway and circulation are the priority interventions.
Cognitive Level: Analysis
Nursing Process: Implementation; *Test Plan:* PHYS

3 **Answer: 1** *Rationale:* The treatment for primary hyperparathyroidism is a parathyroidectomy (surgical removal of parathyroid glands). Options 2, 3, and 4

are incorrect treatments for primary hyperparathyroidism.
Cognitive Level: Application
Nursing Process: Evaluation; *Test Plan:* PHYS

4 **Answer: 2** *Rationale:* Risk for injury related to hypocalcemia is the priority diagnosis as injury may occur as a result of low calcium levels and tetany. The client is at risk for fluid volume deficit, and anxiety and knowledge deficit would not be a priority over injury.
Cognitive Level: Application
Nursing Process: Analysis; *Test Plan:* PHYS

5 **Answer: 3** *Rationale:* The therapeutic effects of mitotane are the results of direct suppression of activity of the adrenal cortex. Modrastane blocks the synthesis of glucocorticoids (option 1), octreotide suppresses ACTH (option 2), and radiation destroys the pituitary gland (option 4).
Cognitive Level: Application
Nursing Process: Analysis; *Test Plan:* PHYS

6 **Answer: 1** *Rationale:* Since the client will have a bilateral adrenalectomy, lifetime corticosteroid replacement is necessary. After the adrenalectomy, the client's aldosterone levels should return to normal; therefore, no dietary restrictions will be necessary.
Cognitive Level: Analysis
Nursing Process: Evaluation; *Test Plan:* PHYS

7 **Answer: 1** *Rationale:* Hydrocortisone is given to replace cortisol in the client with adrenal insufficiency. Abrupt withdrawal of the hormone can precipitate Addisonian crisis. Florinef is given to replace mineralcorticoids. Hyponatremia is caused by aldosterone deficiency, which affects the renal tubules ability to conserve sodium; therefore adding salt to the diet is recommended. Insulin-dependent diabetes is a complication of Addison's disease; however, there is no indication that diabetes precipitated the crisis.
Cognitive Level: Analysis
Nursing Process: Analysis; *Test Plan:* PHYS

8 **Answer: 2** *Rationale:* Because of a deficiency in antidiuretic hormone, diabetes insipidus results in massive diuresis and dehydration. Vasopressin (antidiuretic hormone) is administered to promote fluid retention and achieve fluid balance. Oral fluids are encouraged, and hypotonic fluids are administered.
Cognitive Level: Application
Nursing Process: Implementation; *Test Plan:* PHYS

9 Answer: 1 *Rationale:* Hypertension with systolic blood pressures reaching up to 300 mmHg is possible with pheochromocytoma, making this disorder a life-threatening event. Monitoring blood pressure is a priority. Urine output and neurological status would follow blood pressure, and there is no indication to monitor glucose levels. Treatment of choice for this disorder is an adrenalectomy.
Cognitive Level: Application
Nursing Process: Implementation; *Test Plan:* SECE

10 Answer: 4 *Rationale:* The client should inform the healthcare provider of illness, and then should follow "sick-day rules" as prescribed by healthcare provider, which include taking insulin as prescribed, or increasing insulin as prescribed, consuming extra fluids, resting, and monitoring glucose every 2 to 4 hours. Options 1, 2, and 3 are all correct responses by the client.
Cognitive Level: Analysis
Nursing Process: Evaluation; *Test Plan:* PHYS

References

Bullock, B. A. & Henze, R. L. (2000). *Focus on pathophysiology.* Philadelphia: Lippincott.

Ignatavicius, D., Workman, M., & Mishler, M. (1999). *Medical-surgical nursing across the health care continuum* (3rd ed.). Philadelphia: W. B. Saunders, pp. 1573–1686.

LeMone, P. & Burke, K. (2000). *Medical surgical nursing: Critical thinking in client care* (2nd ed.). Upper Saddle River, NJ: Prentice Hall, pp. 99–162, 671–768.

McCance, K., & Huether, S. (2002). *Pathophysiology: The biologic basis for disease in adults and children* (4th ed.). St. Louis, MO: Mosby, pp. 625–703.

Thomas, C. L. (Ed.). (2001). *Taber's cyclopedic medical dictionary* (20th ed.). Philadelphia: F. A. Davis.

Wilson, B. A., Shannon, M. T., & Stang, C. L. (2001). *Nursing drug guide: 2001.* Upper Saddle River, NJ: Prentice Hall.

CHAPTER 10

Renal and Urinary Health Problems

Julie A. Adkins, RN, MSN, FNP

CHAPTER OUTLINE

OBJECTIVES

■ Define key terms associated with renal and urinary health problems.

■ Identify risk factors associated with the development of renal and urinary health problems.

■ Discuss the common etiologies of renal and urinary health problems.

■ Describe the pathophysiologic processes associated with specific renal and urinary health problems.

■ Distinguish between normal and abnormal renal and urinary findings obtained from nursing assessment.

■ Prioritize nursing interventions associated with specific renal, urinary, and metabolic health problems.

[*Media Link*]

Use the CD-ROM enclosed with this text, or log onto the address given to access the free, interactive Companion Website created for this series. The CD-ROM and Companion Website accompanying this book offer additional practice opportunities and information—NCLEX Review, Case Studies, Glossary, In Depth with NCLEX, and more.

www.prenhall.com/hogan

REVIEW AT A GLANCE

acute renal failure (ARF) *sudden decrease, over days to weeks, in renal function, resulting in retention of urea, nitrogen and creatinine in the blood*

azotemia *increased blood levels of nitrogenous waste products*

calculi *masses of crystals composed of minerals normally excreted in the urine*

chronic renal failure (CRF) *progressive inability, over months to years, of the kidneys to respond to changes in body fluid and electrolyte composition, GFR < 20 percent of normal, serum creatinine > 5 mg/dL*

cystitis *inflammation of the urinary bladder*

glomerulonephritis *inflammation of the capillary loops of the glomeruli*

hematuria *blood in the urine*

nephrolithiasis *stones in the kidney*

oliguria *urine output less than 400 ml in 24 hours*

polycystic kidney disease *a hereditary disease characterized by cyst formation and massive kidney enlargement*

prostatitis *inflammation of the prostate*

pyelonephritis *inflammatory disorder affecting the renal pelvis and functional portion of the kidney*

pyuria *presence of pus in the urine when voided*

uremia *syndrome of renal failure that includes increased blood urea and creatinine levels accompanied by fatigue, anorexia, nausea, vomiting, pruritis and neurologic changes*

urethritis *inflammation of the urethra*

urinary tract infections (UTI) *infection of the urinary bladder, kidney, urethra, or prostrate*

urolithiasis *stones in the urinary bladder*

Pretest

1 A 25-year-old college student is diagnosed with an upper urinary tract infection. Which of the following would be documented on the medical record?

(1) Cystitis
(2) Pyelonephritis
(3) Urethritis
(4) Prostatitis

2 The nurse would expect to see which pathogen on the urine culture and sensitivity (C & S) of a client with a urinary tract infection?

(1) *Streptococcus*
(2) *Staphylococcus*
(3) *E. coli*
(4) *Klebsiella*

3 A urinary tract infection would be considered complicated in which of the following clients?

(1) Teenager who has recently become sexually active
(2) A child, age 2
(3) An elderly, bedridden client
(4) A male client

4 The client with cystitis has a routine urinalysis (UA) done. Pyuria is noted on the report, which means the urine has:

(1) Blood.
(2) Casts.
(3) Excess mucus and white blood cells.
(4) Protein.

5 When assessing the client with urinary calculi, an important subjective finding would be:

(1) Allergies to sulfonamides.
(2) Father of client who has had urinary stones twice.
(3) Last urinary tract infection 2 months ago.
(4) Alcohol intake of two six-packs of beer per day.

6 The presence of red blood cell casts is most likely caused by which disorder?

(1) Urinary tract infection
(2) Pyelonephritis
(3) Renal failure
(4) Glomerulonephritis

7 Which of the following should the nurse suspect as an iatrogenic cause of acute renal failure?

(1) Alcohol
(2) Diet
(3) Nephrotoxic medications
(4) Exercise

8 Glomerular filtration rate is less than 30 percent of normal in which of the following?

(1) Urinary tract infection
(2) Kidney cancer
(3) Acute renal failure
(4) Polycystic kidney disease

9 What laboratory test is a common measure of renal function?

(1) Complete blood count
(2) Blood urea nitrogen/creatinine
(3) Glucose
(4) Alanine amino transferase (ALT)

10 In the second stage of chronic renal failure, what percent of renal tissue is destroyed?

(1) 25 percent.
(2) 30 percent.
(3) 50 percent.
(4) 75 percent.

See pages 336–337 for Answers and Rationales.

I. Risk Factors Associated with Renal and Urinary Health Problems

NCLEX!

A. **Urinary tract infection:** female, geriatric clients; strictures; impaired bladder innervation; chronic disease such as diabetes, prostatic hypertrophy and prostatitis; diaphragm use; instrumentation; and impaired immune response

B. **Urinary calculi:** male, Caucasian race, young and middle adulthood; prior personal or family history of calculi; diseases such as gout, hyperparathyroidism, urinary stasis, repeated infections; medications such as vitamins (A, C, and D), loop diuretics, calcium-containing antacids

C. **Polycystic kidney disease:** genetics; dialysis

D. **Pyelonephritis:** pregnancy; urinary tract obstruction; congenital malformation; urinary tract trauma; scarring; calculi; other kidney disorders; vesicoureteral reflux (urine moves from bladder back toward kidney); diabetes; and sickle cell disease

E. **Glomerulonephritis:** systemic diseases; post-streptococcal infections; staphylococcal or viral infections

F. **Acute renal failure:** major trauma or surgery; African Americans; predominantly males; infection; hemorrhage; diseases such as severe heart failure; severe liver disease; lower urinary tract obstruction; nephrotoxic medications; radiologic contrast dye; and shock

G. **Chronic renal failure:** African Americans, Native Americans, Asians, and European Americans; circulatory failure; urinary tract obstruction; analgesic abuse; diseases such as untreated hypertension (HTN) and diabetes; and cigarette smoking

H. **Bladder cancer:** geographic (heavily industrialized areas and northern regions); men; cigarette smoke; chemicals and dyes used in plastics, rubber and cable industries; substances in work environment of textile workers, leather finishers, spray painters, hair dressers, petroleum workers; and chronic use of phenacetin containing analgesics

   I. Kidney cancer: males, over 50; smoking; obesity; chronic irritation caused by renal calculi; urban environment; industrial chemicals; phenacetin or analgesic abuse

II. Urinary Tract Infection (UTI)

A. Overview

1. **Urinary tract infection is** defined as an infection of the bladder, kidney, urethra, or prostate

2. The urinary tract is normally sterile above the urethra, maintained by a free flow of urine from the kidneys to the meatus and emptying the bladder completely

3. Urinary tract infections are classified according to the region and primary site affected

    a. Lower urinary tract infections include **urethritis** (inflammation of the urethra), **prostatitis** (inflammation of the prostate) and **cystitis** (inflammation of the urinary bladder); cystitis is the most common form of UTI

    b. Upper urinary tract infections include **pyelonephritis** (inflammation of the kidney and renal pelvis)

4. Causes include bowel incontinence, procedures requiring instrumentation, sexual activity, urinary obstruction or calculi, and improper cleaning (especially in children)

B. Pathophysiology

1. Pathogens enter the urinary tract by one of two routes

    a. Ascending from mucous membranes of the perineal area to the lower urinary tract (most common type); gram-negative bacteria, usually *E. coli*, is present in 90% of the cases; it is most frequent in adult females because of colonization of bacteria found in the lower gastrointestinal tract gaining entry by ascending the short, straight female urethra

    b. Hematogenously from the blood; this type is rare and usually associated with previous damage or scarring of the urinary tract

2. A UTI can be categorized as:

    a. *Uncomplicated:* isolated incidence of UTI

    b. *Complicated:* more than two UTIs per year, related to functional, anatomic, metabolic or neurological disorders, related to an antibiotic-resistant pathogen or pregnancy

3. Any UTI in a male client is considered complicated

4. Signs and symptoms include dysuria (painful or difficult urination), urinary frequency and urgency (sudden, compelling need to urinate) and nocturia (two or more awakenings at night to urinate); urine may have a foul odor and appear cloudy; presence of **pyuria** (excess mucus and white cells in the urine) or **hematuria** (bloody urine) caused by bleeding of inflamed bladder wall; older clients may not experience classic symptoms, but instead present with nocturia, incontinence, confusion, behavior change, lethargy, anorexia, or "just not feeling right"

C. Nursing assessment

1. Assessment

   a. Subjective data: duration of symptoms, history of kidney stones, previous urinary, kidney or prostate problems, history of diabetes or hypertension; inquire about last menstrual period (LMP), pregnancy and birth control methods; question the client regarding allergies, medications, and recent antibiotic use; review diet such as increased caffeine, carbonated drinks, and water intake; pain and tenderness (see Box 10-1)

   b. Objective data: vital signs, observe urine (color, consistency, odor), associated symptoms

2. Diagnostic tests

   a. Dipstick urinalysis is usually adequate for the diagnosis and management of isolated acute UTI

   b. A culture and sensitivity (C&S) of the urine should be performed if the UTI is thought to be complicated, caused by recent instrumentation, antibiotic sensitivities, or previous treatment failures

   c. Urinalysis (UA) may show the presence of blood cells or bacteria in the urine; bacteria counts of 100 to 100,000 (normal is negative) are indicative of infection; the urinalysis often shows many red blood cells (RBCs) and may show casts

D. Nursing management

1. Medications

   a. Short term (3- to 5-day) antibiotic therapy for uncomplicated UTI; first-line therapy is trimethoprim-sulfamethoxazole (Bactrim) and nitrofurantoin (Macrobid); alternate first-line therapy includes amoxicillin (Amoxil) and cephalexin (Keflex)

   b. Second-line quinolones are more expensive and can promote resistant strains of bacteria

   c. Phenazopyridine hydrochloride (Pyridium) may be prescribed for comfort measures; clients should be warned that this drug can stain semen or urine orange

2. Instruct to take antibiotics at nighttime if possible as the drug will remain in the bladder longer

3. Instruct to increase fluid intake unless contraindicated

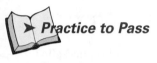

Practice to Pass

A client tells the nurse that she has had frequency and burning on urination. What assessment should the nurse make? What instructions should the nurse give her?

NCLEX!

NCLEX!

Box 10-1		
Common Signs and Symptoms of Urinary Tract Infection	Dysuria	Urinary frequency
	Pyuria	Hematuria
	Nocturia	Suprapubic tenderness

4. Assess pain levels and note any change, which may indicate additional disease processes

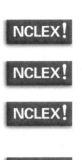

5. Teach the client to avoid caffeinated drinks and alcoholic beverages that can increase bladder spasms and mucosal irritation

6. Teach preventive measures such as emptying the bladder every 2 to 4 hours while awake and maintain fluid intake of 8 to 10 glasses of fluid per day

7. Teach women to cleanse the perineal area front to back, void before and after intercourse, avoid bubble baths, feminine hygiene sprays, douching, and to wear cotton briefs

8. Unless contraindicated, teach the client measures to maintain acidic urine (pH = 5 or less) such as drinking cranberry juice or taking vitamin C daily; avoid excess intake of milk products, fruit juices, and sodium bicarbonate; acidity of the urine inhibits bacterial growth

9. Stress importance of taking all the prescribed medication and keeping follow-up appointments

III. Urinary Calculi

A. Overview

1. **Calculi** are defined as masses of crystals composed of minerals that are normally excreted in the urine; the majority are composed of calcium; other calculi may be made up of magnesium ammonium phosphate, uric acid or cystine

2. Stones may develop and cause obstruction at any point in the urinary system

3. Is termed **urolithiasis** (stones in the urinary tract) or **nephrolithiasis** (stones formed within the kidney)

4. Causes include dehydration, immobility, excess dietary intake of calcium, oxalate, or protein

B. Pathophysiology

1. Urolithiasis involves the precipitation of a poorly soluble salt around a mucoprotein to form a crystalline structure; when the concentration of salt in the urine is high, crystallization or precipitation is minimal

2. Ingesting an increased amount of the involved mineral or decreasing in fluid intake such as during the night, allows an increased concentration where precipitation occurs and stones are formed; when fluid intake is adequate, no stone growth occurs

3. Stone formation is also affected by acidity or alkalinity of the urine and presence/absence of calculus-inhibiting compounds such as pyrophosphate and nephrocalcin in the urine

4. The majority of kidney stones are composed of calcium oxalate or calcium phosphate, which are associated with increased calcium levels in the blood or urine

5. Signs and symptoms vary with their location and size

   a. Renal calculi may be associated with a dull, aching flank pain

   b. Bladder calculi may cause a dull, suprapubic pain

    c. Renal colic causes an acute, severe, intermittent pain of the flank and upper outer abdomen on the affected side; pain may radiate to the suprapubic region, groin and external genitalia; renal colic may be associated with nausea and vomiting, pallor and cool, clammy skin

C. Nursing assessment

    1. Assessment includes symptom analysis, pain (severity, quality, onset, duration, location, and intensity); urinalysis for presence of blood, protein or leukocytes; previous history of stones and treatments and family history of calculi; review dietary intake, milk, calcium-rich foods, and antacids; question the client about hematuria, recent injury or trauma; assess vital signs; inspect, palpate, and auscultate the abdomen and inspect the external genitalia; and assess for vaginal discharge and pelvic pain

    2. Diagnostic tests

        a. Urinalysis is useful in the diagnosis; gross or microscopic hematuria is generally present

        b. Other diagnostic tests may be necessary including urine calcium, uric acid studies, urine oxalate, culture and sensitivity, serum calcium, and phosphorus

        c. Radiographic studies include kidney, ureter, and bladder (KUB), intravenous pyelography (IVP), ultrasound, CT scan and cystoscopy

D. Nursing management

    1. Medications include pain medications as ordered and needed; antiemetics to control nausea

    2. Increase fluid intake to increase urinary output facilitating movement of the stone

    3. Monitor urinary output and strain urine for stones; document the presence of hematuria

    4. Maintain patency and functioning of catheter system if in place

    5. Teach client regarding all diagnostic tests and interventions, such as lithotripsy; and to strain urine, saving all stones for analysis

    6. Maintain frequent telephone contact with client until stone passes if discharged

    7. Instruct client on preventive measures: fluid intake 2,500 to 3,000 mL/day, dietary modifications (low purine, limiting vitamin D and calcium [see Table 10-1]), promote activity level to prevent urinary stasis and to take all medications as prescribed

    8. Teach the client that the presence of a stone increases the risk for developing urinary tract infections; teach the client signs and symptoms of infection and preventive measures

IV. Polycystic Kidney Disease

A. Overview

    1. **Polycystic kidney disease** is defined as a hereditary disease (genetic predisposition) characterized by cyst formation and massive kidney enlargement

---

NCLEX!

NCLEX!

NCLEX!

NCLEX!

Practice to Pass

What self-management instructions should be given to the client with urolithiasis?

NCLEX!

Food Group	Samples of Foods
Acidic	Cheese, cranberries, eggs, grapes, plums, prunes
Alkaline	Green vegetables, fruit except those listed above, legumes, milk products
High calcium	Beans, chocolate, dried fruits, canned fish except tuna, milk products
High purine	Organ meats, sardines, venison, chicken, crab, pork, salmon, veal
High oxalate	Asparagus, beer, colas, celery, cabbage, green beans, nuts, tea, tomatoes

Table 10-1

Foods to Avoid with Urolithiasis

Adapted from: Lemone, P. & Burke, K. (2000). *Medical surgical nursing: Critical thinking in client care* (2nd ed.). Upper Saddle River, NJ: Prentice Hall, p. 914.

2. There are two forms: autosomal dominant (affects adults) and autosomal recessive (typically affects children)

3. Genetics is the primary cause

B. Pathophysiology

1. Adult polycystic kidney disease is a slow, progressive disease that is relatively common, accounting for 10 percent of clients with end-stage renal disease who require dialysis and/or kidney transplant; those individuals with polycystic kidney disease often develop cysts elsewhere in the body including the liver, spleen, and pancreas

2. Of the affected people, 9 to 10 percent experience subarachnoid brain hemorrhage from a congenital aneurysm; there is also an increased incidence of incompetent cardiac valves in clients with polycystic kidney disease

3. Renal cysts are fluid-filled sacs affecting the nephron of the kidney, which may vary in size; as the cysts fill and enlarge, the kidneys will enlarge; renal blood vessels and nephrons become obstructed and functional tissue is destroyed

4. Signs and symptoms include flank pain, hematuria, proteinuria, polyuria, and nocturia; urinary tract infection and calculi are common as the cysts interfere with urine drainage; most clients develop hypertension due to obstruction of the blood vessels; the kidneys become palpable, enlarged, and knobby as fluid-filled cysts replace the functional tissue

C. Nursing assessment

1. Assessment includes presence, location, and duration of symptoms; fluid intake; vital signs; urination practices; polyuria and nocturia; family history and/or previous history of kidney disease and hypertension; review present and past medications and allergies; assess pain levels and intensity

2. Diagnostic tests: renal ultrasonography, IVP, CT scan of kidney, UA

D. Nursing management

1. Medications include angiotensin-converting enzyme (ACE) Inhibitors to control hypertension

2. Instruct and teach the client about diagnostic testing

3. Instruct the client on signs and symptoms of urinary tract infections and obstruction to avoid further damage to the kidney

NCLEX!

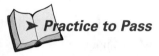

Practice to Pass

A client has just been diagnosed with polycystic kidney disease. How should the nurse explain this disorder to the client?

4. Fluid intake of 2,000 to 2,500 cc/day is encouraged as a preventive measure

5. Stress importance of monitoring blood pressure to identify hypertension for pharmacological intervention

6. Instruct the client to avoid medications that may be nephrotoxic and to check with a healthcare provider before taking any over-the-counter medications

7. Discuss genetics and optional screening of family members especially if renal transplantation is contemplated

V. Pyelonephritis

A. Overview

1. **Pyelonephritis** is defined as an inflammatory disorder affecting the renal pelvis and the functional portion of the kidney tissue

2. Classification

   a. *Acute pyelonephritis,* a bacterial infection of the kidney

   b. *Chronic pyelonephritis,* associated with nonbacterial infections and processes that may be metabolic, chemical or immunological

3. Causes include an ascending bladder infection, blood-borne infections, frequent calculi or other obstructions

B. Pathophysiology

1. The ascending route from the lower urinary tract is the most common pathway; the infection develops in patchy areas spreading to the cortex with WBC infiltration and inflammation

2. The kidney becomes grossly edematous and localized abscesses may form; tissue damage may occur primarily of the tubules; scar tissue replaces the infected/inflamed areas

3. *E. coli* is responsible in 85 percent of the cases; other common pathogens are *proteus* and *klebsiella*

4. The onset of pyelonephritis is typically rapid with chills and fever, malaise, and vomiting along with flank pain, costovertebral tenderness, urinary frequency, and dysuria

5. As with urinary tract infections, older clients may present with behavior changes, confusion, incontinence, or general deterioration

6. Chronic renal failure and end-stage renal disease may develop with chronic pyelonephritis; hypertension may develop as the renal tissue is destroyed

C. Nursing assessment

1. Assessment includes reviewing the onset and duration of symptoms and any associating symptoms including pain (description, severity, frequency); rule out pregnancy; review previous history of urinary tract problems, treatments and testing; review present medications and allergies; vital signs; inspect respiratory and cardiac status; hydration status; inspect external genitalia and abdomen for tenderness, masses, or pain; evaluate urinalysis (preferably by a midstream specimen); intake and output, urinary frequency, urgency, and nocturia; assess urine for blood, odor, and appearance; question the client about family history of kidney disease, infections, diabetes, and hypertension

2. Diagnostic tests: UA (midstream, clean-catch), gram stain of urine, urine C & S, WBC, IVP, voiding cystourethrography (contrast medium into bladder), cystoscopy (direct visualization of urethra and bladder), pelvic/prostrate exam

D. Nursing management

1. Medications

   a. Analgesics

   b. 7 to 10 days of oral antimicrobial therapy: sulfonamides, trimethoprim-sulfamethoxazole (TMP-SMZ, Bactrim, Septra), ciprofloxacin hydrochloride (Cipro)

   c. Urinary anti-infectives: methanamine (Hiprex), nalidixic acid (Neg Gram), nitrofurantoin (Macrodantin)

   d. Urinary analgesics: phenazopyridine (Pyridium)

2. Provide alleviation of pain by medication and nonpharmalogic measures such as heating pads or warm baths, rest, and balanced activity

3. Unless contraindicated, increase fluid intake to 8 to 10 glasses/day to dilute urine, lessening the irritation of the mucosa

4. Teach preventive measures of urinary tract infection such as emptying the bladder every 2 to 4 hours and increased fluids; for women, proper perineal hygiene, voiding before and after intercourse, avoiding bubble baths and douching

5. Teach the client on obtaining a midstream clean-catch specimen

6. Teach to maintain acidic urine (inhibits bacterial growth) by drinking cranberry juice, taking vitamin C, avoiding excess milk products, and avoiding sodium bicarbonate

7. Instruct to complete full course of prescribed medications even if symptoms have resolved

8. Instruct to keep follow-up appointments as scheduled

9. Referral to an urologist may be necessary

10. Teach about common side effects of antibiotics: nausea and superinfections (candidiasis); also teach about others specific to that medication

VI. Glomerulonephritis

A. Overview

1. **Glomerulonephritis** is defined as an inflammation of the capillary loops of the glomeruli

2. It is classified as acute, rapidly progressive, or chronic glomerulonephritis

3. Acute poststreptococcal glomerulonephritis is the most common form

4. Rapidly progressive glomerulonephritis may either be *idiopathic* or *secondary* to an acute infection or a multisystem disease with a greater incidence in males than females

5. Chronic glomerulonephritis is the end stage of glomerular disorders

6. Causes

    a. Acute: systemic diseases such as systemic lupus erythematosus (SLE) or primary glomerular disease, but a *beta hemolytic strep* infection of the pharynx or skin is the most common precipitating factor; *staphylococcal* or viral infections can also lead to post-infectious acute glomerulonephritis

    b. Rapidly progressive: unknown, vasculitis, systemic lupus erythematosus, acute glomerulonephritis

    c. Chronic: unknown, lupus nephritis, diabetic nephropathy, rapid, progressive glomerulonephritis

B. Pathophysiology

1. In *acute* glomerulonephritis, circulating antigen-antibody immune complexes are formed and trapped in the glomerular membrane; these cause an inflammatory response activating the complement system and releasing vasoactive substances and inflammatory mediators; edema and inflammation increase the porosity of the glomerular capillaries allowing plasma proteins and blood cells to escape into the urine; the renin-angiotensin-aldosterone (RAA) system is disrupted, which could lead to hypertension

    a. Symptoms usually subside in 10 to 14 days and 60 percent completely recover

    b. The remaining 40 percent may have persistent impaired renal function, continued proteinuria and/or hematuria leading to chronic glomerulonephritis or renal failure

2. In *rapidly progressive* glomerulonephritis, the glomerular cells proliferate along with macrophages forming crescent-shaped lesions that obstruct Bowman's space

    a. More than 70 percent of the glomeruli is affected with a rapid decrease in the glomerular filtration rate (GFR)

    b. Up to 50 percent of clients will require maintenance dialysis and/or kidney transplant

3. *Chronic* glomerulonephritis involves the slow, progressive destruction of the glomeruli with impaired renal function; the kidneys decrease in size symmetrically and become granular or roughened; eventually, all nephrons are destroyed

4. Signs and symptoms (see Figure 10-1)

    a. Acute: hematuria-brown tinged, proteinuria, salt and water retention, red blood cell casts, hypertension, **azotemia**, fatigue, anorexia, nausea and vomiting, and headache

    b. Rapidly progressive: weakness, nausea and vomiting, flu-like symptoms, oliguria, abdominal or flank pain

    c. Chronic: develop insidiously and are often unrecognized until renal failure is evident

C. Nursing assessment

1. Assessment includes vital signs, remembering that increased fluid volume increases cardiac workload; weight and presence of edema; intake and output (I

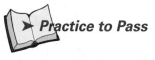

Practice to Pass

A client recovering from Hepatitis B begins to exhibit signs and symptoms of rapid, progressive glomerulonephritis. What is the significance of this disease on the GFR?

NCLEX!

NCLEX!

NCLEX!

Figure 10-1

Critical pathway of glomerulonephritis.

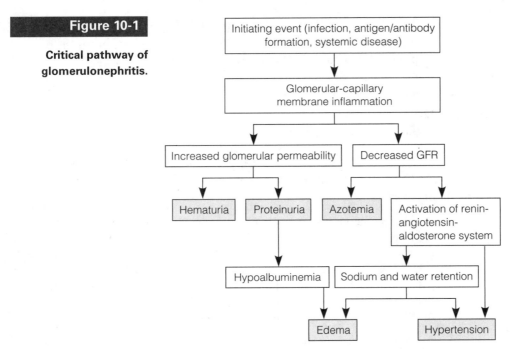

& O); assess energy, activity and fatigue status; signs and symptoms of infections including the skin, throat, and lungs; client's knowledge of the disease, coping abilities, support system, lifestyle changes and need for additional interventions or support

2. Diagnostic tests: throat or skin cultures, antistreptolysin (ASO) titer, sedimentation rate, antinuclear antibody (ANA), blood urea nitrogen (BUN), creatinine, electrolytes, urinalysis, creatinine clearance; x-ray studies including abdominal x-rays, kidney scan, and biopsy

D. Nursing management

1. Medications (treating symptoms since no cure exists)

   a. Immunosuppressive therapy (to decrease risk of end-stage renal disease): cyclophosphamide (Cytoxan), azathioprine (Imuran), chlorambucil (Leukeran)

   b. Glucocorticoids (to decrease remission of nephrotic syndrome): prednisone—these may worsen certain types of glomerulonephritis, such as post-streptococcal

   c. ACE inhibitors and nonsteroidal anti-inflammatroy drugs (NSAIDs) that decrease protein loss

   d. Antibiotics: penicillin

   e. Antihypertensives

2. Educate the client and family regarding the disease process

3. Instruct the client on prescribed medications and side effects of immunosuppressive or steroid therapy

4. Instruct the client and family regarding activity level and dietary restrictions; arrange for a dietary consultation if necessary

5. Teach about the signs and symptoms of improving or declining renal function

6. Instruct on the signs and symptoms of infectious processes

7. Instruct the client to weigh daily and report weight gains to the provider

8. Instruct on fluid restriction if ordered and importance of measuring intake and output

9. Monitor IV fluids and monitor diuretic effect

10. Assess catheter system if indicated

11. Assist with problem solving and support services as needed

VII. Acute Renal Failure

A. Overview

1. **Acute renal failure (ARF)** is defined as a rapid decrease in renal function

2. Acute renal failure is generally recognized by a fall of urinary output and increase in BUN and/or creatinine; oliguria is common but high output failure is possible

3. The most common cause of acute renal failure is ischemia and nephrotoxins; a fall in blood pressure or volume can cause ischemia of the kidney tissue; the exposure of renal tissue is great when nephrotoxins are present in the blood (see Figure 10-2)

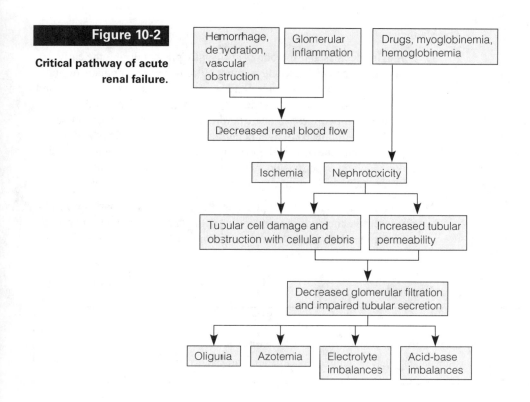

Figure 10-2

Critical pathway of acute renal failure.

NCLEX!

4. ARF may be caused by iatrogenic causes such as nephrotoxic medications, radiologic contrast dye, and surgical shock

5. Causes are categorized into prerenal, intrarenal and postrenal factors (see Box 10-2)

B. Pathophysiology

1. Ischemia is the primary cause of acute renal failure; if allowed to continue longer than 2 hours, ischemia leads to severe and irreversible damage to the tubules with patchy necrosis; GFR is decreased due to ischemia; activation of renin-angiotensin system occurs and tubular obstruction is caused by debris

2. Nephrotoxins destroy tubular cells allowing for the increased permeability caused by necrosis and sloughing; the nephron then has decreased ability to eliminate waste

3. Acute renal failure follows three phases: initiation, maintenance, and recovery

   a. *Initiation phase:* begins with the onset of the event causing tubular necrosis; this phase ends when tubular injury occurs

   b. *Maintenance phase:* begins within hours of the initiation phase and typically lasts 1 to 2 weeks; it is characterized by persistent reduction in GFR and tubular necrosis

   c. *Recovery phase:* begins when the GFR and tubular function have recovered and there is no further elevation of the BUN and creatinine; renal function improves rapidly the first 5 to 25 days and continues up to 1 year

4. Signs and symptoms

   a. Initiation: has few manifestations and often is identified after later manifestations have occurred

   b. Maintenance:

NCLEX!

   1) **Oliguria** (decreased urine output) is usually present during the early maintenance phase; the kidney cannot eliminate waste products during this phase leading to azotemia, fluid retention, electrolyte imbalance and metabolic acidosis; salt and water retention leads to edema and increased risk for congestive heart failure and pulmonary edema; impaired renal elimination leads to hyperkalemia, hyperphosphatemia, and hypocalcemia; infection is the leading cause of death but other complications include hypertension, neurologic symptoms, gastrointestinal manifestations and **uremia,** syndrome of renal failure (see Table 10-2)

NCLEX!

   2) The end of the maintenance phase in oliguric clients is characterized by a progressive increase in urine volume; the damaged tubules are repaired; diuresis indicates the nephrons are sufficiently recovered

---

Box 10-2

Categories of Acute Renal Failure

Prerenal: hypovolemia and cardiovascular failure

Intrarenal: vascular disease, glomerulonephritis, nephritis, and tubular necrosis

Postrenal: extrarenal obstruction, intrarenal obstruction, and bladder rupture

Table 10-2	System	Symptoms
The Multisystem Effects of Uremia	Respiratory	Pulmonary edema, pleuritis, respiratory distress
	Urinary	Hematuria, proteinuria, oliguria, nocturia
	Gastrointestinal	Anorexia, nausea, vomiting, abdominal pain, GI bleeding, uremic fetor
	Endocrine	Hyperparathyroidism, intolerance to glucose
	Musculoskeletal	Bone pain, fractures
	Neurologic	Apathy, lethargy, headache, impaired cognition, insomnia, paresthesias, decreased level of consciousness
	Cardiovascular	Elevated blood pressure, dysrhythmias, congestive heart failure
	Hematologic	Anemia, difficulty clotting
	Reproductive	Females experience amenorrhea, males experience impotence
	Integumentary	Pallor, uremic frost, dry skin, pruritis, ecchymosis

C. Nursing assessment

1. Assessment includes weight; vital signs (watch for orthostatic hypotension due to the diuretics); hydration status; intake and output; identify any underlying causes; assess client's knowledge of disease process, coping methods and needs; pain status and effect of medications; question the client regarding signs and symptoms of illness as well as past medical history, present and past medications, and family history of kidney disease; common signs and symptoms of renal failure include:

   a. Skin: yellow skin, edema, ecchymosis, uremic frost

   b. ENT: urinous breath

   c. Pulmonary: crackles, effusion, tachypnea

   d. Cardiovascular: hypertension, S_3 or S_4, dysrhythmia

   e. Gastrointestinal: GI bleeding

   f. Neurologic: change in level of consciousness (LOC)

   g. Neuromuscular: tremors, hyperreflexia

NCLEX!

2. Diagnostic tests: electrolytes (hyperkalemia, hyponatremia, hyperphosphatemia), BUN (elevated) and creatinine (elevated), ABGs (metabolic acidosis), CBC (anemia), UA (fixed specific gravity, protein, casts), bladder catheterization, renal ultrasonography, tomography, IVP, renal biopsy

NCLEX!

3. Creatinine is more accurate than BUN because it is not affected by proteins in the diet or fluid status; the BUN to creatinine ratio should be 10:1; the creatinine does not increase unless one-quarter of nephrons are not functioning

D. Nursing management

1. Medications

   a. Blood volume expanders: dopamine (Intropin)

   b. Diuretics: furosemide (Lasix) or mannitol (Osmitrol)

   c. Antihypertensives if necessary: ACE inhibitors

   d. Antacids and H_2-receptor antagonists to prevent GI ulcer

    e. Potassium-binding exchange resin: polystyrene sulfonate (Kayexelate)

    f. Specific antacid: calcium carbonate (Tums) to control hyperphosphatemia

NCLEX!

2. Weigh client at the same time daily to document fluid volume status; restrict fluids as ordered

3. Treat infections as soon as possible

4. Record vital signs and monitor for development of congestive heart failure or pulmonary edema; semi-Fowler's position enhances cardiac and respiratory function

5. Monitor lab values

6. Monitor skin status since edema can decrease tissue perfusion and increase the risk for skin breakdown

NCLEX!

7. Administer medications cautiously as ordered and document effectiveness; avoid any medications that are nephrotoxic

NCLEX!

8. Document food intake and arrange for a dietary consultation to incorporate requirements (low protein, high carbohydrate [CHO]), restrictions, and client's preferences

9. Explain and answer questions regarding the disease process and concerns

10. Teach client to monitor weight, blood pressure, and pulse to assess fluid status

11. Educate on medications that are nephrotoxic such as NSAIDs, some antibiotics, x-ray contrast and heavy metals; instruct to avoid magnesium-containing antacids; explain that alcohol ingestion may increase nephrotoxic effects of medications

12. Stress importance of follow-up visits, urinalysis, and bloodwork

VIII. Chronic Renal Failure

A. Overview

1. **Chronic renal failure (CRF)** is defined as the progressive inability, over months to years, of the kidneys to respond to changes in body fluids and electrolyte composition with an inability of the kidneys to produce sufficient urine; GFR is less than 20 percent of normal and serum creatinine is greater than 5 mg/dL

2. There are three stages of renal failure (see Box 10-3)

    a. *Early stage* (renal impairment): unaffected nephrons compensate for the lost nephrons

    b. *Second stage* (renal insufficiency): more than 75 percent of functional renal tissue is destroyed

Box 10-3

Stages of Chronic Renal Failure

Early stage: renal impairment (BUN 20–50 mg/dL)

Second stage: renal insufficiency (BUN > 100 mg/dL; Cr > 4 mg/dL)

Third stage: end-stage renal disease (BUN > 200 mg/dL; Cr > 5 mg dL)

   c. *Third stage* (end-stage renal disease [ESRD]): GFR is less than 20 percent

   3. Ideally, conservative treatment is used; educate the client and family and explore options for long-term management; when conservative treatment is no longer effective, dialysis or renal transplantation is considered

   4. The most common causes of chronic renal failure are diabetic nephropathy, hypertension, glomerulonephritis, cystic kidney disease, and urologic disease

B. Pathophysiology

   1. The pathophysiologic process of chronic renal failure appears as a gradual loss of entire nephron units

   2. The functional capacity of the entire nephron is lost and renal mass is reduced, leading to progressive deterioration of glomerular filtration, tubular secretion and reabsorption; eventually, the kidneys are unable to excrete metabolic waste and regulate fluid and electrolyte balance

   3. Signs and symptoms include (see Table 10-2)

   a. Early stage: clients remain free of symptoms and BUN and creatinine are normal

   b. Second stage: there is a slight rise in BUN and creatinine; few symptoms may be present including oliguria or polyuria

   c. Third stage: there is a sharp increase in BUN (200 mg/dL) and creatinine; symptoms of oliguria and uremia are present; there is usually multisystem effects of chronic renal failure

C. Nursing assessment

   1. Assessment includes vital signs, I & O, edema, daily weight, measurement of abdominal girth daily; fluid and dietary restrictions; client's knowledge of disease and support system; knowledge of treatment options; activity level and fatigibility; medication effect and any side effects; and question client regarding end-of-life care

   2. Diagnostic tests: BUN (elevated), creatinine (elevated), electrolytes (hyponatremia [may be normal], hyperkalemia, hyperphosphatemia, hypocalcemia), CBC (severe anemia and thrombocytopenia), UA (fixed specific gravity, proteins, blood cells, casts), urine C & S, creatinine clearance (decreased), ABGs (metabolic acidosis), renal ultrasonography, and kidney biopsy

D. Nursing management

   1. Medications

   a. Diuretics: usually loop diuretics

   b. Antihypertensives: ACE inhibitors: minoxidil (Loniten), clonidine (Catapress)

   c. Sodium bicarbonate, calcium carbonate (Tums), phosphate-binding agents, calcium supplements, vitamin D

   d. Iron and folic acid supplements; epoitin alfa (Epogen) for anemia

   e. Potassium-binding exchange resin: polystyrene sulfonate (Kayexelate)

   2. Maintain fluid and dietary restrictions; refer for dietary consultation if necessary; limit Na and protein, high CHO

NCLEX!

Practice to Pass

A client with CRF asks why he cannot have a drink with his meal tray and why proteins are limited. How should the nurse respond?

3. Administer and document effects/side effects of medications; meds should be administered cautiously; phosphate-binding agents should be avoided

4. Monitor lab values

5. Use universal precautions and good handwashing at all times to decrease transfer of organisms to the client

6. Provide oral hygiene at least every 4 hours

7. Monitor activity level and fatigibility

8. Arrange mealtime and activities per client preferences and procedures

9. Encourage expression of feelings or concerns and assist the client in development of realistic goals and coping strategies; refer to mental health counselor if necessary

10. Whether client has arteriovenous fistula or peritoneal dialysis, assess site for signs and symptoms of infection, check tubing for kinks

IX. Bladder Cancer

A. Overview

1. Defined as a tumor of the bladder; the majority of tumors affecting the urinary tract arise from epithelial tissue and the most common site for tumor formation is the urinary bladder

2. Bladder cancer is the 5th most common malignancy and the 10th leading cause of cancer deaths

3. Causes include cigarette smoke, exposure to chemicals and dyes, chronic use of phenacetin-containing analgesic agents

B. Pathophysiology

1. Two major factors are implicated in the development of bladder cancer: presence of carcinogens in the urine and chronic inflammation or infection of bladder mucosa

2. Urinary tract tumors begin as nonspecific cellular alterations that develop either as flat or papillary lesions which may be invasive or superficial; papillary lesions are characterized by a polyplike structure attached by a stalk to the bladder mucosa; papillomas are superficial non-invasive tumors and frequently recur; carcinoma in situ is a poorly differentiated flat tumor that invades directly and has a poor prognosis

NCLEX!

3. Signs and symptoms include painless hematuria (most common), which is gross or microscopic, constant or intermittent; symptoms of UTI, and colicky pain

C. Nursing assessment

1. Assessment includes urinary pattern, history of hematuria, pain

   a. Preoperative assessment: assess the client's coping mechanisms and concerns; urinary output and change in color; fluid intake to keep urine dilute; activity level; urinary catheters, tubing and drainage system for patency and obstruction; signs and symptoms of infection

    b. Postoperative assessment: intake and output; color and consistency of urine (bright red blood may indicate hemorrhage); stoma and surrounding skin (with cystectomy); and pain level

  2. Diagnostic tests: UA, urine cytology, IVP, renal ultrasound, CT scan, cystoscopy, and ureteroscopy

D. Nursing management

  1. Medications and treatment

    a. Chemotherapy agents may be used either as primary treatment or prophylactically to prevent recurrence; doxorubicin (Adriamycin), mitomycin C (Mutamycin), calmette guerin (BCG Live)

    b. Radiation can reduce tumor size prior to surgery

    c. Surgical procedures range from simple resection to removal of the bladder

  2. Teach client regarding disease process, interventions and postoperative care

  3. Monitor intake and output carefully, notify healthcare professional if output < 30 cc/hr; irrigate catheter as ordered

  4. Monitor lab values, electrolyte and renal function tests

  5. Encourage fluid intake to 3,000 cc/day to dilute urine and decrease irritation

  6. Teach the family and client about stomal care and catheter care

  7. Discuss family/client concerns about activity, sexual relations, and employment; initiate support group or counseling if necessary

  8. Teach the client/family regarding signs and symptoms of infection and preventive measures

X. Kidney Cancer

A. Overview

  1. Defined as a tumor of the kidney; renal cell cancer is the most common primary tumor; another primary tumor is a tumor of the renal pelvis; these tumors arise in the epithelium of the proximal convoluted tubules

  2. Causes include metastasis from lung and breast cancer, melanoma and malignant lymphoma

B. Pathophysiology

  1. Renal cell tumors metastasize most commonly to the lungs, mediastinum, bone, lymph nodes, liver, and central nervous system

  2. The tumor may produce hormones or hormone-like substances including parathyroid hormones, prostaglandins, prolactin, renin, gonadotropins and glucocorticoids

  3. The classic triad of symptoms (gross hematuria, flank pain, and a palpable abdominal mass) are seen in only 10 percent of the people with renal cell cancer

  4. Signs and symptoms include microscopic or gross hematuria, flank pain, palpable abdominal mass, fever, fatigue, weight loss, and anemia and/or polycythemia

C. Nursing assessment

1. Assessment includes pain (level, location, intensity and character); client's knowledge and understanding of the disease and procedures to be performed; lab values; vital signs; urinary output; fluid intake (oral and intravenous); activity level and fatigue

2. Postoperative assessment includes incision site for signs/symptoms of inflammation or infection; drainage catheters and tubes for patency; respiratory status and GI function to prevent major complications; potential complications of surgery such as paralytic ileus, thrombosis, and embolus

3. Diagnostic tests: renal ultrasound (first diagnostic evidence of a kidney tumor); CT scans (provide information about the tumor density, extension of the tumor and regional lymph node or vascular involvement); chest x-ray, bone scan, and liver function studies are done prior to intervention to evaluate potential metastasis of the disease

D. Nursing management

1. Medications and treatment

   a. Chemotherapy: immunotherapy such as interferon alpha (Roferon-A)

   b. Radiation therapy

   c. Radical nephrectomy (usual treatment)

2. Instruct on signs and symptoms of infection

3. Teach the client to maintain fluid intake 2,000 to 2,500 cc/day and increase during hot weather or exercise

4. Instruct client to void when urge is experienced, and before and after intercourse

5. Teach client to avoid trauma to remaining kidney

6. Continue to encourage the family and client to discuss feelings and concerns

7. Instruct on home medications, wound care, diet, and activity

8. Refer to support services if appropriate

9. Stress importance of follow-up visits and scheduled bloodwork; instruct to report decreased urine output, fever, or abdominal pain

Case Study

L. J. is a 45-year-old construction worker who experienced a large MI with cardiovascular complications. On day 3 of his hospital stay, the nurse notices his urinary output is being maintained at 20 to 25 cc/hr. Another symptom is edema. His potassium (K) is 5.2 mg/L, sodium (Na) is 125 mEq/L, ABGs (pH—7.25, PCO_2—38, HCO_3—21), BUN is 28, Cr is 2.5 mg/dL, lung sounds—soft rales. He is diagnosed with acute renal failure (ARF).

❶ What do L. J.'s ABGs show and is this common with ARF? Why or why not?

❷ What is significant about his electrolytes in relation to his cardiac condition?

❸ What phase of ARF is L.J. in, and what can the nurse tell him is the expected time frame until the kidneys are hopefully working properly again?

❹ Considering his initial diagnosis, presenting signs and symptoms, and the known complications of ARF, what is the greatest cardiovascular concern for L. J.?

❺ Should L. J. be given a low-sodium or high-sodium diet? Why or why not?

For suggested responses, see page 568.

Posttest

1   A urinalysis is ordered for a client with urinary calculi. Which of the following is usually positive on the urinalysis report?

(1) Leukocytes
(2) Nitrite
(3) Protein
(4) Blood

2   A 40-year-old male is at high risk for which of the following, if his dad also had the problem?

(1) Glomerulonephritis
(2) Renal failure
(3) Polycystic kidney disease
(4) Urinary tract infection

3   The client has a urinalysis return showing a high white blood count. Further tests pinpoint the origin in the kidney. The client most likely has:

(1) Acute pyelonephritis.
(2) Renal failure.
(3) Chronic pyelonephritis.
(4) Calculi.

4   It is important to teach clients with chronic pyelonephritis to monitor:

(1) Blood pressure.
(2) Temperature.
(3) Diet.
(4) Stress level.

5   Acute glomerulonephritis is usually caused by which pathogen?

(1) *Group A beta hemolytic streptococcus*
(2) *Staphylococcus*
(3) *E. coli*
(4) *Proteus*

6 Which of the following clients is at highest risk for a urinary tract infection (UTI)?

(1) An elderly client
(2) A male adult
(3) A teenager
(4) A child

7 In rapidly progressive glomerulonephritis, crescent-shaped lesions form and obliterate the:

(1) Bowman's space.
(2) Urinary bladder.
(3) Renal tubules.
(4) Loop of Henle.

8 Sally is diagnosed with an uncomplicated urinary tract infection. The first-line therapy is:

(1) Ciprofloxacin (Cipro).
(2) Trimethoprim-sulfamethoxazole (Bactrim).
(3) Amoxicillin (Amoxil).
(4) Erythromycin (Erythrocin).

9 Which vitamin should the nuse recommend to a client to maintain acidic urine and help with recurrent urinary tract infections?

(1) E
(2) B
(3) C
(4) D

10 Nursing management of the client with a urinary tract infection should include:

(1) Taking medication until feeling better.
(2) Restricting fluids.
(3) Decreasing caffeine drinks and alcohol.
(4) Douching daily.

See pages 337–338 for Answers and Rationales.

Answers and Rationales

Pretest

1 **Answer: 2** *Rationale:* Pyelonephritis is an upper urinary tract infection, involving the kidney tissue. Lower urinary tract infections include urethritis, prostatitis, and cystitis. The most common upper urinary tract infection is pyelonephritis.
Cognitive Level: Knowledge
Nursing Process: Analysis; *Test Plan:* PHYS

2 **Answer: 3** *Rationale:* *E. coli* is the infective organism in over 90 percent of first-time infections. The nurse should check that the organism is sensitive to the antibiotic or notify the healthcare professional.
Cognitive Level: Knowledge
Nursing Process: Analysis; *Test Plan:* PHYS

3 **Answer: 4** *Rationale:* Due to the anatomic structure of the male urethra and bacteriostatic effect of prostatic fluid, all urinary tract infections in the male client should be considered complicated.
Cognitive Level: Application
Nursing Process: Assessment; *Test Plan:* PHYS

4 **Answer: 3** *Rationale:* Urine may have a foul odor and appear cloudy because of mucus and excess white cells present, which is common in cystitis. Casts and proteins are never normal in urine.
Cognitive Level: Knowledge
Nursing Process: Assessment; *Test Plan:* PHYS

5 **Answer: 2** *Rationale:* The greatest risk factor for stone formation is a prior personal or family history of urinary calculi. The other options are important information to know but do not contribute greatly as risk factors.
Cognitive Level: Application
Nursing Process: Assessment; *Test Plan:* PHYS

6 **Answer: 4** *Rationale:* Red blood cell casts are not present in the normal urinalysis but are present in glomerular diseases.
Cognitive Level: Application
Nursing Process: Analysis; *Test Plan:* PHYS

7 **Answer: 3** *Rationale:* Iatrogenic causes result from treatment from a physician or other care

provider. Examples include nephrotoxic medications, radiologic contrast dye, and shock after surgery.
Cognitive Level: Knowledge
Nursing Process: Analysis; *Test Plan:* PHYS

8   **Answer: 3** *Rationale:* In end stage renal failure, 90 percent or more of the nephrons are destroyed. Glomerular filtration rate is < 20 percent normal with increased creatinine and BUN.
Cognitive Level: Knowledge
Nursing Process: Analysis; *Test Plan:* PHYS

9   **Answer: 2** *Rationale:* The blood urea nitrogen is primarily used as an indicator of kidney function because most renal diseases interfere with its excretion and cause blood levels to rise. Creatinine is produced in relatively constant amounts, according to the amount of muscle mass and is excreted entirely by the kidneys making t a good indicator of renal function.
Cognitive Level: Knowledge
Nursing Process: Assessment; *Test Plan:* PHYS

10   **Answer: 4** *Rationale:* In the second stage of chronic renal failure, renal insufficiency, there is at least 75 percent of functional renal parenchyma destroyed.
Cognitive Level: Knowledge
Nursing Process: Assessment. *Test Plan:* PHYS

Posttest

1   **Answer: 4** *Rationale:* Hematuria, either gross or microscopic, is generally present in clients with urinary calculi. Leukocytes and protein may be common with other urinary disorders.
Cognitive Level: Knowledge
Nursing Process: Assessment; *Test Plan:* PHYS

2   **Answer: 3** *Rationale:* Adult polycystic kidney disease is an autosomal dominant disorder. In children, it is caused by an autosomal recessive trait.
Cognitive Level: Application
Nursing Process: Assessment; *Test Plan:* PHYS

3   **Answer: 1** *Rationale:* Acute pyelonephritis is a bacterial infection of the kidney. Chronic pyelonephritis is associated with nonbacterial infections and noninfectious processes that may be metabolic, chemical or immunological.
Cognitive Level: Application
Nursing Process: Assessment; *Test Plan:* PHYS

4   **Answer: 1** *Rationale:* Hypertension may develop as renal tissue is destroyed.
Cognitive Level: Application
Nursing Process: Implementation; *Test Plan:* HPM

5   **Answer: 1** *Rationale:* Infection of the pharnyx or skin with *group-A beta hemolytic streptococcus* is the common precipitating factor for acute glomerulonephritis.
Cognitive Level: Comprehension
Nursing Process: Analysis; *Test Plan:* PHYS

6   **Answer: 1** *Rationale:* Risk factors of urinary tract infections include female, older clients, urinary obstruction or calculi, strictures, chronic disease, prostatic hypertrophy and prostatitis, diaphragm use, instrumentation and impaired immune system. Although children and teenagers can contract UTIs, incontinence and disease conditions in the elderly make them a higher risk population.
Cognitive Level: Application
Nursing Process: Assessment; *Test Plan:* PHYS

7   **Answer: 1** *Rationale:* Glomerular cells proliferate along with macrophages to form crescent-shaped lesions obliterating Bowman's space resulting in a rapid decline in glomerular filtration rate (GFR), which leads to many of the complications.
Cognitive Level: Knowledge
Nursing Process: Analysis; *Test Plan:* PHYS

8   **Answer: 2** *Rationale:* Sulfonamides are considered to be the drug of choice for acute, recurrent, or chronic urinary tract infections when there is no evidence of obstruction or bacteremia.
Cognitive Level: Comprehension
Nursing Process: Analysis; *Test Plan:* PHYS

9   **Answer: 3** *Rationale:* Vitamin C helps to maintain a pH of 5 or less thereby inhibiting bacterial growth. The other vitamins have no proven use in preventing urinary tract infections.
Cognitive Level: Application
Nursing Process: Implementation; *Test Plan:* PHYS

10   **Answer: 3** *Rationale:* Caffeine and alcohol can increase bladder spasms and mucosal irritation, thus increase the signs and symptoms of a urinary tract infection (UTI). Fluids should be taken, and douches will not help a UTI. All antibiotics should be taken completely to prevent resistant strains of organisms.
Cognitive Level: Application
Nursing Process: Implementation; *Test Plan:* HPM

References

Bullock, B. A. & Henze, R. L. (2000). *Focus on pathophysiology*. Philadelphia: Lippincott, pp. 605–611, 621–644.

Corbett, J. V. (2000). *Laboratory tests and diagnostic procedures* (5th ed.). Upper Saddle River, NJ: Prentice Hall.

Lemone, P. & Burke, K. (2000). *Medical-surgical nursing: Critical thinking in client care* (2nd ed.). Upper Saddle River, NJ: Prentice Hall, pp. 453, 895–898, 901–910, 950–958, 979–992.

Meredith, P. & Horan, N. (2000). *Adult primary care*. Philadelphia: W.B. Saunders

Robinson, D. (2000). *Primary care across the lifespan*. St. Louis: Mosby.

Wilson, B. A., Shannon, M. T., & Stang, C. L. (2001). *Nursing drug guide: 2001*. Upper Saddle River, NJ: Prentice Hall.

CHAPTER 11

Male and Female Reproductive Health Problems

Pam Hamre, RN, MS, CNM

CHAPTER OUTLINE

OBJECTIVES

- Define key terms associated with male and female reproductive health problems.

- Identify risk factors associated with the development of male and female reproductive health problems.

- Discuss the common etiologies of male and female reproductive health problems.

- Describe the pathophysiologic processes associated with specific male and female reproductive health problems.

- Distinguish between normal and abnormal male and female reproductive findings obtained from nursing assessment.

- Prioritize nursing interventions associated with specific male and female reproductive health problems.

[*Media Link*]

Use the CD-ROM enclosed with this text, or log onto the address given to access the free, interactive Companion Website created for this series. The CD-ROM and Companion Website accompanying this book offer additional practice opportunities and information—NCLEX Review, Case Studies, Glossary, In Depth with NCLEX, and more.

www.prenhall.com/hogan

REVIEW AT A GLANCE

adenomyosis *condition in which endometrium is present between myometrial cells*

balanitis *infection or inflammation of the foreskin*

benign prostatic hyperplasia (BPH) *enlargement of the prostate gland from non-cancerous hyperplasia*

cryptorchidism *undescended testicle*

dysfunctional uterine bleeding (DUB) *condition causing irregular menstrual bleeding from lack of progesterone*

dysmenorrhea *painful menstruation*

dyspareunia *painful intercourse*

endometriosis *condition in which endometrium implants are present outside the uterus*

epispadias *the urethral meatus is located on the upper (dorsal) aspect of the penis instead of the tip of the shaft; may be located just above the penile tip or anywhere along the shaft*

hypospadias *the urethral meatus is located on the lower (ventral) aspect of the penis instead of the tip of the shaft; may be located just below the penile tip or anywhere along the shaft*

menorrhagia *excessive or heavy menstrual flow*

metrorrhagia *irregular, frequent menstrual bleeding of abnormal amounts*

myoma *uterine muscle tumor*

orchiectomy *removal of a testicle*

pelvic inflammatory disease (PID) *inflammation of the uterus, fallopian tubes, and ovaries*

phimosis *unretractable foreskin that may impede or prohibit urine flow*

prostate specific antigen (PSA) *blood test to measure the antigen produced by prostate cancer*

Pretest

1 The nurse would question a client with balanitis about complaints of which of the following?

(1) Vaginal discharge
(2) Pain with urination
(3) Spontaneous urethral discharge
(4) Back pain

2 The nurse would assess the client experiencing prostatitis for which of the following symptoms?

(1) Spontaneous penile discharge, dysuria, and pain with ejaculation
(2) Painful blisters and crater-like lesions, enlarged groin nodes, fever
(3) Brownish rash on palms, painful crater-like lesions, malaise, and fever
(4) Rectal pain, pain with erection, low abdominal pain, and low back pain

3 A client reports to the clinic with complaints that a sexual partner from last year has been diagnosed with syphilis. The nurse would expect the client to have:

(1) Had a painless sore that healed and a rash on the palms of his hands.
(2) Negative VDRL, negative rapid plasma reagin (RPR), and positive fluorescent treponemal antibody absorption (FTA-ABS).
(3) Night sweats, cough, low-grade fever, and elevated white count.
(4) Vaginal discharge, dysuria, and pain with orgasm.

4 The nurse concludes that teaching has been effective when the mother of an infant born with hypospadias says, "Our son will:

(1) Need surgical correction so that he looks like the other boys."
(2) Require circumcision now to prevent complications later."
(3) Have surgical correction so he will be fertile as an adult."
(4) Likely have other reproductive tract anomalies we can't see."

5 Which medication would the nurse expect the client with dysfunctional uterine bleeding (DUB) be prescribed?

(1) Testosterone
(2) Estrogen
(3) Steroids
(4) Progesterone

6 In preparing to discharge a client with gonococcal pelvic inflammatory disease (PID), the nurse would intervene if the client made which statement?

(1) "I should douche after every episode of intercourse."
(2) "Using condoms will decrease the risk of this happening again."
(3) "My boyfriend and I should be monogamous."
(4) "The sexual position I use won't prevent this infection."

7 A 23-year-old client has been diagnosed with testicular cancer. Which of the following should be included in his teaching plan?

(1) Future fertility is not affected by treatment.
(2) Impotence often results from needed treatments.
(3) Sperm banking should be done prior to treatment.
(4) Sexual interest will increase as a result of treatment.

8 The client with fibrocystic breast disease is most likely to report a diet high in which of the following?

(1) Bacon, sausage, and ground meat.
(2) Fresh fruits and grain cereal.
(3) Cheese and milk.
(4) Coffee and cola.

9 A male client has been diagnosed with *Chlamydia trachomatis* infection. The plan of care should include which of the following?

(1) Instructions to take all of the doxycycline (Vibra-tabs) that was ordered.
(2) Encouragement to use condoms with most episodes of intercourse.
(3) Obtaining the names of sexual contacts if client desires.
(4) Teaching of testicular self-exam (TSE) for diagnosis.

10 The client has a diagnosis of primary dysmenorrhea. Which of the following would likely appear in her history?

(1) Heavy flow and clots for at least 3 months
(2) Irregular menses with breakthrough bleeding
(3) Painful periods since menarche
(4) No periods for the last 7 months

See pages 367–368 for Answers and Rationales.

I. Risk Factors Associated with Male and Female Reproductive Health Problems

    A. Multiple sexual partners increase the risk of sexually transmitted infection and subsequent problems

    B. Smoking creates endothelial cell changes that predispose the cells to more radical changes from viruses such as human papilloma virus (HPV) or pre-cancerous conditions and cancer

    C. Obesity increases the amount of fat-soluble hormones (such as estrogen), chemicals, and illicit drugs in the tissues, which increases the risk of cellular changes in the reproductive tract

    D. Alcohol use is associated with increased numbers of sexual partners and sexual assault

    E. Illicit drug use is also associated with increased numbers of sexual partners and sexual assault, and some drugs (marijuana, cocaine, heroin) are fat-soluble, leading to long-term storage of the drugs in the fatty tissues of the body for weeks to months after the last ingestion of the drug; this can lead to greater effects on the reproductive tract such as decreased spermatogenesis

F. Ionizing radiation can disrupt the normal cell division associated with oogenesis and spermatogenesis, leading to changes in the genetic structure of the gametes

G. Chemical exposure from occupational hazards or misuse of household chemicals can decrease sperm count, motility, and change morphology, as well as cause menstrual cycle changes

H. Specific conditions

1. Uretheral disorders: congenital

2. Prostatitis: urinary catheterization or similar procedures, consumption of alcohol, caffeine, and spicy foods

3. Benign prostatic hyperplasia: age

4. Prostate cancer: age, ethnicity, chemical/environmental exposures

5. Testicular cancer: history of **cryptorchidism** (undescended testicle), trauma, estrogen administration to mother during pregnancy such as diethylstilbistrol (DES), decreased birth weight, prematurity, family history

6. Uterine bleeding: age, family history, stress, weight change, oral contraceptives, intrauterine device (IUD)

7. Dysmenorrhea: smoking, non-use of oral contraception, early menarche

8. Pelvic inflammatory disease (PID): use of IUD, oral contraceptives, and condoms, sexually transmitted diseases (STD), multiple sex partners, previous PID

9. Endometriosis: nulliparity, family history

10. Benign breast disease: age

11. Breast cancer: age, family history (first-degree relative with breast cancer), ethnicity (Caucasian or African American), previous chest area radiation (i.e., treatment for Hodgkin's disease), menarche before age 12 or menopause after age 50, use of hormone replacement therapy over 5 years, nulliparous or first pregnancy after age 30, never breastfed, daily alcohol use, obesity

12. Sexually transmitted diseases: unprotected sex, multipartners, intravenous (IV) drug use, use of street drugs

II. Male Reproductive Health Problems

A. Urethral disorders

1. Overview

   a. **Hypospadias:** the urethral meatus is located on the lower (ventral) aspect of the penis instead of the tip of the shaft; may be located just below the penile tip or anywhere along the shaft

   b. **Epispadias:** the urethral meatus is located on the upper (dorsal) aspect of the penis instead of the tip of the shaft; may be located just above the penile tip or anywhere along the shaft

    c. Phimosis: unretractable foreskin, which impedes or prohibits urine flow

    d. Balanitis: infection or inflammation of the foreskin

    e. Urethritis: inflammation of the urethra

    f. Causes

      1) Hypospadias and epispadias: congenital

      2) Phimosis: congenital or secondary to infection or injury

      3) Balanitis: improper hygiene

      4) Urethritis: insertion of an instrument/catheter, gonococcal infection

2. Pathophysiology

    a. Developmental anomalies

      1) Hypospadias and epispadias develop when the urinary tract forms during embryological development

      2) Eight percent (8 percent) of men have a father or brother with the same condition

      3) Occurs in about 1 in 250 males

      4) Phimosis is an acquired stenosis of the intact foreskin resulting in an inability to retract the foreskin

    b. Inflammatory processes

      1) Balanitis occurs as a result of overgrowth of normal flora under the intact foreskin caused by lack of hygiene

      2) Urethritis is the most common urinary tract infection (UTI)

    c. Signs and symptoms

      1) Hypospadias and epispadias: visual deformity noted

      2) Phimosis: secondary infections and scarring; edema and pain of the glans penis (if constriction occurs); necrosis of glans

      3) Balanitis: redness, swelling, and pain of penis; foul odor and purulent drainage; dysuria

      4) Urethritis: painful urination; discharge from penis

3. Nursing assessment

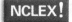

    a. Assessment includes: physical examination of the urethral meatus, color and retractability of the foreskin; characteristics of urine; vital signs (VS) (especially temperature); amount of urine; complaint of discomfort during voiding; presence of discharge

    b. Diagnostic tests: urinalysis or UA (preferably clean catch); culture and sensitivity (C & S)

4. Nursing management

    a. Medications

      1) Urethritis: oral antibiotics, analgesics

2) Balantis: topical or oral antibiotic or antifungal

3) Phimosis: topical steroid application

b. Teach the client the cause of the problem

c. Teach the client hygiene measures to prevent recurrence

d. Males with intact foreskin should be taught to retract the foreskin prior to voiding, wipe the glans dry after voiding, and then replace the foreskin; additionally, the glans of the penis should be retracted, cleansed, dried, and replaced after intercourse and during daily bathing

e. Instruct the client in the proper use of medications, including route, amount, and frequency of use

f. Surgical correction may be undertaken in early childhood if the urethral opening is along the shaft of the penis, primarily to promote fertility in adulthood

g. Treatment of phimosis may consists of stretching under local anesthetic; circumcision may be required

B. Prostatitis

1. Overview

a. Most common form is acute prostatitis, a bacterial infection

b. Chronic prostatitis can be bacterial or non-infectious

c. Can be acute or chronic bacterial or non-bacterial that is chronic in nature

d. Causes include trauma, autoimmune response, gonorrhea, bacterial infection

2. Pathophysiology

a. The prostate gland (see Figure 11-1) secretes a thin, alkaline fluid that is part of the seminal secretion

b. Is not well-understood; bacteria from the rectum or infected urine invade the prostate

---

NCLEX!

▶ *Practice to Pass*

The client with hypospadias asks if his sons will have the condition. How should the nurse respond?

Figure 11-1

Components of the male reproductive system.

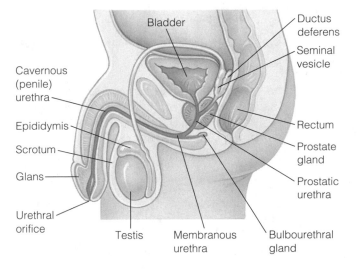

Bladder

Ductus deferens

Seminal vesicle

Cavernous (penile) urethra

Epididymis

Scrotum

Glans

Urethral orifice

Testis

Membranous urethra

Rectum

Prostate gland

Prostatic urethra

Bulbourethral gland

c. Not considered sexually transmitted

d. Signs and symptoms

1) Acute: chills, fever, urinary (dysuria, frequency, urgency, hematuria; pain (suprapubic, perineal, scrotal, lower back, rectal); discharge; enlarged prostate that is tender and warm; palpable seminal vesicles; blood and pus in urine; pain during ejaculation

2) Chronic and nonbacterial: may be asymptomatic; low-grade fever; pain; nocturia; dysuria

3. Nursing assessment

a. Assessment includes obtaining a history on onset, severity, and precipitating factors of symptoms; inspection of urine; VS; symptom analysis of pain

b. Diagnostic tests: urinalysis, physical examination, urine C & S

4. Nursing management

a. Medications include antibiotics

b. Educate client on cause and treatment plan

c. Instruct client to avoid caffeine and alcohol

C. Benign prostatic hyperplasia (BPH)

1. Overview

a. **Benign prostatic hyperplasia (BPH)** is defined as a noncancerous enlargement of the prostate from hyperplasia or hypertrophy (see Figure 11-2)

b. Begins in the 40s but usually not symptomatic until 60s and older

c. Causes include aging process

2. Pathophysiology

a. Results from decreased testosterone and increased estrogen levels

b. Prostate cells increase in size and in number

c. Causes pressure on and decreases the diameter of the urethra

Figure 11-2

Benign prostatic hyperplasia.

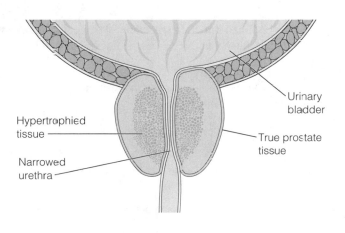

Urinary bladder

Hypertrophied tissue

True prostate tissue

Narrowed urethra

d. Although androgen levels are decreasing as the male ages, the prostate gland is still sensitive to the presence of dihydrotestosterone (DHT), which causes growth of the prostate gland

e. May be asymptomatic until acute onset inhibits opening of the bladder sphincter; excess alcohol intake can be a trigger

f. Signs and symptoms include incomplete bladder emptying, difficulty starting the stream and weak stream; nocturia; feeling of fullness in bladder; increased urinary time; dribbling of urine

3. Nursing assessment

a. Assessment includes client history related to urinating; symptom analysis of urinary problems; characteristics of urine

b. Diagnostic tests: biopsy of the prostate; physical examination; ultrasonography; urinalysis; serum creatinine (CR) and blood urea nitrogen (BUN)

4. Nursing management

a. Medications include finasteride (Proscar), which inhibits testosterone conversion to dihydrotestosterone; gonadotropin-releasing hormone analogues; antiandrogens; alpha-adrenergic antagonist

b. Instruct client to avoid alcohol use, and report increased urinary symptoms

c. If transurethral resection of the prostate (TURP) is indicated, educate client as to

1) The surgical procedure and regional anesthesia

2) Recovery, including continuous bladder irrigation (to prevent clotting) and going home with an indwelling urinary catheter

3) Potential for bladder spasms

4) Avoidance of nonsteroidal antiinflammatory drugs (NSAIDs) use for 10 days pre-operative

D. Prostate cancer

1. Overview

a. Average age at diagnosis is 65

b. Usually slow growing, often asymptomatic in early stages

c. African-American men are 50 percent more likely to develop prostate cancer than Caucasian men; an increased incidence if first-degree relative has prostate cancer

d. Causes include genetic disposition, history of STDs, high-fat diet; hormones; often unknown

2. Pathophysiology

a. Single or multiple areas within the prostate gland develop proliferative cancer and enlarge the gland both outward toward the capsule and then inward toward the urethra (see Table 11-1)

b. Causes are similar to benign prostatic hyperplasia

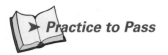

Practice to Pass

The client with benign prostatic hyperplasia with transurethral resection of the prostate (TURP) scheduled in 1 week calls to ask if there are any over-the-counter (OTC) medications that he shouldn't take. How should the nurse reply?

	Table 11-1	Stages of Prostate Cancer		
Stage	**Location of Cancer**	**Symptoms**	**Diagnosis**
1 (A)	Prostate only	Asymptomatic	Accidental discovery (i.e., during trans–uretheral resection of prostate for benign prostatic hyperplasia)
2 (B)	Prostate only	Mild urinary symptoms of enlarged prostate or asymptomatic	Prostate specific antigen (PSA) elevated or palpated during rectal exam
3 (C)	Outside capsule of prostate; may also be in seminal vesicles	Urinary symptoms, rectal or pelvic pain	PSA elevated or palpated during rectal exam
4 (D)	Lymph nodes, bones, liver, lungs	Urinary symptoms, rectal or pelvic pain; plus pain in affected tissue	PSA elevated or palpated during rectal exam
Recurrent	Anywhere in body after previous treatment	Determined by tissue involved	PSA elevated after treatment

    c. Extension of the cancer outside of the prostate gland capsule may also occur, first into the seminal vesicles

    d. Compression of the urethra by the tumor may cause urinary symptoms

    e. Common sites of metastases: lymph nodes, bones, lungs, liver (see Table 11-1 again)

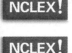

    f. Cancer of the prostate is testosterone-dependent early in the course of the disease

    g. Signs and symptoms include urinary problems (increased frequency, urgency, reduction in stream, nocturia, hematuria); blood during ejaculation; back pain; pain of joints and bone if metastasis occurs; weight loss; fatigue; client may be asymptomatic

  3. Nursing assessment

    a. Assessment includes

      1) History of urinary symptoms as in BPH; question client for known risk factors

      2) Symptom analysis of pain (hips, low back, abdomen, pelvis)

      3) Assess weight, energy level, sexual function/problems

      4) Symptom analysis on urinary status

    b. Diagnostic tests

      1) Screening utilizes **prostate specific antigen (PSA)** blood tests (PSA should be less than or equal to 4.0)

      2) Digital rectal exams recommended yearly for men over 45

      3) Urinalysis

      4) Transrectal ultrasonography (TRUS) if PSA is elevated

        5) Tissue biopsy: diagnosis is through rectal or perineal fine-needle aspiration after increased PSA or rectal exam detects hard nodules on the prostate

        6) Magnetic resonance imagery (MRI) or computerized tomography (CT) for possible metastasis

    4. Nursing management

      a. Medications/treatment

        1) Hormone therapy (via bilateral orchiectomy or monthly injections)

        2) Surgery (transuretheral resection of prostate [TURP] or radical abdominal prostatectomy)

        3) Chemotherapy

        4) Internal or external radiation

NCLEX!

      b. Education needed that most men will be impotent after abdominal prostatectomy, and 40 percent will experience urinary incontinence

      c. Age of the client at diagnosis, concurrent medical conditions, and stage of the cancer determine recommended treatment regimen

NCLEX!

      d. If receiving chemotherapy or radiation therapy, assess mouth for stomatitis, skin condition at radiation site, and signs of dehydration

      e. Educate client as to what their cancer stage means and assess for suicidal tendencies

      f. Provide support for body image disturbance and sexual dysfunction issues, including referral to support groups for client and family

E. Testicular cancer

    1. Overview

      a. Most common cancer in males age 15 to 34

      b. Many forms exist

      c. Types

        1) Germinal cell tumor

        2) Seminomas (most common)

      d. Cause is unknown

    2. Pathophysiology

      a. Types:

        1) Ninety-five percent (95 percent) are germ cell (originating in the sperm producing cells of the testes)

        2) Forty percent (40 percent) are seminomas (slow-growing and remain localized within a teste)

        3) Sixty percent (60 percent) are non-seminoma (more aggressive)

        4) Other forms may be leydig, sertoli, leiomyosarcoma, rhabdomyosarcoma, mesothelioma, or stromal cell

b. Cancer cells grow within the testicle, replacing the parenchymal tissue

c. Spread of the disease is usually by lymphatic (lymph nodes) and vascular channels (to lungs, bone, or liver), even before any large mass appears in the scrotum

d. Signs and symptoms

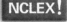

 1) Painless, hard nodule or swelling (usually on only one side of testes), dull ache in the testes

 2) Metastatic symptoms include: respiratory problems (coughing, dyspnea), back of bone pain, gastrointestinal problems

e. There are 3 stages of testicular cancer (see Table 11-2)

3. Nursing assessment

 a. Assessment

  1) Obtain client history of testicular or groin pain, change in size, shape, or consistency of teste, and size and consistency of palpable lumps, presence of cryptorchidism with or without surgical correction

  2) Other: symptom analysis of any pain, respiratory or GI problems

 b. Diagnostic tests

  1) Radioimmunoassay studies for tumor markers (human chorionic gonadotropin [hCG] and alpha-fetoprotein [AFP])

  2) Serum lactic acid dehydrogenase (LDH)

  3) Metastasis: liver function tests, x-ray, and CT scan

  4) Diagnosis made via pathology examination following inguinal **orchiectomy** (removal of a teste) on the affected side

4. Nursing management

 a. Medications include chemotherapy

  1) Cisplatin (Platinol), bleomycin (Blenoxane), and etoposide (VePesid)

  2) Etopside (VePesid) plus cisplatin (Platinol)

 b. Treatment after orchiectomy involves radiation and/or chemotherapy

 c. Monitor vital signs during chemotherapy or radiation treatment and fluid balance assessment because of nausea, vomiting, and diarrhea from treatment modalities

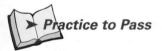

Practice to Pass

The client with a testicular lump is scheduled for an inguinal orchiectomy and asks why the doctor doesn't just remove the lump "like they do with breast lumps." How should the nurse respond?

Table 11-2	Stage	Location
Stages of Testicular Cancer	I	Confined to testicle
	II	Retroperitoneal lymph nodes
	III	Beyond lymph nodes; into lungs, brain, liver, and/or bones

      d. Provide client education on expected client experience with treatment

NCLEX!

      e. If client desires fertility, inform him of sperm banking prior to chemotherapy

NCLEX!

      f. Teach client testicular self-examination (TSE) of remaining teste and to have annual visits to physician

III. Female Reproductive Health Problems

A. Uterine bleeding disorders

1. Overview

   a. Dysfunctional uterine bleeding (DUB) is a nonspecific condition from lack of progesterone, where menstruation is

      1) Irregular, frequent (**metrorrhagia**)

      2) Excessive (**menorrhagia**)

      3) Both (metromenorrhagia)

   b. Occurs mostly in adolescents and in premenopausal women

   c. 25 to 50 percent of women will develop fibroid tumors (**myomas,** leiomyomas), usually in their 30s and 40s, which can also create bleeding disorders

   d. Causes

      1) **Adenomyosis** (a condition in which endometrium is present between myometrial cells) can also cause irregular or heavy menstrual bleeding

      2) Over 90 percent caused by anovulatory cycles

      3) Other: blood dyscrasias, endocrine problems, pelvic inflammatory disease, endometrial cancer or polyps, exogenous estrogen, pregnancy, menopause, athletic training or excessive athletic activity; or no known cause

2. Pathophysiology

   a. Dysfunctional uterine bleeding results from a lack of progesterone

      1) This causes proliferation of fragile endometrium that does not mature into secretory endometrium

      2) Endometrium sheds at irregular times

   b. If the proliferative phase of the menstrual cycle is shortened because of a defect in the follicular phase, spotting and breakthrough bleeding may occur

   c. Excessive flow may be a result of defects during the leutal phase

NCLEX!

   d. Disorders of DUB

      1) Amenorrhea (absence of menstruation)

         a) Primary (by age 17)

         b) Secondary (absence in a previously menstruating woman)

      2) Oligomenorrhea (scant menses)

3) Menorrhagia

4) Metrorrhagia

5) Postmenopausal bleeding

NCLEX!

e. Uterine myomas form in several areas (see Figure 11-3)

1) In the myometrial wall (intramural)

2) Pedunculated and into the uterine cavity (submucosal)

3) Pedunculated (having a stalk) and outwards into the pelvis (subserosal)

f. Adenomyosis is endometrium in the myometrium, which enlarges each month under hormonal influence but is unable to be shed because it is trapped between the myometrial cells

g. Signs and symptoms include change in menstrual cycle (repetitive or long history), fatigue, anemia, hemorrhage, sexual dysfunction, cramping, water retention, anxiety, problems with reproduction; large tumors or the presence of more than one tumor tend to cause more symptoms: enlarged uterus, metrorrhagia, dysmenorrhea, pelvic pressure or fullness, and increased urinary frequency

3. Nursing assessment

a. Assessment

1) Obtain history of bleeding pattern

2) Blood pressure and pulse sitting and standing

3) Symptom analysis of pain or discomforts associated with problem

4) Activity level

5) Sexual and reproductive history

Figure 11-3

**Myomas of the uterus.
A. Intramural;
B. Submucosal;
C. Subserosal.**

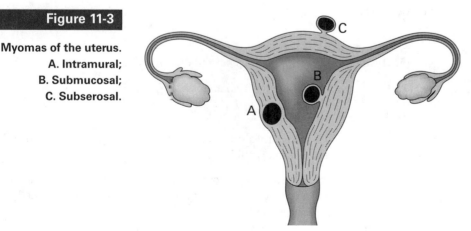

    b. Diagnostic tests

        1) Lab work: complete blood count (CBC), thyroid function studies, endocrine hormones, progesterone level, serum human chorionic gonadotropin (hCG) levels

        2) Pelvic ultrasound

        3) Pap smear

        4) Hysteroscopy

        5) Tumors: diagnosis through ultrasound, CT scan, hysteroscopy, or laparoscopy

        6) Diagnosis of adenomyosis can only be made from microscopic examination of the myometrium after hysterectomy

  4. Nursing management

    a. Medications/treatment includes hormonal agents, oral contraceptives (3 to 6 months), progesterone (Progestaject) or medroxyprogesterone (Provera), iron supplements

NCLEX!

        1) Diagnosis of DUB is confirmed by response to medications or via endometrial biopsy; treatment is aimed at replacing the progesterone through cyclical use of progestins or combination oral contraceptive pills

        2) Treatment of tumors is based on symptoms and includes myomectomy, hysterectomy, fibroid embolization

        3) Treatment of adenomyosis consists of attempting to regulate the menses with hormonal birth control methods, or hysterectomy

    b. Educate the client to use a bleeding calendar to document bleeding each day, noting how much, color, presence of clots, and dysmenorrhea

    c. Provide education on the condition

    d. Instruct in correct use of medications

    e. Pre-operative teaching if surgery is necessary

B. Dysmenorrhea

  1. Overview

    a. Dysmenorrhea is defined as painful menstruation

    b. Is the most common menstrual abnormality

    c. Types

        1) Primary dysmenorrhea (most common), begins with the onset of menses and is usually lifelong; unknown etiology

        2) Secondary dysmenorrhea occurs after the onset of regular menses; usually related to pelvic inflammatory disease, endometriosis, sexually transmitted disease (STD), blockage; fertility problems; use of intrauterine devices (IUD)

2. Pathophysiology

   a. Primary dysmenorrhea

      1) Thought to result from excessive prostaglandin production by the uterus, which causes excessively strong uterine contractions to facilitate shedding the endometrium each menses

      2) The strong contractions cause uterine ischemia and pain

      3) May be exaggerated by anxiety, tension, or stress

      4) Signs and symptoms include pain (abdominal with onset of menses and 12 to 48 hours after menses starts; back, thigh); headache; nausea and vomiting; diarrhea; fatigue; breast tenderness; syncope and collapse; dizziness

      5) Symptoms usually decline or disappear after the first pregnancy or with age

   b. Secondary dysmenorrhea

      1) Scarring or injury from the underlying cause occurs

      2) Signs and symptoms: pain similar to primary dysmenorrhea, but usually after years of a normal menarche

      3) Determination of any underlying condition must be ruled out

3. Nursing assessment

   a. Assessment

      1) Obtain thorough menstrual history including onset of menses and onset of dysmenorrhea

      2) Obtain information on what relief measures have been utilized and their effectiveness

      3) Symptom analysis of pain and discomfort

      4) History of pregnancy and any other female problems

      5) If secondary, determine if **dyspareunia** (painful intercourse) is present

   b. Diagnostic tests

      1) Diagnosis is based on client history for both primary and secondary dysmenorrhea

      2) Pelvic examination

      3) Laboratory tests: follicle-stimulating hormone (FSH), luteinizing hormone (LH), progesterone level, estradiol level, thyroid function tests

      4) Pelvic ultrasonography

      5) MRI or CT

      6) Laparoscopy

      7) Dilation and curettage (D & C) of the uterus

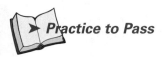

Practice to Pass

An adolescent client asks if her periods will be painful like her friend's are. How should the nurse reply?

4. Nursing management

    a. Medications

        1) Analgesics for discomfort

        2) Nonsteroidal antiinflammatory drugs to inhibit prostaglandins

        3) Oral contraceptives to decrease the length and amount of menstrual flow: norethindrone and ethinyl estradiol (Brevicon)

        4) Antibiotics for secondary form

    b. Educate clients as to the cause of their dysmenorrhea

    c. Teach how to take prescribed or over-the-counter (OTC) medications correctly

    d. Instruct clients to drink plenty of fluids and have an adequate calcium intake

    e. Application of heat to the lower abdomen may help when the discomfort occurs

C. Pelvic inflammatory disease (PID)

    1. Overview

        a. Pelvic inflammatory disease (PID) is defined as an inflammation of the uterus and fallopian tubes (salpingitis), endometrium (endometritis), pelvic peritoneum, and ovaries (oophoritis) usually resulting from infection

        b. Highest incidence occurs among women who have had more than one sexual partner in their lifetime, increasing with greater numbers of partners

        c. 20 percent of women will be infertile after infectious PID; 20 percent will have chronic pelvic pain; ectopic pregnancy occurs 10 times as often after PID

        d. Most prominent in women ages 15 to 24 who are nulliparous

        e. May be acute or chronic

        f. Causes: use of intrauterine devices, oral contraceptives, or condoms; secondary infections are caused by appendicitis, peritonitis, STDs, douching

    2. Pathophysiology

        a. Bacteria invade the uterine and tubal tissues after migrating through the cervix

        b. Migration occurs during ovulation, menstruation, forced through the cervix with douching, childbirth, abortion, or surgery of the reproductive tract

        c. Scar tissue is formed from the infection, which obstructs the uterine tubes

        d. Tubo-ovarian abscesses can form from the obstruction

        e. Bacterial infection causes inflammation, which in turn causes the symptoms

        f. Common infecting organisms include *Neisseria gonorrhea*, *Chlamydia trachomatis*, *E. coli,* or *Gardnerella vaginalis*

g. Signs and symptoms include low abdominal pain, dysmenorrhea, dysparunia, dysuria, and fever; vaginal discharge may be noted (green-yellow, green-gray, or yellow); nausea, malaise

h. Complications of PID include infertility, ectopic pregnancy, pelvic abscess, and dysmenorrhea

3. Nursing assessment

a. Assessment

1) History for onset of symptoms, precipitating factors, known exposure to STDs, number of sexual partners, and amount of douching

2) Assess for VS (fever), activity level, any discharges

3) Symptom analysis of pain and GI symptoms

4) History of menstrual cycle and pregnancies

b. Diagnostic tests

1) Cervical cultures

2) Ultrasound

3) Laparoscopy

4) CBC for elevated white blood count (WBC)

5) Review of client's symptoms

6) Pap smear, visualization of cervix will detect any discharge

4. Nursing management

a. Medications include analgesics for fever and antibiotics (may require inpatient intravenous [IV] form)

1) Tetracycline: doxycycline (Vibramycin)

2) Cephalosporin: cefoxitin (Mefoxin)

3) Aminoglycoside: gentamicin (Garamycin)

4) Fluoroquinolone: ofloxacin (Floxin)

5) Antiprotozoal: metronidazole (Flagyl)

b. Client education

1) Proper timing and use of oral antibiotics

2) Avoiding douching

3) Cause of PID

c. Instruct client to take her temperature three times a day and call if elevation is noted

d. Instruct client to report PID to provider if she becomes pregnant so that ectopic pregnancy can be detected early

D. **Endometriosis**

1. Overview

a. **Endometriosis** is defined as a growth of the endometrium outside of the uterus

b. Most likely sites of growth include the bladder, ovaries, fallopian tubes, bowel, and broad ligament

c. Most often occurs in European-American women of childbearing age

d. Major complication is infertility

e. Causes include unknown, theorized to be caused from embryonic epithelial cells; backflow of menstrual fluid through the uterine tubes during menstruation; and spread of endometrial implants by way of the lymphatic or vascular system

2. Pathophysiology

a. Endometrial tissue is present outside of the uterus, and responds to the hormonal influence of the menstrual cycle

b. However, blood (that normally is shed from intrauterine endometrium) cannot escape and builds up causing scarring and further growth of the endometriosis

c. The bleeding results in inflammation and pain in the tissues

d. Infertility associated with endometriosis may be from mechanical blockage of the tubes from endometrial implants or unexplained

e. Signs and symptoms include dysmenorrhea, dyspareunia, dysuria, constipation, and painful bowel movements during menses, tender masses that are palpable

3. Nursing assessment

a. Assessment

1) Obtain thorough history of symptoms including onset, when in the menstrual cycle symptoms worsen or improve

2) Symptom analysis of pain and related symptoms

3) Assess bowel characteristics

b. Diagnostic tests

1) Diagnosis is made by laparoscopy

2) CBC to identify low hemoglobin and hematocrit (H & H) and rule out infection with WBC

3) Pelvic ultrasonography

4. Nursing management

a. Medications include analgesics for pain, NSAIDS for inhibiting prostaglandin synthesis; hormone therapy such as leuprolide (Lupron); gonadotropin-releasing hormone (GRH) to raise estrogen and progesterone levels to control bleeding

b. Educate the client about endometriosis

c. Provide education on treatment being utilized, including side effects of medications such as hot flashes

d. Provide support and refer to support groups for infertility issues

E. Benign breast disorders

    1. Overview

        a. Fibrocystic disease is defined as benign breast lesions

        b. Common in women 30 to 50 years of age

        c. Causes include hormonal changes, aging, diet high in caffeine

    2. Pathophysiology

        a. Mammary tissue retains fluid and forms a cyst during the latter half of the menstrual cycle, which resolves spontaneously with menstruation

        b. Inflammation from repetition of the filling cause the wall of the cyst to fibrose and become hard, blocking the drainage of the fluid

        c. The cyst remains even after menses

        d. Classification

            1) Nonproliferative lesion: may be cystic or fibrous and may result in a mass in the upper outer breast quadrant after an inflammatory response to irritation of the ducts

            2) Proliferative lesion: lesions without atypical cells

            3) Atypical hyperplasia: lesions that are "borderline," possible morphologic characteristics of cancer cells

        e. Signs and symptoms: painful, mobile, round or oval, smooth lump in the breast tissue that enlarges or becomes more painful premenstrually; nipple discharge (clear, milky, straw-colored, green)

    3. Nursing assessment

        a. Assessment

            1) Obtain history on when the lump was first detected, with size, shape, location, mobility, tenderness, and cyclical changes

            2) Determine if ultrasound or mammogram has been previously performed

            3) Perform breast exam

            4) Identify details of menstrual cycle and previous problems

        b. Diagnostic tests

            1) Mammogram

            2) Ultrasound examination

            3) Needle aspiration may be performed

            4) Excisional biopsy may be done to rule out cancer

            5) Breast examination

    4. Nursing management

        a. Medications include mild analgesics and Vitamin E

        b. There is no cure, but limiting caffeine, smoking, and chocolate usually improves or eliminates the condition

c. Provide education on what is known about fibrocystic breast disease and explain the vagueness of prevention and treatment

d. Reassure client that fibrocystic breast lumps are not precancerous

e. Educate on self-breast exam on a monthly basis and yearly exam by physician; mammograms for women over 40

F. Breast cancer

1. Overview

   a. Defined as growth of abnormal cells in breast tissue that is irregular

   b. Affects 1 out of 9 women over the course of a lifetime; 10 percent of cases linked to mutations in the BRCA1 or BRCA2 gene

   c. Involves the mammary ducts, lobules, or both

   d. Cause: unknown, see risk factors (p. 342)

2. Pathophysiology

   a. Two main locations: lobular (20 percent) and ductal (80 percent)

   b. Breast cancer is hormone-dependent; must have functioning ovaries

   c. Termed

   1) Noninvasive (in situ): proliferation of cancer cells are either ductal or lobular but do not invade surrounding tissue

   2) Invasive (penetration of the tumor into surrounding tissue); arise in the terminal section of ductal tissue; five types

      a) Infiltrating ductal carcinoma: stony hardness when palpated; metastasizes to axillary lymph nodes; most common; poor prognosis

      b) Tubular carcinoma or "well-differentiated"; less common

      c) Medullary carcinoma: bulky, large tumor that is well-circumscribed

      d) Mucinous carcinoma: bulky, slow-growing tumor with sharp edges

      e) Infiltrating lobular carcinoma: uncommon; thick, ill-defined area in breast

   d. May metastasize to bone, brain, lung, liver, skin, and lymph nodes

   e. Tumors are staged according to size of tumor, involvement of lymph node, and metastasis to other sites (see Table 11-3)

   f. Metastasis occurs as small masses of cells break away from the tumor, enter the lymphatic system where they remain, causing swelling of the node or traveling to another node; lymphatic drainage has three pathways

   1) Axillary (most common route of spread)

   2) Internal mammary

   3) Transpectoral

   g. Signs and symptoms include hard, irregular, painless, fixed lump or thickening of a breast area; red, scaly patch of skin on breast; development of nipple inversion or calcifications detected on mammogram; possibly no palpable or visible symptoms initially

Table 11-3	American Joint Committee on Cancer (AJCC) Stages of Breast Cancer		
	Primary Tumor Size	**Regional Lymph Nodes**	**Distant Metastasis**
Stage 0	Microscopic	None	None
Stage I	Less than 2 cm	None	None
Stage IIA	Microscopic up to 5 cm	None or same side mobile nodes	None
Stage IIB	Greater than 2 cm	None or same side mobile nodes	None
Stage IIIA	Microscopic to greater than 5 cm	Same side mobile or fixed nodes	None
Stage IIIB	Any size with or without extension to chest wall	Internal mammary lymph nodes	None
Stage IV	Any size	Any nodes	Present

    h. *Inflammatory carcinoma* is a systemic disease of the breast and the most malignant form of breast cancer

        1) Signs and symptoms include skin erythema, redness, warmth, and induration of the breast; *peau d'orange* sign (edema of skin with orange peel look) is present

        2) Prognosis is poor

    i. *Paget's disease* is a rare type of breast cancer that involves the nipple epithelium

        1) Signs and symptoms include itching, burning of nipple; crusting or ulceration of nipple

        2) Excellent prognosis if confined to nipple

3. Nursing assessment

    a. Assessment includes history on lump: size, shape, location, fixed or mobile, presence of pain, when discovered; obtain family history regarding breast cancer; determine date and location of last mammogram (if any); assess client's fear and knowledge of cancer

    b. Diagnostic tests

        1) Screening mammography

        2) Clinical breast examination

        3) Ultrasonography

        4) MRI

        5) Biopsy (fine needle or excisional); with cytologic examination of fluid

4. Nursing management

    a. Medications include estrogen-antagonist medication (Tamoxifen) may be ordered if the tumor has estrogen receptors; chemotherapy used with large tumors, age less than 50, if nodes are positive, or metastasis present

    b. Treatment: lumpectomy or mastectomy with axillary node dissection followed by radiation

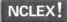

c. Breast reconstruction surgery, if desired by the client, can be performed at the time of mastectomy or later

d. Provide education as to

1) The results of screening and diagnostic tests (mammogram, ultrasound, biopsy, pathology report following lumpectomy or mastectomy)

2) Expected client experience with procedures ordered and anesthesia required for them

3) Appropriate use of home medications

4) Side effects of radiation or chemotherapy if utilized

5) Placement of drains after surgery and their care post-discharge

e. Provide support to client and family, and encourage client to attend support groups such as "Reach for Recovery"

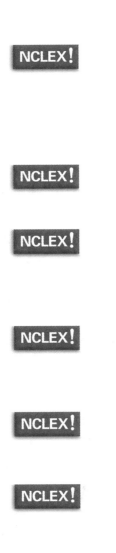

Practice to Pass

A 40-year-old client wants to know when she should start having mammograms. How should the nurse respond?

IV. **Sexually Transmitted Diseases (STDs)**

A. **Gonococcal infection**

1. Overview

a. Defined as infection of the cervix and the male urethra with *Neisseria gonorrhea,* a gram-negative anaerobic diplococci; can also affect mouth, throat and anus

b. Second most common STD; incidence is decreasing, highest incidence in urban areas among men and women 15 to 24 years old

c. Also known as GC or "clap"

d. Cause: direct sexual contact with infected person or by an infected mother to a fetus during delivery

2. Pathophysiology

a. Bacteria present in semen, vaginal, and cervical secretions are distributed during unprotected intercourse to the mucous membranes, causing damage to the cells

b. Damage to the cells triggers the inflammatory response, accounting for the symptoms

c. Infection occurs at site of contact (i.e., vagina, rectum, urethra, oropharynx)

d. Incubation period is 2 to 8 days with symptoms appearing about day 10 after exposure

e. Signs and symptoms

1) Female: thick yellow or greenish-yellow vaginal discharge, new onset of dysmenorrhea and/or dyspareunia, pelvic pain, enlarged groin nodes, rectal pain may be present, urethral discharge may be seen; pharyngitis; purulent exudate from urethra or Bartholin's duct

2) Males: dysuria, thick yellow or greenish-yellow spontaneous penile discharge, pain with ejaculation, rectal pain if engage in rectal intercourse; (oropharynx)—extremely sore throat, reddened oropharynx with copious adherent yellow discharge, fever, enlarged neck nodes

      f. Complications: female—spontaneous abortion if pregnant, premature delivery, salpingitis, PID, infertility secondary to scarring and blockage of fallopian tubes or vas deferens, ectopic pregnancy or chorioamnionitis, abscess of Bartholin's gland

  3. Nursing assessment

    a. Assessment

      1) Obtain sexual history including unprotected intercourse, onset and severity of symptoms, any known exposure to gonorrhea; menstrual history

      2) Assess vital signs, palpate lymph nodes, visually inspect any discharge, perform oral exam

      3) Symptom analysis of any pain

    b. Diagnostic tests

      1) Culture of cervix or urethra

      2) Urine specimen for polymerase chain reaction (PCR) testing

  4. Nursing management

    a. Medications include antibiotic therapy

      1) Oral: ciprofloxacin hydrochloride (Cipro), azithromycin (Zithromax), or doxycycline (Vibra-tabs)

      2) Intramuscular (IM): ceftriaxone sodium (Rocephin)

    b. Client education

      1) Bacterial cause of gonorrhea and transmission through unprotected intercourse

      2) Use of condoms correctly for each episode of intercourse

      3) Limiting number of sexual partners or become abstinent

      4) Use of oral antibiotics including the need to finish all medication

    c. Obtain names of sexual contacts for follow-up testing and treatment

B. Nongonococcal infection

  1. Overview

    a. Defined as a sexually transmitted disease known as chlamydial infection, which causes an acute infection of the reproductive tract

    b. *Chlamydia trachomatis,* a very small anaerobic, obligate intracellular bacteria; the most common STD among men and women 15 to 24 years of age

    c. The incidence is increasing across the United States

    d. Causes: direct sexual contact, perinatally, mother-to-child transmission in delivery

NCLEX!
NCLEX!
NCLEX!
NCLEX!
NCLEX!
NCLEX!

2. Pathophysiology

   a. Bacteria found in semen, vaginal, and cervical secretions are transported during sexual contact; bacteria replicate rapidly and can be spread within 24 hours of becoming infected

   b. Organism usually invades the urethra in men and cervix in women

   c. Can cause conjunctivitis and blindness in the newborn

   d. Incubation period is about 2 weeks after exposure

   e. Permanent tissue scarring can result from the infection

   f. Symptoms: often asymptomatic, and may remain so for years

      1) Females: greenish or yellowish vaginal discharge that will be visualized in the cervical os, sudden onset of dysmenorrhea or dyspareunia, dysuria, or midcycle postcoital bleeding, pelvic pain, pain with orgasm

      2) Males: more likely to be symptomatic than females; dysuria, expressed yellowish penile discharge, pain with ejaculation

   g. Complications include pneumonitis if client is immunocompromised, endocarditis, and meningoencephalitis

      1) Females: PID, endometritis, salpingitis, infertility, ectopic pregnancy

      2) Males: epididymitis, prostatitis, sterility

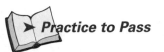

Practice to Pass

When instructing the female client on taking doxycycline (Vibra-tabs) for her *Chlamydia trachomatis* cervicitis, the client states that she thinks she may be pregnant. What should the nurse do?

3. Nursing assessment

   a. Assessment

      1) Obtain sexual history including unprotected intercourse, onset and severity of symptoms, known exposure to chlamydia, menstrual history

      2) Assess vital signs, discharge

      3) Symptom analysis of pain

   b. Diagnostic tests

      1) Cultures of tissue

      2) Antibody tests: direct fluorescent antibody test (DEA), enzyme-linked immunosorbent assay (ELISA)

      3) Urine specimen for polymerase chain reaction (PCR) testing

4. Nursing management

   a. Medications include oral antibiotics such as azithromycin (Zithromax), or doxycycline (Vibra-tabs), erythromycin (EES), or ampicillin (Ampicin)

   b. Client education

      1) Bacterial cause of chlamydia and transmission through unprotected intercourse

      2) Use of condoms correctly with each episode of intercourse

      3) Limiting the number of sexual partners or becoming abstinent

      4) Use of oral antibiotics including the need to finish all medication

   c. Obtain names of sexual contacts for follow-up testing and treatment

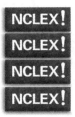

C. Syphilis

   1. Overview

NCLEX!

      a. Defined as a chronic form of STD caused by the spirochete bacteria, *Treponema pallidum*

      b. Four stages: primary, secondary, latent, and tertiary

      c. Often occurs with other STDs such as chlamydial infection or gonorrhea

      d. Highest incidence in African-American men in the southeast United States

NCLEX!

      e. Cause: transmission during sexual contact; through blood; mother to child transfer during childbirth

   2. Pathophysiology

NCLEX!

      a. Distinct stages, onset/timing, symptoms, and transfer are described in Table 11-4

         1) Primary stage: the initial chancre (typical lesion) appears

         2) Secondary stage: development of a systemic illness

         3) Latent stage: period until manifestations of tertiary stage begin; no clinical manifestations occur

         4) Tertiary stage: systemic manifestations occur and complications in this stage may result in death

      b. Infestation can occur in any body tissue or organ

      c. Incubation period ranges from 10 to 90 days

      d. Upon entering the body, the spirochete is spread by way of the blood and lymphatic system

Table 11-4	Syphilis		
Stage	**Onset/timing**	**Symptoms**	**Transfer**
Primary	10 to 90 days after exposure; average 21 days lasts 3 to 5 weeks	Firm, round, small, crater-like chancre at site of bacterial entry that heals spontaneously	Contact with lesion, sexual contact, or blood
Secondary	3 to 6 weeks after chancre appears; may come and go up to 2 years	Brownish rash especially on palms of hands and soles of feet that does not itch; malaise; may have patchy hair loss; mild swollen glands	Contact with rash, sexual contact, blood
Latent	Disappearance of symptoms of secondary stage; lasts for years	None	No
Tertiary	Onset may be several years from initial infection; can be fatal	Depends on site of bacterial invasion: heart valve or aortic stenosis Neurosyphilis leads to CNS involvement, leading to dementia, blindness, paralysis	No

NCLEX!

      e. See Table 11-4 for signs and symptoms

      f. Complications include blindness, paralysis, mental illness, cardiovascular damage, encephalitis, and death; pregnant women with syphilis can transmit the infection to their fetus, resulting in congenital syphilis, causing intrauterine fetal death or numerous central nervous system (CNS) defects

  3. Nursing assessment

      a. Assessment

        1) Obtain sexual history including unprotected intercourse, onset and severity of symptoms, and known exposure to syphilis

        2) Assess for IV drug use

        3) Assess vital signs, mental clarity, lung and heart sounds, activity level

        4) Visual inspection for lesions

      b. Diagnostic tests

        1) Dark field microscopy of scraping from lesion

        2) Blood work: if venereal disease research laboratory (VDRL) or rapid plasma reagin (RPR) are positive, more specific fluorescent treponemal antibody absorption (FTA-ABS) is performed; VDRL will remain positive for life after infection

        3) Immunofluorescent staining

  4. Nursing management

NCLEX!

      a. Medications include long-term IV and/or IM penicillin; weekly then monthly; dose depending on stage

      b. Educate client on cause of syphilis and potentially long duration of the infection

      c. Encourage client to use condoms during every episode of intercourse and to avoid sharing needles

NCLEX!

      d. Obtain names of sexual contacts for follow-up testing and treatment

      e. Instruct on need for compliance with follow-up testing and antibiotic treatment

      f. Assess if allergic to penicillin; educate on expected client experience with desensitization to penicillin in an intensive care unit if penicillin-allergic

D. Herpes

  1. Overview

NCLEX!

      a. Defined as a common STD involving the transmission of herpes virus

      b. Second most common viral STD (*human papilloma* virus or HPV is most common)

NCLEX!

      c. Two types

        1) HSV1 is more likely to be present orally

        2) HSV2 more likely to cause genital infection

NCLEX!

      d. Cause: sexual transmission, blood borne; and mother to fetus during delivery

2. Pathophysiology

a. Retrovirus, infection develops at site of viral entry into the body, virus will travel along dermatome to nerve root and remain dormant there until next outbreak, which will occur at the same site as the primary lesion

b. Transmission can occur during genital contact, oral-genital contact, or digital contact after contact with lesions

c. Asymptomatic viral shedding also occurs

d. Incubation period ranges from 1 to 26 days

e. Reactivation occurs at any time; vesicles will reappear

f. Reactivation is often caused by physical or emotional stress; hormone changes

g. Signs and symptoms

   1) Primary infection symptoms: extremely painful blisters which progress to crater-like lesions lasting up to 3 weeks, malaise, enlarged groin nodes, low-grade temperature

   2) Recurrent infection: extremely painful blisters progressing to crater-like lesions that heal within 10 days

h. Complications include meningitis, encephalitis, arthritis, hepatitis, prostatitis, neonatal transmission can occur transplacentally if primary infection occurs during pregnancy or birth while in primary stage or during recurrent infection, causing systemic neonatal herpes, which has high morbidity (from CNS involvement) and mortality

3. Nursing assessment

a. Assessment

   1) Obtain sexual history including unprotected intercourse or oral-genital intercourse with partner having oral herpes lesions ("cold sores"), onset and severity of symptoms, and known exposure to herpes

   2) Assess vital signs

   3) Symptom analysis of pain

b. Diagnostic tests

   1) Cultures

   2) Diagnosed primarily by symptoms and physical examination

4. Nursing management

a. Medications include: oral antiviral medications: acyclovir (Zovirax) or valacyclovir HCL (Valtrex) started with diagnosis for primary infection, or with onset of symptoms with recurrence; valacyclovir HCL may be used for suppressive therapy

b. Client education

   1) Transmission of herpes simplex virus infections

   2) Appropriate use of medications prescribed

NCLEX!

c. Encourage client with primary infection to report headache or stiff neck immediately

d. Instruct client with urinary hesitancy to run water while trying to void or pour warm water over the perineum or glans of penis

---

Case Study

T. J. is a 45-year-old client that has been diagnosed with prostate cancer. He will be having abdominal prostatectomy surgery next week for the condition.

❶ How should the nurse describe the expected client experience with this surgery?

❷ T. J. asks the nurse how the doctor determines if the cancer has spread beyond the prostate gland. How should the nurse reply?

❸ T. J. asks why his surgery will be abdominal when his 82-year-old uncle had transurethral surgery. What is a correct answer?

❹ Describe the treatments T. J. will most likely undergo after recovering from his surgery.

❺ The pathology report indicates that T. J.'s cancer is stage 3. Describe what this means.

For suggested responses, see page 568.

Posttest

1 When triaging in the clinic, which client should be seen first? The client with:

(1) Genital herpes infection diagnosed yesterday, with a severe headache.
(2) Recurrent herpes infections for 3 years, with burning during urination.
(3) Chlamydia diagnosed yesterday, now with worsening pelvic pain.
(4) Secondary syphilis diagnosed last month, due for penicillin injection.

2 Which of the following statements should be presented in a breast cancer detection for the community?

(1) Mammograms should be started at age 50.
(2) Self-breast exams should be performed weekly.
(3) Birth control pills may prevent breast cancer.
(4) Estrogen replacement may increase breast cancer risk.

3 The client with benign prostatic hyperplasia has undergone transurethral resection of the prostate (TURP) and is asking why he needs continuous bladder irrigation (CBI). The nurse's best response would be:

(1) "The irrigation prevents blood from clotting and blocking the catheter."
(2) "Your bladder needs to be kept full to promote healing after this surgery."
(3) "The urine would be very concentrated without the irrigation."
(4) "The saline running through the bladder helps keep you hydrated."

4 Teaching for the client with endometriosis undergoing leuprolide (Lupron) therapy is effective when she states:

(1) "I may have cold hands and feet while taking this medication."
(2) "It's possible that I'll be heat intolerant while taking these shots."
(3) "My voice may become higher during this therapy."
(4) "Hot flashes are likely while I am taking these shots."

5 Which client is at the highest risk for developing banalitis?

(1) 1-year-old with intact foreskin
(2) Circumcised 40-year-old
(3) 12-year-old with intact foreskin
(4) Circumcised 6-year-old

6 Which client is at lowest risk for developing breast cancer?

(1) Client with BRCA1 gene mutation
(2) Client who had Hodgkin's disease
(3) Client who had first child at age 18, breastfed for 2 years
(4) Client who is a smoker, age 74

7 Female clients with *Chlamydia trachomatis* infections will most likely present with which signs and symptoms?

(1) Painful perineal blisters and sudden high fever
(2) Painless crater-like lesion on the labia that lasts 6 weeks
(3) Rapidly progressing pruritic rash on labia and buttocks
(4) Yellow-green vaginal discharge, dyspareunia, pelvic pain

8 The client with a new diagnosis of genital herpes simplex virus 1 (HSV1) wants to know how she contracted the infection. The nurse's best answer is based on which of the following?

(1) Inanimate objects can harbor HSV1 for several hours
(2) HSV1 is found only in the genital tract and not orally
(3) Sexual contact is the most common mode of transmission
(4) Immune system suppression is needed to contract the infection

9 The client with benign prostatic hyperplasia (BPH) may experience a sudden onset of urinary retention after doing which of the following?

(1) Drinking several cups of coffee in the morning
(2) Having a weekend of binge drinking
(3) Starting a multivitamin supplement
(4) Walking farther than he usually does

10 The client with multiple subserosal uterine myomas for which of the following?

(1) Uterine enlargement, urinary frequency, and pelvic pressure
(2) Uterine enlargement, pain with urination, and vaginal discharge
(3) Uterine atrophy, heavy and painful menses, and decreased libido
(4) Uterine atrophy, pain with intercourse, and vaginal dryness

See pages 368–369 for Answers and Rationales.

Answers and Rationales

Pretest

1 Answer: 2 *Rationale:* Balanitis, or inflammation of the foreskin and prepuce, would cause edema and pain of the penile glans, leading to dysuria. Option 1 is inappropriate for balanitis; a urethral discharge (option 3) may occur in gonorrhea; back pain (option 4) could indicate many diseases, but not balanitis.
Cognitive Level: Application
Nursing Process: Assessment; *Test Plan:* PHYS

2 Answer: 4 *Rationale:* Prostatitis creates pain in the tissues surrounding the prostate gland. Option 1 indicates a gonococcal infection; option 2 herpes virus; and option 3 syphilis (secondary stage).
Cognitive Level: Application
Nursing Process: Assessment; *Test Plan:* PHYS

3 Answer: 1 *Rationale:* Secondary syphilis begins with the healing of the chancre, and ends when the rash disappears, which can take up to 6 months from time of infection. The latent stage of syphilis then starts, which can last for years. VDRL and RPR would need to be positive for syphilis (option 2); option 3 could indicate TB or HIV; option 4 are signs and symptoms of nongonococcal infections in females.
Cognitive Level: Application
Nursing Process: Assessment; *Test Plan:* PHYS

4 Answer: 3 *Rationale:* Hypospadias repair is undertaken using the foreskin to create a channel through the penis to the tip of the glans so that he will deposit his sperm near his partner's cervix. Although option 1 may also be an appropriate answer, it is not the best answer to demonstrate effective teaching. Options 2 and 4 are incorrect.
Cognitive Level: Application
Nursing Process: Evaluation; *Test Plan:* HPM

5 Answer: 4 *Rationale:* DUB most commonly results from a progesterone deficiency that causes a fragile endometrium that fails to mature from proliferative stage to secretory. This causes irregular menstrual bleeding. Treatment is aimed at correcting the cause, thus progesterone supplementation is prescribed.
Cognitive Level: Application
Nursing Process: Analysis; *Test Plan:* PHYS

6 Answer: 1 *Rationale:* Douching should be avoided in order to prevent bacteria present in the lower reproductive tract from being forced upwards into the uterus, potentially causing PID.
Cognitive Level: Application
Nursing Process: Implementation; *Test Plan:* PHYS

7 Answer: 3 *Rationale:* Chemotherapy and radiation used in the treatment of testicular cancer often cause a radically decreased sperm count. If the client desires children, he should consider sperm banking prior to beginning treatment.
Cognitive Level: Application
Nursing Process: Implementation; *Test Plan:* HPM

8 Answer: 4 *Rationale:* Caffeine can precipitate or worsen fibrocystic breast disease. No other dietary factors have been identified.
Cognitive Level: Application
Nursing Process: Assessment; *Test Plan:* HPM

9 Answer: 1 *Rationale:* Doxycycline (Vibra-tabs) is a commonly utilized treatment for chlamydia infections, and like all antibiotics must be taken until the medication is gone. Use of condoms with every sexual encounter decreases the transmission of sexually transmitted diseases. Sexual contacts should be notified of the infection so that appropriate testing can be obtained. This is especially important with Chlamydia because it is so often asymptomatic in women, and early detection can prevent complications such as pelvic inflammatory disease. Testicular self-exam is screening for testicular cancer, not diagnosing.
Cognitive Level: Application
Nursing Process: Implementation; *Test Plan:* PHYS

10 Answer: 3 *Rationale:* Primary dysmenorrhea begins at menarche and is usually a lifelong condition. Options 1, 2, and 4 can occur with secondary dysmenorrhea or endometriosis.
Cognitive Level: Application
Nursing Process: Analysis; *Test Plan:* PHYS

Posttest

1 Answer: 1 *Rationale:* The primary genital herpes infection involves systemic viremia, and encephalitis is a possible complication. Headache and stiff neck may indicate encephalitis, and requires further investigation.
Cognitive Level: Analysis
Nursing Process: Planning; *Test Plan:* PHYS

2 Answer: 4 *Rationale:* Breast cancer detection begins with monthly self-breast exams. Mammograms should be performed yearly after age 40. Birth control pills do not increase or decrease breast cancer risk, but the longer a woman is on estrogen replacement therapy, the greater her risk for developing the disease.
Cognitive Level: Application
Nursing Process: Implementation; *Test Plan:* HPM

3 Answer: 1 *Rationale:* Continuous bladder irrigation serves to flush out the blood that will be oozing from the raw edges of the TURP site before the blood can clot. Clots in the bladder would obstruct the urine flow through the catheter.
Cognitive Level: Application
Nursing Process: Implementation; *Test Plan:* PHYS

4 Answer: 4 *Rationale:* Lupron is a synthetic analog of luteinizing hormone releasing hormone, and acts as an estrogen antagonist, causing the endometriosis deposits to shrink in size, thus decreasing the pain and infertility associated with endometriosis. Hot flashes and night sweats are common side effects while on the medication, and resolve upon discontinuation of the medication.
Cognitive Level: Application
Nursing Process: Evaluation. *Test Plan:* PHYS

5 Answer: 3 *Rationale:* Balanitis, inflammation of the foreskin, occurs due to poor hygiene, and occurs after the foreskin becomes retractable (at about age 3). Options 2 and 4 are incorrect because of the circumcision.
Cognitive Level: Analysis
Nursing Process: Assessment; *Test Plan:* HPM

6 Answer: 3 *Rationale:* Early childbearing with breastfeeding for a total of 2 years or more decreases a woman's lifetime risk of developing breast cancer. BRCA1 or BRCA2 gene mutations increase risk. Hodgkin's disease treatment usually involves chest radiation, which increases breast cancer risk and breast cancer mortality. Aging is another factor: the older a woman becomes, the more likely she is to develop breast cancer.
Cognitive Level: Analysis
Nursing Process: Analysis; *Test Plan:* HPM

7 Answer: 4 *Rationale:* Chlamydia, although often silent and asymptomatic, will eventually present symptoms including new occurrence of dysparunia, dysmenorrhea, low abdominal and pelvic pain, with yellow or yellow-green vaginal discharge.
Cognitive Level: Application
Nursing Process: Analysis; *Test Plan:* PHYS

8 Answer: 3 *Rationale:* HSV1 does not survive more than a few minutes on inanimate objects, and although it is often a genital tract infection it does occur orally. Sexual contact is the most likely method of transmission, and persons with intact immune systems can easily be infected.
Cognitive Level: Application
Nursing Process: Analysis; *Test Plan:* PHYS

9 Answer: 2 *Rationale:* BPH patients may be asymptomatic until large alcohol intake, which relaxes the bladder sphincter, making it impossible to empty the bladder.
Cognitive Level: Application
Nursing Process: Assessment; *Test Plan:* PHYS

10 Answer: 1 *Rationale:* Subserosal uterine myomas are located on the outer surface of the uterus and tend to cause fewer menstrual disorders than submucosal or intramural myomas. However, they do cause mechanical pressure on the pelvic contents from their size and weight, including bladder pressure that results in urinary frequency and urgency.
Cognitive Level: Analysis
Nursing Process: Assessment; *Test Plan:* PHYS

References

American Cancer Society's Cancer Resource Center (1998). Retrieved July 7, 2001 from http://www3.cancer.org/cancerinfo.

Deglin, J. & Vallerand, A. (2001). *Drug guide for nurses* (7th ed.). Philadelphia: F. A. Davis.

Endo-online, the Voice of the Endometriosis Association (2001). Retrieved July 7, 2001 from http://www.endometriosisassn.org/endo.html.

Gonorrhea Fact Sheet. Center for Disease Control and Prevention, National Center for Infectious Diseases, Bacterial STD Branch of the Division of AIDS, STD, and TB Laboratory Research. Retrieved July 8, 2001 from http://www.cdc.gov/ncidod/dastlr/gcdir/gono.html.

LeMone, P. & Burke, K. (2000). *Medical-surgical nursing: Critical thinking in client care* (2nd ed.). Upper Saddle River, NJ: Prentice Hall, pp. 1972, 2048, 2054–2071, 2076–2092.

Lowdermilk, D., Perry, S., & Boback, I. (2000) *Maternity and women's health care* (7th ed.). St. Louis, MO: Mosby, Inc.

McKinney, E., Ashwill, J., Murray, S., James, S., Gorrie, T., & Droske, S. (2000). *Maternal-child nursing.* Philadelphia: W. B. Saunders Company.

National Institute of Health Pelvic Inflammatory Disease Fact Sheet (1998) Retrieved July 7, 2001 from National Institute of Allergy and Infectious Disease website: http://www.niaid.nih.gov/factsheets/stdpid.htm.

Office on Women's Health in the Department of Health and Human Services. *Uterine fibroids.* Retrieved July 5, 2001: http://womenshealth.about.com/library/blfibfaqs.htm.

O'Hara Smith, N. (2001). *Testicular cancer: The pathology report.* Retrieved on July 7, 2001 from Testicular Cancer Resource Center website: http://www.acor.org/TCRC/pathology_report.html.

Pilliteri, A. (1999). *Maternal and child health nursing* (3rd ed.). Philadelphia: Lippincott.

Prostate Cancer (1999). Retrieved July 7, 2001 from Comprehensive Cancer Center of University of Michigan website: http://www.cancer.med.umich.edu/prostcan/staginginfo.htm.

Prostate Enlargement: Benign Prostatic Hyperplasia. (1999) Retrieved July 6, 2001 from National Kidney and Urologic Diseases Information Clearinghouse of the National institute for Health: http://www.niddk.nih.gov/health/urolog/pubs/prostate/#common.

Prostate.org. (2000). Retrieved July 6, 2001 from Prostatitis Foundation website: http://www.prostatitis.org.

Shannon, M., Wilson, B. A., & Stang, C. (1999). *Drug guide: Health professionals edition.* Stamford, CT: Appleton & Lange.

U.S. Department of Health and Human Services, Public Health Service, Centers for Disease Control and Prevention Division of STD Prevention. (1998) *Sexually transmitted disease surveillance, 1997.* Atlanta, GA.

U.S. Preventive Services Task Force, U.S. Department of Health and Human Services, Office of Disease Prevention and Health Promotion. *Guide to Clinical Preventive Services,* (2nd ed.). Genital Herpes Simplex. (1996). Retrieved July 6, 2001 from http://cpmcnet.columbia.edu/texts/gcps/gcps0040.html

Wilson, B., Shannon, M., & Stang, C. (2001). *Nursing drug guide 2001.* Upper Saddle River, NJ: Prentice Hall, pp. 699–701, 783–784, 1181.

CHAPTER 12

Immunological Health Problems

Mical De Brow, RN, PhD

CHAPTER OUTLINE

OBJECTIVES

▮ Define key terms associated with immunological health problems.

▮ Identify risk factors associated with the development of immunological health problems.

▮ Discuss the common etiologies of immunological health problems.

▮ Describe the pathophysiologic processes associated with specific immunological health problems.

▮ Distinguish between normal and abnormal immunological findings obtained from nursing assessment.

▮ Prioritize nursing interventions associated with specific immunological health problems.

[Media Link]

Use the CD-ROM enclosed with this text, or log onto the address given to access the free, interactive Companion Website created for this series. The CD-ROM and Companion Website accompanying this book offer additional practice opportunities and information—NCLEX Review, Case Studies, Glossary, In Depth with NCLEX, and more.

www.prenhall.com/hogan

REVIEW AT A GLANCE

acquired immunodeficiency syndrome (AIDS) *disease syndrome characterized by infection with human immunodeficiency virus (HIV) and opportunistic infections or neoplasms*

allergen *substance, foreign protein, or cell capable of causing alterations in sensitivity*

antibody *immune or protective protein, evoked by an antigen; capable of reacting with a certain antigen*

antigen *substance that as a result of coming in contact with certain tissues induces a state of sensitivity or resistance*

autoimmune disorders *disorders resulting when one's own tissues are subject to the destructive effects of the immune system*

cell-mediated immune response *the immune system response to antigens, which do not evoke the antibody-mediated*

response because they live inside the body's cells (viruses and mycobacterium are examples of such antigens)

cytokines *agents of the lymphoid system (interferons and interleukins) that act to modify the body's response to cancerous cells; they may also be cytotoxic*

graft-versus-host disease (GvHD) *frequent and potentially fatal complication of bone marrow transplant; grafted tissue recognizes host tissue as foreign and mounts a cell-mediated immune response*

humoral immune response *antibody-mediated immune response produced by B-lymphocytes*

hypersensitivity *altered immune response in a client that results in harm to the client*

immunodeficiency *the state in which the client's immune system is incompetent or unable to respond effectively*

immunotherapy *natural and/or synthetic substances used to stimulate or suppress the response of the immune system*

latex allergy *allergic response to latex; common in healthcare workers and others who routinely use latex gloves as barrier protection*

lymphocytes *small, nondescript cells which account for 20 to 40 percent of circulating leukocytes; they are the principal effector and regulator cells of the specific immune response*

macrophage *mature monocytes that actively phagocytize large foreign particles and cell debris*

opportunistic disease *any infection resulting from a deficient immune system*

viral load *the number of circulating human immunodeficiency virus (HIV) particles per milliliter*

Pretest

1 M. J. comes into the Emergency Department and is admitted to the floor because of symptoms of pneumonia. He has not been getting any better and has not responded well to prescription antibiotics. His culture and sensitivity (C & S) for sputum returns, as does his chest x-ray (CXR) with the conclusion that he has *Pneumocystis carinii* pneumonia. The nurse should conclude that he:

(1) Is positive for human immunodeficiency virus (HIV).
(2) Has acquired immunodeficiency syndrome (AIDS).
(3) Has tuberculosis (TB).
(4) Has an infection of unknown origin.

2 A child who contracts chickenpox at age 5 has developed which type of immunity?

(1) Active acquired, natural
(2) Passive acquired, natural
(3) Passive acquired, artificial
(4) Active acquired, artificial

3 A person who is HIV-positive starts to exhibit signs of AIDS. The indication that the client has seroconverted would be partially diagnosed by which of the following?

(1) Low viral load
(2) High CD4 count
(3) High white blood count (WBC)
(4) High viral load

4 A sexually active teenager with flu-like symptoms is given an ELISA test that returns negative. The physician informs her that another ELISA test will be conducted in several weeks. The client wants to know why. The best explanation is that:

(1) The first test may be inaccurate.
(2) The antibodies do not always show up initially.
(3) The test is sensitive and can give false positives.
(4) It is standard practice.

5 A client experiences an anaphylactic reaction after taking an antibiotic for the first time. The results of this Type I hypersensitivity response are caused by:

(1) A histamine precursor causing anaphylaxis.
(2) Antigen-IgE-mast cell interaction.
(3) Cell-mediated response.
(4) Massive numbers of destroyed red blood cells.

6 A client who has recently been diagnosed with diabetes mellitus (DM) Type 1 asks the nurse how she developed this because no one in her family is a diabetic. The nurses' best response is, "DM is an autoimmune disease characterized by:

(1) Failure of the immune system to recognize self."
(2) Exacerbations and remissions."
(3) Accelerated production of killer T cells."
(4) Immunosuppression and altered cortisol levels."

7 A mother of twins calls the office and speaks to the nurse concerning a rash that has developed on both children since taking an antibiotic prescribed 5 days ago. The nurse knows that this is most likely a:

(1) Type I hypersensitivity reaction.
(2) Type II hypersensitivity reaction.
(3) Type III hypersensitivity reaction.
(4) Type IV hypersensitivity reaction.

8 In working with clients with HIV, the nurse knows that the illness is more difficult to manage once AIDS has been diagnosed. Which of the following best characterizes HIV disease?

(1) Individuals who test positive are carriers and considered contagious.
(2) Clinical manifestations have a characteristic and predictable sequence.
(3) The HIV virus invades cells primarily via the bloodstream.
(4) Symptoms result from opportunistic pathology.

9 Which of the following individuals is at highest risk of contact with HIV? An individual who:

(1) Counsels HIV victims and their families.
(2) Works with athletes who perspire a lot.
(3) Collects blood donations via a mobile blood unit.
(4) Performs physicals involving an ELISA test for insurance companies.

10 A client is brought to the Emergency Department after taking a dose of penicillin. Which of the following diagnoses is the highest priority in this client who is demonstrating anaphylaxis?

(1) Ineffective airway clearance
(2) Decreased cardiac output
(3) Risk for injury
(4) Anxiety

See page 395 for Answers and Rationales.

I. Risk Factors for Immunological Health Problems

A. Overview

1. Immunity is the specific response of the body to invasion by microorganisms and foreign protein and, with the other defenses of the body, constitutes an essential protective mechanism

2. The immune system is a complex network of specialized cells and organs that defend the body against attack from foreign pathogens

3. The major **lymphocytes** (a white blood cell [WBC] accounting for 20 to 30 percent of total count) involved in protecting the body against potential infections are B and T cells, which also play an important role in combating tumor growth

4. The cells of the immune system patrol the tissues and organs through both blood and lymphatic vessels

5. Immune system functions

   a. Defending and protecting the body from infection by bacteria, viruses, fungi, and parasites

   b. Removing and destroying damaged or dead cells

   c. Identifying and destroying malignant cells, thereby preventing their development into tumors

6. Immune system components

   a. The human blood is made up of red blood cells (erythrocytes) that transport oxygen, platelets (thrombocytes) that trigger clotting, and white blood cells (leukocytes), which are an important element of the immune system that defend the human body against attack from foreign pathogens

   b. White blood cells (WBCs) originate in the bone marrow from hemocytoblasts (stem cells) that give rise to lymphoid and myeloid stem cells (see Figure 12-1)

      1) *Leukocytes:* white blood cells (WBCs)—are the principal cells involved in the immune response; the normal number of leukocytes is 4,000 to 10,000 cells per cubic millimeter of blood

      2) *Granulocytes* compose 60 to 80 percent of the total number of normal blood leukocytes; have a relatively short life span (hours to days) and are the key defenders in protecting the body from harmful microorganisms during acute inflammation and infection; there are three types

         a) Neutrophils or polymorphonuclear leukocytes (or polys) make up the largest percentage (55 to 70); are phagocytic (responsible for engulfing and destroying pathogens) and arrive first at the site of invasion (because of the release of chemical triggers from damaged tissues and invading pathogens)

         b) Eosinophils account for 1 to 4 percent of the total number of circulating leukocytes; mature in bone marrow shortly before they are released into the circulation where they are very short-lived; are less efficient phagocytic cells than neutrophils; are commonly found in higher numbers in the respiratory and gastrointestinal tracts

         c) Basophils constitute about 0.5 to 1.0 percent of the circulating leukocytes; not phagocytic; granules within basophils contain proteins and chemicals such as heparin, histamine, bradykinin, serotonin, and a slow-reacting substance of anaphylaxis (leukotrienes); these substances are released into the bloodstream during an acute **hypersensitivity** (abnormally sensitive to a stimulus) reaction or stress response

      3) *Monocytes and macrophages*

         a) Monocytes are the largest of the leukocytes and compose 2 to 3 percent of the total circulating leukocytes; released from the bone marrow and circulate for 1 to 2 days before they attach to various tissues where they remain for months to years before they are activated

NCLEX!

Figure 12-1

Production and differentiation of leukocytes from hemocytoblasts.

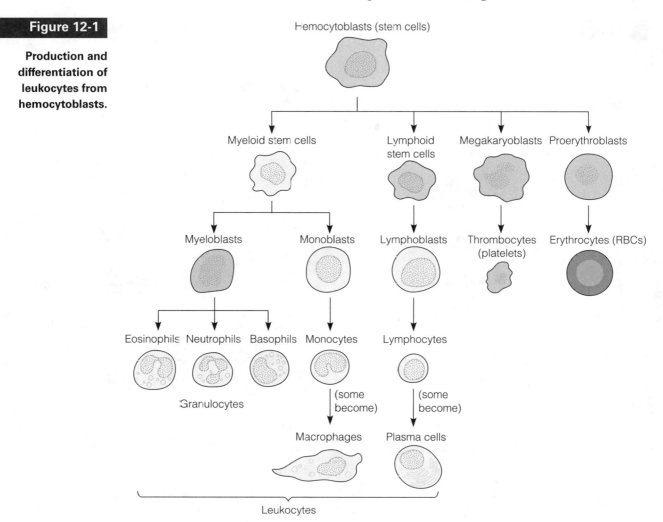

Hemocytoblasts (stem cells)

Myeloid stem cells   Lymphoid stem cells   Megakaryoblasts   Proerythroblasts

Myeloblasts   Monoblasts   Lymphoblasts   Thrombocytes (platelets)   Erythrocytes (RBCs)

Eosinophils Neutrophils Basophils   Monocytes   Lymphocytes

Granulocytes

(some become)   (some become)

Macrophages   Plasma cells

Leukocytes

    b) Monocytes mature into **macrophages** (mature monocytes which actively phagocytize large foreign particles and cell debris) after settling into the tissues

    c) Both types are actively phagocytic with the capacity to engulf large foreign particles and cell debris

    d) Monocytes and macrophages are particularly important in the fight against chronic infections such as viral infections, tuberculosis, and certain intracellular parasitic infections

4) Lymphocytes are small cells that account for 20 to 40 percent of the circulating lymphocytes; are the principal effectors and regulators of the specific immune response (see Figure 12-2)

    a) Monitor the body for cancerous cells in a process known as immune surveillance

    b) Lymphocytes constantly circulate, but in a homing pattern return to lymphoid tissues

Figure 12-2

Development and differentiation of lymphocytes from lymphoblast in bone marrow.

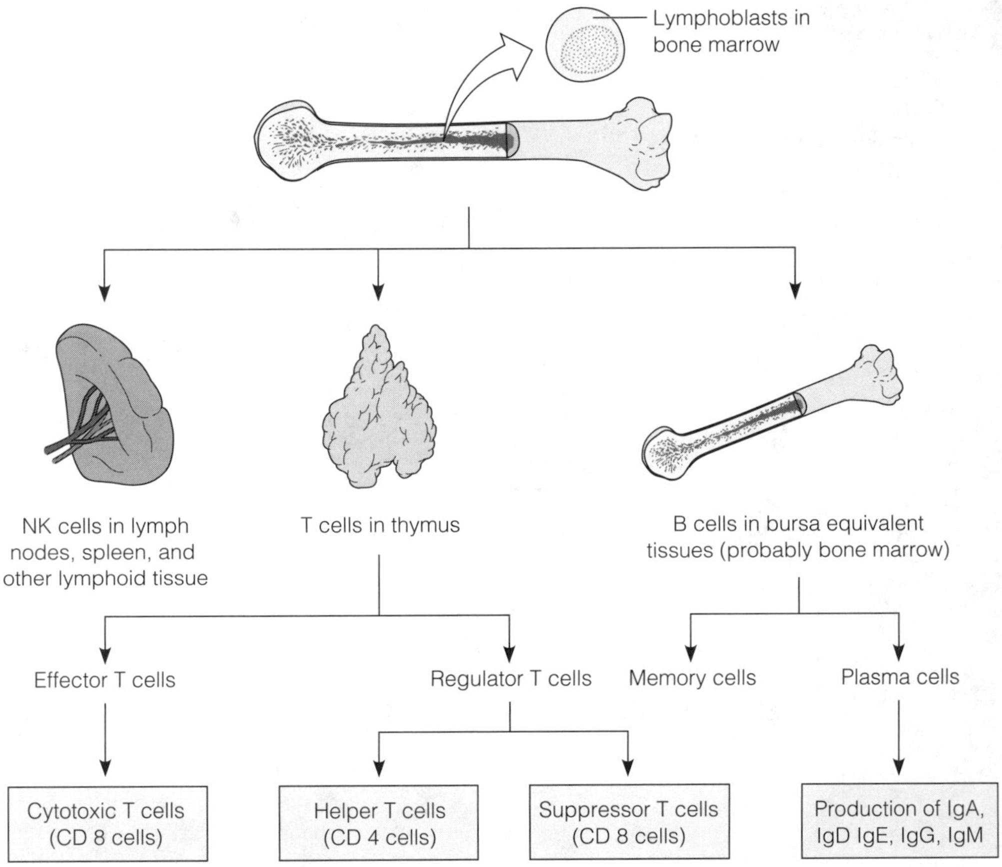

Lymphoblasts in bone marrow

NK cells in lymph nodes, spleen, and other lymphoid tissue

T cells in thymus

B cells in bursa equivalent tissues (probably bone marrow)

Effector T cells

Regulator T cells

Memory cells

Plasma cells

Cytotoxic T cells (CD 8 cells)

Helper T cells (CD 4 cells)

Suppressor T cells (CD 8 cells)

Production of IgA, IgD IgE, IgG, IgM

c) On contact with an **antigen** (substance capable of producing a specific immune response), lymphocytes are activated and mature into either effector cells (plasma cells or cytotoxic cells), which are instrumental in the destruction of antigens, or memory cells

NCLEX!

d) Memory cells activate immediately upon subsequent exposure to the same antigen; are responsible for providing acquired immunity

e) There are three types of lymphocytes: T lymphocytes (T cells), B lymphocytes (B cells), and natural killer cells (NK cells)

f) T and B cells are integral to the specific immune response

g) NK cells are large, granular cells found in the spleen, lymph nodes, bone marrow, and blood that provide immune surveillance and resistance to infection, and play an important role in the destruction of early malignant cells

7. The lymphoid system

   a. Lymphocytes concentrate in lymphoid tissues, which include the lymph nodes, spleen, thymus, tonsils, lymphoid tissue scattered in connective tissues and mucosa, and the bone marrow

   b. The thymus and bone marrow, in which T and B cells mature, are considered primary lymphoid organs

NCLEX!

c. The spleen, lymph nodes, tonsils, and other peripheral lymphoid tissues are considered secondary lymphoid organs

1) Lymph nodes are the most numerous of the lymphoid tissues and are distributed throughout the body as small round or bean-shaped nodules that vary in size from 1 mm to 2 cm, which filter foreign products or antigens from the lymph, storing and supporting proliferation of the lymphocytes and macrophages

   a) Lymph, a clear, protein filled fluid is transported by the lymph vessels

   b) The presence of a foreign protein stimulates lymphocytes and macrophages to proliferate in the lymph nodes

2) The spleen, the largest lymphoid organ in the body, is the only part of the system able to filter blood

   a) Located in the upper-left quadrant of the abdomen

   b) Composed of white pulp, which serves as a site for lymphocyte proliferation and immune surveillance

   c) B cells predominate in the white pulp; blood filtration occurs in the red pulp

   d) The spleen also stores blood and the breakdown products of red blood cells (RBCs) for future use

   e) The spleen is not essential for life; when removed or damaged, the liver and bone marrow assume its functions

3) The thymus gland is located in the superior anterior mediastinal cavity beneath the sternum

   a) It reaches maximum size at puberty and begins to atrophy slowly; in the adult, it is difficult to differentiate from other tissue

   b) The main function of the thymus is to serve as a site for the maturation and differentiation of the T cells

   c) Thymosin, an immunoregulatory hormone, stimulates lymphopoiesis, the formation of lymphocytes or lymphoid tissue

4) Bone marrow is soft tissue found in the hollow cavity of long bones, as well as the flat bones of the skull, sternum, ribs, and vertebrae; produces and stores stem cells (from which all cellular components of the blood are derived)

5) Lymphoid tissues are also located at key sites of potential invasion by microorganisms: the genitourinary, respiratory, and gastrointestinal tracts

8. Bodily response

   a. Nonspecific inflammatory response: when first-line defenses are breached, the resulting damage or invasion produces a nonspecific immune response known as inflammation

b. Specific immune response: the specific immune response occurs with the introduction of foreign substances, or antigens, into the body; the immune response has the following properties:

1) Typically directed against materials recognized as foreign and is not usually directed against the self (because of self-recognition)

2) The response is specific; it is initiated by and directed against particular antigens

3) Response is systemic, not localized

4) The immune response has memory; repeated exposures to an antigen produce a more rapid response

5) Recognition of self: the effectiveness of the immune system depends on its ability to differentiate normal host tissue from abnormal or foreign tissue

  a) The body's components have antigenic properties that are unique and are recognized by the immune system as self

  b) External agents have antigenic properties which are identified by the immune system as non-self

9. Antigens

NCLEX!

  a. Antigens are substances recognized as foreign or non-self and provoke a specific immune response when introduced into the body

  b. Typically, antigens are large protein molecules although other substances (polysaccharides, polypeptides, and nucleic acids) may be antigenic

NCLEX!

  c. Other antigens include transplanted tissue or organs; incompatible blood cells, vaccines, pollen, egg white, and toxins such as snake or bee venom

  d. When an antigen is introduced into the body, it is recognized by a specific receptor on a lymphocyte and an immune response is initiated

B. Humoral immune response

NCLEX!

1. Humoral immune response is defined as an antibody-mediated immune response produced by B lymphocytes

2. Antigens such as bacteria, bacterial toxins, and free viruses usually activate B cells to produce **antibodies** (immune or protective protein evoked by an antigen)

3. The antibody mediated response is characterized by:

  a. Phagocytosis of the antigen by neutrophils

  b. Precipitation: combining of soluble antigens to form insoluble forms (precipitates)

  c. Neutralization: combining with a toxin to neutralize its effects; followed by destruction by phagocytosis

  d. Lysis of antigen cell membrane

  e. Agglutination or clumping of antigens to form a noninvasive aggregate

f. Opsonization: coating of the antigen with antibodies and complement, making it more susceptible to phagocytosis

C. Cell-mediated immune response

1. Cell-mediated immune response is defined as the immune system response to antigens that do not evoke the antibody-mediated response because they live inside the body's cells (viruses and mycobacterium are examples of such antigens)

2. Antigens, such as viral infected cells, cancer cells, and foreign tissue, activate T cells, which are the primary agent of the cell-mediated [cellular] response

3. T cells are antigen specific and are much more complex than B cells

a. Killer T cells bind with cell surface antigens on infected or foreign cells and then either destroy the cell membrane or release cytotoxic substances into the cell

b. Regulator T cells, the majority of which are T helper cells (CD4 cells), play a key role in controlling the immune response by:

1) Stimulating proliferation of other T cells

2) Amplifying the cytotoxic activity of killer T cells

3) Activating B cells to proliferate and differentiate

4) Interacting directly with B cells to promote their conversion into plasma cells capable of producing antibodies

c. The other regulatory T cells (suppressor T cells) provide negative feedback, making the immune response a self-limiting process; they are also important in preventing autoimmune disorders

d. T cells synthesize and release lymphokines, which stimulate:

1) B cells to become plasma cells and produce antibodies

2) Macrophages to become activated macrophages (the most aggressive phagocyte)

3) The proliferation of killer T cells

D. The processes of antibody-mediated and cell-mediated immunity result in the development of acquired immunity or active immunity

1. *Active immunity* occurs when the body produces antibodies or develops immune lymphocytes against specific antigens

a. Memory cells, which can produce an immediate immune response on re-exposure to the antigen, provide long-term immunity

b. Active immunity can be *naturally acquired* resulting from contact with the disease-producing antigen and subsequent development of the disease; this is common for diseases such as chickenpox and hepatitis A

c. Active immunity can be *artificially acquired* through immunization or vaccinations

2. *Passive immunity* provides temporary protection against disease-producing antigens

    a. *Naturally acquired* passive immunity is provided by the transfer of maternal antibodies via the placenta and breast milk to the infant

    b. *Artificially acquired* passive immunity is provided by immune globulins and serums

E. Risk factors

1. Allergies: inherited or acquired sensitivity with repeated exposures; diseases (asthma, AIDS, immunodeficient states); individuals in contact with venomous animals; environment

2. Latex allergy: acquired sensitivity with repeated exposures, employees required to use gloves often (healthcare professionals, rescue workers, firefighters, police officers, food service, housekeeping staff, etc.); clients identifying atopic conditions; spina bifida clients; clients with a history of multiple surgeries when young

3. Anaphylaxis: history of known allergens; injection of antigenic material (allergy shots, serum from a sensitized animal); children receiving immunizations; exercise; blood transfusion

4. Acquired immunodeficiency syndrome (AIDS): healthcare professionals (contact, blood products, needle sticks); homosexual practice; homeless state; blood transfusion; intravenous drug abusers; link to sexually transmitted diseases

II. Allergies

A. Overview

1. An allergy is defined as an abnormal response of the immune system to an **allergen** (substance, foreign protein or cell, capable of causing alterations in sensitivity)

2. When the antigen is environmental or external it is called an allergy, and the antigen is referred to as an allergen

3. Hypersensitivity reactions are classified by the type of immune response that occurs on contact and may also be classified by timing of the response

    a. Anaphylaxis and transfusion reactions are examples of immediate hypersensitivity reactions

    b. Contact dermatitis is a typical delayed reaction

4. Allergens are introduced by contact, inhalation, or ingestion

5. Causes are numerous and include plants, animals, chemicals, molds, grasses, trees, pests, dust, food, drugs, latex, cosmetics, and perfumes

B. Pathophysiology

1. An initial contact or exposure to an allergen is required to produce sensitization

2. Following sensitization, subsequent contact with the allergen produces symptoms; this may occur with the next contact or years later

3. Classified as four types of hypersensitivity responses

a. *Type I* or *IgE-mediated hypersensitivity reaction*

1) Produces an immediate reaction; local or systemic

2) Examples are: immediate—allergic asthma, allergic rhinitis (hayfever), allergic conjunctivitis, and hives; rapid—anaphylactic

3) Occurs when an allergen interacts with IgE bound to mast cells and basophils; this complex prompts release of histamine and other chemicals such as complement, acetylcholine, kinins, and chemotactic factors

4) The histamine is responsible for most of the inflammatory symptoms: peripheral vasodilatation, increased vascular permeability, vascular congestion, and edema

5) The leukotrienes and **cytokines** (agents of the lymphoid system that act to modify the body's response to cancerous cells) involve the T lymphocytes, monocytes, eosinophils, and neutrophils, producing symptoms of contraction of smooth muscle causing bronchiolar constriction and edema

b. *Type II* or *cytotoxic hypersensitivity* reaction

1) Characterized by IgG or IgM type antibodies that react to foreign tissues or cells; are usually immediate responses

2) Examples include hemolytic transfusion reaction of an incompatible blood type or a drug reaction (where the drug forms an antigenic complex on the surface of a blood cell)

3) In this reaction, lysis of blood cells (platelets, erythrocytes, and leukocytes) occurs because of the activation of complement

4) Transfusion reactions: antibodies in the recipient's serum react against antigens in the donor's red blood cells

   a) Results in hemolysis of donor red blood cells, unconjugated bilirubin from the broken down hemoglobin, and precipitation of large amounts of hemoglobin

   b) Symptoms include fever, chills, low back pain, hypotension, tachycardia, nausea, vomiting, urticaria, red-colored urine, shock, and renal failure

5) Other conditions caused by a Type II reaction include erythroblastosis fetalis (Rh incompatibility in mother and child); autoimmune hemolytic anemia and drug induced hemolysis

c. *Type III* or *immune complex-mediated hypersensitivity* reaction

1) Results from the formation of IgG or IgM antibody-antigen complexes that circulate in the blood; are usually immediate responses

2) The complexes adhere to the walls of the vessels and cause inflammation and lead to intravascular, synovial, endocardial, or other organ complications

3) Examples include serum sickness, Arthus reactions, and autoimmune conditions

Practice to Pass

The physician suggests weekly allergy shots for a child with asthma caused by seasonal allergies. How should the nurse explain how the shots will work to the mother?

4) Symptoms are specific to the reaction: serum sickness—fever, joint and muscle pain, urticaria, rash; Arthus reaction—acute, localized edema, tissue inflammation

   d. *Type IV delayed hypersensitivity reaction*

   1) These reactions are cell-mediated rather than antibody-mediated involving T cells of the immune system

   2) Are delayed rather than immediate; with an onset 24 to 48 hours after exposure to the antigen

   3) Result from an exaggerated interaction between an antigen and normal cell-mediated mechanisms

   4) Examples include contact dermatitis, infections, granulomatous inflammation, autoimmune diseases, transplant or graft rejection

   5) Symptoms are specific to the type of response

      a) Contact dermatitis such as poison ivy: redness, induration, lesions, urticaria, weeping

      b) Positive TB skin testing: reddening and induration of > 5 mm at 72 hours

      c) Granulomatous inflammation: leprosy, syphilis, cat-scratch disease

4. Autoimmune disorders

   a. When the immune system's ability to recognize self is impaired and immune defenses are directed against normal host tissue, the result is an autoimmune disorder

   b. Can affect any tissue in the body; some are tissue- or organ-specific and some autoimmune disorders are systemic, with neither antibodies nor the inflammatory lesions confined to any one organ

   c. The mechanism that causes the immune system to recognize host tissue as a foreign antigen is not clear

   d. Known characteristics

   1) Genetics plays a role

   2) More prevalent in females than males

   3) The onset of an immune disorder is frequently associated with an abnormal stressor, either physical or psychological

   4) Are frequently progressive relapsing-remitting disorders characterized by periods of exacerbation and remission

5. Tissue transplants

   a. Transplant success is closely tied to obtaining the best match of tissue antigens to the recipient; an autograft (a transplant of the client's own tissue) is the most successful type of transplantation

   b. *Hyperacute tissue rejections* occur immediately or 2 to 3 days after the transplant of new tissue and are due to preformed antibodies and sensitized

T cells to antigens in the donor organ; this type of rejection is most likely to occur in individuals who have had previous organ or tissue transplants

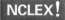

c. *Acute tissue rejection* is the most common and treatable type of rejection episode; it occurs between 4 days and 3 months following transplant

1) It is mediated primarily by the cellular immune response and results in transplant cell destruction

2) The client demonstrates manifestations of the inflammatory process, with fever, redness, swelling, and tenderness over the graft site

3) Signs of impaired function of the transplanted organ may be noted

d. *Chronic tissue rejection* occurs from 4 months to years after transplantation of new tissues or organs

1) It is likely the result of antibody-mediated immune response

2) Antibodies and complement deposit in transplanted tissue vessel walls resulting in decreased bloodflow and ischemia

e. **Graft-versus-host disease** (GvHD) is a frequent and potentially fatal complication of bone marrow transplantation

1) Defined as a disorder occurring when immunocompetent graft cells recognize host tissue as foreign and mount a cell-mediated immune response

2) The host is usually immunocompromised and unable to fight graft cells, and the host's cells are destroyed

3) Other areas affected are the skin, liver, and gastrointestinal tract

C. **Nursing assessment**

1. Assessment includes skin, vital signs (VS), lung sounds, respiratory status, level of consciousness (LOC), fluid status, peripheral perfusion (pulses, capillary refill, temperature of extremities); any complaints of discomfort; mental status (anxiety); history of events leading to allergic reaction

2. Diagnostic tests

a. WBC, high eosinophil level

b. Radioallergosorbent test (RAST), to determine presence of IgE

c. Type and crossmatch

d. Indirect Coombs' test; agglutination occurs if antibodies to an RBC antigen is present

e. Direct Coombs' test; antibodies are present on the client's RBCs

f. Immune complex assays, circulating immune complexes are present

g. Complement assay; complement levels are decreased

h. Skin testing

1) Skin prick test, positive test produces a wheal and erythema

2) Intradermal, wheal of 5 mm or greater and erythema

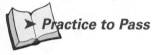

Practice to Pass

Explain in simple terminology how the body develops an autoimmune disease or rejects organ tissue.

3) Patch, mild to severe erythema with papules or vesicles

4) Food allergy testing, presence of symptoms within hours of eating the particular food thought to cause the reaction

D. Nursing management

1. Medications include **immunotherapy** (natural and/or synthetic substances used to stimulate or suppress the response of the immune system such as allergy shots), antihistamines, epinephrine for severe symptoms, cromolyn sodium (Nasalcrom) for allergic rhinitis and asthma, glucocorticoids, over-the-counter (OTC) nasal decongestants such as pseudoephedrine tablets

2. Goal is to minimize exposure, prevent a hypersensitivity response, and provide quick interventions if a response occurs

3. Clients should be instructed to wear a Medic-alert bracelet

4. Airway management is the highest priority if laryngeal edema occurs; administer oxygen; intubate or use nasopharyngeal/oropharyngeal airway if necessary

5. Other therapies consist of plasmapheresis (removal of components in the plasma)

6. Monitor VS

7. Access an intravenous (IV) line and administer fluids as necessary; use of a foley catheter and monitor intake and output (I & O) as indicated

8. Administer blood products following hospital protocol

   a. Have a signed informed consent

   b. Check the blood for type, Rh factor (Rh- must have Rh- and Rh+ must have Rh+), expiration date, crossmatch with another licensed healthcare professional

   c. Monitor VS every 5 minutes for the first 15 minutes and every 30 minutes thereafter until the blood has been infused

   d. Administer the blood with normal saline (NS) only

   e. Stop the transfusion if any reaction occurs, send the blood bag and tubing to the lab for analysis

9. Educate the client on having a bee sting kit or an Epi-pen available at all times

III. Latex Allergy

A. Overview

1. A **latex allergy** is defined as a reaction to contact with latex, producing an allergic contact dermatitis, immediate hypersensitivity, or anaphylaxis

2. Latex is extracted from the tissue beneath the bark of the rubber tree; it is a cloudy white liquid composed of rubber particles, protein, water, and other substances

3. The process used to process the latex affects the amount of protein left in the finished product

4. Produces a type I or type IV reaction

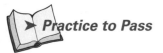

➤ Practice to Pass

Why should the nurse explain to the client who is scheduled for a skin prick test for allergies to avoid antihistamines for 3 days prior to the test?

NCLEX!

NCLEX!

NCLEX!

NCLEX!

5. Prevention of latex allergy reactions should focus on both the client and the staff

6. Causes of latex allergy include exposure through the cutaneous route (gloves, tapes, masks); mucous membranes (anesthesia, rectal examinations, eye and ear droppers); intrauterine devices; intravascular (IV fluids, injectables, IV devices); internal contact through surgery

B. Pathophysiology

1. An allergic reaction is triggered upon contact with the latex (see Section II, Allergies)

2. Reactions usually manifest in three ways

   a. Allergic contact dermatitis (type IV delayed hypersensitivity): most common

      1) An allergic reaction to the residues of the chemical agents used in latex and in manufacturing the plastics

      2) Symptoms include: dry, itchy red rash on the hands and fingers; blistering and weeping of skin; swelling

   b. Immediate hypersensitivity (type I)

      1) The natural latex protein produces an IgE response

      2) Can cause severe, even fatal reactions

      3) Symptoms develop within 5 to 30 minutes from exposure and diminish quickly when exposure removes

      4) Symptoms include immediate itching; intense swelling of fingers and hand; may proceed to anaphylaxis

   c. Anaphylaxis

      1) Occurs when there has been contact with latex through the mucous membranes or body cavities such as in surgery

      2) Symptoms include local or generalized itching; urticaria; angioedema; rhinitis; conjunctivitis; asthma; extreme anxiety; gastrointestinal (GI) complaints (nausea, vomiting, abdominal pain); tachycardia; hypotension; faintness; coma; cardiac arrest

C. Nursing assessment

1. Assessment includes color of skin; degree of moistness of skin; complaints of itching; presence of whelps or urticaria; visual inspection of swelling; history concerning any prior problems (especially if client is going to surgery); history of reaction to fruits (especially banana and kiwi fruit); if anaphylaxis suspected, assess respiratory and cardiac status; LOC; VS; mentation

2. Diagnostic tests

   a. Patch tests or skin prick test: positive for one or more of the latex accelerators

   b. Blood sample for specific IgE test

NCLEX!

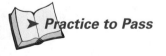

Practice to Pass

What symptoms would be present in a housekeeper who is allergic to latex and why? Why should the gloves not be snapped upon removal?

D. Nursing management

1. Medications include topical steroids, same as for anaphylaxis (see Section IV)

2. Primary treatment is removal of the irritant

3. Educate client on what caused the reaction and to avoid future contact

4. Instruct client to wear a Medic-alert bracelet

5. Instruct client to use a non-irritating soap substitute and emollient creams while affected area is red and irritated

6. Supervise housekeeping practices to reduce latex-containing dust from the environment

IV. Anaphylaxis

A. Overview

1. Anaphylaxis is defined as an allergic response when an antigen is introduced to a highly sensitive individual

2. The response is a type I allergic reaction and is a medical emergency

3. Categorized as local or systemic

4. May lead to anaphylactic shock (see Chapter 17)

5. Multiple causes exist and are individualized: pollens, foods, drugs (antibiotics are common), venom, insect bites, diagnostic agents (dye), antiserum, enzymes, hormones, vitamins, occupational agents

B. Pathophysiology

1. An antigen is introduced and interacts with immunoglobulin E (IgE), which is bound to mast cells and basophils

2. This reaction causes the mast cells to suddenly release histamines and other mediators through the body or locally

3. The mast cells also release packets containing chemical mediators, which attract neutrophils and eosinophils

4. Local reactions include urticaria, vasodilation (warmth), edema, erythema

5. Systemic reactions include respiratory (bronchoconstriction, air hunger, stridor, wheezing, barking cough); cardiovascular (hypotension, tachycardia, impaired tissue perfusion); skin (same as local reaction); gastrointestinal system (nausea, vomiting); angioedema; anxiety

6. Systemic reactions can lead to anaphylactic shock when widespread vasodilation occurs

C. Nursing assessment

1. Assessment includes VS, lung sounds, heart sounds, skin assessment, analysis of complaints, respiratory status, presence of edema, mentation, history of past allergies

2. Diagnostic tests

   a. Initial laboratory tests focus on the acute symptoms: complete blood count (CBC), arterial blood gases (ABG's), type and crossmatch (if blood transfusion

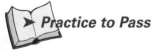
Practice to Pass

Why is an anaphylactic reaction considered an emergency?

involved), RAST, direct and indirect Coombs' Test, immune complex assay, complement assay

    b. Tests to determine the cause of the anaphylaxis would follow, after the client is stabilized (see p. 383)

D. Nursing management

    1. Medications include antihistamines and epinephrine, vasopressors such as dopamine, and corticosteroids

    2. Initial management and airway management are of highest priority

    3. Client teaching

       a. Wear a Medic-alert bracelet

       b. Identify triggers and how to avoid these

       c. Know emergency management until the client can be brought to an emergency room (bee sting kit, Epi-pen)

    4. Initiate and maintain an IV line in order to access emergency drugs

    5. Administer oxygen as needed

    6. Monitor VS frequently, as often as every 15 minutes if needed

V. Acquired Immunodeficiency Syndrome (AIDS)

A. Overview

    1. Acquired immunodeficiency syndrome (AIDS) is defined as the last stage of infection with the human immunodeficiency virus (HIV) (a retrovirus of the lentivirus family)

    2. Immunodeficiency is the state in which the client's immune system is incompetent or unable to respond effectively

    3. The adult classification of HIV disease is based on clinical manifestations and T4 cell counts

       a. Category A: asymptomatic, primary HIV or persistent generalized lymphadenopathy (PGL)

       b. Category B: symptomatic, not category A or C conditions

       c. Category C: AIDS-defining characteristics

    4. Diagnosis is made on the presence of all of the following

       a. CD4 count of less than 200 cells/mm^3

       b. Two opportunistic pathogens

       c. Presence of an AIDS-defining malignancy

    5. Two primary human immunodeficiency viruses

       a. HIV-1, prototype virus, mostly in United States

       b. HIV-2: primarily limited to West Africa

    6. Transmission

       a. Adult to adult: unprotected sexual activity and blood-to-blood contact

       b. Adult to child: perinatal transmission and blood-to-blood contact

     7. Causes

        a. Unprotected sexual activity: vaginal, anal and oral intercourse

        b. Blood to blood: needles, blood transfusions, exposure of healthcare workers

        c. Perinatal transmission: placental or intrapartum transmission and via breast milk

B. Pathophysiology

     1. HIV is a retrovirus, which carries its genetic information in RNA; on entry into the body the virus infects cells which have the CD4 antigen [primarily T helper cells] (see Figure 12-3)

     2. As with any virus, HIV is a parasite and must infect other cells in order to replicate

     3. Many of the target cells used by HIV to replicate are the antigen-presenting cells needed for a normal immune response in the body (CD4 lymphocytes, bone marrow CD 4 precursor cells, monocytic T cell lines, etc.)

     4. Once inside the cell, the virus is transported to lymph nodes and attached by viral gp120 to the host cell

     5. Once attached, the virus enters the host cell, reveals its RNA genome and uses an enzyme, reverse transcriptase, to convert viral RNA to viral DNA by using normal DNA

     6. This viral DNA insinuates itself into the host cell DNA and is replicated during normal cell processes

     7. This process results in two major effects

NCLEX!

        a. The viral number increases (viral load)

          1) **Viral load** is the number of circulating HIV particles per milliliter

          2) Viral loads of less than 10,000 = low risk; 10,000 to 100,000 = moderate risk; greater than 100,000 = high risk

NCLEX!

        b. Infected CD4 cells die

          1) Competent immune system = T4 count of 650 to 1,200 cells/mm^3

          2) Suppressed immune system = T4 count of 500 to 200 cells/mm^3

          3) AIDS: indicator values = T4 count of less than 200 cells/mm^3

     8. The virus may lie dormant or become activated, producing new RNA and virions leading to destruction of host cells

     9. Although the virus may remain inactive, antibodies are produced and detectable between 6 weeks and 6 months of infection; however, these antibodies are not able to fight HIV infection

    10. A client may show negative on antibody test for HIV but still have the virus; a seroconversion time exists (6 to 12 weeks) that allows the HIV-positive client who has no symptoms to start producing antibodies; after seroconversion, antibodies will continue to be produced

Figure 12-3 Pathophysiology of HIV.

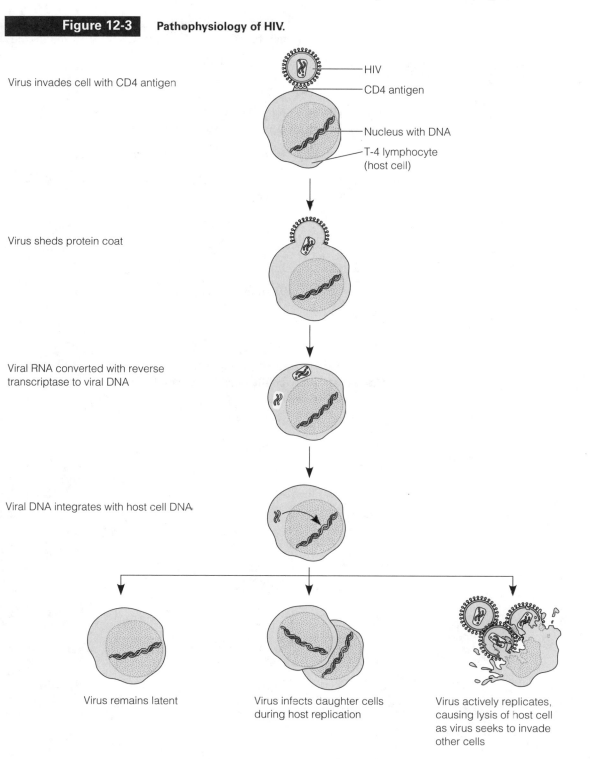

Virus invades cell with CD4 antigen

HIV

CD4 antigen

Nucleus with DNA

T-4 lymphocyte (host cell)

Virus sheds protein coat

Viral RNA converted with reverse transcriptase to viral DNA

Viral DNA integrates with host cell DNA

Virus remains latent

Virus infects daughter cells during host replication

Virus actively replicates, causing lysis of host cell as virus seeks to invade other cells

11. Although T helper cells are primarily infected with HIV, other cells (including macrophages and cells of the central nervous system [CNS]) are also infected

NCLEX!

12. Classification of HIV infection and AIDS

   a. *Category A*

   1) Primary HIV infection: negative HIV antibody tests; influenza-like symptoms; rash; symptoms cease after a few days

   2) Asymptomatic: positive antibody tests, no disease processes

   3) Persistent generalized lymphadenopathy (PGL): positive antibody tests, lymphadenopathy present for more than 3 months

   4) CD4 T cell counts

      a) A1 = greater than or equal to 500/mm^3

      b) A2 = 200 to 499/mm^3

      c) A3 = less than 200/mm^3

   b. *Category B*

   1) Positive antibody tests

   2) Symptomatic: oral thrush, candidiasis, cervical dysplasia, leukoplakia, herpes zoster, pelvic inflammatory disease (PID), fever or diarrhea for more than 1 month

   3) CD4 T cell counts

      a) B1 = greater than or equal to 500/mm^3

      b) B2 = 200 to 499/mm^3

      c) B3 = less than 200/mm^3

   c. AIDS-indicator conditions

   1) Positive antibody tests

   2) AIDS-defining conditions

      a) Pneumocystis carinii pneumonia

      b) Candidiasis

      c) Cytomegalovirus

      d) Mycobacterium tuberculosis

      e) Toxoplasmosis of the brain

      f) Histoplasmosis

      g) Kaposi sarcoma

      h) Lymphomas

      i) AIDS dementia complex

      j) HIV wasting syndrome, weight loss of 10 percent or more of body weight within a 6-month period without intention

3) CD4 T cell counts

a) C1 = greater than or equal to $500/mm^3$

b) C2 = 200 to $499/mm^3$

c) C3 = less than $200/mm^3$

13. Signs and symptoms range from no symptoms to severe immunodeficiency with multiple severe **opportunistic disease** (any infection resulting from a deficient immune system) and neoplasm, including:

a. Flu-like or mononucleosis-like illness lasting days to weeks after contracting HIV

b. Fever, sore throat, joint and muscle pain, headache, rash, and swollen lymph nodes (often first symptom); this presentation is commonly mistaken for influenza, upper respiratory infection, or gastroenteritis

c. Progression from asymptomatic infection to AIDS is not clearly defined; the client may report general malaise, fever, fatigue, night sweats, and unintentional weight loss; diarrhea is common, as are oral lesions of hairy leukoplakia, candidiasis/thrush, and gingival inflammation and ulceration

d. Other symptoms include stiff neck; burning, numbness, and tingling of extremities; headache, lightheadedness, memory loss, mood swings; nausea and vomiting; pain; dyspnea

e. AIDS dementia complex (ADC) is a dementia with cognitive, behavioral, and motor deficits that is common in untreated HIV disease and affects the CNS; it is thought to be caused by infection of HIV in brain cells and symptoms include impaired concentration, mental slowing, forgetfulness, apathy, confusion, hallucinations, personality changes, unsteady gait, leg tremors, motor difficulties

14. There is a long asymptomatic period following initial infection; the host is capable of infecting others during this latent period

15. Seroconversion is when an HIV-infected individual starts producing detectable HIV antibodies; the "seroconversion window" is that time when infection has occurred but HIV antibodies are not detectable; individuals are able to pass the virus to others unknowingly during this period

16. Mean length of time from infection to symptomatology is currently estimated to be 8 to 10 years

C. Nursing assessment

1. Assessment includes common symptoms, weight analysis, GI disturbances, neurological manifestations; gait; mentation; complaints of pain; history of recurring infections; skin assessment; palpation of lymph nodes; VS; lung sounds; oral cavity; vaginal and rectal exam

2. Diagnostic tests

a. Enzyme-linked immunosorbent assays (ELISA) to screen for HIV antibodies; usually will run two different tests

b. Western-blot test, to confirm a positive ELISA finding

Practice to Pass

Explain why an initial ELISA test could be negative in an HIV-positive client and why two ELISA tests are usually conducted, followed by a Western blot?

    c. HIV viral load, high

    d. CBC, anemia, leukopenia, thrombocytopenia

    e. CD4 cell count, low

    f. Immune complex dissociated p24 assay, shows active reproduction of HIV, used for progression of disease

    g. Diagnostic tests for opportunistic infections include:

        1) TB skin tests

        2) Magnetic resonance imagery (MRI) of brain, lymphomas

        3) Cultures

        4) Pap smears

D. Nursing management

  1. Medications

    a. Nucleoside analogs: inhibit action of viral reverse transcriptase, which is necessary for introduction of viral RNA into the cells DNA and replication, resulting in an incomplete viral DNA; example: zidovudine (AZT)

    b. Protease inhibitors: inhibit protease, the viral enzyme necessary for the production of mature viral particles; example: saquinavir (Invirase)

    c. Nonnucleoside reverse transcriptase inhibitors (NNRTIs): block making of DNA by getting on a part of the virus called the reverse transcriptase enzyme; example: nevirapine (Viramune)

    d. Drug cocktails are a combination of the above three types in order to attack the disease more aggressively; close monitoring is necessary

    e. Other agents include chemotherapy, antibiotics for infections, analgesics for pain and discomforts, antiemetics, antidiarrheals

    f. Consult the Center for Disease Control (CDC) for the most accurate information on new drug development (http://www.cdc.gov)

  2. At present, there is a reasonable life expectancy that requires attention to prevention of transmission and avoidance of secondary infections

NCLEX!

  3. All persons should practice safe sex techniques and avoid sharing of or contamination by body fluids

  4. For clients with advanced disease, information about community resources, nonjudgmental care, and health promotion activities are essential

  5. Surgical treatments for abscesses and Kaposi's sarcoma may be indicated

  6. Counseling for psychologic and social effects should be initiated

  7. Maintain clean perianal area if diarrhea is persistent

NCLEX!

  8. Instruct client on foods to avoid that are GI irritants; avoid spicy, acidic foods and those hard to chew

  9. Educate the client on common side effects of medications

NCLEX!

  10. Offer and instruct on proper oral care; avoid toothbrushes; use mouthwash without alcohol

11. Educate the client on symptoms of candida and herpes and when to seek help

12. If blood or body fluid spills occur, instruct the client to use a 1:10 solution of bleach

13. Allow the client and family to talk about the illness and discuss concerns; offer touch

14. Monitor weight and nutritional status; assess caloric intake

15. Encourage ambulation and exercise as tolerated with planned rest periods

16. Offer oxygen as needed for dyspnea

Case Study

A 43-year-old man is brought to the emergency department after being stung multiple times by hornets while cutting grass. He has welts over most of his body, is itching all over, exhibits extreme anxiety, shows tachycardia of 150 on the cardiac monitor and BP 108/65. His frantic wife states that he is allergic to penicillin and has reacted to bee stings in the past.

❶ What immediate assessment should the nurse make?

❷ What additional information is needed from the client or his wife?

❸ What drug therapy would the nurse expect the emergency room physician to institute?

❹ The client's wife asks the nurse to explain to her what is going on. How should the nurse respond?

❺ What discharge instructions should be given to this client, once he is stabilized and able to return home?

For suggested responses, see pages 568–569.

Posttest

1 In addition to a viral load of 25,000, which of the following would indicate that the medications being taken by a client with AIDS are working?

(1) Rare occurrence of symptoms
(2) Negative ELISA test
(3) CD4 cell count of 490
(4) WBC of 1,700 mm^3

2 A child with asthma caused by allergies would be expected to have which of the following findings on a CBC report?

(1) Eosinophils 21.9
(2) WBC 10.9
(3) Monocytes 4.0
(4) Neutrophils 85.7

3 The mother of a child with swollen lymph nodes is extremely panic-stricken that the swelling means cancer. The nurse could calm the mother by stating that:

(1) "The finding is very alarming and could be serious, but you must remember it may be insignificant also."
(2) "The lymph nodes are the organs that filter foreign products and may only be swollen because of an infection."
(3) "The lymph nodes will swell quite often and we may not ever know it."
(4) "The lymph nodes are the major organ indicating a problem with the immune system."

4 Which of the following indicates an example of a nonspecific inflammatory response?

(1) Extreme redness and swelling after being bitten by ants
(2) Anaphylaxis after ingesting a certain food
(3) Developing symptoms of systemic latex allergy
(4) Severe bronchoconstriction after playing football in the grass

5 A client reports to the clinic complaining of itching and weeping along the back of her legs. Upon inspection, wheals are evident that appear to be poison ivy. After talking to the client, it is learned that she broke out a day after sitting on the car seat in shorts. She sat on the same seat as her husband, who had been working in a field of grass all day. This type of reaction is a:

(1) Type I hypersensitivity.
(2) Type II hypersensitivity.
(3) Type III hypersensitivity.
(4) Type IV hypersensitivity.

6 A client with A-negative blood can receive which type of blood transfusion in order to avoid any allergic reaction?

(1) A+
(2) A–
(3) O+
(4) AB+

7 In assessing a client with a suspected latex allergy, the nurse should ask which of the following?

(1) "Are your hands usually moist or dry?"
(2) "What drug allergies do you have?"
(3) "Are you allergic to bananas or kiwi fruit?"
(4) "What types of surgeries have you had?"

8 Which of the following symptoms would be expected in an anaphylactic reaction?

(1) Hypertension
(2) Bradycardia
(3) Rales
(4) Stridor

9 The pathophysiology behind the destructive power of AIDS is that HIV kills the:

(1) B cells that produce antibodies.
(2) T helper cells.
(3) White blood cells.
(4) Platelets.

10 Of the following people, who is at increased risk of acquiring HIV?

(1) A police officer who works the streets and responds to emergencies
(2) A sexually active teenager
(3) A school nurse who examines children
(4) A nurse working on a telemetry unit

See pages 395–396 for Answers and Rationales.

Answers and Rationales

Pretest

1 **Answer: 2** *Rationale: Pneumocystis carinii* pneumonia is the most common opportunistic disease associated with acquired immunodeficiency syndrome (AIDS). The fungus responsible is not pathogenic in individuals with a normal immune system.
Cognitive Level: Analysis
Nursing Process: Assessment; *Test Plan:* PHYS

2 **Answer: 1** *Rationale:* Active acquired immunity occurs when the body produces antibodies or develops immune lymphocytes against specific antigens (chickenpox). Breastfeeding a child would offer passively acquired immunity; immune globulins offer passively acquired artificial immunity; immunizations offer actively acquired artificial immunity.
Cognitive Level: Comprehension
Nursing Process: Analysis; *Test Plan:* PHYS

3 **Answer: 4** *Rationale:* A client with AIDS will usually have a low CD4 count and a high viral load. What is desired is to have a high CD4 count and a low viral load (which should normally be zero). The white blood count will usually show neutropenia.
Cognitive Level: Analysis
Nursing Process: Assessment; *Test Plan:* PHYS

4 **Answer: 2** *Rationale:* The ELISA test may be negative upon initial testing and positive at the time of seroconversion, which takes 6 to 12 weeks after infection. This time period when the antibodies are negative is called the seroconversion window and virally infected individuals may have negative antibody tests.
Cognitive Level: Analysis
Nursing Process: Analysis; *Test Plan:* SECE

5 **Answer: 2** *Rationale:* Type I hypersensitivity reactions are caused by widespread antigen-antibody reactions such as anaphylaxis. These responses are usually immediate and lead to an antigen-antibody complex that causes the release of histamine. Option 4 is an explanation of what occurs with a blood transfusion reaction. Option 3 is an explanation of a Type IV delayed hypersensitivity. Option 1 is false.
Cognitive Level: Knowledge
Nursing Process: Analysis; *Test Plan:* PHYS

6 **Answer: 1** *Rationale:* Recognition of self as foreign is the definition of any autoimmune disease. Further explanation may be needed to explain that the immune system usually recognizes self and identifies

what is foreign, targets foreign cells, and destroys them.
Cognitive Level: Application
Nursing Process: Implementation; *Test Plan:* PHYS

7 **Answer: 3** *Rationale:* You should have recognized this as serum sickness, a reaction a week after ingestion of a drug. Serum sickness is a type III hypersensitivity reaction where formation of IgG or IgM antibody-antigen complexes occurs in the blood.
Cognitive Level: Comprehension
Nursing Process: Analysis; *Test Plan:* PHYS

8 **Answer: 4** *Rationale:* Symptoms of HIV infection are vague and nonspecific. Characteristic manifestations of HIV disease resulting from opportunistic infections and neoplasm make treatment difficult. Invasion may be from sexual contact as well as blood contact. HIV is not always predictable because the virus can lie dormant for many years. There are really no carrier states in HIV.
Cognitive Level: Comprehension
Nursing Process: Analysis; *Test Plan:* PHYS

9 **Answer: 3** *Rationale:* Only fluids containing blood or blood cells have been identified as a mode of transmission for HIV. Collecting blood, especially in a mobile unit (where the population is more diverse) is a risk for any healthcare worker. Appropriate gloving is essential. Counseling may require touch, which isn't a form of transmission; perspiration has not been identified as a form of contact; and the ELISA test requires contact with saliva.
Cognitive Level: Application
Nursing Process: Assessment; *Test Plan:* SECE

10 **Answer: 1** *Rationale:* Because laryngeal spasms and bronchial constriction can occur with anaphylaxis, assessing the client's airway is top priority. The nurse should maintain and establish a patent airway first. Remember the ABCs (airway, breathing, and circulation); cardiac output would come next followed by risk for injury and finally anxiety.
Cognitive Level: Analysis
Nursing Process: Planning; *Test Plan:* SECE

Posttest

1 **Answer: 3** *Rationale:* A client with AIDS will have exacerbations and remissions with opportunistic infections, therefore symptoms may vary. With a diagnosis of AIDS, an ELISA test would remain positive for antibodies. WBC of 1,700 shows neutropenia,

which does not indicate improvement. The CD4 cell count between 200 to 500 is in the "suppressed immune state" but certainly above the 200 mark that is indicative of severe depression of the immune system.
Cognitive Level: Analysis
Nursing Process: Evaluation; *Test Plan:* PHYS

2 **Answer: 1** *Rationale:* Eosinophils are usually elevated in an allergic response. The WBC in option 2 is barely above normal. The monocytes are normal in option 3 and the elevated neutrophils indicate an acute infection (option 4).
Cognitive Level: Analysis
Nursing Process: Assessment; *Test Plan:* PHYS

3 **Answer: 2** *Rationale:* The mother is already alarmed enough, and the nurse needs to be careful with wording of the response. Option 2 is correct and is not alarming so that the mother may be able to focus on a different perspective besides cancer.
Cognitive Level: Application
Nursing Process: Implementation; *Test Plan:* PSYC

4 **Answer: 1** *Rationale:* A nonspecific inflammatory response is usually local and produces inflammation. Options 2, 3, and 4 are all systemic, leading to generalized symptoms.
Cognitive Level: Application
Nursing Process: Analysis; *Test Plan:* PHYS

5 **Answer: 4** *Rationale:* This type of contact dermatitis is commonly a delayed reaction and a type IV hypersensitivity. This reaction is cell-mediated rather than antibody-mediated and delayed 24 to 48 hours.
Cognitive Level: Application
Nursing Process: Assessment; *Test Plan:* PHYS

6 **Answer: 2** *Rationale:* Remember the Rh must also match besides the type of blood (A in this case). Rh matching is not just for mothers and infants to prevent erythroblastosis fetalis.
Cognitive Level: Analysis
Nursing Process: Implementation; *Test Plan:* SECE

7 **Answer: 3** *Rationale:* Clients with a history of allergies to fruit such as bananas or kiwi tend to have latex allergies. The degree of moistness of the skin might need to be assessed but will not determine a latex allergy. Although drug allergies should be asked, this information does not help in determining a latex allergy. Option 4 is also important information for an assessment, but the focus of the question for a latex allergy would be if there were any problems after the surgery similar to the one being exhibited now.
Cognitive Level: Application
Nursing Process: Assessment; *Test Plan:* PHYS

8 **Answer: 4** *Rationale:* A barking cough, wheezing, and stridor are clinical manifestations of the bronchoconstriction and edema that accompanies anaphylaxis. The blood pressure is usually low (hypotension) and the pulse fast (tachycardia).
Cognitive Level: Application
Nursing Process: Assessment; *Test Plan:* PHYS

9 **Answer: 2** *Rationale:* The T helper cells are the primary target for the parasite to infect in order to replicate. The virus destroys the T cells, and along with this destruction, memory cells can also be destroyed, hence opportunistic infections are more prevalent.
Cognitive Level: Knowledge
Nursing Process: Analysis; *Test Plan:* PHYS

10 **Answer: 2** *Rationale:* The police officer and nurse on the telemetry unit should be using standard precautions, which includes gloves anytime body secretions are encountered. Although either of these may encounter blood accidentally, the percentage is low. A school nurse should not be coming into contact with body secretions that would increase the risk factor. A sexually active teenager, especially if the act is unprotected, is at highest risk.
Cognitive Level: Application
Nursing Process: Assessment; *Test Plan:* HPM

References

Bullock, B. A. & Henze, R. L. (2000). *Focus on pathophysiology*. Philadelphia: Saunders, pp. 292–327.

Center for Disease Control. Online at http://www.cdc.gov

Kee, J. L. (1999). *Laboratory and diagnostic tests with nursing implications* (5th ed.). Stamford, CT: Appleton & Lange.

Kidd, P. S. & Wager, K. D. (Eds.), (2001). *High-acuity nursing* (3rd ed.). Upper Saddle River, NJ: Prentice Hall.

Latex Allergy Policy (retrieved September 8, 2001). http://www.smtl.co.uk/MDRC/Latex/Latex-Allergy-Policy/latex-allergy-policy.html, pp. 1–7.

LeMone, P. & Burke, K. M. (Eds.) (2000). *Medical-surgical nursing: critical thinking in client care* (2nd ed.). Upper Saddle River, NJ: Prentice Hall, pp. 270–309.

McKenry, L. & Salerno, E. (2001) *Mosby's pharmacology in nursing* (21st ed.). St. Louis, MO: Mosby, p. 226.

Porth, C. M. (2000). *Concepts of altered health states* (5th ed.). Philadelphia: Lippincott, pp. 213–245.

Venes, D. (Ed.). (2001). *Taber's cyclopedic medical dictionary* (19th ed.). Philadelphia: F. A. Davis.

Wilson, B. A., Shannon, M. T., & Stang, C. L. (2002). *Nurse's drug guide*. Upper Saddle River, NJ: Prentice Hall.

CHAPTER 13

Infectious Health Problems

Barbara Moffett, PhD, RN

CHAPTER OUTLINE

OBJECTIVES

▌ Define key terms associated with infectious health problems.

▌ Identify risk factors associated with the development of infectious health problems.

▌ Discuss common etiologies of infectious health problems.

▌ Describe the pathophysiologic processes associated with specific infectious health problems.

▌ Distinguish between normal and abnormal infectious findings obtained from nursing assessment.

▌ Prioritize nursing interventions associated with specific infectious health problems.

[*Media Link*]

Use the CD-ROM enclosed with this text, or log onto the address given to access the free, interactive Companion Website created for this series. The CD-ROM and Companion Website accompanying this book offer additional practice opportunities and information—NCLEX Review, Case Studies, Glossary, In Depth with NCLEX, and more.

www.prenhall.com/hogan

REVIEW AT A GLANCE

chain of infection *the series of events or conditions that lead to development of a particular communicable disease*

colonization *establishment of an infectious agent in a host*

epidemiology *the study of the distribution of health and illness within the population*

host *organism capable of supporting growth and reproduction of another organism*

iatrogenic infection *disease acquired in a hospital or heathcare setting; also called nosocomial infection*

nosocomial infection *disease acquired in a hospital or healthcare setting; also called iatrogenic infection*

opportunistic infection *disease that occurs only when host defenses are impaired*

pathogen *microorganism capable of causing disease*

pathogenicity *the ability of a microorganism to cause pathologic changes and the process of developing disease*

reservoir *habitat in which a living organism lives and multiplies*

resident (normal) flora *relationship where parasites depend on the host's environment to grow and reproduce but prevent colonization of other microbes and may contribute to synthesis of beneficial substances*

virulence *the ease with which a pathogenic organism can overcome host defenses*

Pretest

1 A client has an opportunistic respiratory infection. Which of the following is most likely correct?

(1) The client has consumed contaminated food or water.
(2) The client has encountered an extremely virulent microorganism.
(3) The client's immune system is compromised.
(4) The client has likely become infected in a healthcare facility.

2 A client presents in the emergency department with fever of 102°F, malaise, and a productive cough. Which of the following should be done first?

(1) Administer the prescribed antibiotic.
(2) Obtain a sputum culture.
(3) Administer acetaminophen to lower fever.
(4) Teach client the importance of handwashing.

3 The drug of choice to treat a "walking" or mycoplasmal pneumonia is:

(1) Mebendazole (Vermox).
(2) Erythromycin (E-mycin).
(3) Chloroquine (Aralen hydrochloride).
(4) Chloramphenicol (Chloromycetin).

4 Which of the following refers to the ability of bacteria to produce pathologic changes or disease in the host?

(1) Virulence
(2) Pathogenicity
(3) Toxogenicity
(4) Latency

5 Which of the following is true concerning human immunodeficiency virus (HIV)?

(1) HIV infection involves CD4 receptor protein on the surface of helper T-cells.
(2) The presence of circulating antibodies that neutralize HIV is evidence that the individual has immunity to HIV.
(3) HIV replication occurs extracellularly.
(4) DNA replication is similar to that of other viruses.

6 Which of the following viruses is most likely to be acquired through casual contact with an infected individual?

(1) Influenza virus
(2) Herpes virus
(3) Cytomegalovirus (CMV)
(4) Human immunodeficiency virus (HIV)

7 A female prostitute enters the clinic for treatment of a sexually transmitted disease. Given that this disease is the most prevalent in the U.S., the nurse can anticipate that the woman has which of the following?

(1) Herpes
(2) Chlamydia
(3) Gonorrhea
(4) Syphilis

8 Endotoxins differ from exotoxins in that exotoxins have which of the following characteristics?

(1) Are composed of lipopolysaccharides
(2) Are found only in Gram-negative bacteria
(3) Are easily destroyed by heat
(4) Are typically not very toxic

9 A client exhibiting symptoms of a rickettsia infection probably acquired it through:

(1) Respiratory droplets.
(2) Mosquitos.
(3) Bites or feces of ticks, lice, or fleas.
(4) Direct skin contact.

10 Nurses should understand the chain of infection because it refers to:

(1) The linkages between various forms of micro-organisms.
(2) The sequence required for transmission of disease.
(3) The clustering of bacteria in a specific pattern.
(4) Increasing virulence patterns among species of microorganisms.

See pages 429–430 for Answers and Rationales.

I. Overview of Infectious Health Problems

A. Introduction

1. **Epidemiology** refers to the study of distribution and patterns of disease in populations

2. Infectious diseases are caused by invasion of **pathogens** (microorganisms capable of causing disease), including bacteria, viruses, fungi, protozoa, rickettsiae, and helminths

3. Types of pathogens

   a. Communicable (such as influenza, hepatitis, tuberculosis)

   b. Noncommunicable (such as cellulitis and endocarditis)

4. Injury of body cells can occur directly by the microorganism, by toxins released from microorganisms, or indirectly from the inflammatory response to the microorganism

B. Risk factors

1. Age (very young or very old)

2. Poor nutrition

3. Immune deficiency (congenital or acquired)

4. Impaired integrity of skin or mucous membranes

5. Circulatory disturbances

6. Alteration of normal flora by antibiotic therapy

   7. Diabetes mellitus

   8. Corticosteroid therapy

   9. Chemotherapy

   10. Smoking

   11. Alcohol consumption

C. Transmission of infection

   1. Occurs through the **chain of infection** (the series of events or conditions that lead to development of a particular communicable disease) (see Figure 13-1)

   2. Causative agents include pathogens listed on p. 401

   3. **Reservoir** (or source) is the environment where the infectious agent can survive

   a. Human: individuals or groups of people

   b. Environment/fomites: contaminated food, water, air, or soil

   c. Animals: such as ticks, fleas, mosquitoes, bats

   4. Portal of exit is the path by which an agent leaves a reservoir

   a. Gastrointestinal (such as ingestion)

   b. Respiratory (such as coughing or sneezing)

Figure 13-1

Steps in chain of infection.

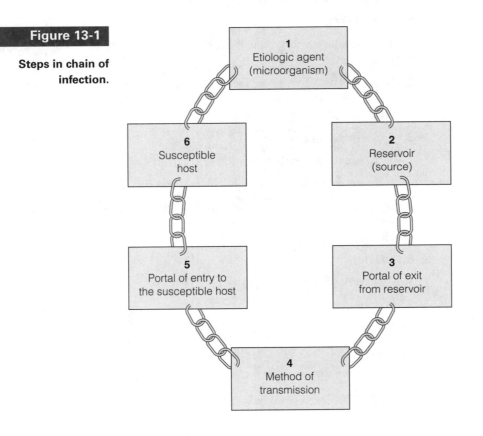

    c. Genitourinary (such as sexual contact)

    d. Blood (such as insect bites, needles)

5. Mode of transmission is the route of transmission of the agent

    a. Contact transmission may be direct or indirect

        1) Direct contact is person-to-person transmission accomplished through body fluids or through contaminated food or water

        2) Indirect contact is transmission accomplished through inanimate objects

    b. Airborne or droplet transmission involves transfer through droplets (from coughing, sneezing, or talking) or through air currents

    c. Vector transmission involves intermediaries such as flies, mosquitos, or other insects or rodents

6. Portal of entry is the location by which an agent enters the body

7. Susceptible **host** (organism capable of supporting growth and reproduction of another organism): individual who lacks resistance to this infectious agent

D. Relationship of host to parasite (host-parasite interaction)

1. **Resident (normal) flora** represent a symbiotic (balanced) relationship where parasites depend on the host's environment to grow and reproduce but prevent **colonization** (establishment of an infectious agent in a host) of other microbes

    a. May contribute to synthesis of beneficial substances

    b. Depends on maintenance of balance

2. **Opportunistic infection** occurs when immunity is compromised and normal flora become pathogenic

3. **Nosocomial** (or **iatrogenic**) **infections** are hospital-acquired and typically are caused by virulent or drug-resistant organisms and are often spread through poor handwashing

E. Factors affecting infection by pathogen

1. Mechanism of action: pathogen can damage normal cells or interfere with cellular metabolism by producing toxins

2. Infectivity: ability of the pathogen to invade and multiply in the host

3. **Pathogenicity** is the origin and process of developing disease

4. **Virulence:** the ease with which a pathogen can overcome host defenses; important components of virulence include invasiveness, adherence, and toxigenicity

5. Toxigenicity refers to the agent's ability to produce endotoxins or exotoxins

6. Defense mechanisms of the body

    a. Physical factors such as skin and mucous membranes

    b. Chemical factors such as the pH of skin, urine, stomach, etc.

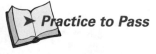

Practice to Pass

Identify conditions that could lead to opportunistic infections.

    c. Normal flora, which helps to prevent colonization by transient organisms by competing for nutrients and contributing to a low pH

    d. Immunity/inflammatory response

    e. Individual factors such as nutrition, genetic make-up, and presence of other illnesses

F. Stages of infectious process

1. Incubation stage: pathogen is present and reproduces but host remains asymptomatic; could last from hours to years

2. Prodromal stage: initial (mild) symptoms appear which may be nonspecific

3. Acute: pronounced symptoms are present; results from toxic by-products of metabolic processes of the microorganism and from tissue damage caused by the inflammatory response

4. Convalescent: diminished symptoms with infection contained

5. Resolution: elimination of pathogen

G. Clinical manifestations

1. General symptoms of systemic infection include malaise, weakness, headache, anorexia, and weight loss

2. Infection may also produce acute inflammatory reactions; the extent of tissue damage is determined by the number and the virulence of the organisms, the site of invasion, and host defenses

3. General manifestations of specific types of infection

    a. Bacterial, viral, and mycoplasma infections

        1) Fever (may be low grade)

        2) Body aches

        3) Regional lymph node enlargement

        4) Site-specific manifestations (i.e., cough, earache, sore throat, etc.)

    b. Fungal infections

        1) Itching/redness of skin

        2) Nail thickening

        3) Thrush in mouth

        4) Vaginal discharge (thick, white)

    c. Protozoa and helminths

        1) Itcing and rash (skin infections)

        2) Diarrhea

        3) Fever (with malaria)

    d. Rickettsiae

        1) Skin rash

        2) Muscles aches

NCLEX!

NCLEX!

NCLEX!

NCLEX!

3) Fever and chills

4) Headache

II. Viral Infections

A. Overview

1. Viruses are tiny intracellular organisms (20 to 100 times smaller than bacteria) that totally depend upon the living host for survival and the necessary materials to replicate

2. Intracellular development allows viruses to bypass many body defense mechanisms

B. Pathophysiology

1. Viral particles are called virions and consist of a single strand of DNA or RNA contained within a protein shell called a capsid

2. Viruses are classified as either DNA or RNA viruses according to their genetic material; also categorized according to mechanism of replication, mode of transmission, or the type of disease produced

3. Viruses produce specific diseases in specific tissues

   a. The protein covering of the virus is type-specific and attaches as a "lock and key" to the host cell membrane

   b. The virus must be able to use the host cell in production of nucleic acid in order to survive since they have no independent metabolism

   c. Mature virions are created within the host cell and released through cell lysis, direct passage to adjacent cells, or through reverse endocytosis

4. Viruses may damage or kill cells they infect, causing disease

5. The viral replication cycle can be relatively brief (minutes or hours) or as long as several days; includes 6 phases of adsorption, penetration, uncoating, replication, assembly, and release

   a. Some viruses enter the host cell and insert their genome into the host chromosome, remaining in a latent, nonreplicating state for long periods of time; examples include the herpes viruses (varicella zoster, chickenpox, genital herpes.) and cytomegalovirus

   b. Influenza virus is transmitted by respiratory droplets

6. Viruses bind to cell membrane receptors, leading to endocytosis of the virus; the virus then uses the cell's resources to synthesize new viral nucleic acids that are released from the host cell to infect other cells

7. Retroviruses replicate in a unique process

   a. The viral RNA is translated into DNA by an enzyme, reverse transcriptase, and is then integrated into the host chromosome

   b. It then exists in a latent state until reactivated

   c. Replication requires reversal of the process

   d. HIV is an example of a retrovirus

8. Bacteriophages are viruses that use bacteria as their hosts; the virus attaches to the bacteria and injects its DNA into the cell for replication

9. Viral infections can be local or systemic and can be either acute or chronic; some viruses are thought to be agents of cancer, although the role of viruses in human cancers is not well understood

10. Viral infection stimulates antibody production primarily through cell-mediated immunity and production of interferon

   a. Antibodies coat particles to make them better targets of macrophages

   b. This coating prevents viruses from entering target cells

   c. Macrophages also secrete cytokines that initiate the inflammatory response

11. Antiviral therapy is difficult to develop because of the large number of variant viruses that cause the same disease and inability of medications to destroy the virus without destroying normal cells

12. Common viral infections and antiviral agents are listed in Table 13-1

C. Nursing assessment

1. Assessment includes identifying factors that increase risk for infection, vital signs (VS), complaints of pain, palpation of lymph nodes, signs and symptoms specific to type of virus

2. Diagnostic tests

   a. Complete blood count (CBC)

      1) Lymphocytes increase in many viral infections; normal lymphocyte count is 25 to 35 percent of the total white blood count (WBC)

      2) T-lymphocytes will decrease with the HIV/AIDS virus, autoimmune disorders, and corticosteroids

      3) Neutrophil counts will decrease in most viral infections

   b. Enzyme-linked immunosorbent assay (ELISA) and Western Blot are positive in diagnosis of HIV

   c. Epstein-Barr nuclear antigen (EBNA) is used to confirm infectious mononucleosis

D. Nursing management

1. Medications

   a. Anti-viral agents (viruses are not sensitive to antibiotics since viruses have no cell wall or cytoplasm and the virus is typically immersed in the host cell); refer again to Table 13-1

   b. Acyclovir (Zovirax) is a popular medication for treating herpes

   c. Anti-pyretic agents to reduce fever

   d. Analgesics to relieve pain and discomfort

2. Instruct client/family concerning infection control measures (good handwashing, etc.)

3. Provide quiet environment, limiting visitors as needed

4. Provide comfort measures to ensure adequate rest

Table 13-1	Common Viral Infections		
Virus	**Transmission**	**Pathological Considerations**	**Nursing Management**
Hepatitis			
Hepatitis A (HAV)	Transmitted through fecal-oral route and through contaminated food and water. Occurs in overcrowded and unsanitary conditions.	Acute onset with incubation of 2 to 6 weeks. Inflammatory process can result in destruction of hepatocytes. Signs and symptoms include anorexia, malaise, jaundice. Liver enzymes likely elevated. A sharp rise in ALT liver enzyme at the time of fever onset is characteristic. Serologic markers include anti-HAV (which may persist for years) and IgM (which is short-lived and may disappear in about 2 weeks). Complete recovery likely.	Disease can be avoided in most cases if immune globulins are administered within 7 days of exposure. Preventive vaccines Havrix and Vaqta are available for those traveling to areas endemic to the disease.
Hepatitis B (HBV)	Transmitted through body fluids from sexual contact or parenterally. May also be transmitted to fetus during pregnancy.	Gradual onset with incubation 6 to 24 weeks. Infection may be acute and self-limiting or may lead to persistent viremia with chronic liver disease or chronic carrier state. There is a gradual and prolonged elevation of ALT liver enzyme. HbsAg is present in early infection. Anti-HBs is present in past infections and anti-Hbe is present in chronic carriers.	Hepatitis B hyperimmune globulin (HBIG) is recommended after exposure to the hepatitis B virus. Recombivax HB and Engerix-B are used prophylactically for prevention in health workers and other high-risk populations. Liver enzymes should be monitored. Clients should be instructed concerning safe sexual practices and to avoid sharing of needles.
Hepatitis C (HCV)	Transmitted through sexual or parenteral routes.	Gradual onset with incubation of 5 to 12 weeks. May produce both acute and chronic hepatitis but is most often chronic. HCV has also been associated with cirrhosis and liver cancer. Causes elevation of ALT. Can be detected with serologic markers anti-HVC but is difficult to determine if infection is current or prior.	Vaccines do not currently exist for HCV. Treatment is symptomatic.
Hepatitis D (HDV)	Transmitted through blood and sexual contact.	Acute onset with incubation 3 to 13 weeks. Clinical manifestations similar to hepatitis B and those with HBV and carriers of HBV are susceptible to infection by HDV.	Vaccines do not currently exist for HDV. Treatment is symptomatic.

(continued)

| Table 13-1 | Common Viral Infections (continued) |

Virus	Transmission	Pathological Considerations	Nursing Management
Hepatitis E (HEV)	Transmitted through fecal-oral route through contaminated food and water.	Rapid onset with incubation 3 to 6 weeks. Results in chronic hepatitis and cirrhosis. A serologic test for anti-HEV has been developed for detection of the virus in the stool.	
Herpes virus			
Simplex (HSV)	Transmitted through direct contact with skin and mucous membrane.	Replicates at site of entry and may pass through regional lymph nodes, enter the blood, and proliferate in the skin and mucous membranes. Most cases are subclinical. May remain latent at site of exposure and be activated by exposure to sunlight, fever or stress. Is characterized by vesicular ulcerations that may appear on the mouth or conjunctiva with HSV 1 or in the genital area with HSV 2; recurrence is common.	Acyclovir (Zovirax) is the drug of choice as an antiviral agent. This drug reduces viral shedding, decreases local symptoms, and decreases severity and duration of acute episodes. It may be used topically, orally, or parenterally.
Varicella zoster (shingles)	Transmitted primarily through the respiratory tract, initially in form of chickenpox. Reactivated in form of shingles.	Primarily seen in the elderly and immunocompromised clients and results from reactivation of latent virus that has remained dormant in sensory cells of the dorsal root ganglion. Exact mechanism is not known. Painful lesions appear to follow a specific dermatome, with lesions appearing on the trunk, chest, forehead, face and neck.	Acyclovir (Zovirax) and vidarabine (Vira-A) have been used for treatment. The vaccine ZIG (zoster immunoglobulin) may be useful for prevention in immunocompromised clients. High doses of interferon alfa (Roferon-A) have also proven useful in reducing viral replication.
Cytomegalovirus (CMV)	Transmitted through saliva, urine, semen, breast milk, and vaginal secretions.	Latent infection usually seen in immunocompromised clients. Highly necrotizing to cells. Fluorescent antibody techniques are used for diagnosis.	Antiviral agents include gancyclovir (Cytovene) and foscarnet (Foscavir). CMV immunoglobulin used in combination with an antiviral has also proven useful.
Epstein-Barr	Transmitted through respiratory droplets or saliva.	Replicates in parotid gland and disseminated through the blood. Incubation 4 to 7 weeks. Associated with mononucleosis. Signs and symptoms include lymphadenopathy, fever, chills, sore throat. Thick tonsillar exudate is often present. Recovery may take up to 4 weeks. WBCs are markedly elevated. Antibodies to the Epstein-Barr nuclear antigen appear during the convalescent period.	Disease is self-limiting and treatment is supportive.

(continued)

Table 13-1	Common Viral Infections (continued)		
Virus	**Transmission**	**Pathological Considerations**	**Nursing Management**
Human immunodeficiency virus (HIV)	Transmitted through blood and body fluids.	Incubation may be 3 to 10 years in adults. CD4 protein of helper T lymphocytes as a receptor for the virus, which attaches by means of its gp 120 surface protein. The virus envelope fuses with the cell membrane and the virus enters the cell. The virus makes a DNA copy of its own RNA using the reverse transcriptase enzyme and the DNA copy is inserted into the genetic material of the infected cell. Infected individuals become immunocompromised and subject to numerous opportunistic infections. A positive ELISA test for presence of antibodies is confirmed through the Western Blot.	Antiviral agents used to treat HIV include nucleoside reverse transcriptase inhibitors (RTIs), non-nucleoside reverse transcriptase inhibitors (NNRTIs), and protease inhibitors. Protease inhibitors are the newest category and have been associated with reduction of viral loads to undetectable levels. Compliance with drug regimens is essential and side effects often make compliance difficult.
Influenza	Transmitted through droplets of upper respiratory secretions.	Incubation period may be 1 to 7 days. Viral replication occurs in epithelial cells of the upper respiratory tract. The virus does not typically enter the blood. Systemic symptoms are derived from endogenous pyrogens and release of interferon. Symptoms include headache, body aches, chills, fever, and rhinitis. Complications may include bronchial pneumonia or secondary bacterial infection. Guillain-Barre and Reye's syndromes have been associated with episodes of influenza.	Amantadine (Symmetrel) is the antiviral agent that prevents penetration of Influenza A into cells and limits replication if administered within 48 hours of onset. Vaccines are formulated each year that can be effective for prevention for up to 6 months. Vaccines are recommended for the elderly and high-risk clients.

Practice to Pass

What are the implications of the presence of latent or recurrent viruses?

NCLEX!

5. Assist with self-care activities as needed

6. Monitor vital signs

7. Institute isolation precautions according to route of transmission

8. Document response to medication

9. Evaluate response to activity, noting weakness, fatigue, or dyspnea

10. Preventive vaccines should be encouraged when available

11. Instruct clients with genital herpes to avoid sexual contact during the acute phase

III. Bacterial Infections

A. Overview

1. Bacteria are single-celled organisms that use the human body as a source for nutrients and environment for growth

2. They contain a single chromosome and are capable of autonomous reproduction

3. Bacteria are classified according to shape, staining characteristics, and requirements related to oxygen

B. Pathophysiology

1. Bacterial growth depends on the body's immune system function and ability of bacteria to resist body defenses

2. Bacteria may produce substances that enhance resistance to host defenses

   a. Production of adherins allows bacteria to strongly attach to structures and penetrate underlying tissues

   b. Development of carbohydrate or protein capsule or slime layers help prevent phagocytosis

   c. Production of leukocidins help destroy phagocytes

   d. Production of enzymes that break down fibrin clots or connective tissue (i.e., streptokinase, hyalurinidase, collagenase, elastase, etc.) and allow bacteria to more easily spread into tissues; production of coagulase causes clotting of plasma and allows bacteria to form a fibrin layer of protection

3. Bacteria may produce toxins that cause damage to cells and tissues

   a. Exotoxins are proteins secreted from tissues that usually have variable specificity and may cause fatal effects

      1) Exotoxins are produced by Gram-positive and Gram-negative organisms and most are denatured by extreme heat

      2) Common examples of the effects of exotoxins are found in botulism and tetanus

   b. Endotoxins are lipopolysaccharides released from bacterial cell membranes with cell division or destruction

      1) They are produced only by Gram-negative bacteria and can withstand high heat

      2) Endotoxins usually cause fever and induce production of cytokines that activate the complement cascade and may cause septic shock

      3) They are generally less toxic than exotoxins

4. Complement proteins may be activated by contact with bacterial cell wall or with release of endotoxins

   a. This activation results in opsonization of microorganisms (to enhance phagocytosis), activation of leukocytes, and destruction of bacterial cells

NCLEX!

(*text continues on p. 415*)

Table 13-2 **Common Bacteria That Cause Infectious Disease**

Bacteria/ Disease Process	Type/ Morphology	Transmission	Pathological Effects	Nursing Management
Clostridium tetani (tetanus)	Gram-positive bacillus; spore-forming	Spores distributed in soil and intestinal tract of humans and animals. Infects wounds from injury.	Clinical manifestations caused by spore generation of exotoxin with affinity for CNS. S/S include neck stiffness, dysphagia, muscle rigidity.	Treated with tetanus antitoxin or immune globulins. Prevention with tetanus toxoid. May require mechanical ventilation.
Clostridium botulinum (botulism)	Gram-positive bacillus; spore-forming	Inhabits soil; frequent contaminant of fruits, vegetables, and fish. Spores are highly heat resistant.	Life-threatening paralytic illness is caused by neurotoxins. Prevents release of ACh from nerve terminals of neuromuscular junction. Damage to cranial nerves causes vision, hearing, and speech difficulties.	Treated with antitoxin from horse serum that only affects circulating toxin; has no effect on toxin bound to nerve cells. Recovery is very gradual over weeks to months.
Corynebacterium diphtheriae (diphtheria)	Gram-positive; nonspore-forming	Airborne droplets colonizing in upper respiratory system.	Produces toxin resulting in epithelial cell necrosis. Inflammatory response causes production of pseudomembrane that may lead to suffocation.	Antitoxin must be administered prior to cell penetration by toxin. Should test for hypersensitivity to horse serum proteins prior to administration. Prevention is through vaccine. Penicillin may be used but is rarely effective when used alone.
Coliform Bacteria *Escherichia coli*	Gram-negative, nonspore-forming rods	Normal resident bacteria of intestines. May spread to urinary tract or wounds directly through fecal contamination or through the blood.	Frequent source of nosocomial infection. S/S include fever and chills. May develop shock from endotoxins. Also frequent bacteria causing urinary tract infections.	Prevention through good handwashing and hygiene practices. Treated with cephalosporins, fluoroquinolones, or aminoglycosides. Should monitor for nephrotoxicity and ototoxicity with aminoglycosides.
Klebsiella pneumoniae	Gram-negative rod, heavily encapsulated	Found in soil, water, food, and intestinal tract.	Also associated with hospital acquired infections. Responsible for severe respiratory tract infections in debilitated clients. S/S include productive cough and weakness.	Treated with aminoglycosides and later generation cephalosporins. Aminoglycosides bind to ribosomes and prevent protein synthesis in bacteria. Cephalosporins interfere with cell wall synthesis.

(continued)

Table 13-2 Common Bacteria That Cause Infectious Disease (continued)

Bacteria/ Disease Process	Type/ Morphology	Transmission	Pathological Effects	Nursing Management
Pseudomonas	Gram-negative rod	Common resident of skin and mucous membranes. Spreads through direct contact.	Major threat to hospitalized and debilitated clients.	Treated with aminoglycosides and later-generation cephalosporins.
Helicobacter pylori	Gram-negative sprial or straight rod	Penetrates gastric mucosa and colonizes gastric epithelium.	Produces enzyme urease that raises pH, allowing bacteria to survive in normally acidic environment. Urea in stomach is converted to ammonia, which is cytotoxic to gastric cells. Causes depletion of gastric mucus, allowing erosion of mucosa.	Treated with macrolides clarithromycin (Biaxin) and metronidazole (Flagyl). Macrolides inhibit protein synthesis while metronidazole disrupts DNA synthesis. Alcohol should be avoided with metronidazole. Macrolides have frequent interactions with drugs.
Haemophilus influenza	Gram-negative bacillus	Occurs only in humans; more common in children than adults. Transmitted person to person through respiratory route.	Virulence enhanced by polysaccharide capsule that resists action of complement. Does not produce exotoxin and endotoxin does not appear to play significant role. Results in otitis media, sinusitis, and respiratory tract infections.	Prevention is through vaccine. Drugs of choice for treatment are ampicillin or cephalosporins.
Gonorrhea (*neisseria gonorrhoeae*)	Gram-negative diplococcus	Transmitted through sexual contact. Primary site of infection is the cervix. Primary site in men is the urethra.	Bacteria contain pili, which aid in attachment to mucosal surfaces in humans and inhibit phagocytosis. Most strains produce extracellular proteases that inactivate immunoglobulins They also produce a cytotoxic factor that damages ciliated epithelial cells. May be asymptomatic in women but result in salpingitis, pelvic inflammatory disease, and infertility; men generally experience purulent discharge and dysuria and may experience urethral stricture.	Drug of choice is a cephalosporin such as ceftriaxone (Rocephin). TMP/SMX (Bactrim) and ciprofloxacin (Cipro) may also be used. Ciprofloxacin inhibits DNA replication while TMP/SMX prevents synthesis of proteins and nucleic acid. Client should be instructed to avoid unprotected sexual contact.

(continued)

Table 13-2	Common Bacteria That Cause Infectious Disease (continued)			
Bacteria/ Disease Process	**Type/ Morphology**	**Transmission**	**Pathological Effects**	**Nursing Management**
Staphylococcus	Gram-positive cocci that grow in clusters in short chains.	Transmitted through hair follicles into the bloodstream or through the urinary or respiratory tract.	Common resident of skin. Hardy non-spore forming bacteria that is heat stable. Anerobes that produce the enzyme catalase. Some forms produce coagulase causing clots in citrated plasma. Pathogenic staph release a number of toxins including hemolysins, leukocidin, enterotoxins, and exfoliatin. They have also been implicated in toxic shock syndrome.	Humans have high resistance to staph due to development of high-antibody titers. Penicillinase-resistant penicillins and cephalosporins are the drugs of choice, however resistant strains have developed. Vancomycin (Vancocin) is the drug of choice for methicillin-resistant strains. It interferes with cell wall synthesis. In cases where resistance has developed to vancomycin, drugs such as quinupristin and dalfopristin (synercid) and linezolid (Zyvox) or combination therapy using vancomycin and gentamycin have been effective.
Streptococcus	Gram-positive cocci that grow in chains or as diplococci.	Transmitted through respiratory droplets or direct contact with secretions.	*Group A beta-hemolytic streptococcus* produces erythrogenic toxin responsible for rash in scarlet fever. Two hemolysins are produced as well as streptokinase that promotes lysis of human blood clots. Diseases produced include pharyngitis, otitis media, peritonsillar abcesses, meningitis, and pneumonia. Glomerulonephritis and rheumatic fever are complications that can result from streptococcal infection.	Penicillin is the drug of choice, with erythromycin used for those allergic to penicillin. Clients should be instructed in the importance of completing the entire course of prescribed antibiotics.

(continued)

Table 13-2	Common Bacteria That Cause Infectious Disease (continued)			
Bacteria/ Disease Process	**Type/ Morphology**	**Transmission**	**Pathological Effects**	**Nursing Management**
Tuberculosis (*mycobacterium tuberculosis*)	Acid-fast and aerobic bacillus (due to large amounts of lipids in cell wall)	Tubercle is transmitted through respiratory droplets from humans, cows, or birds. May also enter blood and lymph system and travel to other parts of the body.	Grows slowly and often results in self-limiting lesion. Initial lesion appears as area of nonspecific pneumonitis. The caseous lesion heals by fibrosis and calcification. This lesion can be reactivated with low host resistance. Exotoxins or endotoxins are not produced. Mycobacteria primarily affect the lungs but may also cause infection in the kidney, liver, and genitourinary tract.	Previous mycobacterial infection can be detected through a PPD skin test, however this does not necessarily establish the presence of active infection. The drugs of choice for treatment of tuberculosis are the antitubercular agents isoniazid (INH) and rifampin (Rifadin). These drugs interfere with protein synthesis or cell wall synthesis. Streptomycin and pyrazinamide (Tebrazid) are also used; It should be noted that standard antibiotics are not effective against mycobacteria. Treatment usually continues for 3 to 6 months and client compliance must be encouraged.

b. Encapsulated bacteria are protected from phagocytosis unless coated with anticapsular antibody

c. Antibiotics are often necessary to assist the immune system in destruction of bacteria

5. Common bacteria causing infectious diseases are identified in Table 13-2

C. Nursing assessment

1. Assessment includes identifying organ system affected by infection; signs and symptoms of infection (fever, malaise, and local or organ-specific indicators); VS; complaints of pain; palpation of lymph nodes

2. Diagnostic tests

   a. CBC

     1) WBC (expressed as number of WBCs per cubic mm) will be elevated ($> 10,000/mm^3$)

     2) Neutrophil count: expressed as absolute neutrophil count (ANC) or percentage of the total WBC; is elevated with most bacterial infections

       a) Both segmented neutrophils (mature) and bands (immature neutrophils) will likely be elevated with infection

       b) With severe or prolonged infection, the percentage of bands will increase to a greater extent than segmented neutrophils (often referred to as a "shift to the left")

       c) Some bacterial infections (typhoid, brucellosis, etc.) may cause neutropenia

   b. Culture and sensitivity: aids in identification of the organism and determination of the antibiotic that can be most effective; collect prior to administration of any antibiotics

   c. Gram stain: allows presumptive identification of the category of bacteria

D. Nursing management

1. Medications include antimicrobial agents, antipyretics, NSAIDs

2. Employ appropriate protective barriers (such as gloves, mask, goggles, gowns) when caring for clients with bacterial infections

3. Instruct client and family in methods to prevent spread of infection

4. Encourage balance of rest and activity

5. Encourage compliance with medication regimen; stress the completion of all medications even though symptoms improve to avoid bacterial resistance

6. Encourage increased fluid intake with most anticrobials

7. Document response to therapy

8. Collect lab specimens as needed to validate resolution of infection

IV. Fungal Infections

A. Overview

1. Fungi may be unicellular (yeasts) or multicellular (hyphae), or may alternate between the two forms

2. Fungi can cause allergic, toxic, and infectious disease in humans

3. Some fungi are part of the normal flora of the skin, mouth, intestines, and vagina

B. Pathophysiology

1. Fungi obtain nutrients by absorption and almost all are aerobic and reproduce by spores

   a. Spores germinate to produce different morphologic forms such as single-celled yeasts or multicelled molds

   b. The cell wall is rigid and composed primarily of polysaccharides external to the cell membrane

2. The plasma membrane contains ergosterol rather than cholesterol, which is useful in antifungal therapy

3. Humans have a high level of innate immunity to fungi, and most infections are mild and self-limiting

4. Factors related to resistance include the fatty acid content of skin, pH of the skin and mucous membranes, normal flora, epithelial turnover, and cilia in the respiratory tract

5. Infections are classified according to three levels

   a. Superficial: limited to outer layers of skin and hair (tinea versicolor)

   b. Cutaneous: extending deeper into keratinized layers of the epidermis (caused by dermaphytes); tinea and candida are the primary examples

   c. Subcutaneous: involves the dermis, subcutaneous tissue, muscle and fascia

      1) Most infections of this type are chronic and visualized as skin lesions

      2) They may be initiated by trauma and may require surgical excision

6. Fungal infections can also be systemic; this form originates primarily in the lung, but may appear as a secondary infection elsewhere; histoplasmosis is a common example

7. Opportunistic mycotic infections are often seen in immunocompromised individuals (those with AIDS, receiving chemotherapy, etc.) or those on long-term antibiotic therapy; the most common forms are candidiasis, aspergillosis, and zygomycosis

8. Transmission is through direct contact with persons or inanimate objects

9. Moisture increases the risk of growth and spread of fungal infection

C. Nursing assessment

NCLEX!

1. Assessment includes location, size, and characteristics of lesions of the skin and mucous membranes; complaints of discomfort (itching); and specific assessment (vagina, mouth, nails)

2. Diagnostic tests

   a. Cultures of skin, nails, or hair

   b. Microscopic examination of scrapings from lesions

   c. Observation under ultraviolent light (spores fluoresce blue-green)

D. Nursing management

1. Medications

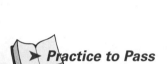

   a. Superficial, cutaneous, and subcutaneous fungal infections are generally treated with topical antifungal agents

   1) These include clotrimazole (Lotrimin), ketoconazole (Nizoral), and nystatin (Mycostatin)

   2) Most commonly reported side effects include burning, pruritis, and local irritation

   b. Amphotericin B (Fungizone) remains the drug of choice for severe systemic mycoses

   1) It is often given along with flucytosine (5-FC) for a synergistic effect

   2) Amphotericin B is associated with many adverse effects including fever, chills, cardiac dysrhythmias, and nephrotoxicity

   c. Other systemic antifungal agents include flucytosine (5-Fluorocytosine), griseofulvin (Grisactin), ketoconazole (Nizoral), and nystatin (Mycostatin)

2. Instruct individuals concerning method of transmission and conditions that increase risk

3. Teach clients importance of using clean articles for personal hygiene each day

4. Teach clients that antifungals often take 7 to 10 days to work

Practice to Pass

How would topical corticosteroids aggravate treatment of a fungal infection?

V. Chlamydial Infections

A. Overview

1. Chlamydial organisms are obligate non-motile intracellular parasites associated with many sexually transmitted diseases (STDs)

2. Chlamydia is the most common bacterial STD in the United States

3. Originally considered a virus, it is now recognized as a bacteria since it contains both RNA and DNA and has a cell wall similar to Gram-negative bacteria

4. Chlamydial infection can lead to pelvic inflammatory disease, infertility, ectopic pregnancy, and chronic pelvic pain

B. Pathophysiology

1. Chlamydia are unicellular organisms that reproduce asexually in the host cells of mammals and birds and transmit directly to humans

2. The cell wall of chlamydia is similar in structure to Gram-negative bacteria with a lipid cytoplasmic membrane; DNA occurs as an irregular mass in cytoplasm and cells lack flavoproteins and cytochromes

3. The cell cycle begins with a highly infectious small cell taken into a host cell by phagocytosis

   a. The cell retains its integrity and is reorganized into a large cell that multiplies by binary fission

b. The large cells then reorganize into small cells capable of infecting new host cells

c. The cell cycle varies between 24 to 48 hours

4. They generally become parasites of epithelial cells, mainly targeting mucous membranes of the eye or genitourinary tract; some forms of chlamydia transmitted by birds can cause infection of the lungs

5. There is generally low pathogenicity except in an immunocompromised host; compromised hosts can easily become reinfected

6. Infection can remain latent or subclinical for years

7. Chlamydia has on its surface a peptide similar to one in heart myosin; this can trigger T cells that attack both chlamydia and heart cells, causing myocarditis

NCLEX!

8. Many clients with chlamydial infection are asymptomatic initially; some may complain of vaginal discharge within 1 to 3 weeks of infection; later signs and symptoms may include lower back pain, nausea, and fever

C. Nursing assessment

1. Assessment includes symptom analysis of pain, VS, inspection of vaginal discharge (females) or penile discharge (males)

2. Diagnostic tests

a. Cell tissue culture is the primary diagnostic tool

b. Enzyme immunoassay (EIA) tests may be used for high-risk clients but result in a fairly high percentage of false positive diagnoses

c. Nucleic amplification tests (usually along with urine tests and cervical swab) have been developed and have been found effective

D. Nursing management

1. Medications

a. Macrolides: erythromycin (E-mycin) or single-dose azithromycin (Zithromax)

b. Tetracyclines: doxycycline (Vibramycin) for 7 days

c. Some fluoroquinolones may also be effective

NCLEX!

2. Instruct clients concerning transmission through sexual contact

3. Instruct clients about need to treat sexual partners

VI. Spirochetal Infections

A. Overview

1. Spirochetes are spiral-shaped bacteria with great motility that live primarily as extracellular pathogens, rarely growing within a host cell

2. Spirochetes possess both DNA and RNA and can penetrate mucous membranes, entering the blood and lymphatic system

B. Pathophysiology

1. Infections may remain latent for years

2. Humoral and cell-mediated immune responses are activated and may decrease spirochete load, but generally will not eliminate disease

3. Most common spirochetes are *treponema pallidum* and *borrelia burgdorferi*

4. *Treponema pallidum* causes sexually transmitted disease (syphilis), the third most common STD in the United States

   a. First signs include indurated, circumscribed, painless ulcer at the site of infection that lasts 10 to 14 days and heals spontaneously

   b. May experience headache, low-grade fever, and lymphadenopathy

   c. Enters period of latency where a certain percentage will develop tertiary symptoms with long term effects in the central nervous system (CNS), blood vessels, and perivascular areas

5. *Borrelia burgdorferi* causes Lyme disease, the most common tick transmitted disease

   a. Lesion expands uniformly from site of bite that is clear in center, with redness at the periphery

   b. Host response often leads to complications such as arthritis and neuropathies; if left untreated may lead to destruction of bone and joints

   c. Symptoms may include fever, neck stiffness, neurological complications such as Bell's palsy or Lyme disease

C. Nursing assessment

1. Assessment includes appearance and location of lesions; VS; signs of lymphadenopathy; sexual history for suspicion of syphilis; complaints of discomfort

2. Diagnostic tests

   a. Cultures (may take 8 to 12 weeks)

   b. Serologic testing for antibodies (may be negative in early stages)

      1) ELISA

      2) Indirect fluorescent antibody tests (IFA)

D. Nursing management

1. Medications include penicillins and tetracyclines (as drugs of choice)

2. Teach individuals to wear protective clothing and/or avoid tick-infested areas

3. Encourage to seek early intervention for suspected tick bites

4. Instruct in use of protective barriers during intercourse for prevention of syphilis

5. Avoid calcium-based products with tetracyclines as they interfere with absorption

VII. Rickettsial Infections

A. Overview

1. Rickettsia are similar to Gram-negative bacteria that can only reproduce within certain susceptible cells

2. They are transmitted to humans by arthropod vectors through bites or feces of ticks, lice, or fleas

3. The most common diseases caused by rickettsia are Typhus and Rocky Mountain spotted fever

B. Pathophysiology

1. Rickettsiae are extremely small rod-shaped, coccoid, or pleomorphic bacteria that are intracellular parasites because of a highly permeable cytoplasmic membrane

2. They typically consist of three layers: an inner cytoplasmic membrane, a rigid cell wall, and an outer layer, and they multiply by binary fission

3. They are primarily found in the endothelium of small blood vessels, particularly the brain, skin, and heart

   a. Hyperplasia of endothelial cells and localized thrombus formation lead to obstruction of blood flow, with escape of red blood cells into surrounding tissue

   b. Inflammation of blood vessels occurs, and is known as angiitis

4. Clinical manifestations are believed to be caused by production of endotoxin

5. Untreated cases result in a 20 to 25 percent fatality

6. Signs and symptoms include skin rash, headache, malaise, muscle aches, chills and nausea and vomiting; fever of sudden onset may last 2 to 3 weeks

C. Nursing assessment

1. Assessment includes VS, skin assessment, symptom analysis of complaints and pain

2. Diagnostic tests

   a. Complement fixation test (may be positive within 14 days)

   b. Indirect fluoroscent antibody test (detects IgM and IgG antibodies)

D. Nursing management

1. Medications include tetracycline (Doxycycline) and chloramphenicol (Chloromycetin)

2. Careful monitoring is required with chloramphenicol due to risk of possible bone marrow suppression

3. Teach individuals importance of prevention through avoidance of arthropod carriers and use of repellent in high-risk areas

4. Sulfonamides should be avoided because they may stimulate rickettsial growth

VIII. Protozoal Infections

A. Overview

1. Protozoa are unicellular organisms that may be spherical, spindle, or cup-shaped

2. Protozoal infections are among the most common infections of humans throughout the world

3. They occur primarily as parasites of the gastrointestinal and genitourinary systems and may result in pneumonia as an opportunistic infection in immuno-compromised clients

B. Pathophysiology

1. Protozoans reproduce asexually by fission, schizogony (multiple fission), or budding

   a. Some also reproduce sexually by fusion of haploid sex cells

   b. Some protozoa produce cysts that enable them to survive outside their host

2. The most common types of infections caused by protozoa are amebiasis, giardiasis, malaria, toxoplasmosis, and *pneumocystis carinii* pneumonia

3. *Amoeba* are transmitted through fecal-oral route

   a. Cysts are excreted in the feces of an infected individual or carrier and ingested through contaminated food, water, or objects

   b. They penetrate the walls of the large intestines causing ulceration and may enter the blood to cause damage to other organs

   c. Certain forms can also be transmitted through mucous membranes via contaminated water

   d. Many individuals serve as carriers without clinical symptoms

   e. Early clinical manifestations include diarrhea with mucous and blood, and flatulence, alternating with constipation

   f. Later manifestations of amebic disorders may include lesions of ulcerative colitis, secondary infection in other parts of the body, and amebic liver abscess

4. *Giardiasis* is the most common protozoan intestinal disease in the United States and is also transmitted through the fecal-oral route

   a. Cysts are ingested through contaminated food or water and result in gastroenteritis

   b. Clinical manifestations include epigastric pain and nausea

5. *Malaria* is caused by a particular genus of protozoa called *plasmodium* and is transmitted through the bite of an infected mosquito

   a. Once infected, a primary exoerythrocytic cycle of asexual reproduction occurs in the human liver and leads to synchronous lysis of large numbers of erythrocytes

   b. Extensive erythrolysis results in anemia and splenomegaly

   c. Since this activity occurs primarily in capillaries, small hemorrhages and ischemia from vascular plugging lead to tissue anoxia

   d. Early symptoms of malaria include headache, anorexia, nausea, vomiting, and photophobia; this may be followed by chills, high fever, and muscle pain

6. *Toxoplasmosis* is acquired through ingestion of cysts from cat feces, by ingesting uncooked meat or unpasteurized dairy products, or through blood transfusions

   a. While healthy individuals often remain asymptomatic, early symptoms may include chills, fever, headache, lymphadenitis, and extreme fatigue

   b. Reactivation toxoplasmosis has become a significant opportunisitc infection in immunocompromised individuals

7. *Pneumocystis carinii pneumonia* results from a protozoan that produces cysts in the lungs of several animal species and is increasingly common in immuno-compromised individuals

   a. The protozoa line the alveolar walls and block gas exchange

   b. Accumulations of lymphocytes, macrophages, and plasma cells, with almost no phagocytosis, results in aggregation of parasites, cellular debris, and plasma proteins that lead to interstitial plasma cell pneumonia

   c. Symptoms include a dry, nonproductive cough and absence of sputum; progressive dyspnea may lead to cyanosis

NCLEX!

C. **Nursing assessment**

   1. Assessment includes gastrointestinal symptoms; risk for protozoal disorders; complaints of pain and/or nausea; VS; intolerance to light; palpation of lymph nodes; activity level; characteristics of sputum if present

   2. Diagnostic tests

      a. Amoeba and giardiasis: note presence and morphology of cysts in fecal smear

      b. Malaria: observe erythrocytic stages on blood smears; CBC

      c. Toxoplasmosis: serologic tests (indirect fluorescent antibody, indirect hemagglutination assay, enzyme-linked immunosorbent assay)

      d. Pneumocystosis: lung tissue biopsy or needle aspiration

D. **Nursing management**

   1. Medications

      a. Amebiasis and giardiasis: drug of choice is metronidazole (Flagyl); disrupts DNA synthesis and synthesis of nucleic acid

      b. Malaria: drugs of choice are chloroquine (Aralen Hydrochloride) and hydroxychloroquine (Plaquenil); interfere with protein synthesis and inhibit DNA and RNA replication as well as nucleic acid synthesis

      c. Toxoplasmosis: pyrimethamine (Daraprim) and pyrimethamine/sulfadoxine (Fansidar); folic acid antagonists

      d. Pneumocystosis: trimethoprim/sulfamethoxazole (Bactrim), a folic acid antagonist

NCLEX!

   2. Instruct individuals to boil water prior to drinking in areas with untreated water

NCLEX!

   3. Instruct on proper handwashing after defecating

IX. **Helminthic Infections**

A. **Overview**

   1. Helminths (worms) are complex organisms that gain entry into humans primarily through ingestion of fertilized eggs or penetration of larvae through the skin or mucous membranes

  2. Helminths are classified as

    a. Cestodes (tapeworms)

    b. Nematodes (roundworms)

    c. Trematodes (flukes)

B. Pathophysiology

  1. Cestode infections are caused by tapeworms living in the intestines

    a. Tapeworms are flat, segmented worms with structures that allow attachment to the intestinal wall

    b. These usually cause little pathology and begin with ingestion of eggs or cysts from infected beef, pork, or fish

    c. The cyst lodges in the intestinal mucosa and can cause symptoms including diarrhea, abdominal pain, nausea, fatigue, anorexia, and paresthesias

    d. The large size of the adult tapeworm results in irritation to the mucosa and infestations can result in intestinal obstruction

    e. Eggs can enter the blood and migrate to various tissues (including the brain)

  2. Nematodes are elongated, unsegmented, cylindrical worms

    a. The eggs develop in the soil, and once ingested, they hatch and larvae undergo migration through the lungs before localizing and maturing in the small intestine

    b. Migration through the walls of the alveoli causes irritation and may result in transient pneumonitis, which may be asymptomatic

    c. This may result in fever, coughing, blood in the sputum, and elevated eosinophil counts

    d. Intestinal nematodes may result in abdominal distention, fever, and obstruction

  3. Trematodes are unsegmented, flat, leaf-shaped worms that require asexual reproduction in a snail intermediate host

    a. Humans become infected by ingesting poorly cooked fish, crabs, or snails

    b. They usually have suckers for attaching to the GI mucosa

    c. Flukes may infect various tissues including blood vessels, intestines, the liver or lungs

    d. Flukes cover themselves with host antigens to avoid antibody response in order to exist in the blood

    e. Inflammatory responses from migrating eggs often lead to scarring and fibrosis in affected organs

    f. Early symptoms include fever, malaise, abdominal pain, itching (rectal), and gastroenteritis

    g. Untreated infections can lead to chronic disorders in affected organs

C. Nursing assessment

  1. Assessment includes complaints of discomfort, weight, bowel patterns, VS, and energy level

2. Diagnostic tests

   a. Examination of stool specimens for ova, cysts, and parasites

   b. CT scan

   c. CBC: eosinophilia

D. Nursing management

1. Medications

   a. All types helminths: drug of choice is albendazole (Albenza), causes degeneration of cytoplasmic microtubules in intestinal wall of helminths, causing decreased ATP production and energy depletion

   b. Other drugs used for cestodes

      1) Mebendazole (Vermox) inhibits uptake of glucose and other nutrients

      2) Niclosamide (Niclocide) inhibits mitochondrial oxidative phosphorylation

      3) Praziquantel (Biltricide) causes loss of intracellular calcium and paralysis of parasites

   c. Other drugs for nematodes

      1) Diethylcarbamazine (Hetrazan) inhibits embryogenesis of nematodes

      2) Ivermectin (Stomectol) inhibits CNS signals, leading to paralysis of nematode

      3) Mebendazole (Vermox) inhibits uptake of glucose and other nutrients

      4) Piperazine (Antepar) and pyrantel (Antiminth) block acetylcholine at neuromuscular junction, resulting in paralysis of the worm

   d. Other drugs for trematodes

      1) Oxamniquine (Vansil) causes loss of intracellular calcium and paralysis of parasites

      2) Praziquantel (Biltricide) causes loss of intracellular calcium and paralysis of parasites

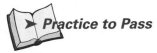

Practice to Pass

What is the most severe and life-threatening complication of infestation with worms?

NCLEX!

2. Instruct individuals in the importance of cooking meat; freezing meat for several days can also destroy infectious eggs

X. Mycoplasmal Infections

A. Overview

1. Mycoplasma species are the smallest known free-living organisms

2. They are pleomorphic organisms with no cell wall (therefore resistant to cell wall–active antibiotics)

3. Mycoplasma pneumonia is also known as atypical or walking pneumonia

B. Pathophysiology

1. Mycoplasma are generally slow growing but vary widely in growth rates; they require fatty acids (sterol) and serum protein for growth and generally adhere to mucosal epithelium

2. Mycoplasma pneumonia occurs most often in children, young adults, and the elderly

   a. It is transmitted by droplets, with an incubation period of 2 to 3 weeks

   b. Individuals may be asymptomatic, however, commons signs and symptoms include headache, low-grade fever, malaise, anorexia, and hacking cough

C. Nursing assessment

1. Assessment includes VS, complaints of pain or discomfort, activity level, nutritional assessment, lung sounds, and presence of cough

2. Diagnostic tests

   a. Cold agglutin antibody titer may be done but is insensitive and nonspecific

   b. Enzyme immunoassay (EIA): positive

   c. Chest x-ray (CXR) will show infiltrates

D. Nursing management

1. Medications

   a. Drug of choice: macrolides—erythromycin (E-Mycin)

   b. Tetracycline hydrochloride (Doxycycline)

   c. Analgesics or NSAIDs for discomfort

   d. Antipyretics for fever

2. Encourage balance of rest and activity

3. Offer fluids unless contraindicated

4. Administer oxygen if needed

XI. Mycobacterial Infections

A. Overview

1. A group of acid-fast bacteria belonging to the *Mycobacteriaceae* family

2. Organisms are slender, Gram-positive rods

3. Common diseases include *M. tuberculosis* (tuberculosis); *M. leprae* (leprosy), and *M. avium-intracellulare* (an opportunistic infection)

B. Pathophysiology

1. The organisms are surrounded by a waxy capsule that is hard to penetrate

2. The organisms may form branches of a fungal nature

3. Are classified as common facultative intracellular parasites; able to survive and grow within a macrophage

4. Humans are the only natural host

5. The response to the cell includes tissue damage as a result of chronic inflammation

6. *M. tuberculosis* (tuberculosis) is an aerobic acid-fast rod

   a. Contagious by respiratory droplets

   b. Incubation is variable, 4 to 8 weeks

   c. Can be reinfected

   d. Signs and symptoms include lung involvement (can be seen on chest x-ray); fever, pleurisy; night sweats; cough; weight loss (see Chapter 1)

7. *M. leprae* (leprosy)

   a. Also known as Hansen's disease; an acid-fast rod–shaped bacillus

   b. Contracted by close contact or prolonged exposure

   c. Skin or nasal mucosa can be portal of entrance

   d. Incubation 3 to 5 years

   e. Signs and symptoms include: lesions of skin that are destructive, as well as involvement of peripheral nerves, upper respiratory passages, testes, hands, and feet; muscle weakness

   f. Erythema nodosum leprosum (ENL) reaction may develop during the end of the first year of therapy with red, painful nodules that become ulcerated and necrotic

8. *M. avium-intracellulare*

   a. An opportunistic organism; acid-fast rod

   b. Contracted by respiratory transmission from soil, water, dairy products, birds, and mammals

   c. Signs and symptoms are pulmonary in nature

C. Nursing assessment

1. Assessment includes lung sounds; symptom analysis; VS; skin assessment; height and weight analysis; nutritional assessment; presence of cough

2. Diagnostic tests

   a. Sputum analysis: culture and sensitivity as well as acid-fast bacillus

   b. CXR

   c. Skin lesion biopsy

   d. Leprosy

     1) Lymphocyte transformation test

     2) Leukocyte migration inhibition test

   e. Tuberculosis: positive TB skin test (PPD or Mantoux), with induration of 10 mm or greater

D. Nursing management

1. Medications

   a. Leprosy

      1) Dapsone (DDS)

      2) Thalidomide (Thalomid): drug of choice for ENL

      3) Corticosteroids

   b. Tuberculosis

      1) Isoniazid (INH), pyrazinamide (PZA), rifampin (RMP)

      2) Combining INH and RMP is most effective

2. Teach the client and family about exposure and proper incubation periods to avoid infecting others

3. Stress the need to continue therapy even if feeling better; avoid alcohol with INH

XII. Prion Infections

A. Overview

1. Prions are mutant forms of protein on the surface of some animal cells that are similar to viruses in ability to cause infection, although smaller in size

2. Prions lack nucleic acid found in viruses

3. They have been linked to chronic degenerative diseases of the central nervous system

B. Pathophysiology

1. Although little is known about the exact mechanism of action, characteristics of the disorders have been identified

2. The disorders are characterized by long incubation periods with a protracted course that usually results in death

3. Pathologic lesions are usually limited to a single organ or tissue system

4. Examples of prion disorders include spongiform encephalopathies such as Creutzfeldt-Jacob disease

   a. This disorder begins with personality changes, memory loss, and altered visual acuity and results in progressive dementia, ataxia, and somnolence and eventually leads to death within 1 to 2 years after onset of symptoms

   b. It is thought to have been transmitted through corneal transplants and contaminated growth hormone

   c. The CNS alterations occur primarily in the cerebral cortex and cerebellum

C. Nursing assessment and management

1. Assess history and pattern of memory loss or changes in personality

2. Document progressive physical and behavioral changes

Case Study

A client has been hospitalized with an intestinal obstruction and undergoes surgery. While recovering from the surgery she develops chills, fever, and malaise and the surgical site is noted as red with purulent drainage. Because of a recent increase in the incidence of methicillin-resistant *staphylococcus aureus* (MRSA) within the hospital unit, the physician suspects MRSA as the source of the wound infection.

❶ What type of infection is this considered, and what is the most important nursing intervention concerning prevention?

❷ What is the most appropriate diagnostic test to determine the causative organism?

❸ What other relevant laboratory findings should be observed?

❹ What is the drug of choice for treating MRSA and what adverse effects should the nurse consider?

❺ If the culture reveals vancomycin-resistant *staphylococcus aureus* (VRSA), what medications are effective?

For suggested responses, see page 569.

Posttest

1   An infection characterized by bacterial resistance may be linked to the fact that the bacterial capsule:

(1) Contributes to the invasiveness of pathogenic bacteria.
(2) Plays a major role in adherence of bacteria.
(3) Does not protect the organism from phagocytosis.
(4) Is always composed of glutamic acid.

2   Which of the following client laboratory test results would likely be elevated with nematode infestation?

(1) Neutrophils
(2) Liver enzymes
(3) Red blood cells
(4) Eosinophils

3   A nurse researcher is interested in the epidemiology of HIV. This means that the researcher is concerned about which of the following?

(1) The causation of the disease
(2) How the disease is transmitted
(3) The most effective treatment regimens
(4) The distribution of the disease in a given population

4   A male college student comes to the clinic after contracting genital herpes. Which of the following interventions would be most appropriate?

(1) Encourage him to maintain bedrest for several days.
(2) Monitor temperature every 4 hours.
(3) Instruct him to avoid sexual contact during acute phases of illness.
(4) Encourage him to use antifungal agents regularly.

5   Which of the following drugs would be most effective in treating genital herpes?

(1) Penicillin (Bicillin)
(2) Rifampin (Rifadin)
(3) Acyclovir (Zovirax)
(4) Ribavirin (Virazole)

6 A young adult male relates to the nurse that he has recently experienced signs and symptoms of infection. His neutrophil count is lower than normal. The nurse concludes that he most likely:

(1) Has a bacterial infection.
(2) Has a viral infection.
(3) Has an immune deficiency disorder.
(4) Is recovering from the illness.

7 A young girl presents with fever and abdominal distention. Her mother states that she has also "coughed up blood" in recent days. Which of the following is compatible with these symptoms?

(1) Mycoplasma pneumonia
(2) Rickettsial infection
(3) Infection with nematodes
(4) Infection with spirochetes

8 Which of the following is correct concerning prion disease?

(1) Prions are opportunistic organisms frequently seen in clients with HIV.
(2) Prions have been linked to chronic degenerative disorders of the central nervous system such as Creutzfeldt-Jacob disease.
(3) Lesions are usually distributed throughout the body.
(4) Prions are similar to viruses in their nucleic acid structure.

9 A client has a WBC of 15,000, of which 60 percent are segmented neutrophils and 3 percent are bands. An antibiotic is prescribed. Three days later the WBC remains at 15,000, 62 percent segs and 10 percent bands. This most likely indicates:

(1) The infection is resolving.
(2) The client is immunocompromised.
(3) The infection is severe or prolonged and not responding to antimicrobial agents.
(4) There is a shift to the right in the differential.

10 Which of the following is incorrect concerning Lyme disease?

(1) The disease is caused by rickettsial pathogens.
(2) Humoral and cell-mediated responses by the body will not generally be sufficient to eliminate the disease.
(3) The disease is transmitted through ticks.
(4) If untreated it may lead to complications of arthritis and destruction of joints.

See pages 430–431 for Answers and Rationales.

Answers and Rationales

Pretest

1 **Answer: 3** *Rationale:* An opportunistic infection is one in which an individual develops a disease from an organism that does not cause disease in healthy individuals. This occurs with compromised immunity.
Cognitive Level: Application
Nursing Process: Assessment; *Test Plan:* PHYS

2 **Answer: 2** *Rationale:* Antibiotics may affect the outcome of the culture. Fever will continue to be present until the bacteria are eliminated, making administration of the antibiotic a priority.
Cognitive Level: Application
Nursing Process: Implementation; *Test Plan:* SECE

3 **Answer: 2** *Rationale:* The erythromycin products are the best for treating mycoplasmal pneumonia or walking pneumonia. Vermox is used for helminthic infections; Aralen hydrocloride is used for protozoal infections; and chloromycetin is used for spirochetal infections.
Cognitive Level: Application
Nursing Process: Implementation; *Test Plan:* PHYS

4 **Answer: 2** *Rationale:* A pathogen is any organism capable of causing disease. Pathogenicity refers to the ability of the organism to cause pathologic changes.
Cognitive Level: Application
Nursing Process: Analysis; *Test Plan:* PHYS

5 **Answer: 1** *Rationale:* The virus makes a DNA copy of its own RNA using the reverse transcriptase enzyme, and the DNA copy is inserted into the genetic material of the infected cell.
Cognitive Level: Knowledge
Nursing Process: Analysis; *Test Plan:* PHYS

6 **Answer: 1** *Rationale:* Influenza virus is transmitted through respiratory droplets. Herpes virus is transmitted by direct contact and HIV through blood and body fluids. Cytomegalovirus is an opportunistic infection.
Cognitive Level: Analysis
Nursing Process: Assessment; *Test Plan:* SECE

7 **Answer: 2** *Rationale:* Epidemiological studies indicate chlamydia as the most prevalent sexually transmitted disease in the United States.
Cognitive Level: Knowledge
Nursing Process: Assessment; *Test Plan:* PHYS

8 **Answer: 3** *Rationale:* Endotoxins are often not destroyed even by autoclaving. Options 1, 2, and 4 are descriptions of endotoxins.
Cognitive Level: Knowledge
Nursing Process: Analysis; *Test Plan:* PHYS

9 **Answer: 3** *Rationale:* Rickettsia are parasites of ticks, fleas, and lice. Influenza is an example of transmission by respiratory droplets, encephalitis is transmitted by mosquitoes; lice and scabies are transmitted by direct contact.
Cognitive Level: Application
Nursing Process: Analysis; *Test Plan:* PHYS

10 **Answer: 2** *Rationale:* Infection occurs in a predictable sequence requiring virulence, movement from a reservoir, and entry into a susceptible host.
Cognitive Level: Knowledge
Nursing Process: Analysis; *Test Plan:* PHYS

Posttest

1 **Answer: 1** *Rationale:* The capsule contributes to the invasiveness of pathogenic bacteria. Encapsulated bacteria are protected from phagocytosis unless coated with anticapsular antibody.
Cognitive Level: Application
Nursing Process: Analysis; *Test Plan:* PHYS

2 **Answer: 4** *Rationale:* Eosinophilia is present with allergies and infestation with parasites. Neutrophils are elevated with acute infections and bacterial organisms. Options 2 and 3 are irrelevant.
Cognitive Level: Application
Nursing Process: Assessment; *Test Plan:* PHYS

3 **Answer: 4** *Rationale:* Epidemiology is the study of how various states of health are distributed in the population.
Cognitive Level: Knowledge
Nursing Process: Assessment; *Test Plan:* HPM

4 **Answer: 3** *Rationale:* Herpes is a virus and is spread through direct contact. An antifungal would not be useful; bedrest and temperature measurement are usually not necessary.
Cognitive Level: Application
Nursing Process: Implementation; *Test Plan:* HPM

5 **Answer: 3** *Rationale:* Acyclovir is the antiviral drug of choice for treating herpesvirus. Penicillin products are used for a wide variety of bacterial infections. Rifadin is used for TB and Virazole is an antiviral agent.
Cogitive Level: Application
Nursing Process: Implementation; *Test Plan:* PHYS

6 **Answer: 2** *Rationale:* Neutrophil counts are often decreased in viral infections and elevated in bacterial infections. Neutropenia can occur because of chemotherapy and immunosuppression. With recovery, his neutrophil count should be returning to normal.
Cognitive Level: Application
Nursing Process: Analysis; *Test Plan:* PHYS

7 **Answer: 3** *Rationale:* Abdominal distention is caused from infestation of worms. Blood in sputum often results from migration of worms through alveoli. Mycoplasma pneumonia has similar side effects as bacterial pneumonia (cough, fatigue, rales, temperature). Spirochetes cause fever, neck stiffness, and lymphadenopathy; rickettsial infections cause headaches, nausea, vomiting, and muscle aches.
Cognitive Level: Analysis
Nursing Process: Assessment; *Test Plan:* PHYS

8 **Answer: 2** *Rationale:* Prions are associated with degenerative encephalopathies. While similar to viruses, they lack nucleic acid and lesions are usually limited to a single organ.
Cognitive Level: Knowledge
Nursing Process: Analysis; *Test Plan:* PHYS

9 **Answer: 3** *Rationale:* With bacterial infection there is an increased need for neutrophils. When the percentage of immature neutrophils (bands) increases at a greater rate than mature neutrophils (segs), it is an indication that the infection is severe or prolonged. This is often referred to as a shift to the left.
Cognitive Level: Analysis
Nursing Process: Analysis; *Test Plan:* PHYS

10 **Answer: 1** *Rationale:* Lyme disease is a spirochetal infection. Examples of rickettsial infections are typhus and rocky mountain spotted fever.

Cognitive Level: Knowledge
Nursing Process: Analysis; *Test Plan:* PHYS

References

Bullock, B. A. & Henze, R. (2000). *Focus on pathophysiology.* Philadelphia: Lippincott, pp. 228–252.

Clark, M. J. (1999). *Nursing in the community* (3rd ed.). Stamford, CT: Appleton & Lange, pp. 740–778, 1051–1053.

Corbett, J. V. (2000). *Laboratory tests and diagnostic procedures with nursing diagnoses* (5th ed.). Stamford, CT: Appleton & Lange.

Doenges, M. E., Moorhouse, M. F., & Geissler, A. C. (2000). *Nursing care plans: Guidelines for individualizing client care* (5th ed.). Philadelphia: F.A. Davis.

Grajeda-Higley, L. (2000). *Understanding pharmacology: A physiologic approach.* Stamford, CT: Appleton & Lange, pp. 223, 237–244, 276.

Inman, W. B. (1999). *Infection control and emerging infectious diseases.* Eau Claire, WI: Pesi Healthcare.

Kee, J. L. (1999). *Laboratory and diagnostic tests with nursing implications* (5th ed.). Stamford, CT: Appleton & Lange.

LeMone, P. & Burke, K. M. (2000). *Medical surgical nursing: Critical thinking in client care* (2nd ed.). Upper Saddle River, NJ: Prentice Hall, pp. 253–259, 488–492, 585, 805, 812–896, 1347, 2078.

Lilley, L. L. & Aucker, R. S. (2001). *Pharmacology and the nursing process* (3rd ed.). St. Louis: Mosby.

Valanis, B. (1999). *Epidemiology in health care* (3rd ed.). Stamford, CT: Appleton & Lange.

VandeWaa, E. A., Henderson, J. D., White, G. L., & Nowatzke, T. J. (1998). Common helminth infections: Battling wormlike parasites in primary care. *Clinician Reviews 8*(5): 75–77, 81–82, 85–90.

Wilkinson, J. M. (2000). *Nursing diagnosis handbook with NIC interventions and NOC outcomes* (7th ed.). Upper Saddle River, NJ: Prentice Hall.

Wilson, B. A., Shannon, M. T., & Stang, C. L. (2001). *Nursing drug guide.* Upper Saddle River, NJ: Prentice Hall.

CHAPTER 14

Integumentary System

Julie A. Adkins, RN, MSN, FNP

CHAPTER OUTLINE

*Risk Factors Associated with
   Integumentary Health Problems*
*Malignant Conditions of the
   Integumentary System*
*Benign Conditions of the
   Integumentary System*

*Bacterial Infections of the
   Integumentary System*
*Viral Infections of the
   Integumentary System*
*Fungal Infections of the
   Integumentary System*

Infestations and Insect Bites
*Allergic Conditions of the
   Integumentary System*
Burns

OBJECTIVES

- Define key terms associated with integumentary health problems.

- Identify risk factors associated with integumentary health problems.

- Discuss common etiologies of integumentary health problems.

- Describe the pathophysiologic processes associated with integumentary health problems.

- Distinguish between normal and abnormal integumentary findings obtained from nursing assessment.

- Prioritize nursing interventions associated with integumentary health problems.

[Media Link]

Use the CD-ROM enclosed with this text, or log onto the address given to access the free, interactive Companion Website created for this series. The CD-ROM and Companion Website accompanying this book offer additional practice opportunities and information—NCLEX Review, Case Studies, Glossary, In Depth with NCLEX, and more.

www.prenhall.com/hogan

REVIEW AT A GLANCE

acne *an androgenically stimulated, inflammatory disorder of the sebaceous glands, resulting in comedomes, papules, inflamed pustules, and occasionally scarring*

atopic dermatitis *an inflammation of the skin from an unknown source in an individual with irritable skin*

basal cell carcinoma *malignant tumor of the skin originating from the basal cells of the epidermis*

burn *tissue injuries caused by the application of heat, chemicals, electricity, or radiation to the tissue*

candidiasis *a fungal infection caused by* Candida albicans, *a yeast-like fungus that most often causes superficial cutaneous infections*

carbuncle (carbunculosis) *aggregates of infected follicles convalesced together to form one large lesion*

cellulitis *a diffuse inflammation of the skin and subcutaneous layers with various presenting lesions including vesicles (small sacs of fluid), bullae (large blisters), abscesses, and plaques*

contact dermatitis *an eruption of the skin related to contact with an irritating substance or allergen*

dermatophyte *a group of fungi that have the ability to infect and survive only on keratin, classified as Tinea infections*

exfoliative dermatitis *an inflammation of the skin characterized by erythema involving loss of exfoliated (peeling) skin*

folliculitis *an inflammation of the hair follicle usually caused by the organism* Staphylococcus aureus *or* Pseudomonas aeruginosa

furuncle (furunculosis) *also known as an abscess or boil, a deep folliculitis consisting of a pus-filled mass that is painful and firm*

herpes simplex *a viral infection that occurs within the keratinolytics and manifests as painful vesicles that often occur in clusters on the skin*

herpes zoster *a viral infection (also known as shingles) that manifests as a cluster of vesicles on the skin; a reactivation of the varicella virus in the dorsal root ganglia that remained in the latent form after the primary infection*

impetigo *a superficial skin infection initially seen as an erythemic vesicle, later changing to a honey-colored crusted lesion*

lentigo *a brown macule resembling a freckle except the border is usually regular*

malignant melanoma *a skin cancer arising from the melanocytes*

molluscum contagiosum *a benign, viral infection of the skin caused by the poxvirus inducing epidermal cell proliferation*

pediculosis *an infestation of the skin or hair by the species of blood-sucking lice capable of living as external parasites on the human host*

psoriasis *a genetically determined, chronic epidermal proliferative disease characterized by erythematous, dry scaling patches, usually with a heavy, silvery surface*

seborrheic dermatitis *an acute inflammation of the skin from an unknown cause that usually begins on the scalp and has rounded, irregular lesions and yellow scales*

seborrheic keratosis *benign plaques, beige to brown or maybe black in color, ranging in size from 3 to 20 mm with a velvety or warty surface*

squamous cell carcinoma *a slow-growing cancer of atypical squamous cells that originates in the epidermis and may metastasize*

Tinea versicolor *common non-inflammatory fungal infection caused by lipophilic yeast*

urticaria *an itchy rash (hives)*

warts *virus induced epidermal tumors*

Pretest

1 The nurse is teaching self-care to a client with psoriasis. The nurse should encourage which of the following for his scaled lesion?

(1) Emollients and moisturizers to soften the scales, and soft brushing of scales
(2) Importance of follow-up appointments
(3) Use of a clean razor blade each time he shaves
(4) Keep occlusive dressings on the lesions 24 hours a day.

2 The nurse teaches a client that the first step in self-management of contact/irritant dermatitis is to do which of the following?

(1) Take antihistamines to control the itch.
(2) Identify and remove the causative agent.
(3) Use over-the-counter (OTC) hydrocortisone cream.
(4) Refer for allergy testing.

3 A mother asks how her second-grade child got head lice. The nurse responds by telling the mother that lice infestation:

(1) Only occurs in socioeconomically deprived people.
(2) Was probably spread by person-to-person contact in the classroom.
(3) Is airborne.
(4) Is due to improper washing of the hair.

4 The nurse conducting a health fair teaches attendees that which of the following groups of people are most at risk for developing malignant melanoma?

(1) Light-skinned people who work indoors
(2) Dark-skinned people who work indoors
(3) Light-skinned people with regular sun exposure
(4) Dark-skinned people with regular sun exposure

5 A client is admitted to the Emergency Department with burns to the chest and arms. The skin is white, dry, and there is no pain. The nurse assesses the type of burn the client has as which of the following?

(1) Superficial thickness
(2) Superficial partial thickness
(3) Deep partial thickness
(4) Full thickness

6 A young boy is brought to the trauma unit with a chemical burn to the face. Priority assessment would include which of the following?

(1) Skin integrity
(2) Blood pressure and pulse
(3) Patency of airway
(4) Amount of pain

7 A 10-year-old female client complains of dandruff. On examination, the nurse notices the dandruff flakes don't brush off the hair, and there is a papular rash on her neck. The nurse suspects which of the following disorders?

(1) Tinea capitis
(2) Dandruff
(3) Seborrheic dermatitis
(4) Pediculosis capitis

8 The nurse is most concerned about a wasp sting for a client who:

(1) Has never been stung before.
(2) Has a history of fever or chills when bitten.
(3) Had hives and shortness of breath with the last sting.
(4) Had a rise in blood pressure to 140/90 when stung.

9 A client who has been on two antibiotics complains of burning on the tongue and doesn't want to eat. Inspection of the tongue reveals a white, milky plaque that does not come off with rubbing. The nurse suspects which condition?

(1) Impetigo
(2) Candidiasis
(3) Burns
(4) Herpes

10 The nurse would include which of the following pieces of information in health teaching for a client with warts?

(1) They are viral and may reappear at the same site or other areas of the skin.
(2) They will not go away without treatment.
(3) They cannot be transmitted.
(4) They only appear in childhood.

See pages 462–463 for Answers and Rationales.

I. Risk Factors Associated with Integumentary Health Problems

A. Malignant conditions

1. Skin pigmentation
2. Preexisting lesions
3. Exposure to chemicals
4. Radiation or excessive sun
5. Trauma
6. Viruses

7. Ethnicity (Caucasian)

8. Fair-skinned complexions

NCLEX!

B. **Individuals with fair skin and light-colored hair** and those with heavy sun exposure are more at risk for malignant melanoma

C. **Benign conditions:** exposure to sun, local trauma, infections, stress, physical disorders, and drugs

D. **Bacterial conditions:** individuals with a compromised immune system, other disorders such as diabetes mellitus, or lack of proper hygiene and nutrition

E. **Viral infections:** depressed immune system, human immunodeficiency virus (HIV), individuals with radiation, chemotherapy, or major organ transplants

F. **Fungal infections:** debilitating disease, poor nutrition, poor hygiene, tropical climates, contact with infected persons or animals, communal showers and pools, occlusive footwear, excessive sweating, sharing of footwear, excessive moisture from clothing, or use of incontinence undergarments with the elderly

G. **Bites and infestations:** living in overcrowded or developing countries, unsanitary conditions, certain geographic regions

H. **Allergic conditions:** immunosuppressed states (such as AIDS), drug therapy, and heredity

I. **Burns:** small children and elderly, high-risk occupations, individuals with decreased sensation to extremities or certain parts of the body

II. Malignant Conditions of the Integumentary System

A. **Overview**

1. Defined as skin cancer from a malignant tumor or neoplasm of the skin

2. There are three types of malignant conditions: basal cell, carcinoma, melanoma, and squamous cell carcinoma

NCLEX!

3. Causes include ultraviolet exposure, extremes in weather, radiological treatment, chemicals, trauma, burns, or chronic infections; fair-skinned people, persons who live in warm climates, and the elderly are at increased risk

B. **Pathophysiology**

1. **Basal cell carcinoma** is an abnormal cell growth of the basal layer of the epidermal skin; it is the least aggressive type and rarely metastasizes to other organs; it is the most common form of skin cancer and may invade surrounding tissue, destroying parts of the body; the tumor takes many forms

   a. Nodular basal cell carcinoma is the most common and appears on the neck, face, and head; it is a pearly colored nodule with well-defined margins and a depressed center or rolled edge

   b. Superficial basal cell carcinoma is the second most common tumor that is located on the trunk and extremities

   c. Other forms include pigmented basal cell (head, neck, and face), rare morpheaform basal cell (head and neck), and keratotic basal cell (pre- and postauricular groove)

2. **Squamous cell carcinoma** is a more aggressive, slow growing cancer of atypical squamous cells that originate in the epidermis and may metastasize via the lymphatic system

    a. Proliferation of keratinizing cells of the epithelium causes the tumor, forming keratin "pearls"

    b. It is most common on sun-exposed areas such as the nose, lips, and hands

    c. The lower lip is a frequent location, especially in smokers

    NCLEX!

    d. It appears as a firm, irregular, flesh-colored papule with a scaly, keratotic surface

    e. It may be erythemic, sore, and/or bleed if touched

3. **Malignant melanoma** is a cancerous tumor arising from the melanocytes (melanin-producing cells in the deepest epithelial layer), which has the ability to metastasize to any organ

    a. The melanoma initially grows superficially and laterally continuing to the epidermis and dermis

    b. It then grows vertically with penetration of the reticular dermis and subcutaneous fat

    c. This type of melanoma frequently affects young people with common sites being the back and legs

    NCLEX!

    d. Melanomas tend to have asymmetry, border irregularity, color variation, and diameter greater than 6 mm (see Box 14-1); key signs include irregular, circular-bordered lesion with hues of tan, black, or blue

    e. Precursor lesions of a malignant melanoma include dysplastic nevi (atypical mole), congenital nevi (present at birth), and lentigo maligna (tan or black patch that has the appearance of a freckle)

    f. Classification of tumors includes superficial-spreading melanoma (about 70 percent) that arises from preexisting nevus, lentigo maligna melanoma, nodular melanoma, and acral lentiginous melanoma

C. **Nursing assessment**

1. Assessment

    a. A symptom analysis about any skin changes or new growths and a history of the amount of sun exposure or sunburn

    b. Assessing any family history of skin disorders, and past history of burns, injury, trauma, or cigarette smoking

---

Box 14-1

ABCDs of Malignant Melanoma

Asymmetry
Border irregularity
Color variegation
Diameter greater than 6 mm

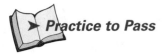

Practice to Pass

A client who regularly suntans states she is not worried about skin cancer. How should the nurse respond?

NCLEX!

NCLEX!

c. Assessing any area/preexisting lesion for change in color, size, or shape, noting any local soreness, oozing or bleeding lesions, pruritis, lymph node enlargement, liver, and spleen

2. Diagnostic tests: shave biopsy (for diagnosis), punch biopsy, incisional biopsy (remove part of tumor), or excisional biopsy (remove all of tumor); for malignant melanoma, a liver profile, complete blood count (CBC), electrolytes, CT scan of liver and brain, chest x-ray (CXR), bone scan, magnetic resonance imaging (MRI) of liver, and biopsy of lymph nodes

D. Nursing management

1. Assess all lesions over the entire body

2. Teach self-monitoring and examination of existing skin lesions and for any new lesions; early diagnosis and intervention are crucial

3. Instruct the client to avoid contact with chemical irritants

4. Educate the client about the importance of sun exposure protection, wearing layered clothing while outdoors, avoiding midday sun, and using sunscreen with a sun protection factor (SPF) over 15

5. Encourage verbalization of client concerns and changes in body image

6. Educate clients on the harmful effects of tanning beds

III. Benign Conditions of the Integumentary System

A. Overview

1. Defined as conditions of the integumentary system that are cutaneous growths with no malignant potential

2. Benign conditions include acne, lentigo, psoriasis, and seborrheic keratosis

3. Causes

a. Acne: oversecretion of sebum and dysfunction of hormones

b. Lentigo: prolonged exposure to the sun

c. Psoriasis and seborrheic keratosis: genetics

B. Pathophysiology

1. **Acne** is an androgen-stimulated, inflammatory disorder of the sebaceous glands resulting in comedones (open form—blackhead; closed form—whitehead), papules (pimples), inflammatory pustules, cysts, and occasional scarring

a. There are three stages of acne

1) Mild: few to several papules, no nodules, and occurring on the face/neck only

2) Moderate: several to many papules or pustules and few to several nodules on the face, back, chest, or upper arms

3) Severe: numerous and/or extensive papules or pustules, many nodules with acne-induced atrophic scarring

    b. Acne involves several factors including increased sebum production, abnormal keratinization of the follicular epithelium, proliferation of propriobacterium acnes, and inflammation

    c. The rate of sebum production is determined genetically; it is increased by the presence of androgens with the earliest changes occurring in the prepubescent years

    d. There are three types of acne: *acne vulgaris* (common adolescent type), *acne conglobata* (causes scarring), and *acne rosacea* (chronic form)

    e. Acne is graded as follows: *Grade 1*—comedonal (open or closed); *Grade 2*—papular with over 25 lesions on the face and trunk; *Grade 3*—pustular with over 25 lesions, mild scarring; and *Grade 4*—nodulocystic, inflammatory nodules, and cysts with extensive scarring

2. Lentigo is a brown macule resembling a freckle except the border is usually regular

    a. There are three types of lentigo: benign lentigo, lentigo maligna, and senile lentigo

    b. *Benign lentigo* may first appear on young children with ultraviolet light exposure and fade in color during the winter months

    c. *Lentigo maligna* is a brown- or black-mottled, irregular bordered, slowly enlarging lesion with an increased number of melanocytes; it is considered pre-malignant in that one-third may progress to a melanoma, usually 10 to 15 years later

    d. *Senile lentigo,* also known as liver spots, occurs on skin exposed to ultraviolet light, especially in older Caucasians

3. Psoriasis is a genetically determined, chronic epidermal proliferative disease that is characterized by erythematous, dry scaling patches and a heavy, silvery surface; there are often recurring remissions and exacerbations

    a. Psoriasis is principally caused by an alteration in cell kinetics of the keratinocytes where the cell cycle is shortened from 311 hours to 36 hours with an increase in epidermal cells

    b. It is often triggered by an infection, most often a streptococcal pharyngitis or a viral upper respiratory infection

    c. There are two types: *Type 1,* which affects the young person who has a strong family history of the disease and is the more aggressive type, and *Type 2,* which affects the older person who generally has no family history of the disease

    d. Type 2 is a more stable type of disease

    e. It is a lifelong process without a cure

4. Seborrheic keratosis is characterized by benign plaques, beige, brown, or maybe black in color, ranging in size from 3 to 20 mm with a velvety or warty surface

    a. Seborrheic keratosis is caused by a proliferation of immature keratinocytes and melanocytes occurring totally within the dermis that is generally seen beginning in middle-age

    b. They appear as "stuck on" spots usually present on the face, neck, scalp, back, and upper chest and may bleed when irritated by clothing or picked

C. Nursing assessment

    1. Acne

        a. Assessment

            1) Symptom analysis regarding onset, type of lesions, and distribution

            2) Inquire about types of cleansers, lubricants/moisturizers, and previous treatments and results

            3) In females, question about flare-ups of acne around menstrual cycle and the use of oral contraceptives

            4) Examine the skin to determine the type of acne (mild, moderate, or severe) and document areas of involvement

            5) Determine the grade of acne present

        b. Diagnostic tests: there are no diagnostic tests for acne; a culture may be taken to differentiate acne from other conditions if pustules are present

    2. Lentigo

        a. Assessment includes symptom analysis regarding onset, location, duration, color changes, and enlargement; ask the client about sun exposure and use of sunscreens

        b. Diagnostic tests: may not require any tests, but a biopsy is suggested for any suspicious lesion

    3. Psoriasis

NCLEX!

        a. Assessment includes determining the location, onset, and duration of the plaques; inquire about previous treatments and results obtained; assess for any triggering factors such as emotional stress, trauma, or seasonal changes

        b. Diagnostic tests: skin biopsy may be needed to differentiate the diagnosis from other conditions, or ultrasonography may be needed to measure skin thickness

    4. Seborrheic keratosis

        a. Assessment includes determining the location, onset, and duration of the plaques; inquire about any changes in the lesion, erythema, or bleeding at the site; assess the client's sun exposure history and any treatments or interventions used in the past

        b. Diagnostic tests: there are no specific diagnostic tests

D. Nursing management

    1. Acne

NCLEX!

        a. Medications

            1) Benzoyl peroxide preparations (over-the-counter), which have an antibacterial, keratolytic, and drying effect

            2) Topical solutions such as clindamycin (Cleocin T solution), erythromycin (A/T/S or EryDerm), tetracycline (Topicycline), isotretinoin

(Accutane), azelaic acid (Azelex), and tretinoin (Retinoic acid, Vitamin A, Retin-A)

    3) Topical antibiotics may assist in decreasing the formation of new lesions even though it is not an infection

    4) Many of these topical solutions are drying to the skin; a small amount should be tested on a hidden area of the skin first, before applying to the entire face

    5) Most of these agents have the side effect of photosensitivity; sun protection should be used

  b. Management is aimed at controlling the disease and is not curative

  c. Instruct the client to use a mild antibacterial soap, avoid cosmetics containing oil, and confine moisturizing lotions to dry patches of skin only

  d. Instruct client not to pick at lesions, which could cause scarring

  e. Educate the client that treatment for 6 to 8 weeks is usual before obvious improvement occurs

  f. Dietary factors have not been shown to effect sebum production, but the client should be counseled on a well-balanced diet

2. Lentigo

  a. Medications include tretinoin (Retinoic acid, Retin-A), however no meds are necessarily required; cosmetics or bleaching solutions may be preferred by clients

  b. Instruct the client on the ABCD method of assessing skin lesions: asymmetry, border, color, and diameter

  c. Teach the client to inspect the skin regularly and to seek medical advice for any noted changes

  d. Instruct to use layered clothing while in sunlight and to use sunscreens with a sun protection factor (SPF) over 15

3. Psoriasis

  a. Medications include topical corticosteroids and tar preparations to decrease inflammation and suppress mitotic activity of psoriasis, anthralin (Dithranol), and calcipotriene (Dovonex)

  b. Photochemotherapy that involves the drug methoxsalen and exposure to ultraviolet-A (UVA) rays has been effective in severe forms and promoting remission; hyperkeratosis is decreased with exposure to UVA and ultraviolet-B (UVB) light

  c. Aveeno baths, tar shampoos, and wet dressings may help alleviate itching

  d. Instruct the client on moisturizing soaps, emollients, and scalp oils to soften scales followed by soft brushing while bathing

  e. Instruct the client on medication treatments and side effects

  f. Emphasize that the disorder is not contagious

g. Provide the client the opportunity to discuss feelings regarding the disorders impact on the individual's life

h. Counsel the client on the importance of maintaining a healthy lifestyle, which includes a well-balanced diet, exercise, moderate alcohol intake, and avoidance of tobacco products

i. Discuss the role of stress in relation to flare-ups of the lesions

4. Seborrheic keratosis

a. Medication treatment is usually not required; treatment is at the preference of the client for cosmetic purposes

b. Educate the client to use sunscreens with a SPF over 15, decrease sun exposure, and avoid tanning; instruct client to wear hats and protective clothing while in the sun

c. Provide assurance that the lesions are benign in nature

d. Teach the client the ABCD of skin lesions; assure client that treatment is not necessary unless requested for cosmetic purposes

IV. Bacterial Infections of the Integumentary System

A. Overview

1. Defined as a break in the skin integrity and invasion of a pathogenic organism

2. Disorders include impetigo, cellulitis, folliculitis; other lesions are the furuncle (furunculosis) and carbuncle (carbunculosis)

3. May be primary (caused by one organism) or secondary (caused by disease process or trauma to the skin)

4. Causes include poor hygiene, deficient nutrition, skin trauma, and excess moisture to the skin; systemic diseases such as diabetes mellitus and malignancies may contribute to furuncles

B. Pathophysiology

1. **Impetigo** is a superficial skin infection initially seen as an erythemic vesicle and later changes to a honey-colored crusted lesion

   a. It is most commonly seen in 2- to 6-year-olds range and may be enhanced by crowded living conditions, poor hygiene, and warm climates

   b. *Staphylococcus aureus* and *Streptococcus pyogenes* (beta-hemolytic) are the most common organisms causing the infection

   c. Impetigo is most often found on the face, arms, legs, and buttocks

   d. Signs and symptoms include extreme itching and red, macular lesions

   e. Impetigo spreads quickly, therefore treatment should be started early

2. **Cellulitis** is a diffuse inflammation of the skin and subcutaneous layers with various presenting lesions including vesicles (small sacs of fluid), bullae (large blisters), abscesses, and plaques

   a. Involved organisms usually are *Streptococcus, Staphylococcus aureus,* or *Haemophilus influenzae*

NCLEX!

Practice to Pass

A client has been diagnosed with acne. What self-care strategies should the nurse explain?

    b. There is usually a preceding wound or trauma to the skin, and it is most common in adults

    c. Signs and symptoms include erythema, warmth, edema, and pain; also frequently present are fever, chills, malaise, and lymphadenopathy

3. Folliculitis is an inflammation of the hair follicle usually caused by the organism *Staphylococcus aureus* or *Pseudomonas aeruginosa*

    a. It can occur at any age, occurs more in males, and is aggravated by shaving

    b. A stye is a folliculitis on the eyelid

    c. Signs and symptoms include red lesions or erythemic pustules that can be painful

4. Furuncles (furunculosis): a furuncle (abscess or boil) is a deep folliculitis consisting of a pus-filled mass that is painful and firm

    a. It is common in children, teens, and young adults

    b. It is caused by *Staphylococcus aureus,* and common sites of infection are the nares, neck, axilla, and genital area

    c. Furnuculosis is the condition resulting from multiple boils

    d. Signs and symptoms are deep, firm, red nodules that are painful and usually drain purulent secretions

5. Carbuncles are aggregates of infected follicles convalesced together to form one large lesion

    a. Carbunculosis is a condition of several carbuncles

    b. Signs and symptoms include painful nodes with pus, chills, fever, and leukocytosis

C. Nursing assessment

1. Assessment includes location, appearance (erythema, swelling, drainage), onset, and duration of lesions; symptom analysis of associated symptoms of fever, chills, and previous outbreaks; vital signs (VS); palpate surface of lesion and adjacent lymph nodes for fluctuance (fluid-filled); assess tetanus prophylaxis status

2. Diagnostic tests: wound culture and sensitivity (C&S) to identify organism and verify antibiotic choice

D. Nursing management

1. Medications include topical antibiotic ointments or oral antibiotics for 10 to 14 days; instruct on the frequent use of antibacterial soaps for preventative therapy

2. Cleanse the site with warm soapy water 2 to 3 times per day; avoid irritating lotions/creams

3. Use warm compresses for comfort

4. Instruct client to use a clean razor each time he/she shaves

5. Incision and drainage of lesion may be necessary

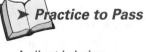

Practice to Pass

A client is being discharged home after hospitalization for cellulitis. What specific discharge instructions should be given?

V. Viral Infections of the Integumentary System

A. Overview

1. Defined as conditions of the skin resulting in a break in the integrity of the skin and the invasion of a virus or intracellular pathogen

2. Disorders include herpes simplex types 1 & 2, herpes zoster, molluscum contagiosum, and warts

3. Causes include drugs with immunosuppressive action such as corticosteroids, birth control pills, and antibiotics; stress and sunlight have been attributed to herpes simplex

B. Pathophysiology

1. **Herpes simplex** is a viral infection that occurs within the keratinolytics and is manifested by painful vesicles that occur in clusters on the skin (HSV type I), also known as fever blister, or genital mucosa (HSV type II)

    a. The virus transverses the afferent nerves to the host ganglion: the trigeminal ganglia are the target of the oral virus (HSV1) and usually affect the lips, face, buccal mucosa, and throat

    b. The sacral ganglia is the target for the genital virus (HSV2); it affects the genital area and is considered a sexually transmitted disease (STD)

    c. The herpes simplex virus occurs in three stages: *primary*—initial outbreak of the virus occurs as blisters; *latency*—virus remains dormant in the ganglia; and *recurrent stage*—the virus is reactivated, travels along the peripheral nerves to the site of the initial infection causing characteristic symptoms

    d. Transmission is by direct contact with the active lesions or by virus-containing fluid such as saliva or cervical secretions with no evidence of active disease; the incubation period ranges from 2 to 14 days; recurrent infections may be triggered by skin trauma, stress, or illness

    e. Signs and symptoms include erythema, vesicles, discomfort (burning, tingling, or pain), fever, and sore throat; there may be associated tenderness, pain, and burning prior to eruption of the lesions and may be associated with fever, myalgia, malaise, or cervical lymphadenopathy; HSV1 infections in infants and children usually appear as a gingivostomatitis with symptoms of pain in the mouth and/or throat and may be accompanied by fever and malaise

2. **Herpes zoster** is a viral infection (also known as shingles) that is manifested as a cluster of vesicles on the skin that usually follows along a dermatome and is unilateral; the vesicles may have purulent fluid in 3 to 4 days, then form crusts which fall off in 2 to 3 weeks

    a. It is a reactivation of the varicella virus in the dorsal root ganglia that remained in the latent form after the primary infection of chicken pox

NCLEX!

    b. Signs and symptoms include erythematous lesions, itching, burning, and pain (may be severe); a complication is visual loss and severe pain along one of the nerves; fever, headache and malaise may precede the rash

    c. It is commonly seen in older adults but can also affect children

3. **Molluscum contagiosum** is a benign viral infection of the skin characterized by white to flesh-colored, shiny dome-shaped papules with a firm, waxy appearance

   a. It is caused by the poxvirus inducing epidermal cell proliferation; it spreads by direct contact and has an incubation period between 2 to 7 weeks and lasts as long as 6 months

   b. It is a common cutaneous manifestation in human immunodeficiency virus (HIV) infection

   c. Humans are the only known source; the lesions occur in groups and are more common in children and adolescents but may affect all age groups

   d. Signs and symptoms include small, waxy, epithelial tumors that may be solid or semiliquid

4. **Warts** are virus-induced epidermal tumors and are commonly seen in children and young adults

   a. The wart virus is located within the epidermal layer proliferating from a mass

   b. They are transmitted by touch and often appear on the hands, periungual regions, and plantar surfaces

   c. Most warts resolve in 12 to 24 months without treatment and are asymptomatic except for plantar warts, which may be very painful

   d. There are several types of warts: common (dome-shaped, above the skin, scaly, irregular surface), filiform (thin projections on a narrow stalk usually on the face), flat (flat-topped, skin-colored papules located on the face and extremities), plantar (occur on weight-bearing surfaces of the feet), and venereal (considered an STD on glans of penis, anal region, and vulva)

   e. Signs and symptoms include lesions, which are round, raised, rough, and gray; genital warts are cauliflower in appearance

C. **Nursing assessment**

   1. Herpes simplex virus

      a. Assessment includes identifying the clinical stage of the disease; the primary stage usually occurs 2 to 14 days following inoculation; lesions are usually grouped vesicles that may rupture, leaving erosions that form crusts; the crusts signal the end of the viral shedding; ask about previous occurrences and exposures to infected persons

      b. Diagnostic tests: viral culture for the most definitive diagnosis

   2. Herpes zoster

      a. Assessment includes questioning the client regarding prior varicella infection and immunocompromised status, examining the skin for characteristic lesions and the distribution of the lesions, and determining if there is ophthalmic involvement

      b. Diagnostic tests: Tzanck smear to identify herpes virus, culture of vesicles, and immunofluorescence to identify varicella

3. Molluscum contagiosum

    a. Assessment includes inquiring about location, appearance, onset, and duration of lesion, past medical history including HIV infection, examination of the skin for lesions, palpating the lesions to determine if firm or fluid-filled in nature

    b. No diagnostic tests are recommended

4. Warts

    a. Assessment includes identifying the type of wart, onset, location, and duration of lesion, and about any previous treatments used

    b. No diagnostic tests are recommended

D. Nursing management

    1. Herpes simplex

        a. Medications during the primary stage include oral viscous xylocaine, Orabase, use of over-the-counter (OTC) products like Blistex to prevent drying, and acetaminophen (Tylenol) for pain; applying ice may help to reduce the swelling

        b. Medications during the recurrent stage of HSV or genital HSV include topical antiviral agents such as penciclovir (Denavir), which is not recommended for children, or acyclovir (Zovirax) ointment applied every 2 hours to speed healing and relieve pain; oral antivirals, such as acyclovir (Zovirax), valacyclovir (Valtrex), or famciclovir (Famvir), may be used in severe cases or for the immunocompromised client with persistent lesions

        c. Instruct client to use sunscreen as a preventative measure

        d. Instruct client about how to decrease the spread of HSV to others

        e. Educate client to avoid sexual activity when active lesions are present and to use condoms with each sexual contact

    2. Herpes zoster

        a. Medications include nonsteroidal antiinflammatory drugs (NSAIDs) or acetaminophen (Tylenol), which may be used for pain and fever; wet compresses of Burow's solution or tap water may be used for comfort measures; systemic therapy with acyclovir (Zovirax), vidarabine (Vira-A), and corticosteroids are indicated for clients when the outbreak is less than 72 hours old or when over 72 hours old with newly developing lesions, when clients are over age 50, and for immunocompromised clients

        b. Suppression of pain, inflammation, and infection is the goal of therapy

        c. Instruct the client of the possibility of post-herpetic pain (pain that persists more than one month after lesions have healed)

        d. Instruct on signs and symptoms of secondary bacterial infections, usually caused from scratching and itching the lesions

        e. Opthalmic involvement requires an emergency referral to an opthamologist

        f. Instruct to avoid clients who may be at risk for infection; such as neonates, pregnant women, and immunosuppressed persons, as well as those who have not previously had chickenpox

g. Stress that follow-up in 1 to 3 days and then again in 7 to 10 days is necessary

h. Educate the client to understand the disease and measures to maintain health

i. Inform the client that scarring at the site of the infection may occur

3. Molluscum contagiosum

a. Medications include liquid nitrogen therapy (client preference), and Duofilm or tretinoin (Retin-A, Avita) for removal of the lesions

b. Instruct the client that these medications are to be used at bedtime; the area should be exfoliated before reapplication and petroleum jelly applied to the surrounding skin

c. For a small number of asymptomatic lesions of molluscum contagiosum, observation for several months is indicated

4. Warts

a. Medications include liquid nitrogen and topical preparations to be used nightly for 6 to 8 weeks; instruct to apply petroleum ointment on surrounding skin to prevent irritation

b. Most clients request treatment/removal of the wart lesion; the filiform wart is usually removed by snip excision

c. Instruct the client on signs and symptoms of infection after removal and on pain relief measures if applicable

d. Educate the client that, since the wart is viral in nature, it may reappear in the same site or on other areas of the skin

VI. Fungal Infections of the Integumentary System

A. Overview

1. Defined as infections caused by fungi (dermatophytes), which are living organisms found on the stratum corneum, hair, and nails

2. Disorders are named for the area of the body involved and include candidiasis, *Tinea versicolor*, and dermatophyte infection; includes Tinea capitis, Tinea corporis, Tinea cruris, Tinea pedis, and Tinea unguium

3. Causes include excess moisture, contact with an infected person or animal, use of broad-spectrum antibiotics, disorders such as diabetes mellitus, malnutrition, iron deficiency anemia, immunosuppressed states, pregnancy, and aging process

B. Pathophysiology

1. **Candidiasis** is an infection caused by *Candida albicans*, a yeast-like fungi that most often causes superficial cutaneous infections

a. *Candida albicans* are part of the normal flora of the skin and mucous membranes; overgrowth is caused when moisture, warmth, and breaks in the epidermal barrier occur

b. Includes oral (thrush), vagina (vulvovaginitis), diaper area (perineal), glans and prepuce of the penis (balantitis), nail folds (paronychia), perineal area, the axilla, umbilical area, and under the breasts

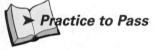

Practice to Pass

A client has been diagnosed with herpes simplex type 2 (HSV2). What explanation should be given about this disease?

c. Candida organisms may also be a causative agent in otitis externa and scalp disorders

d. The fungus needs a host and certain conditions in order to become pathogenic, such as a depressed immune state, debilitation, poor nutrition, moisture, use of antibiotics or steroids (see causes)

e. Signs and symptoms include lesions that are bright red, smooth macules with a macerated appearance and a scaling, elevated border

f. Characteristic "satellite" lesions are small, similar-appearing macules outside the main lesion; specific areas of the body manifest as:

1) Oral thrush: white, milky, non-removable plaques on the oral mucosa that may be associated with a burning sensation or decreased taste

2) Vagina (vulvovaginitis): excessive itching and a thick, white, curdy vaginal discharge

3) Diaper area (perineal): erythema, papules, pustules, and a scaling border

4) Balanitis: flattened pustules, edema, scaling, erosion, burning, and tenderness on the penis

5) Paronychia: erythema, edema and tenderness with possible creamy, purulent discharge with pressure on the nail bed; the nails usually become discolored and have ridging

2. **Tinea versicolor** is a common non-inflammatory fungal infection caused by lipophilic yeast and *Pityrosporum* orbiculare, which is part of the normal flora of the skin

a. Overgrowth occurs for unknown reasons and the infection is not contagious

b. Signs and symptoms include multiple small, circular macules of various colors (white, pink, or brown) usually on the upper trunk, which are usually asymptomatic

3. **Dermatophyte** infections are caused by a group of fungi that have the ability to infect and survive only on keratin; they can affect all age groups

a. These infections include Tinea capitis (ringworm of the scalp), Tinea corporis (ringworm of the body), Tinea cruris (ringworm of the groin and upper thighs), Tinea pedis (ringworm of the foot or athlete's foot), and Tinea unguium (ringworm of the nails or onychomycosis)

b. Dermatophyte infections (tineas) have three causative agents: *Microsporum, Trichophyton,* or *Epidermophyton*

c. Signs and symptoms

1) Tinea capitis: erythema and scaling of the scalp with patchy hair loss

2) Tinea corporis: lesions are generally circular, erythematous, well-marginated with a raised, scaly vesicular border

3) Tinea cruris: lesions are sharply demarcated, scaling patches and usually extremely pruritic

4) Tinea pedis: lesions are fine, vesiculopustular or scaly areas that are usually itchy

5) Tinea unguium: usually involves only 1 to 2 nails; toenails are affected-more often than fingernails; characteristic features include distal thickening and yellowing of the nail plate

C. Nursing assessment

1. Assessment

   a. Symptom analysis about onset, duration, distribution, and presence of symptoms

   b. Possible contact with others (including animals) with similar lesions

   c. Previous treatments used and results

   d. Any underlying chronic conditions and past or present medications

   e. Examination of skin to determine type and distribution of lesions and associated symptoms

2. Diagnostic tests: a culture of scraping (skin, hair, or nails) or microscopic examination of scaling using a 10 percent potassium hydrogen (KOH) preparation; a Wood's lamp, which uses ultraviolet (UV) light; area fluoresces blue-green in the presence of a fungal infection

D. Nursing management

1. Medications

   a. Antifungals that are available in various forms (creams, powders, shampoos, vaginal suppositories, and oral tablets) containing the following drugs: clotrimazole (Mycelex), nystatin (Mycostatin, Nilstat), miconazole (Monistat), undecylenic acid (Desenex), ketoconazole (Nizoral), fluconazole (Diflucan), and amphotericin B (Fungizone)

   b. Topical treatment is preferred, but some cases require oral medications such as miconozole (Monistat), nystatin (Nilstat), ketoconazole (Nizoral), and fluconazole (Diflucan)

   c. Systemic therapy is necessary for moderate to severe disease that occurs in immunocompromised persons

2. Instruct clients to avoid sharing linens or personal items

3. Instruct clients to dry all skin folds and use a clean towel and washcloth daily

4. For Tinea pedis, put socks on before underwear to prevent spread of infection from feet; wear light cotton socks and change frequently; wear sandals or open-toed shoes when possible but avoid plastic footwear and occlusive shoes

5. Apply drying or dusting powders and topical antiperspirants to decrease moisture

6. For vaginal candida, avoid tight clothing and pantyhose, bathe frequently and dry genital area thoroughly; treatment of the sexual partner may be necessary to avoid reinfection or have partner use condoms until resolved; avoid douching and change perineal pads frequently

NCLEX!

NCLEX!

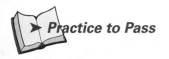

Practice to Pass

A client returns to the clinic with recurrent Tinea pedis. What should the client be told regarding preventative measures?

7. Reducing the risk of fungal infections can occur with weight loss by obese clients and maintenance of normal serum glucose levels in diabetic clients to decrease risk of infection

NCLEX!

8. Instruct clients that relief of symptoms may occur quickly with topical medication but stress the need to use topical applications for 7 to 10 days

9. Follow-up visits should be scheduled every 2 to 4 weeks for clients receiving long-term oral antifungal treatment to monitor liver function profile and complete blood count (CBC)

VII. Infestations and Insect Bites

A. Overview

1. Defined as an invasion of the skin by an insect or parasite

2. Disorders include common insect bites (stings) and pediculosis

3. Causes include living in infested areas and contact with an infected person or clothing/material

B. Pathophysiology

1. An insect sting or bite occurs when there is secretion of venom into the skin by an insect or spider; arthropods affect many by being pests, inoculating poison, invading tissues, or transmitting disease

   a. Stings by yellow-jackets, hornets, honeybees, and wasps result in generalized allergic reactions of varying severity in approximately 0.4 percent of the population

   b. Honeybees, wasps, hornets, and yellow-jackets embed a firm, sharp stinger in the skin and the venom is secreted; the injected venoms are proteins with enzyme activity that cause local or general reactions classified as toxic or allergic

   c. There are many species of spiders, but the brown recluse spider and the black widow are the two species capable of producing severe reactions

      1) The brown recluse spider is small and light brown and lives in dark areas such as closets, basements, and under porches

      2) The spider bite can cause local or general reactions, even death; the venom is similar to that of a rattlesnake

      3) The black widow bite resembles a pinprick, injecting a neurotoxin that causes an ascending motor paralysis

      4) The potent toxin is rapidly absorbed, causing necrosis at the site

   d. IgE-mediated hypersensitivity to the insect venom may be confirmed by skin testing with suitable dilutions of available venom—usually done by an allergist

   e. Signs and symptoms

      1) Brown recluse spider: a large area of necrosis at the site, pain, itching and swelling; after a week, the area has extreme swelling with a white or black center (appearing to erupt)

2) Black widow spider: pain at the site, which lasts only briefly, rigid abdominal muscles with extreme abdominal pain, and motor paralysis

3) General reactions to insect bites: redness, itching, swelling, warmth, and extreme pain

4) Systemic symptoms such as fever, chills, nausea, vomiting, and weakness may occur

5) Anaphylactic reactions such as shortness of breath and wheezing may appear if the client is allergic to the sting

2. **Pediculosis** is an infestation of the skin or hair by the species of blood-sucking lice capable of living as external parasites on the human host

   a. Pediculosis capitis is the head louse, the size of a sesame seed ranging in color from clear to red/brown

   b. Pediculosis pubis ("crabs") infests the genital area and is one of the most common sexually transmitted diseases

   c. Pubic lice can be spread by sexual contact

   d. Head lice is common among schoolchildren of all socioeconomic backgrounds and is spread by close contact as well as sharing combs, hats, and scarves

   e. Scabies is the infestation of the skin by the mite *Scarcoptes scabier hominis*

   f. In scabies, the fertilized female mite burrows into the skin and remains there laying 2 to 3 eggs per day

   g. The eggs hatch in 3–4 days, reach maturity in 4 days, migrate to the skin surface, mate, and repeat the cycle

   h. Scabies is more common among people who don't have access to bathing or laundry facilities as the lice can live in clothing and be transmitted by contact of infected clothing or bed linens

   i. Signs and symptoms

      1) Pediculosis corporis: macules, wheals, and papules, pruritus, excoriation from scratching; lines in the folds of the skin are common, representing the burrowing of the mite; the lesions may be erythematous papules or purplish nodules accompanied by raised burrows which are thread-like linear ridges with a minute black dot at one end

      2) Pediculosis pubis: pruritus, irritation of genital area, and blue- or slate-colored macules

      3) Pediculosis capitis: itching, eczematous dermatitis, inflammation caused by scratching, pustules, crusts, matted, odorous hair

C. Nursing assessment

   1. Insect stings and bites

      a. Assessment includes symptom analysis regarding type of bite or sting, when occurred and location of bite or sting; assess for anaphylactic reactions and refer for immediate treatment; assess the site for symptoms specific to the type of bite

      b. Diagnostic tests: there are no tests indicated unless a severe allergic reaction is noted; a CBC and IgE may be performed if necessary

  2. Pediculosis

     a. Assessment

       1) Questions about intense pruritis—the most common symptom in pediculosis

       2) Appearance: head lice may resemble dandruff flakes; however they are not easily brushed off

       3) A papular urticaria, which may be present at the neck or pubic area

       4) Severity of itching: nocturnal itching, which is a classic symptom of scabies, as well as during exposure to hot water or steam

       5) Inquire about onset of symptoms; client becomes itchy approximately 10 to 14 days after exposure

     b. Diagnostic tests: skin scraping of the scabies nodule may be recommended to reveal portions of the mite but clinical diagnosis is usually made by presentation

  D. Nursing management

    1. Insect stings and bites

     a. Medications include local analgesics such as ibuprofen and antihistamines such as diphenhydramine (Benadryl) that are used for mild reactions; epinephrine 1:1000 may be administered for mild symptoms also

     b. Outpatient or inpatient treatment for stings and bites depends on the individual response

       1) First aid treatment may include removal of the stinger by scraping; do not squeeze or use a tweezer; then clean the wound

       2) Apply ice packs to the bite, 10 minutes on/10 minutes off

       3) Elevate the affected part, maintain adequate airway, and transport to emergency facility if warranted

       4) The wound from a brown recluse spider should not be opened but cleansed daily and allowed to erupt on its own

     c. If the history suggests a severe anaphylactic reaction, initiate emergency treatment immediately; if the client is stable, assess the client's vital signs, examine the site for erythema and edema

     d. For severe and potentially life-threatening reactions, immediately transport to the local emergency department.

     e. Educate the client to prevent re-exposure and about the risks of increasing severity of responses in the future

     f. Instruct the client to use insect repellants when outdoors or in infected areas

     g. For clients allergic to insect bites, an Epi-pen should be available at all times; educate on the proper use of the Epi-pen if prescribed

    h. Client may need referral for allergy testing if a mild to severe anaphylactic reaction occurs

    i. For sensitive individuals, a medical alert tag should be obtained and worn at all times

  2. Pediculosis

    a. Medications to kill the nits include lindane (Kwell), which comes in a lotion or shampoo; gamma benzene hexachloride, malathion (Prioderm lotion) or permithrin (NIX), corticosteroids for itching, and antibiotics as needed for infections

    b. Nits on the hair must be mechanically removed

    c. Instruct the client as to the proper way to treat the condition; some medications such as NIX take only one treatment, while others (Lindane) take two treatments, 7 days apart in order to kill the eggs; advise that olive oil or a solution of 50 parts white vinegar to 50 parts water may loosen nits

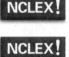

    d. Educate clients about mode of transmission (person to person) and preventative measures such as not sharing personal items

    e. Instruct the client/family to machine wash all washable clothing and dry in a hot dryer at least 20 minutes; upholstered furniture, pillows, and stuffed animals may be ironed with a hot iron or vacuumed

    f. Stress importance that all family members must be treated at the same time

VIII. Allergic Conditions of the Integumentary System

A. Overview

  1. Allergic conditions are those that cause inflammation (dermatitis) as a result of contact with an allergen, infection, or disease; these can be acute or chronic

  2. Disorders include contact dermatitis, atopic dermatitis, seborrheic dermatitis, exfoliative dermatitis, and urticaria

  3. Causes include plants such as poison oak, poison sumac, or poison ivy; harsh chemicals; dyes; perfumes; latex gloves; metals; insecticides; soaps; detergents; foods; drugs such as methyldopa for hypertension, diseases such as AIDS, leukemia, and lymphoma; transfusion reactions; insect bites or stings; heat; cold; stress; sunlight; and serum sickness

B. Pathophysiology

  1. Contact dermatitis is an eruption of the skin related to contact with an irritating substance or allergen (see Box 14-2)

    a. *Irritant contact dermatitis* affects individuals exposed to specific irritants producing an immediate response

    b. *Allergic contact dermatitis* is an allergic reaction mediated by IgE and affects only individuals previously sensitized to the irritant, thus it is a delayed hypersensitivity reaction; a sensitizing antigen is formed on initial contact, which is taken to the T cells; these T cells become sensitized and this creates the initial sensitizing effect; upon subsequent exposures, skin reactions will occur (see Figure 14-1)

Box 14-2	
Common Causes of Contact Dermatitis	• Acids
	• Alkalis: soaps, detergents, household cleaners
	• Cosmetics: perfumes, dyes, oils
	• Hydrocarbons: lubricating oil, mineral oil, paraffin
	• Insecticides
	• Fabrics
	• Metal salts: such as zinc, copper, nickel, silver
	• Plants: ragweed, poison oak, poison ivy, poison sumac, pine
	• Rubber products: latex

Adapted from LeMone, P. & Burke, K. (2000). *Medical-surgical nursing: Critical thinking in client care* (2nd ed.). Upper Saddle River, NJ: Prentice Hall, p. 590.

c. The location of the rash helps provide clues about the offending agent

d. Signs and symptoms include acute contact dermatitis, presents as papules, vesicles, bullae with surrounding erythema; crusting, oozing, and pruritis may be present; chronic contact dermatitis may present with an erythematous base, thickening of the skin, scaling and fissuring

Figure 14-1

An antigen binds with a killer T cell or helper T cell in order to remember the event through the development of memory T cells or antibody production through B cells.

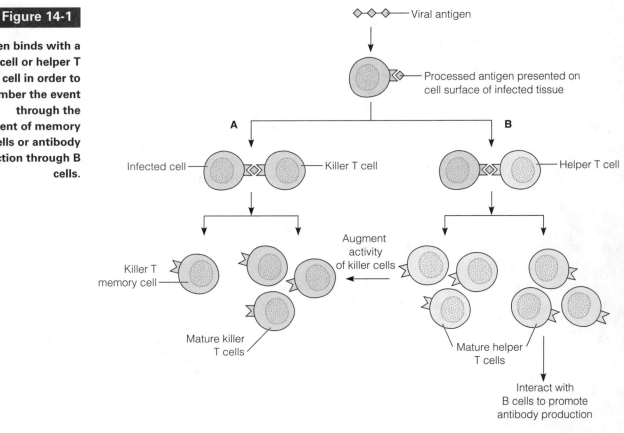

2. **Atopic dermatitis** (eczema) is a common inflammatory skin disorder of unknown cause and is seen frequently with children and adults

   a. Although the cause is unknown, a cell-mediated immunity, excess sensitivity to histamine, and increased levels of IgE are related to the disorder

   b. The condition has allergic, heredity, and/or psychological components

   c. The initiation of the immune response triggers an inflammatory reaction

   d. A complication is secondary infection

   e. Signs and symptoms include erythema, scaling, pruritis, and lesions on the hands, feet, arms, and legs

3. **Seborrheic dermatitis** is an acute inflammatory condition with an unknown cause

   a. It affects the scalp (cradle cap), forehead, postauricular regions, eyebrows, eyelashes, nasolabial folds, axillary, and genital areas; all ages can be affected

   b. Signs and symptoms include yellow or white plaques that may scale, crusts with a greasy appearance, pruritus, oozing, and loss of hair

4. **Exfoliative dermatitis** is an inflammation of the skin characterized by erythema involving loss of exfoliated (peeling) skin

   a. Local and systemic effects may occur and have either an unknown cause or may be associated with other diseases or causes

   b. A complication of the generalized form is debilitation, dehydration and secondary infection

   c. Signs and symptoms

      1) Local effects: scaling, erythema, pruritus, loss of hair and nails

      2) Systemic effects: weakness, malaise, hypothermia or fever, lymphadenopathy, hepatomegaly, eosinophilia, and depression

5. **Urticaria** (hives) is described as an itchy rash that may be recurrent

   a. *Acute urticaria* usually subsides over several hours; examples include solar urticaria (exposure to sun), delayed pressure urticaria (produced by pressure, occurs after delay of 1 to 4 hours), aquagenic urticaria (ordinary water), and occurs because of an allergic reaction

   b. *Chronic urticaria* persists over 6 weeks; examples include cold urticaria (from cooling to rewarming), cholinergic urticaria (heat urticaria), and induced urticaria (extreme exercise)

   c. Urticaria is caused by a massive release from mast cells in the superficial layers of the skin and is a vascular reaction of the skin

   d. True urticaria lesions do not remain in the same area over 24 hours; if present longer than 72 hours, cutaneous vasculitis must be considered a possible cause

   e. Signs and symptoms include single or multiple areas of raised, blanched central wheals surrounded by a red flare that is highly pruritic; it may occur anywhere on the body with size ranging from 1–2mm to 15–20cm

C. Nursing assessment

1. Assessment for dermatitis conditions

    a. A symptom analysis regarding location, duration, and associated symptoms

    b. Ask about occupation or recreational activities

    c. Review exposures to any irritants or allergens and previous treatments

    d. Examine the skin to determine location and distribution

2. Assessment for urticaria includes a symptom analysis of the onset, duration, and possible causes and skin examination to determine distribution

3. Diagnostic test: scratch or intradermal tests for allergy testing, IgE level, eosinophil level, and skin biopsy for diagnostic purposes

D. Nursing management

1. Contact/irritant dermatitis

    a. Medications include aluminum acetate for drying, antihistamines or calamine lotion for pruritus, cortisone if needed, and topical emollients

    b. The first step in the management of contact/irritant dermatitis is to identify and remove the causative agent

    c. Wet dressings and oatmeal baths may aid in alleviating oozing and pruritic lesions

    d. Instruct the client on signs and symptoms of secondary bacterial infections

2. Atopic dermatitis

    a. Medications include antihistamines, softening lotions, cortisone lotion, and oral antibiotics if needed

    b. Instruct client to avoid soaps and ointment, keep bathing to a minimum; bath oils may help soften skin

    c. Clothing should be of a soft texture and wool should be avoided

    d. Clip fingernails to decrease damage while scratching

3. Seborrheic dermatitis

    a. Medications include selenium containing shampoos, keratolytic agents, topical and systemic cortisone lotions

    b. Frequent shampooing is suggested if on the scalp

    c. Scrupulous skin hygiene and keeping the skin dry is imperative

4. Exfoliative dermatitis

    a. Medications include corticosteroids, emollients, and antihistamines

    b. Treatment is the same as contact dermatitis

5. Urticaria

    a. Medications include antihistamines and H_2 receptor antagonists to reduce itching and prevent prolonged symptoms; corticosteroids may be used for pressure urticaria and topical sunscreens are recommended for solar urticaria

    b. Instruct the client on proper use of medications for urticaria

    c. If urticaria occurred as a result of an allergic reaction, stress that possible life-threatening reactions may occur on reexposure

    d. Cool moist compresses help to control itching; increasing fluids and use of skin lubricants is recommended; avoidance of harsh soaps, frequent bathing, and products with alcohol should be recommended

    e. Referrals to an allergist or dermatologist should be considered for unresolved itching

IX. Burns

A. Overview

    1. **Burns** are defined as alterations in skin integrity resulting in tissue loss or injury caused by heat, chemicals, electricity, or radiation

    2. A superficial thickness burn (first degree) involves a minimal depth of the skin and is limited to the outer layer of the epidermis

    3. Superficial and deep partial thickness burns (second degree) involves damage extending through the epidermis and dermis; regeneration of the epidermis is not impaired

    4. A full thickness burn (third degree) involves the epidermis and dermis with damage into the underlying tissue

    5. Causes include thermal, chemical, electrical, and radiation

        a. *Thermal burns* are the result of dry heat (flames) or moist heat (steam or hot liquids) and are the most common type of burn; they cause cellular destruction that results in vascular, bony, muscle, or nerve complications

        b. *Chemical burns* are caused by direct contact with either acidic or alkaline agents; they destroy tissue perfusion, leading to necrosis

        c. *Electrical burns* follow the path of least resistance (muscles-bones-blood vessels-nerves); the severity of the burn depends on the type and duration of current and amount of voltage; electrical burns include sources such as direct current, alternating current, and lightning

        d. A *radiation burn* is usually associated with sunburn or radiation treatment for cancer; it is usually superficial; extensive exposure may lead to tissue damage and multisystem involvement

B. Pathophysiology

    1. A burn from any source is a major insult to the entire body, involving an altered integrity of the skin, which could lead to infection, as well as many systemic effects

    2. Within several hours, capillary integrity is lost due to the release of several mediators of inflammation, primarily histamine and prostaglandin, which are vasodilators

    3. Fluid passes from the intravascular system (causing hypotension) to the interstitial system (causing massive edema)

NCLEX!

NCLEX!

4. This fluid will begin to shift back within 24 to 48 hours and intravascular overload will then be a concern

5. The loss of intravascular volume causes an increased blood viscosity (with a risk for clots), decreased cardiac output (possibly leading to shock or pulmonary congestion), decreased blood flow to the kidneys (causing hypoxia and decreased urinary output), and an increase in the renin-angiotension-aldosterone (RAA) system to increase volume which leads to retention of Na and water and further edema

6. Cells cannot maintain adequate electrolyte shifts and results in the following: excess sodium (Na) intracellularly, excess potassium (K) extracellularly; these effects as well as shifts in magnesium (Mg) and phosphorus (P) can lead to cardiac dysrhythmias and altered central nervous system function

7. Cortisol is released because of the stress and depresses the immune system, which intensifies the risk for infection

8. The sympathetic nervous system is activated, along with the stress factor, increasing metabolic rate and oxygen demands; this hypermetabolism, the increased energy needed for healing, and the release of cortisol and epinephrine lead to a breakdown of tissue, protein metabolism, and fat wasting

9. Glucose is released as a result of the stress and causes hyperglycemia

10. Complications are numerous (see Table 14-1)

11. Signs and symptoms

NCLEX!

    a. Superficial thickness burn: erythema of the tissue, the skin may be tender and blanches under pressure

    b. Partial thickness burn: the skin is red and blistered and very tender or painful; appearance may vary depending on whether burn is superficial partial thickness or deep partial thickness; the deeper the burn, the more it begins to resemble full thickness

NCLEX!

    c. Full thickness burn: skin is tough and leathery but not tender; may also appear waxy or pearly white

Table 14-1	System	Major Complication
Complications of Burns	Immune	Infection with *Staphylococcus aureus* or methcillin resistant *staphylococcus aureus* (MRSA), septic shock
	Cardiovascular	Blood clots leading to cerebrovascular accident or myocardial infarction, heart failure, cardiac arrest, pulmonary edema
	Gastrointestinal	Peptic ulcer (decreased blood flow to gut), impaction
	Respiratory	Adult respiratory distress syndrome (ARDS), lung damage if inhalation, hypoxia
	Hematological	Burn shock, disseminated intravascular coagulopathy (DIC), anemia
	Renal	Oliguria, renal failure
	Fluids and electrolytes	First 24 to 48 hours: hyponatremia, hypokalemia, hypoproteinemia, hypochloremia After 24 to 48 hours: hypernatremia, hyperkalemia, hypovolemic shock, and dehydration

C. Nursing assessment

1. Assessment

   a. A symptom analysis of the cause of the burn, time occurred, past medical history, and present medications and allergies

   b. Assess overall general appearance for distress and amount of pain

   c. Assess the depth of burn

   d. Assess the extent of the burn (% total body surface area or TBSA) using the Rule of Nines (see Figure 14-2)

   e. Assess cardiac status, respiratory status, airway patency, and hydration status

   f. Airway status is essential whenever the burn has the capability of compromising the airway because of edema

   g. Keep in mind possibilities of abuse and neglect; inquire about past injuries and burns

NCLEX!

| Figure 14-2 | The "Rule of Nines" is a method of quickly estimating the percentage of total body surface area of the burn injury. |

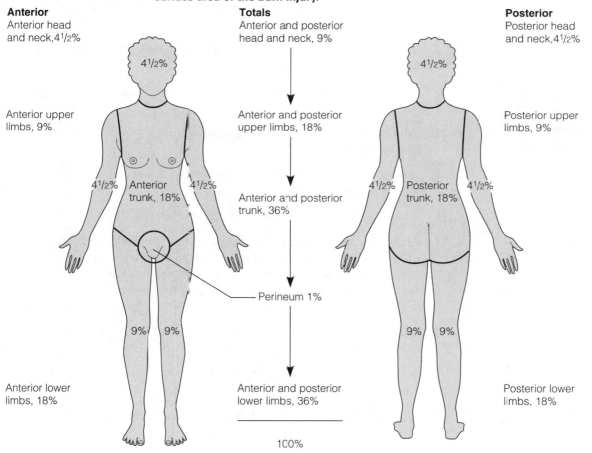

Anterior
Anterior head and neck, 4 1/2%

Totals
Anterior and posterior head and neck, 9%

Posterior
Posterior head and neck, 4 1/2%

4 1/2%   4 1/2%

Anterior upper limbs, 9%

Anterior and posterior upper limbs, 18%

Posterior upper limbs, 9%

4 1/2% Anterior trunk, 18% 4 1/2%

Anterior and posterior trunk, 36%

4 1/2% Posterior trunk, 18% 4 1/2%

Perineum 1%

9% 9%

9% 9%

Anterior lower limbs, 18%

Anterior and posterior lower limbs, 36%

Posterior lower limbs, 18%

100%

2. Diagnostic tests: Rule of Nines to estimate burn size; blood urea nitrogen (BUN), creatinine clearance, urine output, urinalysis to avoid shock; CBC, electrolytes, albumin, bilirubin, alkaline phosphatase, arterial blood gases (ABGs), type and crossmatch (TXM), chest x-ray (CXR), electrocardiogram (ECG); C & S (if indicated); pulmonary function tests

D. Nursing management

1. Medications include narcotics, sedatives, analgesics for pain, tetanus (if not current), antibiotics, antacids or H_2-blockers, topical antimicrobials such as silver nitrate, silver sulfadiazine, polysporin, etc.

2. Remove all rings and jewelry to avoid a tourniquet effect of the affected site

3. Flush a chemical burn copiously with water and apply cold compresses; remove affected clothing and cover the area with a dry sheet

4. Administer oxygen if necessary for any type of burn

5. Maintain proper hydration and encourage high-protein, high-calorie diet; monitor intake and output (I & O)

6. For superficial thickness burns, topical anesthetic creams or spray may be used several times a day to relieve pain and no dressings are needed

7. For partial thickness burns, leave blisters intact

8. Small burns may be covered with antibiotic ointment and a non-adherent dressing to absorb drainage

9. For larger burns, cover the area with silver sulfadiazine 1%, non-adherent dressing and bulky dressing to absorb any drainage

10. Full thickness burns will not heal on their own and require skin grafting to heal

11. Use of sterile technique (and possibly protective isolation) is required to decrease the risk of infection

12. Monitor pain management needs and treat pain before debriding episodes and around the clock if needed

13. Assess for tetanus prophylaxis and administer tetanus toxoid if needed

14. Educate the client on use of sunscreens, accessing electrical cords/outlets, isolating household chemicals, use of low temperature setting for hot water heater, use of household smoke detectors with emphasis on proper maintenance, risks of smoking in bed, and proper storage and use of flammable substances

15. Instruct the client and family regarding care of the burn at home, and signs and symptoms of infection

16. Evaluate need for counseling and family support, physical, vocational or occupational rehabilitation

17. Encourage the client to verbalize feelings of despair or depression if disfigurement has occurred

Case Study

J. M. is an 80-year-old female who has noticed a blistery rash on her abdomen for the past several days. The healthcare provider informs her that she has herpes zoster.

❶ What history should the nurse ask J. M. about?

❷ What assessment should the nurse perform?

❸ How should the nurse explain the disease?

❹ What medication instructions are necessary?

❺ What home instructions should be given to J. M. regarding her disease?

For suggested responses, see pages 569–570.

Posttest

1 A 70-year-old female complains of burning and itching for several days in her right abdominal area. She thinks she has been bitten by something because she can feel small bumps at the site. The nurse suspects which of the following conditions based on this assessment data?

(1) Insect bite
(2) Herpes zoster
(3) Scabies
(4) Warts

2 A 23-year-old male presents with a pustular inflammation of his neck. Which of the following would the nurse use as an important management strategy?

(1) Squeeze the area periodically
(2) Keep the area moist
(3) Changing razors each time he shaves
(4) Strict dietary changes

3 A client asks the nurse in the dermatologist's office about what characteristics folliculitis, furunculosis, and carbunculosis all have in common. The nurse replies that all three disorders are:

(1) Viral infections involving the epidermal layer of the skin.
(2) Fungal infections caused by poor hygiene.
(3) Bacterial infections that are highly contagious.
(4) Bacterial infections involving the hair follicles.

4 A 2-year-old child has been sick with a cold and has developed a honey-colored lesion on her chin within the past 3 days. The nurse determines that this clinical picture is consistent with which of the following?

(1) Impetigo
(2) Scabies
(3) Herpes simplex
(4) Contact dermatitis

5 The nurse would include which of the following in the nursing management of the client with psoriasis?

(1) Emphasize that the disease can be transmitted by skin-to-skin contact
(2) Emphasize the importance of keeping the areas dry
(3) Medications can be tried but may not be effective
(4) Educate the client on healthy lifestyle changes

6 A client presents to the clinic with thick, white flaky skin. The nurse knows that these symptoms occur when the cell cycle is shortened, such as occurs with which of the following diseases?

(1) Psoriasis
(2) Herpes
(3) Impetigo
(4) Acne

7   The nurse working at a community health fair in the booth for skin assessment should be teaching the ABCD rule as a definitive measurement for which diagnosis?

(1) Basal cell carcinoma
(2) Squamous cell carcinoma
(3) Malignant melanoma
(4) Acne

8   A man suffers from burns to the arms and chest when a fire got out of control. The nurse removes jewelry from the affected burn site in order to do which of the following?

(1) Be able to assess the fingers more accurately
(2) Prevent a tourniquet effect at the site
(3) Prevent infection
(4) Avoid interference with the first aid treatment of the burn

9   A 9-year-old child plays three baseball games on a hot, humid summer day. The child is at high risk for dehydration and which of the following conditions?

(1) Skin cancer
(2) Full thickness burn
(3) Partial thickness burn
(4) Superficial thickness burn

10   When evaluating a client with a new skin lesion, it is most important to ask the client about which of the following?

(1) What foods they eat
(2) What cosmetics they use
(3) Sun tanning habits
(4) Allergies

See pages 463–464 for Answers and Rationales.

Answers and Rationales

Pretest

1   **Answer: 1** *Rationale:* Emollients will ease dry skin that increases pruritus and causes the psoriasis to be worse. Washing and drying the skin with rough linens or pressure may cause excoriation. Constant occlusion may increase the effects of the medication and increase the risk of infection.
Cognitive Level: Application
Nursing Process: Implementation; *Test Plan:* HPM

2   **Answer: 2** *Rationale:* In order to plan the appropriate management of contact/irritant dermatitis, the cause of the inflammation should be identified. Removal of the cause may be all the treatment needed. Antihistamines and hydrocortisone creams are treatment options. Skin testing may be helpful to determine the allergen if not evident in the history.
Cognitive Level: Application
Nursing Process: Assessment; *Test Plan:* PHYS

3   **Answer: 2** *Rationale:* Lice are transmitted by direct contact with infested persons or by sharing hats, brushes, or combs of infected persons. Classrooms are excellent areas for close contact, and children

often do not know when other classmates have lice. Options 1, 3, and 4 are incorrect.
Cognitive Level: Application
Nursing Process: Assessment; *Test Plan:* PHYS

4   **Answer: 1** *Rationale:* The disease is ten times more common in fair-skinned people who work indoors. This population often experiences severe sunburns and blistering in childhood and tends to vacation in areas of intense sun exposure. Remember, episodic intense sun exposure is more damaging than constant exposure.
Cognitive Level: Application
Nursing Process: Assessment; *Test Plan:* HPM

5   **Answer: 4** *Rationale:* There is no sensation of pain to light touch in full thickness burns because the pain and touch receptors have been destroyed. There may not be pain with some partial thickness degree burns, but the appearance described is characteristic of full thickness.
Cognitive Level: Application
Nursing Process: Assessment; *Test Plan:* PHYS

6   **Answer: 3** *Rationale:* A burn involving the face, neck, or chest may cause airway closure because of

the edema that occurs within hours. Remember the ABCs: airway, breathing, and circulation. Airway always comes first, even before pain. The nurse will also assess skin integrity (option 1), blood pressure and pulse (option 2), and pain (option 4), but these are not the highest priority assessments.
Cognitive Level: Analysis
Nursing Process: Assessment; *Test Plan:* PHYS

7   **Answer: 4** *Rationale:* Pediculosis capitis is head lice, and nits are cemented to the hair shaft. They are most commonly seen on hair on the back of the head near the nape of the neck. A papular excoriation may be present at the nape of the neck secondary to scratching.
Cognitive Level: Application
Nursing Process: Assessment; *Test Plan:* PHYS

8   **Answer: 3** *Rationale:* If the client previously had a reaction to a wasp sting, immediate treatment must be administered. If a reaction is anticipated, do not complete the exam or wait for symptoms to develop, be proactive. Pain often causes the blood pressure to rise. The client who has never been stung should be monitored closely.
Cognitive Level: Analysis
Nursing Process: Assessment; *Test Plan:* PHYS

9   **Answer: 2** *Rationale:* Candidiasis (oral thrush) often develops as a result of the overgrowth of bacteria after a client has been on an antibiotic.
Cognitive Level: Application
Nursing Process: Assessment; *Test Plan:* PHYS

10   **Answer: 1** *Rationale:* Since a wart is a virus-induced epidermal tumor, it may reappear at the original site or another body area despite the fact that the original wart was removed. Immunity may develop to further warts after 5 years.
Cognitive Level: Application
Nursing Process: Planning; *Test Plan:* PHYS

Posttest

1   **Answer: 2** *Rationale:* Dermatomal pain, itching, or burning may be severe and often begins 4 to 5 days before eruption occurs. The trunk is affected in the majority of cases. An insect bite usually manifests immediately, warts do not burn or itch, and scabies usually do not burn. Scabies form lines in the folds of the skin.
Cognitive Level: Application
Nursing Process: Analysis; *Test Plan:* PHYS

2   **Answer: 3** *Rationale:* Folliculitis is an inflammation of the hair follicle caused by infection, chemical irritants or injury. It is most commonly caused by *Staphylococcus aureus.* Using a clean razor each time he shaves will decrease the risk of reinfection.
Cognitive Level: Application
Nursing Process: Implementation; *Test Plan:* HPM

3   **Answer: 4** *Rationale:* All three diagnoses are a bacterial infection of the skin arising from the hair follicle, where bacteria can accumulate, grow, and cause a localized infection. Options 1–3 are incorrect.
Cognitive Level: Application
Nursing Process: Analysis; *Test Plan:* PHYS

4   **Answer: 1** *Rationale:* Impetigo is an infection of the skin typically beginning with a vesicle or pustule. The lesion ruptures, leaving an open area that discharges a honey-colored serous liquid that hardens into a crust. Impetigo spreads quickly if not treated.
Cognitive Level: Application
Nursing Process: Assessment; *Test Plan:* PHYS

5   **Answer: 4** *Rationale:* Psoriasis is a chronic disease with factors such as stress precipitating an exacerbation. A healthy lifestyle is recommended and includes a well-balanced diet, frequent exercise, moderate alcohol intake, and avoidance of tobacco products. The disease cannot be transferred to another person; keeping the skin moist relieves the itching; and medications can be effective.
Cognitive Level: Application
Nursing Process: Implementation; *Test Plan:* HPM

6   **Answer: 1** *Rationale:* Normally, the keratinocyte migrates to the outer layer of the skin in 14 days. Psoriatic skin cells complete this journey in 4 to 7 days producing an abnormal keratin that forms thick, flaky scales at the surface of the skin. Options 2, 3, and 4 do not have white, flaky skin as a characteristic.
Cognitive Level: Application
Nursing Process: Assessment; *Test Plan:* PHYS

7   **Answer: 3** *Rationale:* Melanomas tend to have asymmetry (A), border irregularity (B), color variegation (C), and diameter (D) greater than 6 mm. The ABCD rule can be applied to any skin condition, but malignant melanoma is the most severe and has changes in all four of the rules.
Cognitive Level: Comprehension
Nursing Process: Assessment; *Test Plan:* PHYS

8 **Answer: 2** *Rationale:* Restrictive jewelry and clothing are removed immediately from the burn victim to prevent circumferential constriction of the torso and extremities. Assessment of the fingers and interference with treatment may require removal of jewelry, but the primary reason is option 2.
Cognitive Level: Application
Nursing Process: Implementation; *Test Plan:* SECE

9 **Answer: 4** *Rationale:* A superficial thickness burn, such as a sunburn, involves only the epidermal layer of the skin. The color ranges from pink to bright red and small painful blisters may form.
Cognitive Level: Application
Nursing Process: Assessment; *Test Plan:* PHYS

10 **Answer: 3** *Rationale:* Tanning and sun exposure can increase susceptibility to skin cancer and not all individuals use a sunscreen or consider tanning as having serious consequences.
Cognitive Level: Application
Nursing Process: Planning; *Test Plan:* HPM

References

Barker, L. (1999). *Principles of ambulatory care.* Baltimore: Williams and Wilkins.

Cash, J. & Glass, C. (2000). *Family practice guidelines.* Philadelphia: Lippincott, Williams & Wilkins.

Dambro, M. (1999). *Griffith's five minute clinical consult.* Philadelphia: Lippincott.

Fauci, A. et al. (1998). *Harrison's principles of internal medicine* (14th ed.). New York: McGraw-Hill.

Hall, J. (1999). *Saver's manual of skin diseases* (8th ed.). Philadelphia: Lippincott.

LeMone, P. & Burke, K. (2000). *Medical-surgical nursing: Critical thinking in client care* (2nd ed.). Upper Saddle River, NJ: Prentice Hall, pp. 554–670.

Meredith, P. (2000). *Adult primary care.* Philadelphia: W. B. Saunders.

Robinson, D., Kidd, P., & Rogers, K. (2000). *Primary care across the lifespan.* St. Louis, MO: Mosby.

Singleton, J. (1999). *Primary care.* Philadelphia: Lippincott.

Uphold, C. & Graham, M. (1998). *Clinical guidelines in family practice.* (3rd ed.). Gainesville, FL: Barmarrae Books.

Weber, J. (2001). *Nurse's handbook of health assessment* (4th ed.). Philadelphia: Lippincott, Williams & Wilkins.

CHAPTER 15

Hematological and Oncological Health Problems

Susan K. Steele, MN, RN, AOCN

CHAPTER OUTLINE

OBJECTIVES

■ Define key terms associated with hematological and oncological health problems.

■ Identify risk factors associated with the development of hematological and oncological health problems.

■ Discuss the common etiologies of hematological and oncological health problems.

■ Describe pathophysiological processes associated with specific hematological and oncological health problems.

■ Distinguish between normal and abnormal hematological and oncological health findings obtained from nursing assessment.

■ Prioritize nursing interventions associated with specific hematological and oncological health problems.

[Media Link]

Use the CD-ROM enclosed with this text, or log onto the address given to access the free, interactive Companion Website created for this series. The CD-ROM and Companion Website accompanying this book offer additional practice opportunities and information—NCLEX Review, Case Studies, Glossary, In Depth with NCLEX, and more.

www.prenhall.com/hogan

REVIEW AT A GLANCE

achlorhydria *the absence of free hydrochloric acid in a pH maintained at 3.5*

cheilosis *cracks in the corners of the mouth*

hemoglobin electrophoresis *a blood test that causes the hemoglobin molecule to migrate in solution in response to electric currents to determine the presence and percentage of hemoglobin S*

intrinsic factor *a substance secreted by the parietal cells of the gastric mucosa that promotes absorption of vitamin B_{12}*

factor VIII *an alpha globulin that stabilizes fibrin clots*

factor IX *a vitamin-dependent beta globulin essential in stage 1 of the intrinsic coagulation system as an influence on the amount of thromboplastin available*

ferritin *an iron-phosphorus-protein complex that contains about 23 percent iron*

mean corpuscular hemoglobin (MCH) *a measurement of the average weight (concentration) of hemoglobin in red blood cells (RBCs)*

mean corpuscular hemoglobin concentration (MCHC) *the ratio of the weight of hemoglobin to the volume of erythrocytes*

mean corpuscular volume (MCV) *a measurement of the size (volume) of the red blood cells (RBCs)*

neutropenia *a decrease in neutrophils*

nadir *the lowest level of bone marrow suppression following chemotherapy*

paresthesias *altered sensations such as numbness or tingling in the extremities*

pernicious anemia *the body's inability to absorb vitamin B_{12} because of a lack of intrinsic factor, a substance secreted by the parietal cells of the gastric mucosa*

petechiae *small, flat, purple or red spots on the skin or mucous membranes caused by minute hemorrhage in the dermis or submucous layer*

Philadelphia chromosome *characteristic chromosomal abnormality present in chronic mylogenous leukemia (CML)*

pica *craving to eat unusual substances such as clay or starch*

plethora *engorged or distended blood vessels causing a ruddy color of the face hands, feet, ears, and mucus membranes*

proprioception *ability to identify one's position in space; problems may include difficulty with balance and spinal cord damage*

purpura *hemorrhage into the tissues as evidenced by bruising*

Schilling test *a vitamin B_{12} absorption test that indicates lacks of intrinsic factor by measuring excretion of orally administered radionuclide labeled B_{12}*

Pretest

1 A client with anemia has a hemoglobin of 6.5 g/dL. The client is experiencing symptoms of cerebral tissue hypoxia. Which of the following nursing interventions would be the most important in providing care?

(1) Providing rest periods throughout the day
(2) Instituting energy conservation techniques
(3) Assisting in ambulation to the bathroom
(4) Checking temperature of water prior to bathing

2 The nurse observing manifestations of complications in a client with multiple myeloma concludes that they are caused by which of the following?

(1) Systemic effects of substances secreted by malignant plasma cells.
(2) Increased white blood cells and platelet production
(3) Increased red blood cells and immunoglobulin production
(4) Increased platelet production and bone marrow destruction

3 A client has a diagnosis of myelodysplastic syndrome. The nurse planning care keeps in mind that this condition:

(1) Is one of a group of hereditary bone marrow conditions.
(2) May progress to acute myelogenous leukemia.
(3) Is referred to as pre-lymphoma.
(4) Responds well to treatment.

4 A 40-year-old client is referred to a hematologist with a tentative diagnosis of acute myelogenous leukemia (AML). The client's only complaint is fatigue. Which of the following diagnostic tests would the nurse expect to be ordered first?

(1) Liver function studies
(2) Uric acid
(3) Lumbar puncture
(4) Bone marrow biopsy

5 Which of the following dietary recommendations should the nurse make to increase the intake of nutrients needed for erythropoiesis?

(1) Milk, eggs, liver, and green leafy vegetables
(2) Apples, peanuts, oats, and cottage cheese
(3) Cantaloupe, lima beans, and sweet potatoes
(4) Dry yeast, grapefruit, and tuna fish

6 A client has an order for an iron preparation to be given by the parenteral route. The nurse plans to give the medication by which of the following routes?

(1) Intermittent infusion.
(2) Deep gluteal intramuscular (IM) injection, using the Z-track method.
(3) Intramuscular in the deltoid to promote medication dissipation through muscle contraction.
(4) Subcutaneous injection with weekly site rotation.

7 In the normal blood clotting cycle, the final formation of a clot will occur at which of the following times?

(1) During the platelet phase.
(2) During the vascular phase.
(3) When fibrin reinforces the platelet plug.
(4) When the plasmin system produces fibrinolysis.

8 The client is given radioactive vitamin B_{12} in water for a Schilling test. The nurse instructs the client that the primary purpose of this test is to measure his body's ability to do which of the following?

(1) Store vitamin B_{12}.
(2) Digest vitamin B_{12}.
(3) Absorb vitamin B_{12}.
(4) Produce vitamin B_{12}.

9 A client with a history of sickle cell anemia begins to complain of pain. The nurse expects that the client is going into sickle cell crisis because of the pain, which signals which of the following?

(1) Vasoocclusion by sickled cells.
(2) Viscosity of the blood.
(3) Spasms caused by thickened blood.
(4) Cells in the marrow causing bone pain.

10 The nurse diligently assesses a leukemic client with neutropenia for signs of infection, anticipating that they will be absent or muted because:

(1) Most infections are caused by organisms that are part of the body's normal flora.
(2) The white blood cells (WBCs) drop rapidly and recovery time is slow.
(3) Neutrophils are necessary to produce an inflammatory response.
(4) The immunoglobulins are reduced.

See page 486 for Answers and Rationales.

I. **Risk Factors Associated with Hematological and Oncological Health Problems**

A. **Lifestyle factors** such as smoking and alcohol consumption

B. **Dietary and nutritional factors** such as decreased intake of B vitamins and iron

C. **Leukemia:** occupational and physical environment risk factors such as exposure to chemicals (benzene and arsenic), exposure to large amounts of radiation, genetic factors, Down syndrome, viral etiology, chemotherapeutic agents

D. **Lymphoma:** viral exposure, genetics, ethnicity, and/or immune system compromise

E. **Hematological cancers:** iatrogenic agents such as immunosuppressive agents as well as chemotherapy

F. **Anemia:** socioeconomic factors, such as poverty and inadequate nutrition

II. Leukemia

A. Overview

1. Defined as a malignant neoplasm of the blood-forming tissues of the bone marrow, spleen, and lymph system

2. Characterized by an abnormal proliferation and accumulation of immature white blood cells (WBCs or leukocytes) and their precursors that infiltrate the bone marrow and peripheral blood as well as body organs and tissues

3. Types: categorized by the type of WBC affected by the disease (granulocytic, lymphocytic, monocytic) and the course and duration of the disease (acute or chronic)

   a. Acute lymphocytic/lymphoblastic leukemia (ALL)

      1) Immature lymphocytes proliferate in the marrow

      2) Abnormal leukemic cells resemble immature lymphocytes or lymphoblasts

      3) Most common in children between the ages of 2 and 10

      4) A second rise in incidence occurs in middle age and in older adults

   b. Acute myelogenous/myelocytic leukemia (AML) or acute granulocytic leukemia (AGL)

      1) Immature granulocytes proliferate and accumulate in the marrow

      2) Rate of incidence increases with age (especially over 50 years)

      3) Auer rods may be present in the cytoplasm of the myeloblasts; a standard diagnostic criterion for AML is that over 30 percent of hematopoietic cells must be myeloblasts

      4) Myelodysplastic syndrome, a hematological disorder of the bone marrow, is referred to as pre-leukemia and may progress to AML; this syndrome has abnormal hematologic cell production and low peripheral blood counts

   c. Chronic lymphocytic leukemia (CLL)

      1) Abnormal incompetent lymphocytes proliferate, accumulate, and spread to other lymphatic tissue

      2) More common in men

      3) Occurs most frequently between the ages of 50 and 70; more gradual onset

   d. Chronic myelogenous leukemia (CML)

      1) Abnormal stem cells lead to an uncontrolled proliferation of granulocyte cells resulting in a marked increased in circulating blast cells, which can then lead to leukostasis and intracerebral hemorrhage

      2) In most cases, the characteristic chromosomal abnormality is present; referred to as the **Philadelphia chromosome** (an abnormal chromosome 22)

      3) Occurs primarily between the ages of 30 to 50, incidence is slightly higher in men; more gradual onset

Practice to Pass

A client is being discharged following induction therapy for acute myelogenous leukemia (AML). He is in his nadir period. What type of education will be needed? What type of clinical follow-up should be expected over the next 7 to 10 days?

4. Cause is usually unknown, but may be related to risk factors (see p. 467.)

B. **Pathophysiology**

NCLEX!

1. Abnormal or immature WBCs form and do not function properly; as a result of the massive proliferation of abnormal immature cells, fewer normal WBCs are produced; the abnormal cells can continue to multiply and infiltrate causing damage to the bone marrow, spleen, lymph nodes, liver, kidneys, lungs, gonads, skin, and central nervous system (CNS)

2. Normal bone marrow becomes diffusely replaced with abnormal or immature WBCs, interfering with the bone marrow's ability to produce other types of cells such as erythrocytes and thrombocytes; bone marrow becomes functionally incompetent with resulting bone marrow suppression

3. Acute leukemia has a rapid onset, progresses rapidly, with a short clinical course; left untreated, death will result in days or months; symptoms relate to a depressed bone marrow, infiltration of leukemic cells into other organ systems, and hypermetabolism of leukemia cells

NCLEX!

4. Chronic leukemia has a more insidious onset with a more prolonged clinical course; asymptomatic early in the disease; life expectancy may be more than 5 years; symptoms relate to hypermetabolism of leukemia cells infiltrating other organ systems; cells are more mature and function more effectively

NCLEX!

5. Signs and symptoms include anemia, infection from inadequate numbers of mature, functioning WBCs to defend the body against pathogens, hemorrhage from thrombocytopenia, shortness of breath, fatigue, malaise, weakness, weight loss, decreased activity tolerance, bone or joint pain, headaches, visual disturbances, anorexia, fever, anemia, thrombocytopenia, petechiae or other ecchymosis, gingival bleeding, epistaxis, pallor, generalized lymphadenopathy, hyperuricemia, splenomegaly, increased WBCs, hepatomegaly

C. **Nursing assessment**

1. Assessment includes breath sounds, activity tolerance, pain, nutrition, vital signs, signs of bleeding or infection, lymph node enlargement, spleen, liver, and oral mucosa

NCLEX!

2. Infection is a common presenting factor in acute leukemia, but signs and symptoms may be absent because of **neutropenia** (a decrease in neutrophils); CNS manifestations are most common in lymphocytic leukemia

3. Hemoglobin, hematocrit, platelet count, and granulocyte count will drop consistently during chemotherapy administration reaching its lowest point 5 to 7 days after the initiation of therapy; counts will remain low for 7 to 10 days and will slowing begin rebounding, platelets first, then WBCs, then red blood cells (RBCs)

NCLEX!

4. Diagnostic tests: bone marrow biopsy and aspirate is the only definitive diagnostic test, complete blood count (CBC), electrolytes, cultures (if infection present)

D. **Nursing management**

1. Medications include analgesics to control pain; antiemetics for nausea; alkylating agents such as cisplatin (Platinol); antimetabolites such as fluorouracil

(5-FU); mitotic inhibitors such as vincristine (Oncovin); and radioactive drugs such as sodium radioiodine (Iodotope)

2. Massive amounts of chemotherapy are often given at one time (called induction therapy) for certain types of leukemia such as AML

3. Bone marrow biopsy

   a. Assess coagulation factors before procedure

   b. Posterior iliac crest, anterior iliac crest, and sternum are preferred locations

   c. After procedure, apply firm pressure for 5 minutes and observe puncture site for hemorrhage hourly for at least 4 hours

NCLEX!

4. Protect from infection (see Box 15-1 for neutropenic precautions), especially in **nadir** period (lowest level of bone marrow function from suppression following chemotherapy); identify risk of infection by calculating the client's absolute neutrophil count (ANC): WBC (% bands + % segs) = ANC (needs to be 1,000 or greater)

NCLEX!

5. Prevent bleeding; (soft tootbrush, fall prevention, safety with razors)

6. Prevent fatigue secondary to anemia, plan adequate rest periods, limit visitors if necessary

7. Maintain hydration and nutrition, evaluate weight loss

8. Stomatitis (inflammation of mouth) is common, therefore oral assessments and good oral hygiene should be initiated daily or more frequently as needed

9. Encourage and assist client and family to discuss concerns and fears

10. Discuss hair options early in the event alopecia occurs from chemotherapy

III. Lymphoma

A. Overview

1. Defined as a group of malignant neoplasms that affect the lymphatic system

NCLEX!

2. Hodgkin's disease is a malignant disorder of the lymph nodes that is characterized by the presence of the Reed-Sternberg cell

---

Box 15-1	
Neutropenic Precautions	• Use meticulous handwashing.
	• Provide oral hygiene after meals and at hour of sleep.
	• Screen all visitors and staff for colds or infections.
	• Monitor vital signs every four hours.
	• Prohibit fresh fruit or flowers.
	• Change intravenous (IV) tubing every 24 hours.
	• Avoid certain medications that may mask fever, such as acetaminophen (Tylenol) and ibuprofen (Advil).
	• Avoid rectal temperatures and suppositories.
	• Administer antibiotic/antifungal/antiviral therapy as prescribed.

3. Non-Hodgkin's lymphomas are a broad group of neoplastic disorders that affect the lymphatic system and include all lymphomas except Hodgkin's disease

4. Cause is unknown or associated with predisposing factors

B. Pathophysiology

1. *Hodgkin's disease (HD)*

   a. Reed-Sternberg cells (malignant cells) replace normal cellular structure; these are giant cell mutations of the T-lymphocyte that are present in the lymph node when diagnosed with HD

   b. Originates in one lymph node and then spreads to adjacent structures through the lymph system

   c. Eventually infiltrates other tissues including the liver, spleen, lungs, bone marrow, and ureters

   d. Peaks in two age groups: 15 to 35 years of age, and then again from 55 to 75 years of age; occurs twice as often in men than women

2. *Non-Hodgkin's lymphoma*

   a. Cells that make up lymphoid tissue become abnormal and eventually crowd out normal cells within specific regions of the lymph nodes; there are no Reed-Sternberg cells

   b. Lymphoma usually originates outside lymph nodes and becomes disseminated rapidly

   c. Incidence increases between the ages of 50 and 70; men are more frequently affected than women

3. Insidious onset, diagnosis usually occurs from pressure exerted by large nodes on surrounding tissues and/or obstruction/infiltration of lymphoma into vital organs such as the kidney, lung, or spleen

4. Staging based on Ann Arbor classification

   a. Stage I: limited to a single lymph node or single extra-lymphatic organ

   b. Stage II: involvement of two or more lymph node areas on the same side of the diaphragm or local involvement of an extra-lymphatic organ

   c. Stage III: involvement of lymph node regions on both sides of the diaphragm, with involvement of extra-lymphatic region and/or spleen

   d. Stage IV: diffuse involvement of one or more extra-lymphatic regions or tissues

NCLEX!

5. Signs and symptoms include painless lymph node enlargement; (unilateral or bilateral); cervical generally involved first, then axillary and inguinal (most easily assessed since they are more superficial); clients with more advanced disease often present with: weight loss, night sweats, malaise, chills, pruritus, anorexia, non-productive cough, dyspnea, and renal failure

C. Nursing assessment

1. Assessment includes lymph nodes, presence or absence of pain, nutritional status, weight, activity level and tolerance, respiratory status, and kidney function

2. Diagnostic tests: CBC, blood urea nitrogen (BUN), creatinine, lymph node biopsy is the only definitive diagnosis of either Hodgkin's or non-Hodgkin's lymphoma (either through surgical incision or needle aspirate); lymphangiogram (radiologic examination of the lymphatic system using a blue oil-based dye infused via the lymphatic vessels to determine the extent of involvement)

D. Nursing management

1. Medications

   a. Hodgkin's disease: alkylating agents such as cisplatin (Platinol); antibiotics such as doxorubicin (Adriamycin)

   b. Non-Hodgkin's lymphoma: alkylating agents, mitotic inhibitors such as vincristine (Oncovin)

2. Post-procedure care following lymphangiogram

   a. Instruct client that urine, veins of the lower extremities, and dorsal skin of the feet may have a blue-green discoloration from dye excretion for 2 to 5 days

   b. Monitor for signs of dye-based complications: cough, dyspnea, pleuritic pain, hemoptysis

3. Protect from infection

4. Maintain normal body temperature

5. Prevent/decrease pain

6. Maintain adequate nutrition and hydration

IV. Multiple Myeloma

A. Overview

1. Defined as plasma cell neoplasms or related disorders comparable with proliferation and collection of immunoglobulin or plasma cells

2. Affects mostly men 50 to 69 years of age; more prominent in African-Americans

3. Cause is unknown, however some studies suggest that multiple myeloma reflects an inappropriate response to an antigen or a virus like particle; genetics may be involved

B. Pathophysiology

1. Malignant plasma cells arise from one clone of B cells, proliferate within the hematopoietic tissue, and then infiltrate the rest of the bone to produce osteolytic lesions; substances secreted by the malignant plasma cells produce systemic effects and involve the bone marrow causing major complications

2. Subsequent bone destruction leads to hypercalcemia and pathologic fractures

3. Proliferation of plasma cells crowds the marrow space, usually inhibiting the production of RBCs

4. Plasma cells also synthesize and secrete an abnormally small number of immunoglobulins, increasing the risk of infection

5. In some cases, a marked increase in IgG or occasionally IgA increases the blood's viscosity, leading to occlusion of small blood vessels

6. The hallmark of multiple myeloma is the production of an abnormal immunoglobulin (the M component) indicated by elevated blood levels and the presence of Bence Jones protein in the urine

7. Signs and symptoms

   a. Gradual, insidious onset with clients suffering from recurrent infections, especially pneumonia

   b. Pain is a major problem for these clients as bony destruction begins to occur and lytic bone lesions occur

   c. Cord compression may occur from vertebral collapse

   d. Diffuse osteoporosis with a negative calcium balance may also be seen

   e. Renal stones occur with demineralization

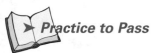

   f. Hypercalcemia can also cause neurological disturbances (confusion, depression), gastrointestinal (GI) distress, altered musculoskeletal status, fluid and electrolyte imbalance, and altered cardiopulmonary function

   g. Renal disease may develop as a result of renal calculi and the toxic effect of Bence Jones protein on the renal epithelial cells

C. Nursing assessment

1. Assessment includes symptom analysis of pain, history of fractures, recurring pneumonia, kidney problems, musculoskeletal problems, or cardiovascular complications

2. Diagnostic tests: electrolytes, chest x-ray (CXR), CBC, BUN, creatinine, computerized tomography (CT) scan, IgE, urinalysis

D. Nursing management

1. Medications

   a. Analgesics to manage pain

   b. Antimicrobial therapy in the presence of positive blood cultures

   c. Melphalan (Alkeran) and cyclophosphamide (Cytoxan), the most common chemotherapeutic agents used to manage the condition

   d. Management of hypercalcemia through the use of steroids, IV hydration, diuretics, and medications, calcitonin (Calcimar), etidronate disodium (Didronel), gallium nitrate (Ganite), and pamidronate disodium (Aredia)

2. There is no cure for multiple myeloma, so the treatment is palliative

3. Maintaining adequate hydration is of primary concern; fluids are administered to attain a urinary output of 1.5 to 2 L/day

4. Weight-bearing, range of motion (ROM), and ambulation helps the bone reabsorb calcium; ambulation is most significant in lowering the calcium level

5. Radiation therapy is usually limited to clients with disabling pain or those with spinal cord compression

> **➤ Practice to Pass**
>
> A client with multiple myeloma has recently been diagnosed with bone metastasis. She was started on long-acting morphine sulfate (MS Contin) tablets while in the hospital. In preparation for discharge, what important information should the nurse review with the client and significant other?

6. Blood transfusions are often indicated to manage the resultant anemia

7. Autologous and allogenic bone marrow transplants are also an option

8. Gallium nitrate (Ganite) is contraindicated with renal insufficiency (creatinine greater than 2.5 mg/dL)

9. Manage pain if metastasis occurs, instructing the client on how to take the medications prior to severe pain and possible side effects

IV. Thrombocytopenia

A. Overview

1. Defined as a platelet count less than 100,000/mm^3

NCLEX!

2. Is the most common cause of abnormal bleeding

3. Hemorrhage from minor trauma and spontaneous bleeding can occur when platelet count falls below 20,000/mm^3

4. Fatal gastrointestinal, cerebral, and pulmonary hemorrhage can occur if the count drops below 10,000/mm^3

5. Causes include unknown reasons, diseases (anemias, systemic lupus erythematosus, acquired immunodeficiency syndrome [AIDS]), after viral infections, chemotherapy or radiation, hypersplenism or splenomegaly, coronary bypass or autotransfusion, heparin therapy

B. Pathophysiology

1. Related to three basic mechanisms: accelerated platelet destruction or consumption, defective platelet production, or disordered platelet distribution

2. *Idiopathic thrombocytopenia purpura* (ITP) occurs when the destruction of platelets is greatly accelerated

NCLEX!

   a. The destruction is believed to be caused by the body's immune system and is therefore categorized as an autoimmune disorder

   b. Acute ITP is more common in children, while chronic ITP is more common in adults

   c. Platelets become coated with antibodies as a result of the autoimmune response mediated by the B lymphocytes; although the platelets function normally, the spleen sees them as foreign, and destroys them

   d. Platelet circulation time is decreased to 1 to 3 days

3. *Secondary thrombocytopenia* is a condition in which there is a defect in platelet production; this defect may occur as a result of:

   a. Medication use, such as thiazide diuretics, acetylsalicylic acid (ASA), ibuprofen (Advil), indomethacin (Indocin), naproxen sodium (Anaprox), sulfonamides, quinidine sulfate (Quinidex), cimetidine (Tagamet), digitalis (Lanoxin), furosemide (Lasix), heparin sodium, morphine sulfate, vitamins C and E

   b. Spices: ginger, cumin, turmeric, cloves, garlic

   c. Viral or bacterial infections

   d. Bone marrow disorders

     e. Chemotherapy and radiation therapy

  4. *Disordered platelet distribution* occurs when large numbers of platelets are sequestered in the spleen; occurs as a result of lymphoma, portal hypertension, and hypothermia during heart surgery

  5. Signs and symptoms include decreased platelet count; prolonged bleeding time; **purpura** (hemorrhage into the tissues as evidenced by bruising); ecchymosis (flat or raised areas of discoloration of the skin or mucous membrane caused by subcutaneous bleeding); **petechiae** (small, flat, purple or red spots on the skin or mucous membranes caused by minute hemorrhage in the dermis or submucous layer); weakness and fatigue

C. Nursing assessment

  1. Assessment

     a. Evaluation of skin for signs of hemorrhage and symptom analysis of any bleeding episodes; look for petechiae and purpura on the most common areas (anterior thorax, arms, and neck); other common types of bleeding are epistaxis, menorrhagia, hematuria, and gastrointestinal bleeding

     b. Activity tolerance (may be reduced from a secondary anemia)

     c. Home medications used, including herbal products

     d. Recent infections

  2. Diagnostic tests: CBC, platelet count, coagulation studies including prothrombin time (PT) and partial thromboplastin time (PTT), bone marrow exam

D. Nursing management

  1. Medications include steroids to suppress the immune response in ITP; immunoglobulin has been shown to have a temporary therapeutic effect in immune response disorders

  2. Thrombocytopenic precautions should be initiated (see Box 15-2)

  3. Focus of client education is primarily on the risk for bleeding

  4. Platelet transfusions may be given when platelet counts fall below 20,000/mm^3, but are of little benefit in ITP

Box 15-2	
Thrombocytopenic Precautions	• Avoid intramuscular (IM) or subcutaneous (SQ or SC) injections. • Avoid use of acetylsalicylic acid (aspirin) or aspirin-containing products. • Avoid use of toothbrushes and razors. • Avoid invasive or traumatic procedures. • Assess for signs of bleeding (skin, mouth, nose, feces, urine). • Guaiac all stool, urine, and emesis. • Pad side rails if necessary. • Avoid venipuncture (clients usually have a triple-lumen central line in place for blood sampling, medication administration, and blood product transfusion). • Administer stool softeners as necessary.

5. Clients should be educated about the Cushingoid side effects of steroid therapy, such as adiposity, edema, capillary fragility, and excessive hair growth

6. Treatment may consist of a spleenectomy, especially in ITP

V. Hemophilia

A. Overview

1. Defined as a group of hereditary clotting factor disorders characterized by prolonged coagulation time that results in prolonged and sometime excessive bleeding

2. Hemophilia A and B are X-linked recessive disorders transmitted by female carriers, displayed almost exclusively in males (see Figure 15-1)

3. Cause is genetics

B. Pathophysiology

1. *Hemophilia A* (classic hemophilia) is a deficiency in **factor VIII** (an alpha globulin that stabilizes fibrin clots); deficiency is determined by first performing a PTT on the client's plasma; a factor VIII deficient plasma substrate is then mixed with the client's plasma and the degree of correction in the PTT is determined and compared to the degree of correction obtained by normal plasma

2. *Hemophilia B* (Christmas disease) is a deficiency in **factor IX** (a vitamin-dependent beta globulin essential in stage 1 of the intrinsic coagulation system as an influence on the amount of thromboplastin available); deficiency is determined by first performing a PTT on the client's plasma; a factor IX deficient plasma substrate is then mixed with the client's plasma and the degree of correction in the PTT is determined and compared to the degree of correction obtained by normal plasma

   a. Despite the difference in factor deficiency, hemophilia A and B are clinically identical

   b. Clients with hemophilia A and B form platelet plugs at the site of bleeding, but the clotting factor deficiency impairs the coagulation response and the capacity to form a stable clot

   c. With a factor level greater than or equal to 5 percent, bleeding is the result of trauma or surgery

   d. Spontaneous bleeding can occur with factor level activity below 1 percent resulting in hemoarthrosis with joint deformity and potential disability

Figure 15-1

Genogram illustrating inheritance pattern for hemophilia A and B, which are X-linked recessive characteristics. Females carry the gene, but males express the gene and develop the disorder.

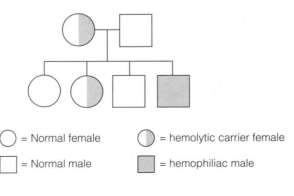

○ = Normal female   ◐ = hemolytic carrier female

□ = Normal male   ▨ = hemophiliac male

3. *Von Willebrand's disease* is a deficiency of the von Willebrand factor (vWF) and platelet dysfunction

   a. Factor VIII has three properties, pre-coagulant activity, antigenic activity, and von Willenbrand factor activity

   b. It is classified as an autosomal dominant trait factor VIII defect; in hemophilia A, vWF is normal, but in von Willebrand's disease, vWF is characteristically low (less than 40 percent of control sample activity)

   c. This disorder is seen in both genders

4. Signs and symptoms

   a. Prolonged clotting times

   b. Subcutaneous ecchymosis and hematomas

   c. Bleeding from the gums

   d. Gastrointestinal bleeding, evidenced by hematemesis (vomiting blood), occult blood in the stools, gastric pain, or abdominal pain

   e. Urinary tract bleeding evidenced by hematuria

   f. Pain or paralysis resulting from pressure of the hematomas on nerves

   g. Hemarthrosis (joint bleeding, swelling, and damage)

   h. Slow oozing of blood from minor cuts, with the onset of bleeding being delayed for several hours, or even days after the injury

C. Nursing assessment

1. Assessment includes assessment of bleeding, pain, skin, and oral mucosa; perform a symptom analysis of any bleeding episodes, infections, or difficulty in controlling bleeding; question home medications and use of herbal products

2. Diagnostic tests: PT (normal); PTT (prolonged); fibrinogen (normal); platelet count (normal); prolonged bleeding time in von Willebrand's disease, CBC, guaiac stool, and urinalysis (UA)

D. Nursing management

1. Medications include replacement of deficient factor

   a. Hemophilia A: cryoprecipitate containing 8 to 100 units of factor VIII per bag at 12-hour intervals until bleeding ceases

   b. Hemophilia B: plasma or factor IX concentrate given every 24 hours or until bleeding ceases

   c. Von Willebrand's disease: cryoprecipitate containing 8 to 100 units of factor VIII per bag at 12-hour intervals until bleeding ceases

2. Referral for genetic counseling is essential

3. Acetylsalicylic acid (aspirin) should never be given to a client with hemophilia

4. Stop topical bleeding as quickly as possible by applying direct pressure or ice, packing the area with gel foam or fibrin foam, and applying topical hemostatic agents such as fibrin

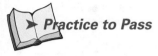

Practice to Pass

Both the client with hemophilia and the client with thrombocytopenia have a nursing diagnosis of Risk for injury: hemorrhage. How do these two medical diagnoses differ in their nursing interventions? How are they similar?

NCLEX!

NCLEX!

5. When joint bleeding occurs, totally rest the joint, apply ice, and administer hemophilia factors

6. Treatment may consist of plasmapheresis and/or prothrombin complexes for the development of antibody inhibitors against the specific coagulation factor

VII. Anemia

A. Overview

1. Defined as a condition where the hemoglobin content of the blood is insufficient to satisfy bodily needs

2. Caused by decrease in circulating RBCs, but may also be caused by accelerated hemolysis, decreased production, or high numbers of reticulocytes; other causes include side effects of medications, menstruation, GI bleeding

B. Pathophysiology

NCLEX!

1. Anemia reduces the oxygen carrying capacity of the blood, producing tissue hypoxia

2. Basic classifications of anemia are nutritional, hemolytic, and bone marrow depression; see Box 15-3 for types of anemias within each classification

3. Nutritional anemia results from nutrient deficiencies that disrupt erythropoiesis or hemoglobin synthesis

   a. *Iron-deficiency anemia*

      1) Supply of iron is inadequate for optimal formation of RBCs related to excessive iron loss caused by bleeding, decreased dietary intake, or malabsorption

      2) Adequate iron in the RBC is essential since the oxygen molecule attaches to it

      3) Considered a microcytic-hypochromic anemia (RBC diameter less than 6 with decreased pigmentation) with an increase in the red cell size distribution width (RDW)

      4) Erythrocytes are small (microcytic) and pale (hypochromic); **mean corpuscular volume (MCV**; measures size) is decreased and **mean cor-**

Box 15-3

Classification of Selected Anemias

Nutritional Anemias
- Iron-deficiency anemia
- Vitamin B_{12} anemia
- Folic acid anemia

Hemolytic Anemias
- Sickle cell anemia
- Thalassemia
- Acquired hemolytic anemia
- Glucose-6-phosphate dehydrogenase anemia

Bone Marrow Depression Anemia
- Aplastic anemia

puscular hemoglobin (MCH) or **mean corpuscular hemoglobin concentration** or **MCHC** (calculated value of the hemoglobin present in the RBC compared to its size), will be decreased; the MCV, MCH, and MCHC should be analyzed only when the hemoglobin is low

5) An average diet supplies the body with 12 to 15 mg/day of iron, of which only 5 to 10 percent is absorbed

6) Iron is stored in the body as **ferritin,** an iron-phosphorus-protein complex that contains about 23 percent iron; it is formed in the intestinal mucosa, when ferritin iron joins with the protein apoferritin; ferritin is stored in the tissues, primarily in the reticuloendothelial cells of the liver, spleen, and bone marrow

7) Normal iron excretion is less than 1 mg/day through the urine, sweat, bile, feces, and from desquamated cells of the skin; the average woman loses 0.5 mg of iron daily or 15 mg monthly during menstruation; menstruation is the most common cause of iron deficiency in women while gastrointestinal bleeding is the most common cause in men

8) Develops slowly through three phases: body's stores of iron used for erythropoiesis are depleted; insufficient iron is transported to the bone marrow; and iron deficient erythropoiesis begins, allowing small hemoglobin deficient cells to enter the peripheral circulation in large numbers; iron is needed on the hemoglobin so the oxygen molecule will attach

9) Signs and symptoms develop gradually with the client not seeking attention until the hemoglobin drops to 7 to 8 g/dL; manifestations include fatigue, weakness, shortness of breath, pallor (ear lobes, palms, and conjunctiva), brittle spoon like nails; **cheilosis** (cracks in the corners of the mouth); smooth sore tongue; dizziness, hypoxia, and **pica** (craving to eat unusual substances such as clay or starch)

b. *Vitamin B₁₂ deficiency anemia*

1) Impairs cellular division and maturation especially in rapidly proliferating RBCs

2) Macrocytic (megaloblastic) anemia (RBC diameter greater than 8)

3) **Pernicious anemia** is the body's inability to absorb vitamin B_{12} because of a lack of **intrinsic factor,** a substance secreted by the parietal cells of the gastric mucosa

4) Laboratory examination shows an increase in the MCV and MCHC

5) Gastric secretion analysis reveals **achlorhydria:** the absence of free hydrochloric acid in a pH maintained at 3.5

6) Inevitably develops after total gastrectomy, with 15 % of clients developing pernicious anemia after partial gastrectomy or gastrojejunostomy

7) Lack of vitamin B_{12} alters the structure and disrupts the function of the peripheral nerves, spinal cord, and brain

8) Clients with this anemia tend to have fair hair coloring or become prematurely gray

9) Signs and symptoms include pallor or slight jaundice with a complaint of weakness, smooth sore beefy red tongue, diarrhea, **paresthesias** such

as numbness or tingling in the extremities), impaired **proprioception** (ability to identify one's position in space) which may progress to difficulty with balance and spinal cord damage)

  c. *Folic acid deficiency anemia*

    1) Required for DNA synthesis and the normal maturation of RBCs

    2) Macrocytic (megaloblastic) anemia (RBC diameter > 8); MCV high with low hemoglobin

    3) Causative etiology: poor nutrition, malabsorption syndrome, medications that impede absorption (oral contraceptives, anticonvulsants, methotrexate [MTX]), alcohol abuse, and anorexia

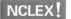

    4) Signs and symptoms include pallor, progressive weakness, fatigue, shortness of breath, and palpitations; GI symptoms are similar to B_{12} deficiency, but usually more severe (anemia, glossitis, cheilosis, and diarrhea); neurological symptoms seen in B_{12} deficiency are not seen in folic acid deficiency and therefore assist in differentiation

C. Nursing assessment

  1. Assessment includes symptom analysis of activity tolerance, skin color, nails, oral assessment, GI and nutritional assessment; neurological assessment is indicated in Vitamin B_{12} anemia

  2. Diagnostic tests: CBC, MCV, MCH, MCHC

  3. Collect 24-hour urine for **Schilling test,** a vitamin B_{12} absorption test that indicates if a client lacks intrinsic factor by measuring the excretion of orally administered radionuclide labeled B_{12}

D. Nursing management

  1. Iron-deficiency anemia

    a. Medications include administration of oral iron preparations before meals if tolerated and nausea does not occur; vitamin C enhances absorption, while antacids inhibit absorption; intramuscular (IM) dextran (Gentran 75) should be administered using the Z-track technique to prevent tattooing of the skin

      1) Parenteral iron is given to clients that have an intolerance to iron preparations, habitually forget their medications or continue to suffer blood loss

      2) Because of the high risk of allergic reaction, a physician should be present when the first dose is administered

    b. Increase the number and amount of iron-rich foods, such as beef, chicken, egg yolk, pork loin, turkey, and whole grain breads and cereals

    c. Monitor for safety and injury if severe anemia occurs due to the possibility of tissue and cerebral hypoxia

  2. Vitamin B_{12} deficiency anemia

    a. Medications include parenteral replacement of vitamin B_{12} IM; required for life for clients lacking the intrinsic factor

    b. Clients with insufficient dietary intake are instructed to increase intake of foods such as eggs, meats, and dairy products

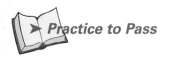

Practice to Pass

What is the primary difference between pernicious anemia and anemia caused by a folic acid deficiency? How are the two similar?

3. Folic acid deficiency anemia

   a. Medications include oral folic acid supplements indefinitely with malabsorption or impaired folic acid metabolism

   b. In malnourishment, foods containing folic acid should be added, such as green leafy vegetables, broccoli, organ meats, eggs, and milk

VII. Sickle Cell Anemia

A. Overview

1. Defined as a hereditary, chronic form of hemolytic anemia

2. Eight percent of African Americans are heterozygous (carriers) for sickle cell anemia thereby inheriting one affected gene or the sickle cell trait

3. One percent of African Americans are homozygous (identical genes) for the disorder, thereby inheriting a defective gene from both parents or sickle cell anemia with likelihood to experience sickle cell crisis

4. Caused by an autosomal genetic defect (one gene affected) that results in the synthesis of hemoglobin S (see Figure 15-2)

B. Pathophysiology

1. Produced by a mutation in the beta chain of the hemoglobin molecule though a substitution of the amino acid valine for glutamine in both beta chains

2. When there is decreased oxygen tension in the plasma, hemoglobin S causes RBCs to elongate, become rigid, and assume a crescent sickled shape causing the cells to clump together and obstruct capillary blood flow, causing ischemia and possible tissue infarction

   a. Conditions likely to trigger a sickle cell crisis include hypoxia, low environmental and/or body temperature, excessive exercise, high altitudes, or inadequate oxygen during anesthesia

   b. Other causes include elevated blood viscosity/decreased plasma volume, infection, dehydration, and/or increased hydrogen ion concentration (acidosis)

Figure 15-2

Inheritance pattern for sickle cell anemia.

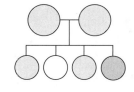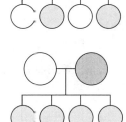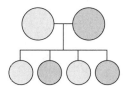

Key:

◯ Normal

◯ Sickle cell trait: heterozygous defective genes

◯ Sickle cell anemia: homozygous defective genes

3. With normal oxygenation, the sickled RBCs resume their normal shape

4. Repeated episodes of sickling and unsickling weaken the cell membrane, causing them to hemolyze and be removed

5. A vasoocclusive crisis begins with sickling in the microcirculation and leads to the following cascade:

   a. Vasospasm creates a logjam effect, which brings blood flow through the vessels to a stop

   b. Thrombosis and infarction of local tissue occur

   c. Crisis results, which is extremely painful and can last from 4 to 6 days

6. Sickle cell trait is a generally mild condition that produces few, if any, manifestations

7. Signs and symptoms include anemia with sickled cells noted on a peripheral smear; general manifestations similar to those of hemolytic anemia (pallor, jaundice, fatigue, and irritability); large joints and surrounding tissue may become swollen during crisis; priapism (abnormal, painful continuous erection of the penis) may occur if penile veins are obstructed

C. **Nursing assessment**

1. Assessment includes symptom analysis of activity tolerance, skin color, swelling of joints, and degree of pain if any

2. Diagnostic tests: **hemoglobin electrophoresis,** a blood test that causes the hemoglobin molecule to migrate in solution in response to electric currents is done to determine the presence and percentage of hemoglobin S and is used for a definitive diagnosis; CBC

D. **Nursing management**

1. Medications include folic acid supplements (to meet the increased metabolic demands of the bone marrow) and analgesics

2. Hydration therapy as well as scheduled transfusions will decrease painful crisis episodes

3. During a crisis, hydration therapy is essential to improve blood flow, reduce pain, and prevent renal damage

4. For clients experiencing a pain crisis, treatment includes rest, oxygen, analgesia, and hydration

XI. **Polycythemia (Polycythemia Vera)**

A. **Overview**

1. Defined as an increase in the number of circulating erythrocytes and the concentration of hemoglobin in the blood; also known as polycythemia vera, PV, or myeloproliferative red cell disorder

2. Bone marrow stimulates an overproduction of erythrocytes, leukocytes, and thrombocytes thereby increasing blood viscosity, blood volume, and congestion of tissues and organs with blood

3. Can be a primary or secondary disorder

4. Causes include primary—unknown; secondary—erythropoietin-secreting tumors, Cushing's syndrome, end-stage renal disease, hypoxemia, and long-term dialysis

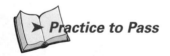

Practice to Pass

The nurse sees a client with sickle cell anemia in the outpatient clinic. He is planning to fly to Orlando, Florida, for vacation with his parents during spring break. What education should the nurse give the client and his parents to prevent the client from experiencing a crisis while away?

B. Pathophysiology

1. *Primary polycythemia*

   a. Most common in Caucasian men of European Jewish ancestry

   b. Is a neoplastic stem cell disorder characterized by the overproduction of RBCs, certain WBCs, and platelets

   c. Erythrocytosis causes increased blood volume and viscosity with liver and spleen congestion

   d. Thick, slow-moving blood becomes an ideal environment for acidosis and clotting, with resultant tissue and organ infarction secondary to thrombi

2. *Secondary polycythemia*

   a. Most common form of PV

   b. Excess of erythropoiesis that arises as a response to an abnormal increase in erythropoietin

   c. Abnormally high levels of erythropoietin may also be produced because of hypoxemia, in turn caused by:

   1) Prolonged exposure to high altitudes

   2) Systemic disorders that affect oxygenation (chronic obstructive pulmonary disease [COPD], congestive heart failure [CHF])

   3) Hypoventilation secondary to morbid obesity

   4) Long-term smokers: "smokers erythrocytosis"

3. Signs and symptoms

   a. Plethora (engorged or distended blood vessels causing a ruddy color of the face, hands, feet, ears, and mucous membranes)

   b. Engorgement of the retinal (bloodshot eyes) and sublingual veins

   c. Splenomegaly (primary PV only)

   d. Hepatomegaly; headache, a feeling of fullness in the head, dizziness, weakness, fatigue on exertion, visual disturbances, hypertension, hypermetabolism, epigastric distress and backache

   e. Pruritis that does not respond to antihistamines

   f. Manifestations of vascular disease (angina, intermittent claudication, cerebral insufficiency)

C. Nursing assessment

1. Nursing assessment includes symptom analysis of pain, itching, skin color, palpation of spleen or liver

2. Diagnostic tests: high erythrocyte count (high, 8 to 12 million/mm^3); decreased MCHC; increased leukocytes, thrombocytes, and total blood volume

D. Nursing management

1. Medications include antineoplastic agents (but their side effects are often worse than the disease); radioactive phosphorus (may cause generalized suppression of hematopoiesis with resultant anemia, leukopenia, or thrombocytopenia)

2. Encourage smoking cessation in clients who smoke

3. Manage underlying chronic condition (COPD, CHF) with supportive measures and appropriate drug therapy

Case Study

M. L. is a 62-year-old married retired schoolteacher with three grown children who live in various parts of the United States. Her husband is a pharmaceutical representative and travels frequently for his job. M. L. has been a diabetic since age 25 and takes 30 units of insulin at breakfast and 10 units of insulin at bedtime. Over the last 2 months, the client has had difficulty getting over a cold, experienced periods of extreme fatigue, lost 10 pounds, and has low-grade temperature of 100°F. Her physician conducted blood studies and a bone marrow biopsy and aspirate, which led to the diagnosis of acute lymphocytic leukemia (ALL). Currently the client is hospitalized, has a triple-lumen Hickman catheter in place, and is undergoing chemotherapy with vincristine (Oncovin), methotrexate (MTX), and prednisone.

Assessment finds the client oriented to person, place, and time; complaining of headache, dizziness upon standing; slight numbness, tingling of her lower extremities; petechiae cover her arms, chest, and upper thighs; skin color pale; recoil is less than 6 seconds, with dry mucous membranes. Small ulcerated area is present on outer aspect of right ankle; Hickman site is clean and dry but slightly red; no obvious dyspnea but complains of shortness of breath upon exertion; lung sounds clear; sputum slightly yellow in color; vital signs: pulse 90; blood pressure 140/84 lying and 128/72 standing; respirations 20 and regular; lab work: white blood count (WBC) 9,000/mm^3; red blood count (RBC) 2.23; hemoglobin 8.8g/dL; hematocrit 26%; platelets 12,000/mm^3; WBC differential: segs 10%; bands 1%; lymphocytes 60%; glucose: 250 mg/dL; albumin 2.4g/dL; calcium 8.0 mEq/L.

❶ What are the most important nursing diagnoses, and how should they be prioritized?

❷ What is the relationship between the client's absolute neutrophil count (ANC) and the risk for infection?

❸ How will the nurse know the client is developing infection?

❹ What effect will the client's diabetes have on her treatment course?

❺ How should the nurse prepare the client for discharge from the hospital?

For suggested responses, see page 570.

Posttest

1 A client with anemia due to chemotherapy has a hemoglobin of 7.0 g/dL. Which of the following complaints would be indicative of tissue hypoxia related to anemia?

(1) Dizziness
(2) Fatigue relieved by rest
(3) Skin that is warm and dry to the touch
(4) Apathy

2 A client's medical record indicates that the client has a positive Philadelphia chromosome. The nurse plans care for which of the following disorders?

(1) Acute myelocytic leukemia (AML)
(2) Hairy cell leukemia
(3) Chronic myelogenous leukemia (CML)
(4) Chronic lymphocytic leukemia (CLL)

3 A nurse caring for a client who has experienced a bone marrow biopsy and aspiration should assess for which of the following as the most serious complication?

(1) Hemorrhage
(2) Infection
(3) Shock
(4) Splintering of bone marrow fragments

4 For the client diagnosed with iron-deficiency anemia, the nurse should recommend an increased intake of which of the following foods?

(1) Fresh citrus fruits
(2) Milk and cheese
(3) Organ meats
(4) Whole grain breads

5 The nurse would interpret that a client is most severely at risk for bleeding when which of the following is noted on laboratory test results?

(1) Neutrophils are 50 percent
(2) Lymphocytes are 30 percent
(3) Platelets are less than 20,000
(4) Basophils are 0

6 The common feature of leukemia is which of the following?

(1) A compensatory polycythemia stimulated by thrombocytopenia.
(2) An unregulated accumulation of white blood cells in the bone marrow.
(3) Increased blood viscosity resulting from an overproduction of white cells.
(4) Reduced plasma volume in response to a reduced production of cellular components.

7 The nurse would teach a client with sickle cell trait that he or she:

(1) Should avoid fluid loss and dehydration.
(2) Can expect to experience hemolytic jaundice.
(3) Can expect to experience chronic anemia.
(4) Is protected from sickle cell crises under normal circumstances.

8 A client with pancytopenia enters the clinic with excess ecchymosis. The client should be cautioned to avoid which of the following, since medications can alter platelet function?

(1) Acetylsalicylic acid (aspirin), digitalis (Lanoxin), and quinidine sulfate (Quinidex)
(2) Milk of magnesia, heparin, and quinidine sulfate (Quinidex)
(3) Senna (Senokot), furosemide (Lasix), and phenytoin (Dilantin)
(4) Acetaminophen (Tylenol), sulfonamides, and penicillins

9 The nurse would explain to a client newly diagnosed with hemophilia that it is a hereditary bleeding disorder that:

(1) Has a higher incidence in females.
(2) Is associated with joint bleeding, swelling and damage.
(3) Is related to genetic deficiency of the von Willebrand factor.
(4) Can be caused by lack of vitamin B_{12}.

10 A client enters the clinic with complaints of a sore mouth. Physical assessment reveals a beefy red tongue. These symptoms are most suggestive of which of the following disorders?

(1) Pernicious anemia
(2) Hemolytic anemia
(3) Sickle cell anemia
(4) Polycythemia vera

See pages 486–487 for Answers and Rationales.

Answers and Rationales

Pretest

1 **Answer: 3** *Rationale:* Cerebral tissue hypoxia is commonly associated with dizziness. The greatest potential risk to the client with dizziness is injury, especially with changes in position. Planning for periods of rest and conserving energy are important with someone with anemia because of his or her fatigue level, but most important is safety.
Cognitive Level: Anaylysis
Nursing Process: Implementation; *Test Plan:* SECE

2 **Answer: 1** *Rationale:* Major complications of multiple myeloma include bone pain, hypercalcemia, renal failure, anemia, and impaired immune responses that are a result of bone marrow involvement and the systemic effects of substances secreted by the malignant plasma cells.
Cognitive Level: Comprehension
Nursing Process: Analysis; *Test Plan:* PHYS

3 **Answer: 2** *Rationale:* Myelodysplastic syndromes often progress to acute myelogenous leukemia. They are often refractory to treatment and are associated with a poor prognosis. They are not hereditary and are often referred to as pre-leukemia.
Cognitive Level: Comprehension
Nursing Process: Analysis; *Test Plan:* PHYS

4 **Answer: 4** *Rationale:* Bone marrow biopsy and aspirate is the only definitive diagnosis of AML. The presence of Auer rods is diagnostic for AML. The presence of leukemic cells in the spinal fluid is more common in acute lymphocytic leukemia (ALL). Uric acid and lactic dehydrogenase levels may be elevated in AML, but this is not diagnostic for the disease.
Cognitive Level: Application
Nursing Process: Assessment; *Test Plan:* PHYS

5 **Answer: 1** *Rationale:* Option 1 contains foods high in protein, folic acid, iron, and B_{12} that are needed for erythropoiesis. Options 2, 3, and 4 contain lesser amounts.
Cognitive Level: Application
Nursing Process: Implementation; *Test Plan:* PHYS

6 **Answer: 2** *Rationale:* IM administration is recommended over intravenous infusion because of the potential for anaphylaxis. The gluteal muscle is the best route for administration since the muscle is large and highly vascular. The Z-track method is preferable to prevent tattooing of the skin and tissue necrosis caused by infiltration into the subcutaneous tissue.
Cognitive Level: Application
Nursing Process: Implementation; *Test Plan:* PHYS

7 **Answer: 3** *Rationale:* Platelet aggregation forms a platelet plug at the site of bleeding, but fibrin reinforces the platelet plug. The absence of clotting factors impairs the coagulation response and the capacity to form a stable clot.
Cognitive Level: Application
Nursing Process: Analysis; *Test Plan:* PHYS

8 **Answer: 3** *Rationale:* Pernicious anemia is caused by the body's inability to absorb vitamin B_{12}. This is caused by a lack of intrinsic factor in the gastric juices. The Shilling test helps diagnose pernicious anemia by determining the client's ability to absorb vitamin B_{12}.
Cognitive Level: Application
Nursing Process: Analysis; *Test Plan:* PHYS

9 **Answer: 1** *Rationale:* Pain from sickle cell crisis is primarily related to obstructed capillary blood flow causing ischemia and possible tissue infarction. While dehydration often causes increased viscosity, the primary cause of pain is vasoocclusion of the blood vessels from sickled red blood cells.
Cognitive Level: Application
Nursing Process: Assessment; *Test Plan:* PHYS

10 **Answer: 3** *Rationale:* The client with neutropenia is unable to mount an inflammatory response. Fever is usually the first sign of infection. Options 1, 2, and 4 are all true, but they explain why the neutropenic client is at greater risk for infection.
Cognitive Level: Analysis
Nursing Process: Analysis; *Test Plan:* PHYS

Posttest

1 **Answer: 1** *Rationale:* Cerebral tissue hypoxia is commonly associated with dizziness. Recognition of cerebral hypoxia is critical since the body will attempt to shunt oxygenated blood to vital organs.
Cognitive Level: Application
Nursing Process: Assessment; *Test Plan:* PHYS

2 **Answer: 3** *Rationale:* Approximately 95 percent of clients with CML are Philadelphia chromosome-positive. This represents a translocation of the long arms of chromosomes 9 and 22.
Cognitive Level: Application
Nursing Process: Analysis; *Test Plan:* PHYS

3 **Answer: 1** *Rationale:* The risk for hemorrhage is of greatest risk since a large-bore needle is used to perform the biopsy and aspiration. Many of these clients often have an altered clotting capability. While the risk of infection is also a consideration, the procedure is performed under sterile conditions and is less of a concern than hemorrhage.
Cognitive Level: Application
Nursing Process: Assessment; *Test Plan:* PHYS

4 **Answer: 3** *Rationale:* Organ meats such as liver are a good source of iron as well as green leafy vegetables and egg yolks. Whole grain breads also contain iron, however not in as high a quantity as organ meats.
Cognitive Level: Application
Nursing Process: Implementation; *Test Plan:* HPM

5 **Answer: 3** *Rationale:* Options 1, 2, and 4 relate to the white blood cells. A platelet count below 20,000 increases the client's risk for severe bleeding because of reduced platelets to assist in the clotting cascade to form a clot.
Cognitive Level: Analysis
Nursing Process: Analysis; *Test Plan:* PHYS

6 **Answer: 2** *Rationale:* Leukemia is a result of erratic production of white blood cells by the bone marrow, which replace normal marrow components. It can arise from both a lymphatic and a myelocytic etiology. White blood cells are often immature and incapable of performing their expected function(s).
Cognitive Level: Knowledge
Nursing Process: Analysis; *Test Plan:* PHYS

7 **Answer: 4** *Rationale:* Sickle cell trait is generally a mild condition that produces few if any manifestations. These clients are considered carriers of the disease and require genetic counseling to determine presence of the hemoglobin S. Certain stressors result in a sickle cell crisis.
Cognitive Level: Application
Nursing Process: Planning; *Test Plan:* HPM

8 **Answer: 1** *Rationale:* All of the medications in the first option can affect platelet aggregation and should be avoided in a client with bleeding tendencies. A thorough review of all medications taken at home should be done whenever clients are issued new medications.
Cognitive Level: Application
Nursing Process: Implementation; *Test Plan:* PHYS

9 **Answer: 2** *Rationale:* Hemophilia is a group of hereditary clotting factor disorders characterized by prolonged coagulation time that results in prolonged and sometime excessive bleeding. It is a X-linked recessive characteristic transmitted by female carriers, displayed almost exclusively in males often resulting in spontaneous bleeding into the joints resulting in hemoarthrosis with joint deformity and potential disability. Option 3 is a specific form of hemophilia, von Willebrand's disease. Option 4 is pernicious anemia.
Cognitive Level: Comprehension
Nursing Process: Implementation; *Test Plan:* PHYS

10 **Answer: 1** *Rationale:* Assessment findings in pernicious anemia include a smooth red beefy tongue, altered sensations such as numbness or tingling in the extremities, and difficulty identifying one's position in space, which may progress to difficulty with balance and spinal cord damage.
Cognitive Level: Application
Nursing Process: Assessment; *Test Plan:* PHYS

References

Alexander, J. (1998). Nursing care of the client with lymphoma and multiple myeloma. In J. K. Itano & K. N. Taoka (Eds.), *Core curriculum for oncology nursing* (3rd ed.). Philadelphia: W. B. Saunders, pp. 496–504.

Camp-Sorrell, D. (1998). Myelosuppression. In J. K. Itano & K. N. Taoka (Eds.), *Core curriculum for oncology nursing* (3rd ed.). Philadelphia: W. B. Saunders, pp. 207–222.

Fitzgerald, M. A. (1999). Hematologic disorders. In E. Q. Youngkin, K. J. Sawyer, J. F. Kissinger, & D. S. Israel (Eds.), *Pharmacotherapy: A primary care clinical guide*. Stamford, CT: Appleton and Lange, pp. 605–620.

Green, C. (2000). *Critical thinking in nursing: Case studies across the curriculum*. Upper Saddle River, NJ: Prentice Hall, pp. 19–22.

LeMone, P. & Burke, K. M. (2000). *Medical-surgical nursing: Critical thinking in client care* (2nd ed.). Upper Saddle River, NJ: Prentice Hall, pp. 1264–1324.

Mansen, T. J. & McCance, K. L. (1998). Alterations of erythrocyte function. In K. L. McCance & S. E. Huether (Eds.), *Pathophysiology: The basis for disease in adults and children* (3rd ed.). St. Louis: Mosby, pp. 878–898.

Mansen, T. J., McCance, K. L., & Field, R. B. (1998). Alterations in leukocyte, lymphoid, and hemostatic function. In K. L. McCance & S. E. Huether (Eds.), *Pathophysiology: The basis for disease in adults and children* (3rd ed.). St. Louis: Mosby, pp. 899–934.

McCance, K. L. (1998). Structure and function of the hematologic system. In K. L. McCance, & S. E. Huether (Eds.), *Pathophysiology: The basis for disease in adults and children* (3rd ed.). St. Louis: Mosby, pp. 845–877.

Moran, M. J. & Ezzone, S. A. (1998). Nursing care of the client with leukemia. In J. K. Itano & K. N. Taoka (Eds.), *Core curriculum for oncology nursing* (3rd ed.). Philadelphia: W. B. Saunders, pp. 484–495.

Olsen, S. J., Morrison, C. H., & Ashley, B. W. (1998). Prevention of cancer. In J. K. Itano & K. N. Taoka (Eds.), *Core curriculum for oncology nursing* (3rd ed.). Philadelphia: W. B. Saunders, pp. 681–694.

Wagner, K. D. (2001). Acute hematologic dysfunction. In P. S. Kidd & K. D. Wagner (Eds.), *High acuity nursing*. Upper Saddle River, NJ: Prentice Hall.

Wilkinson, J. M. (2000). *Nursing diagnosis handbook* (7th ed.). Upper Saddle River, NJ: Prentice Hall.

Wilkes, G. M., Ingwersen, K., & Burke, M. B. (1999). *Oncology nursing drug handbook*. Boston: Jones and Bartlett.

CHAPTER 16

Genetic and Developmental Health Problems

Lynn H. Doyle, RN, MS, CPNP

CHAPTER OUTLINE

OBJECTIVES

▮ Define key terms associated with genetic and developmental health problems.

▮ Identify risk factors associated with the development of genetic and developmental health problems.

▮ Discuss the common etiologies of genetic and developmental health problems.

▮ Describe the pathophysiological processes associated with genetic and developmental health problems.

▮ Distinguish between normal and abnormal genetic and developmental health findings obtained from nursing assessment.

▮ Prioritize nursing interventions associated with specific genetic and developmental health problems.

[Media Link]

Use the CD-ROM enclosed with this text, or log onto the address given to access the free, interactive Companion Website created for this series. The CD-ROM and Companion Website accompanying this book offer additional practice opportunities and information—NCLEX Review, Case Studies, Glossary, In Depth with NCLEX, and more.

www.prenhall.com/hogan

REVIEW AT A GLANCE

autosomal *all chromosomes other than the sex (XX or XY) chromosomes; in normal human cells, there are 22 pairs of autosomal chromosomes and 2 pairs of sex chromosomes*

carrier *a person who has one affected autosome and one unaffected autosome; they have no clinical disease but can pass on the gene to offspring*

choreiform *a rapid and jerky body motion that is involuntary*

chromosome *protein structures consisting of DNA that map out the functions of cells within the body; 23 pairs*

congenital *a condition present since birth; causes are genetic, environmental, or multifactorial*

gamete *one of two cells created by meiosis; male (spermatozoon) and female (ovum)*

gene *genetic material (DNA) responsible for programming body function and characteristics—the basic unit of inheritance*

genotype *the entire genetic makeup of an individual, such as the pattern of the genes on the chromosomes*

heterozygous *distribution of zygote for autosomal dominant presentation; only one abnormal autosomal has to be present (e.g., Marfan's syndrome)*

homozygous *malformation created with autosomal recessive presentation; both abnormal chromosomes must be present (e.g., cystic fibrosis)*

karyotype *the pictorial analysis of the chromosomes of an individual*

malformation *abnormal development process in utero leading to defect in organ or region of body*

meiosis *the two stages of separating to create two gametes that can then combine to have both parent traits within the new zygote*

mitosis *the stages of separation to create a new daughter cell in order to replace the older cells for normal growth and replacement*

mosaicism *an individual with the presence of cells from two different genetic materials*

multifactorial *combination of causes for congenital defect, i.e.; environmental plus gene abnormality*

nondisjunction *an abnormal separation during meiosis; instead of a pair of gametes there is a trisomy (3) or monosomy (1) combination*

prototype *genes responsible for observable expression of an individual's traits, such as brown hair or blue eyes*

steatorrhea *foul-smelling stool containing undigested fat*

syndrome *a congenital defect associated with a characteristic set of anomalies (e.g., Down syndrome)*

translocation *after a chromosome breaks, a transfer of part or the entire chromosome to another chromosome leading to a severe or fatal defect*

trisomy *a condition in the chromosome where there are three instead of a chromosome pair in the cell (e.g., trisomy 21)*

X-linked *an inherited gene disorder located on the X-chromosome (e.g., Duchenne's muscular dystrophy)*

zygote *the end product of parent cells (male/female) joining during reproduction*

Pretest

1 Which of the following responses is best when a nurse is asked by the family about why a client with Huntington's chorea should be given thickened liquids?

(1) The client is at risk for dehydration.
(2) The client is at risk for aspiration.
(3) The client may have difficulty chewing.
(4) The client may have pain on swallowing.

2 The infant with Down syndrome should go through which of Erikson's developmental stages first?

(1) Initiative vs. self doubt
(2) Industry vs. inferiority
(3) Autonomy vs. shame and doubt
(4) Trust vs. mistrust

3 The adolescent with Marfan's syndrome should be monitored for which potentially lethal complication?

(1) Aortic rupture
(2) Retinal detachment
(3) Hyperextended joints
(4) Seizure

4 The parent of a child born with albinism type I asks the nurse how this happened. The nurse's best response is that the disorder is:

(1) Autosomal dominant.
(2) Autosomal recessive.
(3) X-linked.
(4) Multifactorial.

5 A priority nursing intervention for the infant with cleft lip is which of the following?

(1) Monitoring for adequate nutritional intake
(2) Teaching high-risk newborn care
(3) Assessing for respiratory distress
(4) Preventing injury

6 The child with cystic fibrosis should take pancrelipase (Pancrease) how often?

(1) Three times daily
(2) After each loose stool
(3) As ordered
(4) With each meal and snack

7 A child is noted to have lymphedema, webbed neck, and low posterior hairline. Which of the following diagnoses is most appropriate?

(1) Turner's syndrome
(2) Down syndrome
(3) Marfan's syndrome
(4) Klinefelter's syndrome

8 A child with cleft palate begins pulling on his left ear, is irritable, and begins to run a temperature of 102°F. The nurse knows the child is at risk for which of the following based on these symptoms?

(1) Pneumonia
(2) Urinary tract infection (UTI)
(3) Otitis media
(4) Cellulitis

9 A child with a karyotype showing XXY is a candidate for which of the following?

(1) Turner's syndrome
(2) Klinefelter's syndrome
(3) Down syndrome
(4) Marfan's syndrome

10 The child with phenylketonuria (PKU) must maintain a low phenylalanine diet to prevent which of the following complications?

(1) Irreversible brain damage
(2) Kidney failure
(3) Blindness
(4) Neutropenia

See pages 514–515 for Answers and Rationales.

I. Risk Factors Associated with Genetic and Developmental Health Problems

    A. Miscarriage: genetic defects cause 60 percent of spontaneous abortions (miscarriages)

    B. Maternal and paternal influences

        1. Familial: tends to run in certain families or ethnic groups

        2. With each subsequent offspring, the incidence may increase although each pregnancy should be viewed as an independent event

            a. Endocrine: higher incidence of non-insulin dependent diabetes mellitus (NIDDM) in Native American families

            b. Cardiac: ventral septal defect increased reoccurrence among siblings

            c. Hematology: Mediterranean descent increases risk for glucose-6-phosphate dehydrogen deficiency (G6PD), thalassemia

    C. Age

        1. Increased age of sperm, ova, or **gametes** (one or two cells created by meiosis)

            a. Parents over 35 years of age; both mother and father increase incidence of abnormal **zygote** (end product of parent cells joined during reproduction)

such as trisomy (a condition in the chromosome where there are three instead of a chromosome pair in a cell)

    b. Autosomal (all chromosomes other than the sex [XX or XY]): dominant disorders such as Marfan's syndrome

  2. Adolescent: younger age of mother leads to increase risk

    a. Factors related to hormonal changes

    b. Dietary insufficiency of protein, iron

    c. Risk-taking behaviors: smoking, drugs

D. Nutrition

  1. Malnutrition leads to poor cell formation

  2. Folic acid deficiency is a known factor in spina bifida

  3. Low protein increases risk of congenital heart disease

  4. Iron-deficiency anemia and small for gestational age (SGA)

E. Environment

  1. Teratogens: interfere with fetal development

    a. Drugs

      1) Tobacco increases incidence of congenital defects

      2) Alcohol exposure leads to fetal alcohol syndrome (FAS)

      3) Drugs, i.e., phenytoin (Dilantin) has a higher incidence of congenital malformation

    b. Radiation leads to increase risk of **nondisjunction** (an abnormal separation) during **meiosis** (two stages of separating to create two gametes)

    c. Infection

      1) Can interfere with fetal development

      2) Rubella leads to increased risk of microcephaly

      3) Cytomegalovirus (CMV) leads to increased risk of optic atrophy

  2. Oxygen deprivation

    a. Smoking leads to increased possibility of prematurity

    b. Maternal hypertension can lead to birth complications and cerebral palsy

F. Multifactorial (combination of causes for a congenital defect)

  1. Combination of all of the above: disruption in utero plus hereditary predisposition, example: cleft lip/palate

  2. Genetic predisposition that leads to **malformation** (abnormal development process in utero leading to defect in organ or region of body)

    a. Approximately 5 to 10 percent of cancers have a **gene** (genetic material [DNA]) marker

    b. Positive human leukocyte antigen-B (HLA-B) allele in children with diabetes type 1

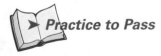

Practice to Pass

What is the rationale for developing a family tree (pedigree) as a part of family planning?

II. Trisomy 21 (Down Syndrome)

A. Overview

1. Defined as a chromosome disorder involving the 21st chromosome

2. **Syndrome** (a congenital defect associated with a characteristic set of anomalies) is a predisposition for:

   a. Congenital heart disease: atrial ventricular canal; 40 to 50 percent have improper development of separate atria and ventricles on left and right, which can cause congestive heart failure (CHF)

   b. Leukemia, 30 times higher incidence

   c. Hypothyroidism, 20 times higher incidence

   d. Hirschsprung's disease, higher incidence

B. Pathophysiology

1. Malformation involves 21st **chromosome** (23 pairs of protein structures consisting of DNA that map out the functions of cells within the body)

   a. Trisomy

   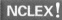

   1) Nondisjunction: causes 92 to 95 percent of Down syndrome; zygote contains 3 chromosomes instead of normal pair at chromosome #21; increased incidence with paternal/maternal age

   2) **Mosaicism** (presence of cells from two different genetic materials in the same individual)—causes 1 to 3 percent of Down syndrome; trisomy occurs during **mitosis** (stages of separation to create a new daughter cell); leads to some normal and abnormal cell lines; milder form of the syndrome

   b. **Translocation** (a transfer of part or the entire chromosome to another chromosome leading to a severe or fatal defect)

   1) Causes 3–5% of Down syndrome

   2) Zygote has exchanged materials from break in chromosome #21

   3) No increased risk with age, but does have a 5 to 15 percent risk of reoccurrence

2. Signs and symptoms

   a. Physical characteristics

   1) Hypotonia: lack of general muscle tone

   2) Hyperflexibility: able to flex joints beyond 180 degrees

   3) Wide space between first and second toe

   4) Transverse palmar crease: (horizontal crease across palm) or plantarcreane in foot is present in all clients with Down syndrome (see Figure 16-1)

   5) Low-set ears: normal is along an imaginary line from eye to top of ear

   6) Epicanthal folds: folds of skin along external to internal edge of eye

   7) Depressed nasal bridge

   8) High, arched, narrow palate and protruding tongue

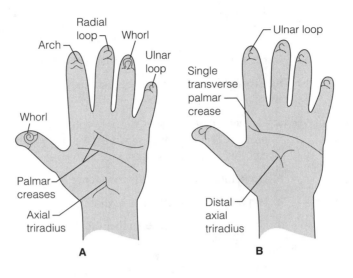

Figure 7-1

Characteristic palm markings. A. Normal individual. B. Individual with Down syndrome.

b. Intellectual characteristics

1) Moderate to severe mental retardation

2) Emphasis is on concrete and individualized operations

c. Sensory deficits

1) Myopia

2) Hyperopia

3) Strabismus

C. Nursing assessment

1. Assessment

a. Early detection (look for physical attributes in newborn nursery)

b. Family assessment

1) Use tool to measure family strengths Apgar, family profile

2) Assess grieving process: denial, nonacceptance of diagnosis; depression; unable to care for self or others; withdrawal, not speaking with family; anger; being unreasonable with nursing staff

c. Physical characteristics: muscle strength and flexibility, appearance and distinguishing features, growth and development, sensory status, respiratory and cardiac status for possible complications

2. Diagnostic tests include genetic screen to detect cause of abnormal chromosome 21

a. Prenatal: amniocentesis to identify #21, chronic villi sampling

b. Postnatal: chromosome #21, detection of trisomy

D. Nursing management

1. Development

a. Goal: promote optimal development; the infant may develop at a slower rate with smaller steps; involve family in setting goals for child

NCLEX!

    b. Interventions should be planned according to developmental level

        1) Infant

            a) Cognition: Piaget's sensorimotor: Denver Developmental Screening Test (DDST) or comparable developmental screening tool to determine baseline level; monitor progression; enroll in infant stimulation program

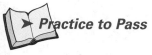

            b) Social: Erickson's trust vs. mistrust: assessment of family, cultural, and feeding interaction to reinforce a positive family bond; refer to social services if suspect abuse/neglect

        2) Toddler

            a) Cognition: Piaget's sensorimotor, continue to promote sensory stimulation; reinforce realistic expectations/goals

NCLEX!

            b) Social: Erickson's autonomy vs. shame and doubt, unsuccessful toilet training can lead to child abuse; anticipatory guidance in relation to temper tantrums

        3) Preschool

            a) Cognition: Piaget's preoperational support; involvement in the child's early education program

            b) Social: Erickson's initiative vs. self-doubt, allow for successes within an integrated school program

        4) School-age

            a) Cognition: will usually remain in Piaget's concrete formations; give simple, visual cues for any teaching during hospitalizations

Practice to Pass

Why is it important to understand child development in the client with Down syndrome?

            b) Social: Erickson's industry vs. inferiority; inclusion programs are beneficial for schools and the child; after school activities

        5) Adolescence: social, Erickson's identity vs. role confusion; must involve in teen activities; information on reproduction and puberty at their level

        6) Adult: job placement; level of living independence; parent or guardianship and living will issues need to be resolved

NCLEX!

2. Monitor for respiratory infections (especially in the infant); because of large protruding tongue and hypotonia, child has an increased incidence of respiratory complications/compromise

    a. Vital signs: increased respiratory rate, fever

    b. Congestion

    c. Inability to tolerate feedings

    d. Prevent infection

NCLEX!

        1) Liquify secretions with humidifier

        2) Use saline and bulb syringe to suction secretions

3. Cardiac defects: monitor for congestive heart failure

    a. Monitor for urine output, minimum 1 to 2 cc/kg/hr

    b. Monitor for edema

Practice to Pass

Why is it important to determine the cause of trisomy 21?

    c. Activity and feeding tolerance

    d. Note change in color, cyanosis

  4. Post-operative care for the child with heart defect correction

  5. Priority nursing diagnoses: Altered development, Altered parenting, Potential for ineffective airway clearance, Altered tissue perfusion, and Decreased cardiac output

III. Turner's Syndrome

A. Overview

  1. Defined as a deletion or abnormal X on chromosome 45; there are a total of 45 chromosomes with 22 somatic pairs and only 1 sex chromosome (45, XO)

  2. Syndrome predisposition for:

    a. Hypothyroidism

    b. Aortic coarctation

    c. Renal structure anomalies

    d. Behavior and learning disturbances

B. Pathophysiology

  1. Female phenotype with incidence 1:2,500 female births

  2. Not clear but thought to be nondisjunction or fragmented X

  3. The only monosomy that is viable; 99 percent are nevertheless spontaneously aborted

  4. Signs and symptoms

    a. Newborn

      1) Low posterior hairline

      2) Lymphedema of feet and legs

      3) Webbed neck

    b. Child: short stature; growth slows after age 3; below 3 percent on growth chart

      1) No development of secondary sex characteristics during puberty

      2) Lack of or nonfunctioning ovaries

      3) Wide-spaced nipples

      4) Short 4th metacarpals

      5) "Shield-like" chest with underdeveloped breasts

      6) Normal intellectual development

      7) Frequent urinary tract infections (UTI's)

C. Nursing assessment

  1. Assessment includes any signs symptoms of renal, cardiac, or thyroid dysfunction

a. Renal: note any urinary tract infections

    b. Cardiac: aortic coarctation, decrease in lower extremity blood pressure

    c. Hypothyroidism: intolerance to cold, weight gain, lethargy, hair loss, enlarged thyroid gland

  2. Early recognition: note physical characteristics in newborn nursery

  3. Assessment of family and cultural characteristics, noting strengths of family

  4. Additional assessment: growth charts (height and weight), observance of sex characteristics, physical characteristics

  5. Diagnostic tests

    a. Labs: blood urea nitrogen (BUN), creatinine (CR) for kidney function

    b. Radiology: voiding cystourethrography (VCUP), cystoscopy

    c. Prenatal genetic testing before birth

    d. Genetic **karyotype** (pictorial analysis of the chromosomes of an individual after birth

D. Nursing management

  1. Medications include (as appropriate)

    a. Estrogen prior to age 12 years

    b. Progesterone for secondary sexual characteristics

  2. Monitor nonverbal and verbal suggestion of hopelessness

  3. Encourage teen support group

  4. Encourage verbalization

  5. Early detection: note characteristics at birth in order to initiate genetic counseling for family

  6. Genetic counseling

    a. Educate on defect, sex-linked chromosome disorder

    b. Family planning; determine if possible the type of malformation

  7. Nursing priority diagnoses: Body image disturbance; Altered sexuality patterns; Altered family processes; Risk for fluid volume imbalance

IV. Klinefelter's Syndrome

A. Overview

  1. Defined as a polysomic **X-linked** (an inherited gene disorder located on X-chromosome) chromosome defect with one or more extra X-chromosomes in the **genotype** of the entire genetic make-up of individual male

  2. Associated with increased parental age; maternal/paternal

  3. Incidence: 1:850 male births

> **▶ Practice to Pass**
>
> How is it possible for the client with Turner's syndrome to not be diagnosed until adolescence?

B. Pathophysiology

1. During meiosis, nondisjunction of the X- and Y-chromosome causes the disorder

2. With an increase in Xs, there is an increase in mental retardation

3. Usually occurs as presence of extra chromosome #47; additional X and possibly Y chromosomes 47-XXY 48-XXYY, etc.

4. Signs and symptoms

   a. Tall, lean body with disproportionately long legs to trunk

   b. Small or undescended testicles

   c. Gynecomastia

   d. Sterility

   e. Sparse facial hair

   f. Voice does not change at puberty

   g. Normal intellectual development, may have delay in language

   h. Abnormalities

      1) Scoliosis

      2) Dental abnormalities

      3) Cardiac abnormalities

      4) Pulmonary disease

C. Nursing assessment

1. Assessment includes sexual characteristics, growth chart (height and weight), reproductive history

2. Early recognition of physical characteristics that may be delayed until puberty

3. Family and cultural assessment

D. Nursing management

1. Medication including testosterone

2. Support child and family through diagnosis

   a. Verbalize positive attributes

   b. Demonstrate parenting

   c. Provide anticipatory developmental and safety guidance

   d. Support constructive discipline

3. Early child development program

   a. Use face position and eye contact

   b. Stimulate cognitive development

   c. Monitor for achievement of physical, cognitive, and psychosocial milestones

4. Genetic counseling

   a. Family planning

   b. Family support/referral

5. Encourage teen support

   a. Identify effective ways to express anger/frustration

   b. Identify community resources

   c. Education on sterility

   d. Encourage peer support

6. High priority nursing diagnoses: Body image disturbance, Altered family processes, Risk for altered development

V. Phenylketonuria (PKU)

A. Overview

1. Defined as a metabolic disorder defective in the enzyme phenylalanine hydroxylase that metabolizes phenylalanine, leading to accumulation of phenylalanine and other metabolites

2. Autosomal recessive disorder with **homozygous** presentation (malformation created with autosomal recessive presentation; both chromosomes must be present) (see Table 16-1)

3. If untreated, will lead to severe mental retardation, seizures, and death

4. Incidence 1:15,000, carrier state can be detected; more common in Caucasians

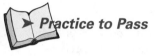

Practice to Pass

Explain nondisjunction as the cause of Klinefelter's syndrome.

Table 16-1
Phenylketonuria: Autosomal Recessive Gene Pattern (Both Chromosomes Present)

A.   Carrier father

		D	d
Carrier mother	D	DD	Dd
	d	dD	dd

B.   Carrier father

		D	d
Disease mother	D	DD	Dd
	D	DD	Dd

C.   Normal father

		d	d
Disease mother	D	Dd	Dd
	D	Dd	Dd

D.   Normal father

		d	d
Carrier mother	D	Dd	Dd
	d	dd	dd

DD = Disease   D = disease gene
dD, Dd = Carrier   d = normal gene
dd = No risk

B. Pathophysiology

1. Enzyme phenyl hydroxylase is absent, which converts phenylalanine to tyrosine

2. Tyrosine is needed by the body for melanin pigment and for the hormones epinephrine and thyroxin

3. Phenylalanine is responsible for growth; the accumulation of serum phenylalanine leads to irreversible central nervous system damage and mental retardation

4. Increased metabolites in the blood (phenylpyruvic acid and phenylacetic acid) are excreted in urine, causing a musty odor and phenylketonuria (PKU)

5. Signs and symptoms

   a. Musky odor to urine

   b. Neuromuscular development delay

   c. Failure to thrive

   d. Mental retardation by age 6 months

   e. Acute episodes

      1) Possible seizures

      2) Vomiting

      3) Eczematous rashes

C. Nursing assessment

1. Assessment includes growth and development, urine, nutritional status, skin, signs of dehydration

2. Diagnostic tests (done after 24 hours of protein-containing fluids)

   NCLEX!

   a. Newborn screen: blood specimen taken within 7 days of birth; phenylalanine levels over 10 to 15 mg/dL leads to brain damage

   b. Electroencephalography (EEG)

D. Nursing management

1. Diet maintained from infancy to adolescence

   a. Breast-feeding possible if phenylalanine levels are monitored

   NCLEX!

   b. Phenylalanine level must be maintained between 2 to 8 mg/dL

   c. Dietary products: Pro-Phree or Phenex-1 are examples of low phenylalanine products

   d. Avoid meats, which are highest in phenylalanine

   e. Older child can exchange some vegetables, but should maintain minimal meat consumption

2. Monitor growth and development

   a. Must maintain adequate nutrition with an extremely limited diet

   b. Educate family on importance of maintaining routine primary healthcare visits for screening and growth assessment

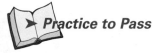

Practice to Pass

A client and her husband are carriers of the phenylketonuria (PKU) allele. She asks the nurse what the risk is that their children will present with the disease. How should the nurse respond?

3. Monitor phenylalanine levels

   a. Phenylalanine at dangerous levels if greater than 15mg/dL

   b. Increased stress, illness, growth spurts will trigger increased phenylalanine levels

   c. Most common sign/symptom is vomiting leading to dehydration

   d. Maintain seizure precautions

4. Plan for genetic counseling with the family

   a. Genetic screening to assess offspring **carrier** (one affected and one unaffected autosome)

   b. Future pregnancy planning (see Table 16-1 again)

5. Female with PKU at puberty

   a. Counseling on secondary sexual developmental

   b. Counseling on family planning if mother has the disorder

      1) If partner is carrier, 2:4 chance of reoccurrence if partner is not a carrier, all offspring will be carriers (see Table 16-1 again)

      2) Instruct on strict control of diet if planning pregnancy

      3) Treated as an inpatient for strict control of diet if client becomes pregnant

6. Priority nursing diagnoses: Risk for injury related to seizure activity and increased phenylalanine levels; Knowledge deficit related to diet therapy; Risk for altered development related to CNS damage

VI. Huntington's Disease

A. Overview

1. Defined as a rare, inherited disease caused by degeneration in the cerebral cortex and the basal ganglia; defect on chromosome #4

2. An autosomal dominant disease with **heterozygous** (only one abnormal autosomal has to be present) presentation (see Table 16-2)

3. Usually evident between 25 and 55 years of age

4. 5/100,000 occurrence, occurs in all ethnic groups, life expectancy about 10 years

5. Also called Huntington's chorea

B. Pathophysiology

1. Degeneration in the cerebral cortex and basal ganglia causes a deficient inhibitory neurotransmitter system and neurotransmitters are lost; especially gamma-aminobutyric acid (GABA)

2. GABA is an inhibitory transmitter of the central nervous system (CNS) that inhibits specific target pathways to slow increased activity in these pathways

   a. A deficiency of GABA causes increased neural excitation

   b. Associated with epilepsy, anxiety disorders, depression

Table 16-2		

Huntington's Disease: Autosomal Dominant Gene Pattern (Only One Chromosome Present)

A.   Normal father

		d	d
Disease	D	Dd	Dd
mother	d	dd	dd

B.   Disease father

		D	d
Disease	D	DD	Dd
mother	d	dD	dd

DD, Dd, dD = Disease   D = disease gene
dd = No risk   d = normal gene

    c. Receptors are concentrated in two areas

        1) Limbic system, controlling emotional behaviors

        2) Locus cerulues, controlling arousal

3. An imbalance in basal ganglia occurs between dopamine and acetylcholine, and GABA

    a. Acetylcholine is decreased

    b. Dopamine not affected (unlike Parkinson's disease)

NCLEX!

    c. **Choreiform** (rapid and jerky body motion that is involuntary) movements result from deficient neurotransmitter inhibition

4. Degeneration in cerebral cortex leads to progressive increase in labile emotions caused by decrease in GABA

    a. Violent behavior changes

    b. Dementia

5. Alleles inherited from the father results in onset later in life than if inherited from the mother

6. Other physiologic changes

    a. Lesions may occur in the putamen, corpus striatum, and thalamus

    b. Frontal lobes of brain atrophy, enlarge, and change the lateral ventricle structure

NCLEX!

    c. Neurons in certain areas of the brain are reduced

7. Symptoms begin between the age of 25 to 55 years

8. Signs and symptoms

    a. Movement

        1) Choreiform movements

        2) Athetosis: slower movements than choreiform

    b. Intellect: progressive degeneration, impaired memory and judgment

    c. Severe dementia

        1) Impulsiveness

        2) Paranoia

        3) Neurosis

        4) Outbursts verbally and emotionally

        5) Irritability

        6) Delusions and hallucinations

        7) Suicidal tendency

        8) Personality changes

C. Nursing assessment

    1. Assessment includes memory, ability to follow commands, assessment of ability to perform activities of daily living (ADLs) and degree of movement problems, mental status, history of recent changes in personality and level of consciousness, ability to stay on-task

    2. Diagnostic tests

        a. Diagnosis made by clinical manifestations and family history

        b. No prognostic lab studies to treat or predict the disease

        c. Positive gene marker on DNA testing for conclusive diagnosis

        d. Magnetic resonance imagery (MRI) to assess brain involvement

D. Nursing management

    1. Medications

        a. Haloperidol (Haldol)

            1) Block dopamine and restore neurotransmitter balance

            2) Treat dyskinesia and modify behavior

            3) Major side effects: extrapyramidal reaction, sedation

        b. Reserpine (Serpalan)

            1) Treat behavior problems and decrease dyskinesia

            2) Major side effects: respiratory depression, bronchospasms, bradycardia, thrombocytopenia

    2. Genetic counseling

        a. Autosomal dominance needs only one affected autosome

            1) 2:4 reoccurrence if one parent has Huntington's (see Table 16-2)

            2) 3:4 reoccurrence if both parents have Huntington's (see Table 16-2)

        b. Ethical considerations in testing gene presence

            1) The variance in age of presentation

            2) Currently no cure

            3) Family planning issues

3. Nutrition

   a. Establish baseline and monitor for weight loss; increase calories and protein to support increased activity level

   b. Maintain good oral hygiene

   c. Altered swallowing could lead to aspiration

      1) Maintain in upright position during eating

      2) Give small amounts

      3) Give thickened liquids

4. Long-term care

   a. Monitor family for issues related to behavior control

   b. Suicide precautions may be necessary

   c. Drug and alcohol abuse common and should be monitored

   d. Institutionalization when home care no longer possible

5. Controversial therapies: fetal brain tissue transplants have been moderately successful, but ethical issues exists related to source of transplant

6. Future therapies

   a. Gene replacement therapy: replaces the abnormal gene on chromosome #4

   b. No medication available to cure the disease

7. Priority nursing diagnoses: Knowledge deficit, Altered nutrition: less than body requirements, Risk for aspiration, Ineffective family coping

VII. **Marfan's Syndrome**

   A. **Overview**

   1. Defined as a connective tissue disorder caused by atrophy of neurons in specific areas of brain; involves chromosome #15

   2. An autosomal dominant disorder with heterozygous presentation; no carrier status

   3. A **congenital** (present since birth) disorder with 25 percent spontaneous mutations

   4. Incidence 1:10,000

   B. **Pathophysiology**

   1. A mutation of frillin-1, a connective tissue protein that is found in body tissue, occurs

   2. Defect is in the elastic fibers of connective tissues causing long, thin extremities; hyperextendable joints; and spinal deformities

   3. Associated defects

      a. Aortic aneurysm: most common cause of early death; weakness within the aorta leads to dilatation and rupture

      b. Optic lens disorders: dislocated optic lens, retinal detachment, cataracts, glaucoma, and myopia

Practice to Pass

What are the ethical implications of early diagnosis by identifying gene marker #4 in offspring of the client with Huntington's chorea?

NCLEX!

4. Signs and symptoms

   a. Tall, lean body with thin fingers (arachnodactyly) and winged scapula

   b. Vision disturbances

   c. Musculoskeletal deformities: pectus excavatum, curvature of thoracic spine, hyperextensibility of joints, scoliosis

5. Often associated with sports-related cardiac arrest

C. Nursing assessment

1. Assessment includes growth and development, proportioned body, visual examination, range of motion, scoliosis screening, auscultation of abdomen for pulse, blood pressure, cardiac status

2. Diagnostic tests: genetic screening, MRI if aneurysm suspected

D. Nursing management

1. Medications include beta blockers for cardiac problems

2. Community and school education

   a. Support automated external defibrillator (AED) implementation

   b. Health physical prior to participation in athletic events

   c. Scoliosis screening

3. Sensory

   a. Note any change in vision

   b. Encourage yearly eye exams

4. Cardiac

   a. Monitor cardiac status: auscultation of abdomen, pulse, vital signs

   b. Aortic valve replacement may be indicated

   c. Maintain blood pressure within normal limits

5. Genetic counseling

   a. Discuss family planning and risk of reoccurrence

   b. Parent and child education on risks for associated anomalies

6. Priority nursing diagnoses: Potential for decreased cardiac output; Sensory/perceptual alterations: visual; Body image disturbance; and Knowledge deficit related to dysrhythmias

VIII. Albinism

A. Overview

1. Defined as a lack of skin pigmentation caused by the absence of tyrosinase, which is needed for melanin synthesis

2. An autosomal recessive chromosomal disorder with homozygous presentation

3. Incidence is 1:17,000 individuals

4. Two types

    a. Type I: oculocutaneous

    b. Type II: less pigmented

B. Pathophysiology

1. Autosomal recessive disorder; both parents are carriers

    a. 25 percent chance of mutation

    b. 25 percent chance not carrying gene

    c. 50 percent chance of having carrier status

    d. Risk is unchanged with each subsequent pregnancy

2. Individuals are deficient in tyrinase, an enzyme needed to synthesize melanin, but have a normal number of melanocytes

3. Type I: *oculocutaneous*

    a. Defect in tyrosinase

        1) Unable to convert tyrosine to dopa

        2) Results in lack of melanin synthesis

    b. Associated visual problems

        1) Foveal hypoplasia can occur; abnormal retinal development because of lack of pigment

        2) Transillumination: the iris lacks sufficient pigment to screen light coming into eye

        3) Associated vision disturbances: nystagmus, strabismus, myopia, hyperopia, photophobia

4. Type II: *less pigmented*

    a. May have slight pigmentation

    b. No ocular or integument variations

5. Syndromes associated with albinism; Hermansky-Pudlak syndrome (HPS)

    a. Syndrome of albinism including bleeding tendencies

    b. Can include lung (pulmonary fibrosis) and bowel (inflammatory bowel disease)

    c. Bleeding problems result from malfunction of platelets and include nosebleeds, bruising or severe bleed during surgery or childbirth

    d. Client will have normal results in prothrombin time (PT), partial thromboplastin time (PTT); may lack Von Willebrand factor (less than 70 percent occurence, higher risk of bleed)

6. Signs and symptoms

    a. Lack of pigment in skin, hair, eyes

        1) Skin (pale or pink)

        2) Hair (white or yellow)

        3) Eyes (light-colored or pink)

 b. Vision assessment

   1) Low vision 20/50

   2) Legally blind 20/200

   3) VEP: visually evoked potential for young infant

C. Nursing assessment

 1. Nursing assessment includes visual exam and inspection of color in the skin, hair, eyes, ability to read because of nystagmus; any extraocular eye movement

 2. Diagnostic test: none

D. Nursing management

 1. Symptomatic care

   a. Screen vision

   b. Avoid sun exposure; use maximum sunscreen

   c. Wear sunglasses

   d. Frequent checks for potential melanoma

   e. Corrective visual wear/aids

 2. Genetic counseling

   a. Teach parent/child potential for future children with albinism

   b. Genetic screening of family

 3. Cultural competency

   a. Dispel myths related to mixed ethnicity or inbreeding as the cause

   b. Educate about genetics as the cause

 4. Priority nursing diagnoses: Knowledge deficit; Risk for impaired skin integrity; Risk for sensory/perceptual alterations

IX. Cystic Fibrosis (CF)

A. Overview

 1. Defined as an autorecessive chromosome disorder with exocrine gland dysfunction, which manifests in multiple body systems

 2. Multisystem involvement: respiratory, pancreatic, liver, gastrointestinal (GI)

   a. Severity of symptoms varies on an individualized basis

   b. Goal is to increase longevity

 3. Incidence is 1:2,000; affects mostly Caucasians

B. Pathophysiology

 1. Homozygous presentation: chromosome #9 defect with multiple variations, but most common is alteration in the ^F508 gene; different gene abnormalities result in variations in the disease symptoms

2. Primary feature is lack of function of chloride channels: failure to open or absence of channels

3. Defective protein inhibits transport of sodium/chloride, leading to an increased viscosity of secretions and an increase of sodium chloride (NaCl) in sweat

4. System pathophysiology

   a. Respiratory tract

      1) Decreased ciliary function and increased thickness of mucous secretions occurs

      2) Decreased function of alveoli and alveolar plugs leads to repeat infections and chronic obstructive pulmonary disease (COPD)

         a) COPD leads to cor pulmonale (right-sided CHF caused by respiratory problems) and chronic hypoxemia

         b) *Pseudomonas aeruginosa* and *Staphylococcus aeureus* are common organisms that resist antibiotics, leading to drug-resistant pneumonia

      3) Sinus tract disease with polyps and chronic thick mucus

   b. Gastrointestinal

      1) Thick secretions block the ducts leading from pancreas to duodenum

      2) Malabsorption occurs because digestive enzymes don't reach food

         a) Predominantly fats and fat-soluble vitamins A, D, K, E

         b) Leads to malnutrition if untreated

   c. Pancreas: damage to Islets of Langerhans causes an increased incidence of insulin-dependent diabetes mellitus (IDDM)

   d. Liver: biliary obstruction leads to cirrhosis and gallbladder disease

5. Signs and symptoms

   a. Respiratory

      1) Frequent pneumonias (methcicillin resistant staphylcoccus aureus [MRSA] leads to high mortality)

      2) Productive cough with thick, foul-smelling secretions

      3) Clubbing of nails from chronic hypoxemia

      4) Persistent sinusitis for the adolescent

      5) COPD leads to chronic high CO_2 level

   b. Nutrition

      1) Large protruding abdomen

      2) Infant: failure to thrive

      3) Older child: osteomalacia (rickets), abnormal clotting times, and malnourishment

NCLEX!

c. Newborn: ileus related to thick mucus from meconium

d. Infant

   1) Rectal prolapse because of thick stools

   2) **Steatorrhea** (foul-smelling stool containing undigested fat)

e. Older child

   1) Diabetes-related disorders if diabetic ketoacidosis unchecked

   2) Delayed secondary sexual characteristics

f. Young adult

   1) Female: thick cervical secretions lead to decreased fertility

   2) Males: sterile or minimal sperm production related to blocked seminal ducts

C. Nursing assessment

  1. Nursing assessment includes: respiratory status, vital signs, auscultation of lung sounds, abdominal size, stool characteristics, sexual characteristics, reproductive history, analysis of sputum, daily weight, growth chart

  2. Diagnostic tests

    a. Classic NaCl sweat test (2 to 5 times greater than normal)

    b. Newborn screen: decreased trypsin (enzyme produced by pancreas) level in stool indicates CF, normal is positive in small amounts (required in most states)

    c. Prenatal and carrier status screening: available for ^F508 (70 percent of CF)

    d. Arterial blood gases (ABGs) or pulse oxymetry

    e. Chest x-ray (CXR)

    f. Pulmonary function studies (PFS)

D. Nursing management

  1. Medications

    a. Bronchodilators: albuterol (Ventolin)

    b. Antibiotic aerosol: tobramycin (Tobrex)

    c. Corticosteroids: beclomethasone (Vanceril)

    d. Dornase alfa (Pulmazyme) to alter mucous viscosity (aerosol)

    e. Antibiotics for respiratory infection

    f. Annual immunizations

    g. Pancrelipase (Pancrease) by mouth

  2. Nursing interventions

    a. Respiratory

      1) Administer oxygen as needed: use caution with O_2 administration; chronically high CO_2 can alter respiratory drive

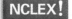

2) Assess for respiratory status

3) Educate on the proper administration of inhalers and oxygen: separate corticosteroids by 20 to 30 minutes from other inhalers; administer the corticosteroids last

NCLEX!

4) Monitor for side effects of medications, particularly tachycardia

5) Increase fluids to liquefy secretions

6) Chest physiotherapy: postural drainage and percussion/vibration to loosen and clear secretions; flutter device and huffing procedure used to assist in increasing expectoration; perform after bronchodilation

NCLEX!

7) Treat pulmonary infections; there is increased risk for antibiotic-resistant microorganisms; it is important to monitor therapeutic response

b. Pancreas

NCLEX!

1) Pancreatic enzyme replacements such as pancrelipase (Pancrease) must be given before each meal or snack

2) Note stool characteristics (steatorrhea) to determine absorption

3) Assess growth while hospitalized; monitor daily weights at same time and using same scale

3. Chronic degenerative disease

a. Lung/heart transplant current trend to treat irreversible lung/heart disease

b. Developmental issues

1) Support adolescents who struggle with sexuality and chronic illness

2) Monitor parental characteristics of overprotection

3) Discuss end-of-life issues as they arise

4. Genetic counseling

a. Provide anticipatory guidance for the parents of the child with CF for future pregnancies

b. Encourage genetic counseling for the client with CF

c. Update client on therapies for gene replacement as they become available

5. Priority nursing diagnoses: Failure to thrive r/t malabsorption; Altered growth and development r/t chronic illness; Impaired gas exchange r/t increased mucous secretions; Risk for infection r/t decreased alveolar function; Altered family processes r/t chronic disease; Knowledge deficit r/t care of child with CF

X. Cleft Lip/Palate

A. Overview

1. Cleft lip is defined as a vertical opening (cleft) in the upper lip

2. Cleft palate is defined as a fissure in the roof of the mouth creating a passageway between the mouth and nose

3. Is the most common craniofacial malformation

4. Cleft lip and palate can be:

   a. Together or separate

   b. Unilateral or bilateral

   c. Complete or incomplete

5. The cause is multifactorial and is associated with various syndromes (i.e., Pierre Robbin's)

B. Pathophysiology

1. Interruption in development, leading to lack of fusion or rupture of palate or lip

   a. 6 to 8 weeks gestation for cleft lip (CL)

   b. 8 to 12 weeks gestation for cleft palate (CP)

2. Cleft lip may involve external nares, nasal cartilage, nasal septum, and alveolar process

3. Cleft palate may involve uvula and soft palate

4. Signs and symptoms include visual defect, crusting on cleft, swallowing air, vomiting, difficulty sucking, expulsion of formula through nose (cleft palate), aspiration, difficulty with speech, otitis media

C. Nursing assessment

1. Cleft lip apparent at birth: unilateral, bilateral, or complete

2. Cleft palate needs more thorough assessment in newborn

   a. Biuvula or split uvula is indicative of a cleft

   b. Note any feeding difficulties

3. Overall assessment: nutritional status, abdominal distention, lung sounds (aspiration), signs of infection at site, weight, speech and dental (when older), hearing

D. Nursing management

1. Cleft lip: surgical repair recommended and can occur as a young infant (approximately 2 months)

2. Cleft palate

   a. Team approach with stages of repair occurring as young infant through adolescence

   b. Coordination of team

      1) Orthodontist: oral-pharyngeal development and dentition

      2) Speech: develop sucking and treat altered speech

      3) Otolaryngologist: assesses and treats chronic otitis related to abnormal connection between Eustachian tube and posterior oropharynx

      4) Audio: chronic otitis leads to hearing loss

      5) Plastic surgeon: repairs craniofacial anomalies

      6) Social worker: monitors financial and emotional needs

3. Preoperative nursing interventions

   a. Nutrition

   1) Assess adequate intake

   2) Encourage parent with modified nipple or supplemental tube feeding

   3) Assess if child can adequately suck

   4) Monitor to prevent aspiration of formula or breast milk

   b. Oropharyngeal (CP)

   1) Understand and educate family on orthodontic hardware for the infant/child

   2) Monitor effectiveness of speech therapy for coordinating speech/adequate sucking

   c. Hearing

   1) Frequent monitoring for hearing loss

   2) Listen to family for reports of delayed or altered speech

4. Postoperative nursing interventions

   a. Prevent damage to surgical site

   1) Child with repair of cleft lip is not to be placed prone

   2) Keep objects away from mouth

   3) Elbow restraints: monitor for skin breakdown to area restrained

   4) Educate family to keep child's hands away from face if restraints off

   5) Cleanse area with prescribed solution, usually peroxide (H_2O_2) and sterile water (H_2O)

   6) Lubricate lip with antibiotic ointment

   7) Devices such as Logan bar or bow to relieve tension on incision site

   b. Monitor for adequate fluid/nutrition intake, weigh daily

   c. Monitor for incisional pain

5. Growth and development

   a. Monitor family for positive bonding with infant

   1) Important to bring child with cleft to parent soon after delivery

   2) Connect families early with support group and repair team

   b. Monitor child for positive self-image

   c. Genetic counseling for familial tendencies

6. Priority nursing diagnoses: Altered nutrition r/t poor sucking ability; Altered parenting r/t child with a disability, Pain r/t surgical correction; Risk for aspiration r/t open communication within oropharyngeal cavity; Risk for infection

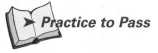

Practice to Pass

Why is it important to assess for a biuvula in the newborn?

Case Study

J. P. is a 6-month-old client admitted to the unit with the diagnosis of recurrent pneumonia. On admission, the nurse notes that the client has a respiratory rate of 50, heart rate of 170, and a temperature of 102°F. The client is retracting substernally with bilateral wheezes and rhonchi. The mother states that this is her son's third admission since birth for pneumonia. She also mentions that he hasn't been gaining weight like her older child had at 6 months of age.

❶ How is this consistent with cystic fibrosis?

❷ What tests could be ordered to confirm the diagnosis?

❸ What nursing interventions could alleviate the respiratory distress?

❹ What is the rationale behind the poor weight gain?

❺ What teaching needs to be done with the family about the respiratory component of cystic fibrosis before the child goes home? What genetic counseling should occur for the family?

For suggested responses, see pages 570–571.

Posttest

1 A client comes into the clinic for a physical examination, a required prerequisite for him to participate with his high school basketball team. He is a tall, lean male with long, slender fingers. His mother mentions that he will have his first game next week, and she is concerned about his health. The parent has heard about high school athletes dying on the basketball court during games. What congenital anomaly could the parent be referring to and what is the associated life-threatening defect?

(1) Down syndrome and atrial-ventricular (AV) canal
(2) Marfan's syndrome and aortic dilatation
(3) Phenylketonuria (PKU) and seizures
(4) Turner's syndrome and hypothyroidism

2 The parent of a client with albinism would need to be taught which preventive healthcare measure by the nurse?

(1) Ulcerative colitis diet
(2) Use of a high-SPF sunblock
(3) Hair loss monitoring
(4) Monitor for growth retardation

3 The nurse involved in genetic counseling for the family of a mother with Huntington's is asked if they have a chance of developing the same disorder. What is the best response?

(1) If the mother alone has the disease, they have a 2:4 chance of inheriting the same disorder.
(2) Both parents must have the disease for the offspring to inherit the same disorder.
(3) The disorder is a spontaneous disruption of the neurotransmitters with no inheritance principles
(4) If the mother has the disease, they have a 1:4 chance of inheriting the same disorder.

4 The symptoms in a client with cystic fibrosis have progressed rapidly over the past 2 years. Presently, the client is in the Emergency Department with significant respiratory distress. What physical characteristics should the nurse expect to see in the client?

(1) Low-set ears
(2) Gray appearance
(3) Clubbed fingernails
(4) Jaundice

5 The foul-smelling, frothy characteristic of the stool in cystic fibrosis results from the presence of large amounts of which of the following?

(1) Sodium and chloride
(2) Undigested fat
(3) Semidigested carbohydrates
(4) Lipase, trypsin, and amylase

6 The nurse has considered oxygen administration because of a client's obvious respiratory distress and circumoral cyanosis. What factor should the nurse consider when administering oxygen in a client with cystic fibrosis?

(1) Children with cystic fibrosis respond poorly to oxygen administration.
(2) Administration of oxygen can decrease the respiratory drive.
(3) Oxygen would antagonize the cosmic field.
(4) Oxygen should only be administered via facemask.

7 Mr. and Mrs. W. are the parents of a baby with Down syndrome. Through genetic counseling, the baby has been identified as having a chromosome 21 translocation. Which of the following represents the risk that this couple will conceive another child with trisomy 21?

(1) 5 to 15 percent
(2) 10 percent
(3) 25 percent
(4) No increased risk

8 Nursing care of the client with Klinefelter's syndrome focuses mainly on which of the following areas?

(1) Fluid and electrolyte balance.
(2) Body image.
(3) Preventing complications.
(4) Development of fine motor skills.

9 A gene that produces the same characteristics when it is either presented as a homozygous or heterozygous chromosome is called which of the following?

(1) Autosomal dominant.
(2) Autosomal recessive.
(3) Familial.
(4) Multifactorial.

10 Why is it important to keep the post-operative client in elbow restraints following a cleft-lip repair?

(1) The client could pull out the nasogastric tube.
(2) The client might dislodge the intravenous catheter.
(3) The client may experience aspiration of formula.
(4) The client may disrupt the lip suture line.

See pages 515–516 for Answers and Rationales.

Answers and Rationales

Pretest

1 Answer: 2 *Rationale:* An individual with Huntington's develops chorea (rapid, jerky movements) and might have difficulty swallowing liquids, which could lead to the potential of aspiration of nonthickened liquids.
Cognitive Level: Application
Nursing Process: Implementation; *Test Plan:* PHYS

2 Answer: 4 *Rationale:* The child with Down syndrome will go through the same first stage, trust vs. mistrust, only at a slower rate. Therefore, the nurse should concentrate on developing a bond between the primary caregiver and the child.
Cognitive Level: Application
Nursing Process: Assessment; *Test Plan:* HPM

3 **Answer: 1** *Rationale:* The connective tissue disorder of Marfan's syndrome can include aortic insufficiency, which can lead to aortic rupture or dissection, which is the primary cause of death for the disorder.
Cognitive Level: Application
Nursing Process: Analysis; *Test Plan:* PHYS

4 **Answer: 2** *Rationale:* Albinism type I is an autosomal recessive disorder. Both parents must be carriers for the child to inherit the congenital disorder.
Cognitive Level: Application
Nursing Process: Analysis; *Test Plan:* PHYS

5 **Answer: 1** *Rationale:* The infant with cleft lip is unable to create an adequate seal for sucking. The child is at risk for inadequate nutritional intake as well as aspiration.
Cognitive Level: Application
Nursing Process: Implementation; *Test Plan:* PHYS

6 **Answer: 4** *Rationale:* Pancrease or pancreatic enzyme increases absorption of fats and proteins via the pancreatic duct. It should be given before food enters the duodenum.
Cognitive Level: Application
Nursing Process: Implementation; *Test Plan:* PHYS

7 **Answer: 1** *Rationale:* These are the three key assessment features in Turner's syndrome. If the child is diagnosed early in age, proper treatment can be offered to the family. All newborns should be screened for possible congenital defects.
Cognitive Level: Application
Nursing Process: Assessment; *Test Plan:* PHYS

8 **Answer: 3** *Rationale:* The child with cleft lip has communication between the oropharynx and the Eustachian tube. The child is at high risk for recurrent ear infections. The symptoms described are common with otitis media.
Cognitive Level: Analysis
Nursing Process: Assessment; *Test Plan:* PHYS

9 **Answer: 2** *Rationale:* The child with Klinefelter's has an extra "X" and possible replication of "Y." The karyotype shows the pictorial analysis of the chromosomes of an individual.
Cognitive Level: Application
Nursing Process: Analysis; *Test Plan:* PHYS

10 **Answer: 1** *Rationale:* The child with PKU must maintain a strict low-phenylalanine diet to prevent

central nervous system damage, seizures, and eventual death.
Cognitive Level: Application
Nursing Process: Implementation; *Test Plan:* PHYS

Posttest

1 **Answer: 2** *Rationale:* The physical characteristics of the client are consistent with Marfan's syndrome. The connective tissue disorder can involve the heart and specifically the aorta and can lead to a fatal aortic aneurysm.
Cognitive Level: Analysis
Nursing Process: Assessment; *Test Plan:* PHYS

2 **Answer: 2** *Rationale:* Without melanin production, the child with albinism is at risk for severe sunburns. Maximum sun protection should be taken, including use of hats, long sleeves, minimal time in the sun, and high-SPF sunblock, to prevent any problems.
Cognitive Level: Application
Nursing Process: Implementation; *Test Plan:* SECE

3 **Answer: 1** *Rationale:* Huntington's is an autosomal dominant disorder needing only one chromosome to be present. The risk of transmission of the chromosome 4 defect is 2:4 incidence if one parent has the disease, meaning 2 children will have the disorder and 2 will be normal. If both parents have it, 3 of the 4 children will have the disease and 1 will be normal.
Cognitive Level: Analysis
Nursing Process: Assessment; *Test Plan:* HPM

4 **Answer: 3** *Rationale:* The child with cystic fibrosis is chronically hypoxic because progression of chronic obstructive pulmonary disease (COPD). Clubbing of nailbeds occurs after 6 months of inadequate oxygenation.
Cognitive Level: Application
Nursing Process: Assessment; *Test Plan:* PHYS

5 **Answer: 2** *Rationale:* The client with cystic fibrosis absorbs fats poorly because of the thick secretions blocking the pancreatic duct. The lack of natural pancreatic enzyme leads to poor absorption of predominantly fats in the duodenum. Foul-smelling frothy stool is termed steatorrhea.
Cognitive Level: Application
Nursing Process: Analysis; *Test Plan:* PHYS

6 **Answer: 2** *Rationale:* Clients with chronic carbon dioxide retention (hypercapnia) are dependent on oxygen to drive the respiratory system. Too much oxygen will decrease the body's desire to breathe. Therefore, the nurse should monitor the respiratory

status/rate of a client with cystic fibrosis for potential apnea.
Cognitive Level: Application
Nursing Process: Analysis; *Test Plan:* PHYS

7 **Answer: 1** *Rationale:* Translocation has an increase risk of 5 to 15 percent for subsequent births to be trisomy 21. Nondisjunction is the most common and has a minimal increase in risk of reoccurrence. This information is important to disclose to the family in genetic counseling.
Cognitive Level: Application
Nursing Process: Analysis; *Test Plan:* HPM

8 **Answer: 2** *Rationale:* The adolescent client with Klinefelter's syndrome is a tall, lean male with no

secondary sex characteristics. Body image is the appropriate nursing diagnosis for the adolescent.
Cognitive Level: Application
Nursing Process: Implementation; *Test Plan:* PSYC

9 **Answer: 1** *Rationale:* An autosomal dominant trait can be present alone or as a pair and lead to a significant congenital disorder. As a result, the disorder has a higher incidence and there is no "carrier" status.
Cognitive Level: Application
Nursing Process: Analysis; *Test Plan:* PHYS

10 **Answer: 4** *Rationale:* For optimal appearance and healing of the suture line for cleft lip repair, the client should not be allowed to touch the mouth.
Cognitive Level: Application
Nursing Process: Implementation; *Test Plan:* SECE

References

Ball, J. & Bindler, R. (1999). *Pediatric nursing: Caring for children* (2nd ed.). Stanford CT: Appleton & Lange, pp. 447–455, 593–603, 899–901.

Bindler, R. & Ball, J. (1999). *Pediatric clinical skills* (2nd ed.). Upper Saddle River, NJ: Prentice Hall, pp. 58–59, 104–108.

Denk, M. J. & Magee, W. P. (1996). Cleft palate closure in the neonate: Preliminary report. *Cleft Palate-Craniofacial Journal* 33(1): 57–66.

LeMone, P. & Burke, K. M. (2000). *Medical surgical nursing. Critical thinking in client care* (2nd ed.). Upper Saddle River, NJ: Prentice Hall, pp. 1232, 1846–1850.

Pillitteri, A. (1999). *Maternal and child health nursing* (3rd ed.). Philadelphia: Lippincott, pp. 142–164, 266–272.

Porth, C. (1998). *Pathophysiology: Concepts of altered health states* (5th ed.). Philadelphia: Lippincott.

Thomas, C. L. (Ed.). (1999). *Taber's cyclopedic medical dictionary* (19th ed.). Philadelphia: F. A. Davis.

Wilkinson, J. M. (2000). *Nursing diagnosis handbook with NIC interventions and NOC outcomes* (7th ed.). Upper Saddle River, NJ: Prentice Hall, pp. 148–156, 184–188, 540–542.

Wilson, B. A., Shannon, M. T., & Stang, C. L. (2001). *Nursing drug guide 2001*. Upper Saddle River, NJ: Prentice Hall.

Wong, D. L. (1999). *Whaley and Wong's nursing care of infants and children* (6th ed.). St. Louis, MO: Mosby, pp. 177, 257, 1084–1090.

CHAPTER 17

Multisystem Health Problems

Jana G. Brannan, MN, RN, CNAA

CHAPTER OUTLINE

Risk Factors Associated with
Multisystem Health Problems

Shock
Trauma

Disseminated Intravascular
Coagulopathy (DIC)

OBJECTIVES

▮ Define key terms associated with multisystem health problems.

▮ Identify risk factors associated with the development of multisystem health problems.

▮ Discuss etiologies of multisystem health problems.

▮ Describe the pathophysiological processes associated with specific multisystem health problems.

▮ Distinguish between normal and abnormal multisystem findings obtained from nursing assessment.

▮ Prioritize nursing interventions associated with multisystem health problems.

[*Media Link*]

Use the CD-ROM enclosed with this text, or log onto the address given to access the free, interactive Companion Website created for this series. The CD-ROM and Companion Website accompanying this book offer additional practice opportunities and information—NCLEX Review, Case Studies, Glossary, In Depth with NCLEX, and more.

www.prenhall.com/hogan

REVIEW AT A GLANCE

anaphylactic shock *shock resulting from an immune response to the presence of antigens; a form of distributive shock*

antigen *a foreign substance introduced into the body that causes the body to produce antibodies and can cause allergic reactions*

bacteremia *the presence of bacteria within the bloodstream*

cardiac tamponade *compression of the heart muscle by excess fluid or blood within the pericardial sac*

cardiogenic shock *shock caused by abnormal cardiac functioning or "pump" failure*

contusion *a bruising of tissue*

disseminated intravascular coagulopathy (DIC) *a disorder of coagulation in which the body alternately hemorrhages and clots in response to injury; the body's*

clotting reservoirs are overwhelmed resulting in massive hemorrhaging

fibrinolysis *process in which thrombi (clots) are broken down*

hypovolemic shock *shock caused by a decrease in the circulating volume as a result of actual fluid or blood loss*

laceration *any tearing or slicing of the flesh and possibly underlying fleshy structures*

metabolic acidosis *a condition caused by the abnormal decrease in bicarbonate concentrations within the body; the body's pH becomes acidic*

neurogenic shock *shock that results from a decrease in sympathetic control of vasomotor responses, usually as a result of spinal injury; a form of distributive shock*

obstructive shock *shock in which the ventricles are not able to fill or empty*

appropriately because of a block in the flow of blood from the heart

pulse pressure *the difference between systolic and diastolic pressure readings; normally about 30 to 40 mmHg*

pulsus paradoxus *a notable decrease in the pulse upon inspiration*

shock *the state of inadequate perfusion and oxygenation to vital organs and tissues throughout the body*

septic shock *shock that occurs in response to the release of endotoxins from bacteria, generally Gram-negative; a form of distributive shock*

toxic shock syndrome *a form of septic shock that occurs most commonly in women who utilize tampons while menstruating; staphylococcus aureus is generally thought to be the bacteria involved*

trauma *a physical injury caused by outside forces*

Pretest

1 A client involved in a motor vehicle accident presents with vital signs of BP 120/62, pulse 100, respirations 28 to 32 and labored, and temperature 98.4°F orally. On examination of the chest, obvious rib fractures to the anterior chest are discovered, and breath sounds are absent in this area. The client's trachea is deviated to the left side of the neck. The client is probably experiencing which diagnosis?

(1) Spontaneous pneumothorax
(2) Tension pneumothorax
(3) Iatrogenic pneumothorax
(4) Open pneumothorax

2 A client presents after a near-drowning incident in which he was submerged for an undetermined amount of time. The client has since regained consciousness and is alert and oriented, but anxious. Vital signs are BP 120/72, pulse 92, respirations 26, temperature 98.0°F orally. Pulse oximetry indicates an SaO$_2$ of 93 percent on 4 L/min of oxygen via nasal cannula. Which of the following is the client at greatest risk to develop?

(1) Cardiogenic shock
(2) Spontaneous pneumothorax
(3) Renal failure
(4) Acute respiratory distress syndrome (ARDS)

3 A client has been involved in a motorcycle accident and on presentation is alert and oriented with intermittent periods of confusion and is complaining of moderate to severe thirst and left thigh pain. Vital signs are BP 100/60, pulse 112, respirations 28, and temperature 98.4°F orally. Capillary refill is 3 seconds and urinary output is 30 cc/hour. On examination there is an obvious pelvic deformity and the left thigh is distended. A diagnosis of hypovolemic shock is established. Which phase of shock is the client experiencing?

(1) Initial phase
(2) Compensatory phase
(3) Progressive phase
(4) Irreversible phase

4 A client presents complaining of difficulty breathing and generalized weakness after having suffered chest pain for approximately 1 hour the previous night. On exam, the client's skin is pale and diaphoretic, breath sounds are equal with crackles noted throughout all lung fields, capillary beds are dusky, and jugular venous distention is present. Vital signs are BP 98/50, pulse 118 and thready to palpation, respirations 26 and labored, temperature 98.6°F orally. Which condition is the client suspected of suffering upon presentation?

(1) Obstructive shock
(2) Neurogenic shock
(3) Hypovolemic shock
(4) Cardiogenic shock

5 A client presents who has ingested the third dose of an antibiotic prescribed for a urinary tract infection. The client is weak, diaphoretic, complaining of difficulty breathing, appears flushed, and has generalized itching. Which of the following forms of shock is suspected?

(1) Septic
(2) Anaphylactic
(3) Hypovolemic
(4) Iatrogenic

6 A client presents after a fall from approximately 10 feet. The initial body point of contact was the upper-middle back, and he is complaining of sharp pain in this area with movement. What type of injury is suspected with the presenting complaint?

(1) Head injury
(2) Renal injury
(3) Cervical/spine injury
(4) Pelvic injury

7 A client presents with the complaint of chest pain, tachycardia, and dyspnea. On exam, heart sounds are muffled. Which of the following assessment findings would support a diagnosis of cardiac tamponade?

(1) A deviated trachea
(2) Pulse 40 with inspiration
(3) Absent breath sounds to the lower lobes
(4) Blood pressure 140/76

8 A client who has suffered a penetrating bowel injury has several concerns to be addressed for future care that require prioritizing. Which of the following conditions would receive priority in developing the client's care?

(1) Constipation
(2) Peritonitis
(3) Paralytic ileus
(4) Intestinal adhesions

9 A client presents with a laceration to the forehead sustained in a fight and reports no loss of consciousness. The client is confused and has a strong alcohol smell to the breath. Which of the following diagnostic procedures would be paramount?

(1) Skull x-ray and urine alcohol
(2) CAT scan of the brain and blood alcohol
(3) Blood alcohol and glucose
(4) Electroencephalography (EEG) and blood alcohol

10 A client has a suspected femoral fracture. There is gross swelling to the left thigh, and the skin is tight and bruised. The client complains of numbness and tingling in the toes. On examination, the toes are cool and dusky with diminished sensation. The client is most probably suffering from which of the following pathologies?

(1) Deep vein thrombosis
(2) Fat embolism
(3) Wound infection
(4) Compartment syndrome

See pages 552–553 for Answers and Rationales.

I. Risk Factors Associated with Multisystem Health Problems

A. Shock

1. Hypovolemic shock

   a. Hemorrhagic: trauma (internal and external), aneurysm dissection, disseminated intravascular coagulopathy (DIC)

   b. Nonhemorrhagic: burns, vomiting, diarrhea, inadequate intake, excessive sweating, severe third-spacing

2. Cardiogenic shock: myocardial infarction (most common), dysrhythmias (heart block, supra-ventricular tachycardia [SVT], atrial fibrillation), electrolyte imbalances, cardiac tamponade, cardiomyopathy, cardiac valve disease, cardiac surgery, pericarditis, genetic anomalies

3. Obstructive shock: cardiac tamponade, pulmonary embolism, obstructive valve disease, tension pneumothorax, pulmonary hypertension

4. Distributive (*normovolemic*)

   a. Anaphylactic shock: antibiotic therapy, immunization, food, animal or chemical exposure (sensitization must occur prior to event), allergies, new drug therapy, insect bites, venomous bites

   b. Septic shock: trauma, surgical procedures of the gastrointestinal and urinary tract, therapy involving invasive devices and procedures (IVs, urinary catheter, tracheal intubation), burns, immunosuppresive states (cancer, human immunodeficiency virus [HIV], acquired immunodeficiency syndrome [AIDS], steroidal therapy), diabetes, tampon usage, elderly

B. Trauma

1. Factors predisposing an individual to traumatic injury are limitless

2. Certain lifestyle patterns, professions, and hobbies greatly increase the risk such as fire and police personnel, motorcycling, farmworkers, construction workers, electricians; high impact sports such as football, skiing, racing; and ingesting alcohol or controlled substances while operating equipment

3. Exposure to forces of acceleration, deceleration, or various forces of thrust and energy upon an inadequately protected individual because of neglect to utilize safety devices such as seat belts or harnesses or lack of following standard safety procedures

C. **Disseminated intravascular coagulopathy (DIC):** shock, complications of pregnancy, hemolytic reactions, trauma, metabolic acidosis

II. Shock

A. Overview

1. **Shock** is the state of inadequate perfusion and oxygenation to vital organs and tissues throughout the body; it cannot be defined as one specific disease

2. Manifests itself as a syndrome within many diseases or traumatic injuries that may be life-threatening

3. The body normally maintains perfusion to the cellular level by cooperation of:

   a. The pumping mechanism of the heart

   b. An intact vascular "highway" that facilitates blood flow

   c. An adequate amount of oxygenated blood that is exchanged at the capillary level with metabolic wastes

4. Any disruption of any component within this system results in an algorithmic attempt to compensate, which manifests itself in the classic signs and symptoms of shock

5. Types of shock

   a. Hypovolemic: hemorrhagic and nonhemorrhagic

   b. Cardiogenic

   c. Obstructive

   d. Distributive: anaphylactic and septic

6. Cause is usually related to a major insult to the body

7. Hemodynamic concepts that are the basic components of vascular homeostasis are important in identifying and treating shock states (see Figure 17-1)

   a. Stroke volume (SV): the amount of blood that is ejected from the left ventricle into the aorta with every contraction of the ventricle

   b. Cardiac output (CO): the amount of blood pumped from the left ventricle every minute; calculated by the equation *Stroke volume × Heart rate*

   c. Systemic vascular resistance (SVR): the amount of resistance provided by the vascular bed against the flow of blood being ejected from the left ventricle; when the sympathetic system is stimulated in response to a threat, vasoconstriction occurs, increasing the SVR

   d. Mean arterial pressure (MAP): the average pressure maintained within the arterial system of the body; calculated by *Cardiac Output × Systemic Vascular Resistance*

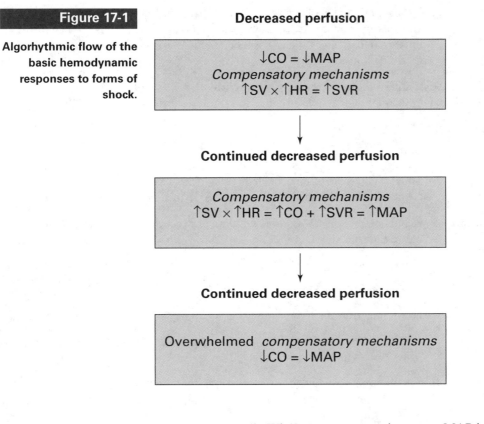

Figure 17-1

Algorhythmic flow of the basic hemodynamic responses to forms of shock.

Decreased perfusion

$\downarrow CO = \downarrow MAP$
Compensatory mechanisms
$\uparrow SV \times \uparrow HR = \uparrow SVR$

Continued decreased perfusion

Compensatory mechanisms
$\uparrow SV \times \uparrow HR = \uparrow CO + \uparrow SVR = \uparrow MAP$

Continued decreased perfusion

Overwhelmed *compensatory mechanisms*
$\downarrow CO = \downarrow MAP$

1) When any component increases, MAP increases

2) Conversely, with any decrease, there is a drop in MAP

3) An increase or decrease in the intravascular volume effects MAP in a parallel manner

NCLEX!

8. Whatever the cause of a shock state, the reactions and symptoms will generally follow the same course with a few notable signs defining the particular type of shock or the underlying cause

NCLEX!

9. It is important to *first* identify that a state of shock is occurring rather than identifying the particular type

B. Pathophysiology

1. Shock is a syndrome that manifests itself as a result of attempts by the body to achieve homeostasis in direct response to a perfusion and oxygenation insult

2. Origination of the insult may differ, but the compensatory mechanisms for all types will progress through similar stages (see Box 17-1)

   a. *Initial phase of shock* (mild)

   1) A decline in circulating blood volume (500 cc or less) activates baroreceptors in the vascular system to note the decline in MAP; sympathetic activity is activated; beta receptors are stimulated to increase oxygen consumption of the cardiac muscle

Box 17-1

Systemic Effects and Compensatory Response of Shock

Neurologic

- Hypoxia with decreasing volume and systemic pressure
- Cerebral edema with severe, continuing hypoxia
- Circulatory collapse as sympathetic stimulation is lost

Respiratory

- Bronchodilation and increase in respiratory rate in response to hypoxic status at cellular level
- Diminished respirations as a result of continued hypoxia to pulmonary tissue

Cardiac

- Increase in rate and contractility as a result of sympathetic stimulation in response to decreasing volume
- Decreasing blood pressure as shock progresses
- Diminished perfusion to the heart itself as a result of continued hypoxia

Gastrointestinal

- Ischemia as a result of the shunting of blood to the heart, lungs, and brain
- Ulcer and paralytic ileus may form as a result of prolonged ischemia

Renal

- Ischemia as a result of compensatory shunting to heart, lungs, and brain
- Release of renin in response to decreased renal perfusion and decreased glomerular filtration, which results in decreased urine production in an effort to raise BP
- Tubular necrosis with prolonged renal hypoxia and renal failure

Integumentary

- Vasoconstriction with sympathetic stimulation
- Edema occurs in late shock as a result of fluid shifting to the interstitial spaces

2) Catecholamines (epinephrine and norepinephrine notably) are released, creating vasoconstriction in areas that can more easily undergo periods of ischemia, such as fat, bone, and skin; SVR is increased as a result

3) Bronchodilation and increased cardiac output occurs as a result of beta receptor stimulation

4) Few objective physical assessment findings are noted because vasoconstriction is minimal and little anaerobic activity occurs

b. *Compensatory phase of shock* (moderate shock)

1) With volume loss of 25 to 30 percent, more intense compensatory measures are initiated; MAP continues to decline

2) Cardiac contractility, rate, and peripheral vasoconstriction increase

3) In an attempt to shunt blood flow to organs most vital for survival (heart, lungs, brain), there is diminished blood flow to the kidneys, liver, and gastrointestinal tract

4) Capillary pressure decreases allowing fluid shifts from interstitial spaces into the vascular compartment in order to expand the circulating volume

NCLEX!

5) Decreased renal perfusion initiates the renin-angiotensin-aldosterone (RAA) process, causing thirst and an increased reabsorption of water and sodium

6) Objective findings become apparent

c. *Progressive phase of shock* (severe or decompensated)

1) As shock continues to progress, compensatory mechanisms from the previous phase continue unchecked, worsening the status

2) Volume loss of 35 to 50 percent occurs because of hemorrhage or fluid leakage

3) Continued vasoconstriction enhances the already hypoxic state of cells and tissues

4) As cells die because of the hypoxic state, they release destructive enzymes and proteins into the surrounding tissues, increasing the oncotic pressure into the interstitial space, and decreasing the circulating volume even further

NCLEX!

5) The body shifts from aerobic to anaerobic respiration at the cellular level and lactic acid is produced as a byproduct; an acid-base imbalance occurs in the form of **metabolic acidosis** (a disorder that is caused by an abnormal decrease in bicarbonate concentrations in the blood, the pH of the body shifts to an acidic state)

6) Dramatic physical changes in assessment parameters occur

d. *Irreversible phase of shock*

1) Despite restoration of circulating volume or the stabilization of vital signs, death will occur

2) Microcirculation has been compromised beyond repair, resulting in widespread cellular death that eventually encompasses the tissues of vital organs

3) Symptoms displayed during shock are part of the "survival" physiology the body initiates in response to a disease or injury

4) Systemic changes are closely correlated with advancing sympathetic stimulation and the byproducts of that stimulation

3. The overall course of shock states is very similar; however, the underlying cause may vary the pathological processes

a. Six types of shock: hypovolemic, cardiogenic, obstructive, anaphylactic, septic, and neurogenic

b. Anaphylactic, septic, and neurogenic are known as *distributive* forms of shock in that there is an adequate intravascular volume available; however, it is distributed in a manner within the body that does not sustain perfusion and oxygenation

    c. Hypovolemic shock

        1) **Hypovolemic shock** is caused by a decrease in circulating volume greater than 15 percent

        2) Loss of volume is from obvious hemorrhaging, extracellular fluid and/or plasma loss from burns, peritonitis, or ruptured aneurysms

        3) Loss of fluids can also be from the gastrointestinal tract because of severe vomiting, diarrhea, or gastric suctioning

        4) Inadequate intake, excessive sweating, diuretic usage, and interstitial shifting (third-spacing) associated with processes such as liver disease and severe protein wasting may cause this form of shock

        5) Loss of circulating volume causes an inadequate MAP, activating the sympathetic system and initiating compensatory mechanisms

        6) Signs and symptoms (see Table 17-1)

    d. Cardiogenic shock

NCLEX!

        1) **Cardiogenic shock** is caused by abnormal cardiac functioning or "pump failure"

        2) There is adequate volume within the intravascular space, however, perfusion and oxygenation at the cellular level is inadequate because of the inability of the heart to move blood throughout the body with acceptable force

NCLEX!

        3) The most common and dangerous cause of cardiac failure is myocardial infarction; cardiomyopathy, cardiac tamponade, valve disease, and dysrhythmias are contributing factors

        4) A decrease in MAP stimulates the sympathetic system; beta receptors within the heart are stimulated as a result, creating a dangerous scenario in that oxygen consumption is increased in the very organ that is compromised, thus placing greater stress on cardiac tissue

Table 17-1   **Clinical Manifestations of Hypovolemic Shock**

	Initial	Compensatory	Progressive	Irreversible
Subjective	c/o pain and thirst; sensorium intact	Anxious; restlessness; c/o greater thirst; episodes of confusion	Confused; restless; agitated	
Objective	Tachycardia; respirations baseline; normotensive; fleshtone or pallor of extremities; skin dry or slightly moist; refill < 3 sec; normal or slightly decreased output; ABGs normal	Hypotension; tachycardia; tachypnea; skin cool, pale, and dry/diaphoretic; refill < 4–6 sec; output less than 300 cc/hr; ABGs indicate encroaching or present metabolic acidosis	Profound hypotension; tachycardia with weak or nonpalpable peripheral pulses; cardiac dysrhythmias; tachypnea; skin pale and/or cyanotic; capillary beds without refill, dusky or blanched ABGs— metabolic acidosis; diminished or absent output; no purposeful movement	Severe hypotension; tachypnea with shallow depth; diminishing air exchange with crackles; cardiac dysrhythmias; skin mottled; ABGs— profound metabolic acidosis; anuria; comatose

c/o = complains of
WNL = within normal limits

5) Distal vascular beds become congested with deoxygenated blood creating the hallmark nail bed cyanosis with this form of shock

6) Increased SVR occurs from the pooling that occurs in the periphery

7) Pressure is then exerted on the left ventricle, causing pulmonary congestion as fluid "backs" into the lungs

8) Signs and symptoms (see Table 17-2)

e. Obstructive shock

1) **Obstructive shock** results from an inability of the ventricles of the heart to fill or empty appropriately because of an obstruction in the blood flow from the heart; cardiac preload is decreased and severely compromised; may be difficult to diagnose

2) There is an increased pressure on the right side of the heart and an inadequate blood return

NCLEX!

3) This form of shock is differentiated from cardiogenic shock in that the heart itself has adequate pumping capabilities and is not necessarily diseased; it is the presence of some "obstruction" outside of the heart that compromises perfusion; trauma may create obstructions

4) Pulmonary embolism (PE) is the most common cause of obstructive shock; damage to the alveolar from the "explosion" of the embolus in the lung creates an increasing pressure on the right side of the heart because of an inability of the blood to enter easily into the lung from the right ventricle; in the presence of a suspected pulmonary embolus, signs and symptoms of shock should be correlated to obstruction

5) Signs and symptoms often correlate with right-sided heart failure: jugular venous distention, hepatomegaly, edema (see Table 17-3)

f. Anaphylactic shock

NCLEX!

1) **Anaphylactic shock** results from an overwhelming immune response to the presence of an allergen or **antigen** (a foreign substance introduced into the body that causes the body to produce antibodies)

2) This form of shock is particularly catastrophic and requires aggressive and immediate intervention as circulatory collapse is rapid

Table 17-2		Signs and Symptoms
Clinical Manifestations of Cardiogenic Shock	**Subjective**	Restless Agitated
	Objective	Hypotension Tachycardia with weak, thready pulse Cardiac dysrhythmias Decreased pulse pressure Tachypnea with labored depth and crackles Jugular venous distention (JVD) Skin cool and moist Circumoral cyanosis Nail beds dusky

Table 17-3		Signs and Symptoms
Clinical Manifestations of Obstructive Shock	**Subjective**	Anxiety Somnolence
	Objective	Hypotension Tachycardia Tachypnea with dyspnea Jugular venous distention (JVD) Pallor Pericardial friction rub Muffled heart sounds or gallop (S$_3$) Chest pain Decreased to absent urinary output Signs and symptoms of a pneumothorax Open chest wound or fractured ribs Diminished or absent breath sounds Whistling or rushing sounds with inspiration Tracheal deviation

3) Associated with the administration of antibiotics or exposure to a foreign protein; parenteral medication administration routes are more prone to cause true anaphylaxis than oral routes

4) On exposure to an antigen, the body's immune system produces an antibody specific to the allergen

5) With subsequent exposure, a reaction occurs wherein large amounts of histamines are released into the blood stream in response to the foreign body

6) Histamines cause marked dilation in the arterioles as well as increasing capillary permeability

7) There is a profound fluid shift into the interstitial spaces from the intravascular compartment, creating edema

8) Overwhelming vasodilation and pooling of circulating blood in the periphery causes a precipitous drop in MAP; vasodilation produces the characteristic skin flushing and warmth

9) Laryngeal edema may occur, and bronchospasms further compromise pulmonary function and airway clearance

10) Signs and symptoms (see Table 17-4)

g. Septic shock

1) **Septic shock** that is most often associated with the endotoxic release of Gram-negative bacteria into the bloodstream, although it may also be caused by some Gram-positive bacteria; massive vasodilation occurs in response to the pathogen's release of toxins into the bloodstream

2) An initial infection occurs and progresses to frank **bacteremia,** (presence of bacteria in the blood); sepsis follows in most instances

Table 17-4		Signs and Symptoms
Clinical Manifestations of Anaphylactic Shock	Subjective	Marked restlessness Anxiety Severe itching and difficulty swallowing
	Objective	Hypotension Tachycardia Tachypnea with wheezing and possible stridor Diminished breath sounds Hypersalivation and/or drooling Generalized urticaria Edema (focusing on orbital and facial components) Cardiac dysrhythmias Skin cool and moist Flushing Abdominal cramping Emesis

3) Some shock states may be present without obvious bacteremia if there is a localized infection large enough to generate a sufficient toxic release

4) **Toxic shock syndrome** is a form of septic shock that occurs most commonly in menstruating women who use tampons and is most commonly produced by the *staphylococcus aureus* organism; blood cultures may not always be positive with this form of septic shock

5) As pathogens release their poison into the blood stream, the inflammatory process responds to the destruction of blood cells and the presence of bacteria with the help of the immune system

6) Initial presentation is generally with a fever and flushing that is not seen in other forms of shock

7) Disseminated intravascular coagulation (DIC) is associated with this form of shock and will be reviewed later in this chapter

8) Signs and symptoms (see Table 17-5)

h. Neurogenic shock

1) **Neurogenic shock** occurs as a result of decreased sympathetic control of vasomotor responses; parasympathetic stimulation is unchecked, allowing peripheral vasodilation to occur, thereby decreasing MAP

2) This form of shock is somewhat rare and generally associated with significant spinal trauma

3) Because neurogenic shock is often associated with trauma, it is important to remember to rule out hypovolemic shock initially, even in the absence of obvious volume loss or bleeding

4) Signs and symptoms (see Table 17-6)

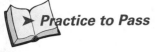

Practice to Pass

A 23-year-old woman who has suffered no apparent injury or recent illness is diagnosed as being in shock. What predisposing risk factor would be investigated and why?

Table 17-5		Early Shock	Late Shock
Clinical Manifestations of Septic Shock	**Subjective**	Sensorium intact with restlessness and agitation Nausea Possible abdominal tenderness	Hypotension Tachycardia Cardiac dysrhythmias
	Objective	Normotensive Tachycardia Tachypnea Skin flushed Warm and moist Moderate to severe hyperthermia Shivering Emesis Exudate from wound sources	Tachypnea with laboring and shallow depth Skin cool and pale Normothermic to hypothermic (indicates decreasing basal metabolic rate) Somnolence to coma Decreased to absent urinary output

4. Acute respiratory distress syndrome (ARDS) (see Chapter 1)

   a. Acute respiratory distress syndrome (ARDS) is a form of respiratory failure that generally occurs in otherwise healthy individuals following a catastrophic injury or disease state; formerly known as "shock lung"

   b. The exact mechanism of development for this syndrome is unknown, however, the end result is a significant increase in the capillary permeability within the lungs, allowing proteins and water to collect

   c. There is a diminished production of surfactant, causing a decreased elasticity of the alveoli and subsequent alveolar collapse that worsens the edema

   d. Exact mechanism for development is unknown, but predisposing conditions would include all forms of shock, sepsis, chemical or fluid aspiration, hemolytic reactions and trauma

   e. Supplemental oxygen does not improve the condition, a hallmark of diagnosing ARDS

5. General signs and symptoms are common to all forms of shock (see Figure 17-2)

Table 17-6		Signs and Symptoms
Clinical Manifestations of Neurogenic Shock	**Subjective**	Level of consciousness varies according to the underlying cause
	Objective	Hypotension Bradycardia followed by tachycardia (especially in brain and spinal trauma) Skin flushed followed by pallor and coolness Possible hypothermia Decreased to absent urinary output Respiratory rate is dependent on cause of shock

Note: Traumatic injuries and central nervous system depressants vary the objective findings accordingly.

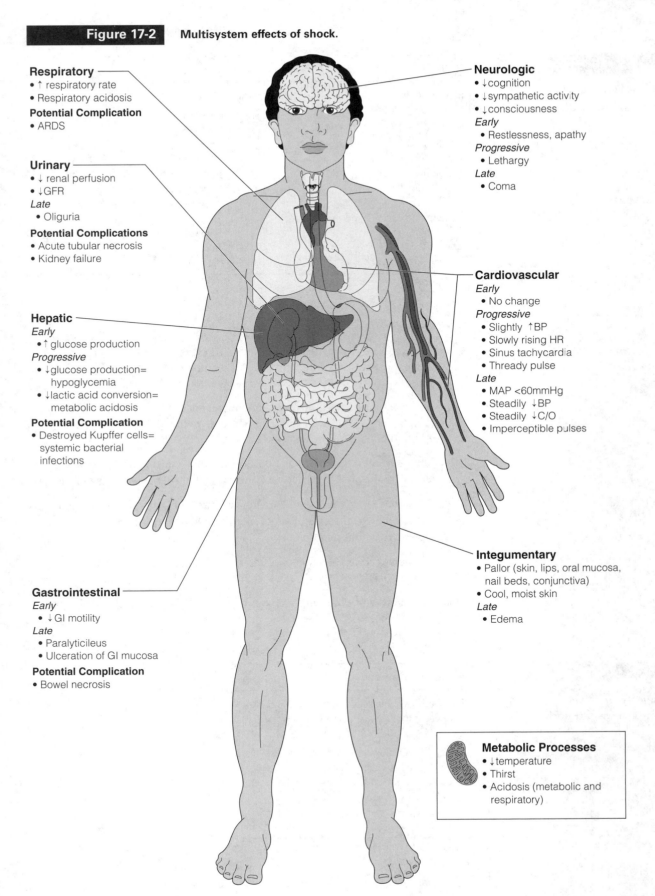

Figure 17-2 Multisystem effects of shock.

Respiratory
- ↑ respiratory rate
- Respiratory acidosis

Potential Complication
- ARDS

Urinary
- ↓ renal perfusion
- ↓GFR

Late
- Oliguria

Potential Complications
- Acute tubular necrosis
- Kidney failure

Hepatic
Early
- ↑ glucose production

Progressive
- ↓glucose production=
  hypoglycemia
- ↓lactic acid conversion=
  metabolic acidosis

Potential Complication
- Destroyed Kupffer cells=
  systemic bacterial
  infections

Gastrointestinal
Early
- ↓GI motility

Late
- Paralyticileus
- Ulceration of GI mucosa

Potential Complication
- Bowel necrosis

Neurologic
- ↓cognition
- ↓sympathetic activity
- ↓consciousness

Early
- Restlessness, apathy

Progressive
- Lethargy

Late
- Coma

Cardiovascular
Early
- No change

Progressive
- Slightly ↑BP
- Slowly rising HR
- Sinus tachycardia
- Thready pulse

Late
- MAP <60mmHg
- Steadily ↓BP
- Steadily ↓C/O
- Imperceptible pulses

Integumentary
- Pallor (skin, lips, oral mucosa,
  nail beds, conjunctiva)
- Cool, moist skin

Late
- Edema

Metabolic Processes
- ↓temperature
- Thirst
- Acidosis (metabolic and
  respiratory)

C. Nursing assessment

    1. Assessment criteria for each category

        a. *Hypovolemic shock*

            1) Assessment includes symptom analysis of pain and thirst, level of consciousness, vital signs (VS), skin color and temperature, capillary refill, urinary output, evidence of coping (or lack of), cardiac rhythm, heart and lung sounds, movement, peripheral pulses, assess for risk factors

            2) Diagnostic tests

                a) Hemoglobin and hematocrit (H&H): baseline levels should be obtained and serial measurements performed to reflect changes; H&H levels with whole blood loss will reflect a decrease; an increase of the H&H levels will be noted when the majority of fluid lost is within the vascular system such as occurs with dehydration and third-spacing

                b) Urinalysis may indicate the presence of blood secondary to direct injury or indirect "shaking" of the kidney during the traumatic incident

                c) Arterial blood gases (ABGs): normal to metabolic acidosis

                d) Type and cross match: in preparation for blood administration

                e) Coagulation studies such as partial thromboplastin time (PTT), prothrombin time (PT)

        b. *Cardiogenic shock*

            1) Assessment includes preexisting cardiac dysfunction such as myocardial infarction or trauma and other risk factors; VS; heart rhythm; pulses; lung sounds; heart sounds; presence of edema; skin color and temperature; capillary refill and color of nailbeds; mentation; urinary output (note: damage from myocardial infarction versus cardiac tamponade may be differentiated by observing for signs and symptoms of tamponade such as jugular venous distention (JVD) without symptoms of pulmonary congestion and by auscultating for a pericardial friction rub; this is an important distinction because treatment for tamponade must be instituted immediately)

            2) Diagnostic tests

                a) Hemoglobin and hematocrit levels may be decreased with a long medical history of heart disease from chronic renal hypoperfusion

                b) Cardiac enzymes and isoenzymes may be elevated as a result of cardiac tissue damage

                c) Chest x-rays (CXR) may indicate cardiomegaly and pulmonary edema

                d) Electrocardiogram (EKG) 12-lead

                e) ABGs: metalbolic acidosis

        c. *Obstructive shock*

            1) Assessment includes risk factors and predisposing diagnoses such as thrombophlebitis, deep vein thrombosis (DVT) and risk factors for

DVT such as smoking and contraceptive use; VS; presence of edema; skin color and temperature; complaints of respiratory or cardiac problems; lung sounds; heart sounds; trachea midline

2) Diagnostic tests

   a) Cardiac enzymes and isoenzymes may be elevated secondary to myocardial tissue damage

   b) Chest x-rays may indicate the presence of pneumothorax

   c) Echocardiogram may indicate presence of pericarditis or valve disease

   d) ABGs

   e) 12-lead EKG

   d. *Anaphylactic shock*

   1) Assessment includes preexisting exposure to medication, foods associated with high allergic reactions (iodine containing foods, coarse wheat products, various nuts), animals or insects and other risk factors; perform a thorough head-to-toe assessment to locate source of bite/sting (only after aggressive treatment has been initiated); assess for mentation; complaints of itching and difficulty swallowing; VS; lung sounds; heart sounds; presence of edema; gastrointestinal (GI) complaints; respiratory status; in many instances anaphylactic shock progresses to circulatory collapse and coma within minutes

   2) Diagnostic tests

      a) Complete blood counts (CBC) may indicate an overall increase in white blood cells (WBC) in response to the inflammatory process

      b) Eosinophil counts may also be elevated in response to the presence of allergens

      c) Other laboratory or radiology tests are noncontributory for anaphylaxis

      d) ABGs

   e. *Septic shock*

   1) Assessment includes preexisting signs or symptoms of infection even if current treatment for an infection is in progress; assess for other risk factors; VS; mentation; skin color and temperature; GI complaints; signs of infection/inflammation; urinary output

   2) Diagnostic tests

      a) Complete blood counts indicate an elevated white blood cell count initially; as shock progresses, the body's immune response is overwhelmed and there is a decrease in the overall white blood cell count; monocytes may be increased in response to macrophage activity in the presence of bacteria

      b) *Blood and wound culture and sensitivity* (C&S) testing indicates the presence of a specific bacteria or multiple bacteria; testing of spinal fluid may be performed to diagnose neurological infections

c) Radiology testing may include the use of ultrasound, magnetic resonance imaging (MRI), or computerized tomography (CT) to identify sources of infection or abscesses

d) Coagulation studies

f. *Neurogenic shock*

1) Assessment includes risk factors to include traumatic injury, central nervous system (CNS) depressants, and anesthesia; VS; skin color and temperature; urinary output; mentation

2) Diagnostic tests: laboratory testing is limited in its ability to assist in the diagnosis of this form of shock; radiology studies may reveal spinal or cranial trauma

2. Primary diagnostic tests (common to most forms)

a. Arterial blood gases (ABGs): reflect metabolic acidosis (lowering of pH) that develops as a result of increasing carbon dioxide levels in the blood stream secondary to hypoxia

b. Urinalysis: indicates an increasing specific gravity and osmolality as the urine becomes more concentrated

c. Blood urea nitrogen (BUN): levels increase in response to diminishing renal function

D. Nursing management

1. Organization

a. Pre-hospital: baseline history to include vital signs, mechanism of injury, machinery involved if traumatic situation, environmental factors surrounding an accident; in the event that no pre-admission report is available, information must be obtained simultaneously with physical assessments and interventions

b. Specialty personnel within the hospital should be organized prior to the arrival of a trauma victim suffering from shock if possible; these health care providers include respiratory, radiology (to include CT), additional nursing support, surgeons, anesthesiologists, orthopedists, and radiologists

c. Ancillary units such as intensive care unit (ICU) and operating room (OR) need to be notified of a potential admission

d. In many facilities a trauma protocol is initiated within the emergency unit itself wherein a team approach is followed so that care is delivered in an organized manner; nurses may be assigned to an anatomical area or to a procedure, becoming the "intravenous (IV) nurse" or the "thoracic nurse"

2. General treatment measures

a. Maintain life support by instituting ABC (airway, breathing, circulation) guidelines

b. Supine position with spinal alignment maintained

c. Airway should be secured, protected, and supplemental oxygen should be initiated through the appropriate delivery device dependent on the client's overall assessment

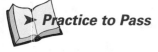

Practice to Pass

A client presents with a diagnosis of cardiogenic shock. What diagnostic value is the most accurate for gauging the severity of shock and why?

NCLEX!

    d. Initiate an intravenous (IV) access appropriate to the specific form of shock; usually an 18-gauge for peripheral IV line

    e. Initiate continuous cardiac and SaO_2 (pulse oximetry) monitoring and prepare for frequent, repetitive vital sign assessments

    f. Maintain stabilization to all deformities and prevent hypothermia by covering the client

    g. All clients suspected of experiencing shock should have an indwelling urinary catheter inserted for accurate output recordings; do not attempt to place in the presence of obvious pelvic deformity or active bleeding from the urethra

    h. Sympathomimetic medications may be administered for their inotropic and vasoconstrictive effects; epinephrine hydrochloride (Adrenalin), dopamine hydrochloride (Intropin), isoproterenol hydrochloride (Isuprel)

        1) A positive inotropic effect provides for increased cardiac contractility

        2) Sympathomemetic medications stimulate beta-one receptors (heart and lung), creating an increase in oxygen consumption by heart

        3) Sympathomimetics may not be given to those in cardiogenic shock or with serious heart disease secondary to the cardiac stress they create

  3. *Hypovolemic shock*

    a. Medications include sympathomimetics, vasopressors, and medications to treat acid-base and electrolyte imbalances

    b. Place the client in a supine position with legs elevated to increase blood flow to the brain with consideration given to stabilize the neck and obvious deformities; avoid this, however, if a head injury is suspected

    c. Prepare for the potential application of antishock trousers (inflatable pant-like devices that compress the lower half of the body to enhance circulation to the heart, lungs, and brain)

    d. Gain intravenous access through the initiation of at least two large-bore cannulas (18-gauge or larger)

        1) Prepare to assist in percutaneous insertions in cases of severe shock for rapid fluid resuscitation, avoiding the jugular and subclavian veins if possible

        2) Intraosseous infusions may need to be initiated in cases of severe burns or pediatric clients

    e. Initiate IV fluids

        1) Crystolloids (isotonic or balanced solutions such as normal saline [NS] and lactated Ringer's [LR]) may be initiated in cases of mild shock

        2) Moderate to severe shock may indicate the administration of colloidal solutions to expand the volume of plasma, however, these should be given with the understanding that coagulation disorders may develop as well as hypersensitivity reactions

        3) Colloidal solutions also increase oncotic pressure in the intravascular space, which may predispose the client to circulatory overload, pulmonary edema, and allergic reactions

f. Blood, a type of colloid, is also given with caution

   1) Infection, as well as hemolytic reactions are a concern

   2) Obtain a type and crossmatch lab specimen for donor specific unit retrieval, however, universal O-negative blood should be requisitioned if time does not allow for specific matching and hospital protocol allows

   3) Monitor vital signs every 15 minutes, a febrile reaction (fever) usually indicates a reaction

g. In severe, unremitting shock, autotransfusions may be administered, wherein the client's own blood is collected through special measures and reinfused

4. *Cardiogenic shock*

   a. Medications include agents to correct acid-base and electrolyte imbalances; typically, sympathomimetic agents that stimulate alpha and beta receptors indiscriminately are avoided due to the increased oxygen demand they place on cardiac tissue

   b. Place the client in a supine position or with a slight elevation of the legs if the systolic pressure is low; this position is contraindicated in those clients experiencing signs and symptoms of pulmonary distress associated with pleural effusion

   c. Initiate an intravenous access, however, client's experiencing this form of shock may have fluids restricted

5. *Obstructive shock*

   a. Medications include vasopressors such as norepinephrine bitartrate (Levophed)

   b. Prepare for the insertion of a thoracostomy tube to relieve a tension pneumothorax

   c. Prepare for pericardiocentesis to relieve cardiac tamponade

   d. Provide supportive treatment with fluids

6. *Septic shock*

   a. Medications include inotropics and broad spectrum antibiotics; empirical antibiotic therapy is generally initiated prior to receiving results of culture and sensitivity testing, however, all cultures should be collected prior to the initiation of antibiotic therapy

   b. Prepare to administer fluid in the form of crystolloids

7. *Anaphylactic shock*

   a. Medications include crystolloids, sympathomimetics (specifically epinephrine) as well as antihistamines, vasopressors, and glucocorticoids; sympathomimetic agents should be used with great caution in those clients with heart disease

   b. Aerosol treatments for bronchodilation may be given in the presence of bronchospasms

   c. Maintain the client in a supine position and do not overheat with covering

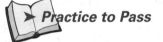

Practice to Pass

A client presents with a diagnosis of septic shock. When would antibiotics be initiated and what classification of therapy would be given?

8. *Neurogenic shock*

    a. Medications include crystalloid solutions and vasopressors

    b. Place the client in a supine position, maintaining skeletal alignment in the presence of suspected spinal trauma

9. Reassessment

    a. Nursing management of all forms of shock requires continuous and accurate monitoring of the client's status to identify improvement or deterioration

    b. Vital signs, urinary output, and laboratory parameters are fundamental

    c. Clients experiencing shock are also at great risk to develop gastrointestinal ulcers secondary to GI ischemia, and ARDS

    d. Various monitoring devices may include central venous pressure, capillary wedge pressure or intracranial pressure

    e. Signs of resolution with a shock state include stable vital signs that provide adequate perfusion, improved and/or adequate urinary output, appropriate orientation and alertness, a hematocrit and hemoglobin level within normal parameters or improving, and a pH within normal limits

III. Trauma

A. Overview

1. **Trauma** is defined as the physical injury to the body from external forces; there are many predisposing factors and all parts of the body are vulnerable

2. Trauma may range from simple to complex, depending on the organs and systems involved

3. Injury is generally a result of

    a. Accelerating forces: gunshot wound is an example

    b. Decelerating forces: impact from motor vehicle accident (MVA)

4. Injuries may be blunt, penetrating, or shearing in nature

5. Body organs and tissues may also experience traumatic injury as a result of medical procedures and treatment

6. It is impossible to predict with certainty the effects that one type of injury may have on an individual, so care must be approached in an algorithmic, organized, and rapid manner

B. Pathophysiology

1. *Skull/brain trauma*

    a. Trauma to the skull may take the form of soft tissue or bone injury and is often associated with acceleration and deceleration of great velocity

    b. The scalp and face have an extensive vascular system so that wounds may bleed in copious amounts; if this is combined with other areas of hemorrhage, a hypovolemic state may occur

    c. Intracranial hemorrhages may be classified according to their location to the protective meningeal coverings of the brain; the dura (outer), the arachnoid (middle), and the pia mater (internal); hemorrhaging may also occur within any other area within the brain itself forming an intracerebral hematoma

    d. Subdural (below the brain's lining) or epidural (above the brain's lining) hematomas may develop; these may be acute in nature or develop over the course of hours

        1) Subdural are common and usually from venous tissue bleeding

        2) Epidural are usually from arterial bleeding

    e. The symptoms of brain injury are closely related to the amount and locale of damage and may be diffuse or specific in nature

    f. *Closed* trauma to the head may occur with or without a fracture to the skull; there is no passage formed by the injury from the brain to the atmosphere

        1) Hemorrhaging within the brain creates pressure; as this pressure elevates, more damage from the force created by the bleeding results in more injury; hypoxemia increases cerebral blood flow in response to the elevating carbon dioxide levels creating more swelling

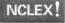

        2) The brain injury itself may suppress vital functions such as ventilation, worsening the hypoxic state

        3) Depending on the location of the injury, sensory and motor function may be impaired, reflected in paresthesias, paralysis, and an altered sensorium (leaving the client open to further injury)

        4) Injuries that hemorrhage rapidly and profusely may cause a "shift" of the brain as pressure is exerted

    g. *Open* head injuries are those in which the integrity of the cranial cavity has been compromised, leaving a passage for material (such as bacteria) to move from the atmosphere to the brain

        1) This type of trauma may also result in brain tissue swelling and hemorrhage; many of the same symptoms will be present as those involved with a closed head injury depending on the locale and extent

        2) Open head injuries tend to be more focal in nature rather than diffuse

    h. Injuries to the protective tissues of the brain pose a unique problem of infection in that a bacterium may be introduced, resulting in the infectious process of meningitis

    i. Trauma to the ear, sinus and eye may also provide potential routes for infection to the brain and must be investigated

    j. Facial bone injury may be isolated or complicate a skull injury

        1) Mandibular and maxillary fractures are generally a result of blunt or crushing forces to the facial area and pose a unique problem to airway management

        2) Trauma to facial nerves may also be present

    k. Orbital fractures, often seen with fractures of the zygomatic bones, may also involve damage to the eye sphere itself

    l. All fractures of the face, with or without the presence or hemorrhaging, should be viewed with suspicion, and cranial integrity should be verified

2. *Cervical/neck trauma*

    a. Cervical and neck trauma should automatically be suspected with head injuries, falls, or injuries to the chest and upper back

    b. May involve soft tissue and/or the cervical portion of the spinal column

    c. Great vessel injury to the carotid arteries or jugular veins is life-threatening in nature, and a hypovolemic state may be immediate and profound

    d. Damage to the trachea may occur simultaneously with great vessel injury and may result in either mechanical blocking of air, or diminished air exchange secondary to the presence of active hemorrhaging

    e. Cervical spinal injuries involve the vertebrae from C1 to C8; these injuries should be suspected in the presence of head injuries as well as injuries that may result in hyperflexion (bending back) of the neck, such as car accidents that "whip" the head back

    f. Traumatic injuries that strike the top of the head and push the head down into the body (axial loading) should also be suspected of creating spinal injuries (see Figure 17-3)

NCLEX!

NCLEX!

NCLEX!

Figure 17-3   **Spinal injury mechanisms. A. Compression of cord. B. Stretching of cord. C. Compression fracture.**

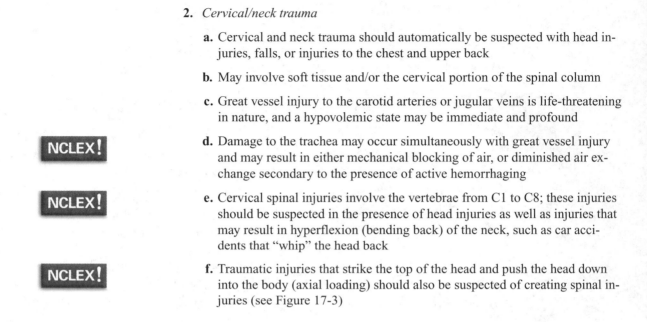

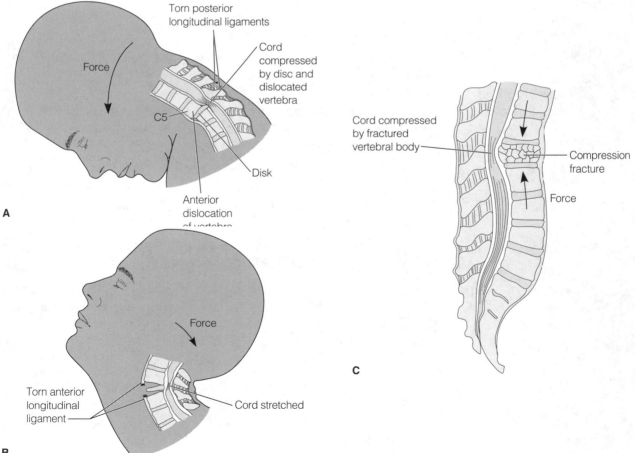

g. Depending on the specific location and whether the cord itself has been transected (complete severance), a variety of symptoms may occur as innervation of various organs and structures is disrupted

h. Higher cord damage may result in the cessation of vital life functions such as respiration

i. Lower cervical cord injury may also mimic higher lesions because of the paralysis of other functions; therefore, a specific determination of the location of the injury should not take precedence over interventions

3. *Chest trauma*

a. Injuries to the chest are most often the result of blunt or penetrating trauma

b. Bone injury may occur to the surrounding protective cage of the chest, with or without trauma to the underlying tissues and organs; however, cardiac and pulmonary injury should always be ruled out when there is enough force to injure the bony structures encasing these organs

c. With significant chest injuries, air exchange and tissue perfusion may be profoundly impaired; a hypovolemic state may be created as a result

d. Great vessel injury is another potential complication of chest trauma and may result in the severance or tearing of these structures

e. Significant heart problems

1) **Cardiac tamponade** results when the heart is compressed by excess fluid or blood in the pericardial sac

   a) The ensuing decrease in output results in cardiogenic or obstructive shock

   b) This condition progresses rapidly

   c) A hallmark sign of cardiac tamponade is the finding of **pulsus paradoxus** or paradoxical pulses, a notable decrease in the pulse upon inspiration

   d) The **pulse pressure** (difference between systolic and diastolic pressure, about 30–40 mmHg) also begins to diminish in tamponade

2) In differentiating a myocardial infarction versus cardiac tamponade in the initial assessment, it is important to assess for the presence of jugular venous distention that will occur in tamponade without the concurrent pulmonary congestion that is seen with heart failure from myocardial infarction; a friction rub may also be auscultated in tamponade

3) A **contusion,** or bruising of tissue, is assigned differently in that cardiac tissue itself is injured as opposed to the pericardial area; contusions should always be suspected with cardiac tamponade

4) A preexisting cardiac condition may further complicate the scenario as a result of the diseased heart's inability to tolerate the additional stress

    f. Significant lung problems

        1) Pneumothorax: a pneumothorax is an emergent condition in which air leaks into the pleural space, either through the lung itself (closed) or from the outside atmosphere (open)

            a) The negative pressure within the pleural space becomes equal to the atmosphere, resulting in the collapse of the area of the lung involved

            b) A pneumothorax may be spontaneous in nature and not evolve from an injury, however, most occur as the result of blunt or penetrating trauma to the pleural space

        2) Tension pneumothorax: in the event that the pleural cavity becomes open to the outside atmosphere through penetrating trauma to the chest, a tension pneumothorax may result

            a) The wound itself becomes a valve, allowing air to enter the chest cavity and none to escape

            b) The increasing pressure may cause a shift of the mediastinum away from the side of the injured lung

NCLEX!

            c) The trachea also deviates to the side of the unaffected lung, a hallmark sign of tension pneumothorax

            d) Increasing pressure on the unaffected lung compromises the already impaired gas exchange

        3) Hemothorax: pneumothorax where blood collects into the pleural space as a result of blunt or penetrating trauma; hemorrhaging into the pleural cavity impairs gas exchange as well as potentially causing a significant source of hypovolemia

        4) Flail chest: a flail chest results when two or more ribs are fractured, in line, resulting in chest wall instability

NCLEX!

            a) With inspiration and expiration, this segment moves paradoxically with the other areas of the chest

            b) On inspiration the involved area moves inward, while on expiration, the area may appear to bulge

            c) This paradoxical movement mechanically impairs the normal expansion of the lungs and is often associated with underlying pulmonary injuries such as a contusion or pneumothorax

  4. *Abdominal trauma*

    a. Injury to the abdomen may cause a multitude of complications in the trauma client because of the numerous organs and major blood vessels located within the cavity

    b. In the event that a specific determination of the organ involved cannot be made initially, basic life support and shock management should take precedence

    c. After a specific diagnosis is made to the injured organ, the functional limitation of the organ(s) should be considered and included in the continuing plan of care

d. Any rupture of an abdominal organism should include focus on the spillage of organ contents into the abdominal cavity that may result in infectious or chemical peritonitis

1) Liver: injuries to this organ may result through blunt or penetrating trauma

    a) The liver is a large reservoir of blood, so significant injury to this organ may cause a hypovolemic crisis

    b) Contusions and hemorrhaging within this organ may be insidious in nature and signs and symptoms may not initially appear

    c) Liver injury should be suspected in the presence of lower rib fractures, pulmonary trauma, and thoracic and abdominal injuries

2) Pancreas: injury to the pancreas from trauma carries a high risk of other associated injuries because of its location; hypovolemia may result as well as injury to the surrounding organs from released pancreatic fluids and its digestive enzymes

3) Spleen: injury to the spleen may result from blunt or penetrating sources and is a significant source of hemorrhaging

    a) As a part of the lymph system, the spleen is not essential to maintenance of vital life functions and may be removed

    b) Acute injury may result in hypovolemia

    c) Injury in clients that have previously enlarged spleens, such as pregnant women and those suffering from mononucleosis, occurs with greater ease

4) Bowel: bowel injury may be specific to the small or large intestines

    a) Both areas may be injured by blunt or penetrating sources, however, the large bowel, or colon, is more often associated with abdominal trauma

    b) Trauma to the colon is frequently associated with peritonitis from the introduction of intracolonic bacteria being released into the abdominal cavity

5) Stomach: injury to the stomach is a rare finding in trauma, probably as a result of its location within the protective shell of the rib cage

    a) Penetrating injuries, such as gun shots, comprise the majority of gastric injuries associated with trauma

    b) Because of its anatomical location, injury to the spleen is very often associated with stomach trauma

    c) Damage may cause the spillage of gastric juices and air into the surrounding cavities

5. *Genitourinary trauma* (closely associated with abdominal trauma)

a. Renal trauma: the kidneys are well protected by the spinal column and ribs, however, traumatic injury may result from blunt or penetrating forces

1) Because the kidneys are somewhat "free-floating" in nature they can be jostled, resulting in hematuria with minimal trauma

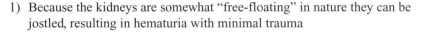

2) The renal system is also prone to significant damage as a result of diminished blood flow secondary to shock

3) In the presence of identified abdominal, thoracic, or pulmonary trauma, injury to the renal system should be highly suspected even without the finding of hematuria

4) Most renal injuries are minor in nature, but profound blood loss may occur with vessel tearing or rupture

5) Injuries to the ureter are very rare and are usually penetrating in nature

b. Bladder trauma: bladder trauma is most often associated with blunt trauma, however, penetrating injury may result from external forces as well as from fractures of the pelvis

1) Rupture of the bladder occurs most often in the presence of a distended, full bladder at the time of injury

2) While the bladder is not viewed as a significant source of bleeding, injury to this organ should be analyzed in conjunction with pelvic injuries that may cause gross hemorrhaging; its location near the great pelvic vessels warrants high levels of attention in assessment

c. Urethral trauma: trauma to the urethra is somewhat uncommon and usually associated with blunt injury in males

1) "Saddle"-type injuries may occur in both females and males wherein the pubis symphysis impacts an object while decelerating, such as a steering column or cross beam

2) Pelvic fractures are often associated with urethral injury

6. *Fractures*

a. A break in the continuity of any bone is considered a fracture

b. Fractures result when the bone cannot withstand the exertion of mechanical forces being exerted upon it; the force may be direct or indirect in nature, such as spontaneous fractures that occur when body weight upon standing alone is enough to injure weakened bony matter

c. When the integrity of the bone is broken, there is hemorrhaging within the site that begins the inflammatory process

d. Swelling causes pain and influences movement of surrounding muscles and tissues

e. Severe fractures may impinge on neurological innervation and/or may compromise blood flow to the extremity involved

NCLEX!

1) Compartment syndrome can occur: any excess swelling or pressure that constricts blood flow to the muscles and nerves

2) Hypoxemia and cellular death may result at the site and distal to the injury, creating a potential loss of limb

f. Fractures near great vessels that tear or rupture as a result of the injury may also cause secondary hemorrhaging creating a hypovolemic state

g. Large bone fractures such as the pelvis or femur may create a hypovolemic state due to the blood loss from the bone itself

h. *Spinal fractures*

1) Fractures to the spinal column at the cervical level are generally the result of deceleration and acceleration which flex, hyperextend, or rotate the neck

2) Penetrating or crushing injuries are more common below the cervical spine

3) Vertebral fractures may completely sever the spinal cord, resulting in paralysis below the site of the break

4) Disruption of the blood supply to the cord may also cause permanent damage

5) The extent and location of the fracture determines the degree of system impairment and results from damage to the pathways extending from the spinal cord to the organs and tissues they control

6) Injury to the spine may also be seen in post-traumatic states when ligaments and bones are unstable and subsequent maneuvering occurs

i. *Pelvic fractures*

1) Pelvic fractures occur most frequency in the elderly from low-velocity falls; these are generally closed, non-displaced

2) In younger, healthier individuals, high-velocity, deceleration injuries to the pelvis are seen as a result of motor vehicle accidents and falls

3) These injuries may be a significant source of hemorrhaging in and of themselves and may indicate a source of trauma for other systems such as the abdominal and urinary organs

4) Pelvic fractures and other long bone fractures are prone to the release of fat, potentially forming a life-threatening fat embolus

j. *Acetabulum, hip, and proximal femur fractures*

1) The proximal portion of the femur meets the pelvis at the acetabulum and forms the hip; this area of the body is prone to fracture within the geriatric population from falls or pathologic fractures, which occur as a result of porous bone density

2) The femur is the largest bone in the body and contains a significant amount of blood stored in the shaft; a great amount of force is needed to break this bone, and as such, assessment for other pelvis and knee injuries should be done

3) Because of their close location to the femoral vessels, injuries to these bones may also result in injury to arteries, veins, and innervation; hypovolemia may be of significant concern

4) Peripheral blood flow and neurological function to the lower extremities may be severely compromised

k. *Soft tissue injuries*

1) Soft tissue injuries are those injuries resulting in damage to tissues and their underlying vasculature

NCLEX!

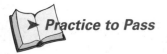

A client presents with a small caliber gunshot wound to the lower left lateral chest with signs and symptoms suggesting a pneumothorax and shock. No other injury is noted. What type of shock and pneumothorax is suspected and why?

NCLEX!

NCLEX!

NCLEX!

2) These may be crushing in nature or as a result of a puncture or **laceration** (injuries to soft tissue that result in a tearing or slicing of the skin and possibly the underlying fleshy structures)

3) These injuries may also be seen within industrial settings where liquid or air is utilized under high pressure

   a) The substance is introduced to the tissues at great volumes and under tremendous pressure

   b) Tissues are crushed, altering circulation in the area

4) Bone or ligament and tendon involvement are usually not seen in the presence of a primary diagnosis of tissue injury

5) Hemorrhage into the surrounding tissue at the site of the injury results in diminished perfusion to the area that may cause tissue necrosis or delayed healing

C. Nursing assessment

1. Multisystem injury that endangers the loss of life or limb requires rapid and sequential assessment and intervention for a successful outcome

2. Each primary assessment phase will correspond with an immediate intervention in the event that a deviation is discovered

   a. It must also be remembered that there are generally multiple members of a trauma team who will be assessing and intervening almost simultaneously

   b. A secondary assessment occurs after life-threatening injuries are maintained and airway, breathing, and circulation (ABC's) are restored

3. Treatment for a "higher" level system, such as the airway, should never be postponed in order to complete the entire sequence

4. Many hospitals utilize rapid assessment forms that allow for a determination of the intensity or severity of a trauma client's condition; these tools provide great assistance in organizing the most common needs of the clients found at differing levels of acuity

5. Assessment

   a. Pre-arrival

      1) Vital signs

      2) Focused injury findings

      3) Neurological status (to include if victim has lost consciousness)

      4) Machinery involved (includes type and caliber of weapon)

      5) Current medications, medical history, allergies

      6) Safety belt usage

      7) Mechanism of injury, time of injury

      8) Environmental factors such as chemical spills

      9) Tetanus immunization status if wounds are present

b. If there is no report available prior to the client's arrival, pertinent information should be gathered simultaneously with assessment of client's condition; *treatment should never be delayed secondary to an absent or incomplete history*

c. Information regarding the circumstances of the injury is important to rule out secondary and delayed manifestations of an injury, however, life support is carried out in the same and consistent manner for all victims of trauma

d. Upon arrival

NCLEX!

1) Assess airway and adequate ventilation through observation and auscultation; note deviations such as absence of breathing or inadequate ventilations and irregular depth or rate

2) Assess for vomitus or debris in the mouth

3) Assess for flail segments of the chest, diminished or absent breath sounds, presence of a deviated trachea (trachea is "pushed" to one side rather than the midline in the anterior neck), and the sounds of any air movement through a wound

4) Assess cardiac activity through gentle palpation of the carotid pulse and/or auscultation

5) Assess cardiac rhythms via a cardiac monitor for dysrhythmias

6) Assess for distant cardiac sounds, pericardial rub and the presence of distended jugular veins

7) Assess for obvious sources of hemorrhaging, to include the urethral meatus and the rectum

8) Be sure to include an assessment of the client's back while maintaining spinal alignment

9) Assess for signs and symptoms of shock, specifically hypovolemic or cardiogenic shock (close attention should be given to diminishing urinary output, as pulse and blood pressure may not alter dramatically until late shock is reached)

10) Assess neurological status for the level of responsiveness to include peripheral posturing, sensation and mobility

11) Assess pupillary size and response

12) Assess for paralysis and symmetry of movement

13) Rectal tone may be assessed for the presence of spinal cord injury

14) Assess for fractures with special attention provided to the thoracic, pelvic, and femoral areas

15) Assess for pain, shortening, and rotation of the legs commonly found in hip fractures

16) Assess peripheral pulses and extremity temperature and color

17) Assess for fracture variations and locations, numbering sites in the event there are multiple injuries; crushing injuries may mask displaced

bones, but may be threatening in and of themselves; areas of gross distention may produce a *compartment* or tourniquet effect at the site and distal to the injury, blocking blood flow and producing a limb-threatening emergency

6. Diagnostic tests

   a. Hemoglobin and hematocrit: hypovolemic shock is always a significant potential for the trauma client; decreasing levels and the rate of deterioration may indicate severe hemorrhaging

   b. White blood count: may elevate as a result of the inflammatory response to trauma or as a response to the presence of blood in the abdominal cavity, indicating a source of hemorrhage

   c. Arterial blood gases (ABGS): indicates respiratory failure and acid/base imbalances; used to direct supplemental oxygen therapy

      1) Respiratory failure is indicated by a $PO_2 < 50$ mmHg or a $PCO_2 > 50$ mmHg

      2) If the failure is acute in nature, the pH (normal 7.35 to 7.45) will fall as CO_2 is retained

   d. EKG: may reveal dysrhythmias requiring treatment or procedural interventions

   e. Cardiac enzymes: an elevation determines whether cardiac tissue damage has occurred

   f. Urinalysis: urine with microscopic hematuria may indicate minor to significant genitourinary trauma

   g. Blood alcohol: traumatic injuries are often associated with alcohol ingestion

      1) Severe intoxication compromises airway clearance and respiratory effort

      2) The client is at more risk for injury and it is important to differentiate diminished mentation from injury versus that brought on by intoxication or an abnormal glucose

   h. Glucose testing: hyperglycemia may be mistaken for alcohol intoxication upon presentation secondary to the pungent, fruity smell of the breath and the confusion clients typically exhibit

D. **Nursing management**

   1. Pre-arrival

      a. Organize ancillary staff such as additional nursing support, respiratory and radiology personnel and any other medical consultants based upon the client's status

      b. Equipment: organize equipment to include resuscitative equipment (crash cart with airway management equipment and medications), intravenous access equipment and fluid, urinary catheterization equipment, bandaging supplies, sterile water and basins, and lab specimen collectors and other supplies as needed for procedures such as cricothyrotomy, thoracostomy, thoracotomy, peritoneal lavage, and pericardiocentesis

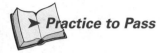

Practice to Pass

A client presents with a cast on the lower left arm because of a fracture from falling. The upper-left arm is severely bruised and distended, and the client is complaining of severe "pressure" to this area. What emergent condition could be related to the client's injuries?

2. Standard interventions

NCLEX!

NCLEX!

NCLEX!

    a. Trauma clients should receive assistance with ventilation in the form of supplemental oxygen

    b. Establishment of a venous access with a gauge appropriate to the intended fluids and treatment

    c. Cardiac monitoring and continuous/intermittent vital sign monitoring to include pulse oximetry

    d. Trauma clients should have alignment maintained at all times in the supine position; obvious deformities should be splinted and supported; slight elevation of the legs may be performed in the absence of head injury, cardiac decompensation or pulmonary edema/congestion

    e. Accurate observation of intake and output

        1) A urinary catheter should be inserted when accurate values are required

NCLEX!

        2) Do not insert a catheter when bleeding from the urethral meatus is noted or there is obvious hip and pelvic deformity until bladder injury is ruled out

    f. Document all assessments, interventions, and responses

    g. Maintain airway, circulation, and neurological assessment (see Table 17-7)

    h. Manage shock state

3. Fractures

    a. Medications include antibiotics, which may be given prophylactically for open wounds, and analgesics

    b. Support and split obvious fractures without manipulating or "reducing" (bending a fracture into alignment) the bone, utilizing pillows, folded linens, and tape

    c. Release any constricting garments or splints without manipulating the fractured area, frequently performing neurovascular checks distal to the site of injury

> **▶ Practice to Pass**
>
> A pre-hospital report by emergency medical personnel indicates a near-drowning victim who dove head first into shallow waters. What preparations, including department contacts, would be made prior to the client's arrival?

Table 17-7   **Nursing Management of Trauma**

Airway	Circulation	Neurological
• Establish and maintain adequate airway • Use supplemental oxygen • Remove debris with tongue depressor and suction • Utilize airway supplements such as oropharyngeal or endotracheal tubes • Utilize nasal intubation if cervical injury suspected • Prepare for thoracostomy (chest tube) if needed	• Monitor for cardiac dysrhythmias • Prepare to administer medications and perform procedures specific to arrhythmia, such as defibrillation • Prepare for a thoracotomy if necessary • Pericardiocentesis may be needed if cardiac tamponade is evident • Monitor vital signs every 5 to 15 minutes	• Assess neurological status every 15 minutes as needed • Medications include osmotic diuretics and steroids for cerebral edema; antibiotics for open head injury • Maintain immobile and aligned cervical spine while neurological assessment is unstable • Restrict fluids if level of consciousness is changing and shock is not evident • Use hyperventilation to lower cerebral edema • Control seizures

    d. Ice may be applied to cool the area, avoiding direct contact with the skin or injured area

    e. In the presence of an open or suspected open fracture, sterile, saline-soaked gauze should be applied until a through cleansing of the area is accomplished

  4. Hemorrhaging

    a. Obvious sources of external hemorrhaging should be gentle, direct pressure applied through moist, sterile bandaging

    b. A hemothorax may contain over one liter of blood and may constitute a significant source of volume loss; a thoracostomy tube may be inserted and an autotransfusion may be performed

    c. Bleeding from within the abdomen and retroperitoneum may occur with or without abdominal distention and rigidity until late into the shock sequence; peritoneal lavage may be performed to determine the presence of blood

    d. Fractures of the pelvis and femur are also capable of producing profound hypovolemic states; as with all states of hypovolemia, treatment is guided by restoration of the intravascular volume through administration of crystalloids or colloids, to include blood, and by administration of sympathomimetics

IV. Disseminated Intravascular Coagulopathy (DIC)

A. Overview

  1. **Disseminated intravascular coagulopathy (DIC)** is a complex and abnormal process of the body's normal clotting mechanisms in response to an injury

  2. Clotting processes are overwhelmed, resulting in the depletion of normal clotting mechanisms, leaving the organism open to massive hemorrhaging

  3. DIC may become a complicating side effect in some forms of shock, most commonly with septic shock; it is secondary to other disorders

  4. High mortality rate

  5. Causes of DIC include sepsis, shock, malignant neoplasms, liver disease, metabolic disorders, circulatory disorders, gynecological conditions, spinal or brain injuries, transfusion reactions and immune disorders including venomous bites

B. Pathophysiology

  1. In healthy individuals, homeostasis is maintained between vessel injury and bleeding with appropriate and encapsulated areas of clot formation; clotting only becomes a problem when no injury has been sustained or when hemorrhaging depletes the organism's reservoir of clotting factors

  2. The intrinsic and/or extrinsic clotting pathways are activated in response to a traumatic injury

  3. Thromboplastin is released from damaged cells and as a result, platelets begin to adhere to the damaged vessel or blood cell forming a "barrier" to prevent further hemorrhaging and injury

  4. A plug of fibrinogen and fibrin is stabilized at the site of the injury through the processes of normal clot formation; the clot or plug is then removed through a process called **fibrinolysis** (process by which a clot is broken down)

5. The process of fibrinolysis may occur immediately or days after an injury and causes the release of fibrin degradation products (FDPs) and fibrin degradation fragments (FDFs); in healthy individuals or those suffering only minor injuries, the process is restricted to the area of injury

6. Clients suffering from massive tissue and cellular damage, such as traumatic or shock states, deplete the clotting factors as they are used up in an attempt to prevent further hemorrhaging

7. This cycle becomes self-defeating in that circulating fibrin clots become widespread throughout the body's intravascular volume, often causing widespread thrombosis (blood clots in the bloodstream)

8. Thrombi indicate to the body that further damage is occurring and the body responds by releasing more clotting factors until, finally, massive hemorrhaging occurs; circulating FDPs also have an anticoagulant affect, exacerbating the scenario

9. The client is hemorrhaging at a life-threatening level, while at the same time clotting extensively in an unrelenting cycle

10. Signs and symptoms

   a. Decreased blood pressure and peripheral pulses

   b. Purpura, ecchymosis, petechiae

   c. Cyanosis and bleeding that may range from mild oozing around catheter/IV sites and oral mucosa to profound volume loss noted by occult blood in the stool or vomitus and hematuria

   d. Intraabdominal bleeding may manifest itself with pain, distention, and rigidity

   e. Hypoxemia

   f. Dyspnea, air hunger

   g. Neurologic symptoms: confusion, decreased level of consciousness (LOC), seizures

   h. Renal symptoms: oliguria

   i. GI symptoms: nausea, vomiting

   j. Epistaxis

   k. Seizures

   l. Pain: chest, muscles, back, and abdomen

C. Nursing Assessment

1. Assessment

   a. Risk: any client who presents with obvious signs and symptoms of frank hemorrhaging without obvious injury; or conditions that predispose an individual such as shock, septicemia, or those receiving blood products

   b. Assessment includes VS, pulses, cardiac status, respiratory status, assessment of all orifices and venipuncture sites, symptom analysis of pain, skin color, capillary refill, mentation, urinary output, GI complaints

2. Diagnostic tests

   a. Prothrombin (PT) and partial thromboplastin time (PTT): both elevated

   b. Fibrin degradation products (FDP) and fibrin degradation fragments (FDF): both elevated

Practice to Pass

A client presents with frank hematuria, bleeding from the gums, and an elevated prothrombin time and partial thromboplastin time. What other diagnostic test may be ordered to support a diagnosis of disseminated intravascular coagulopathy (DIC) versus another coagulation abnormality and why?

    c. D-dimer test will be elevated

       1) Serial testing is very important and assists in determining the diagnosis of DIC as opposed to other bleeding disorders

       2) A steady increase in these values indicates ongoing, massive clot breakdown rather than a lack of clotting factors

    d. CBC

    e. Electrolyte panel

    f. BUN, creatinine (CR)

D. Nursing management

NCLEX!

    1. Medications include heparin (in some clients) to neutralize the effects of circulating thrombin

      a. However, the administration of heparin should be utilized with great care and only when extreme circumstances warrant its use

      b. Generally this anticoagulant is administered when DIC is not rapidly reversed through treatment of the underlying cause or in those individuals who are threatened by bleeding or massive thrombis formation

    2. It is important to treat the underlying cause of DIC as quickly as possible and treat for a shock state that has precipitated the crisis

NCLEX!

    3. Fresh frozen plasma and cryoprecipitate are administered to replace coagulation factors

    4. Monitor coagulation tests not only for diagnosis, but for treatment

---

Case Study

A trauma victim presents after a motor vehicle accident in which the pre-hospital report indicates that the steering wheel in the car was broken and no seat belts were worn. Vital signs are BP 100/58, pulse 116, respirations 26 and labored, temperature 97.2°F oral. The client is intermittently confused and is lethargic. There is a 6-inch laceration to the frontal scalp. Pupils are equal and reactive. Upon exam, there is a large ecchymotic area to the right anterior chest and paradoxical movement is noted. Breath sounds are absent to the right base, anteriorly and posteriorly. The right leg is externally rotated and shortened.

❶ What fundamental interventions would be initiated immediately upon arrival based on this information?

❷ What procedures would potentially be performed?

❸ What phase and type of shock is suspected on presentation? What diagnostic values would contribute to determining the phase and type?

❹ What are the potential injuries that are most highly suspected of contributing to the shock state?

❺ What physical finding would cause concern when determining whether to place a urinary catheter for accurate output monitoring?

For suggested responses, see page 571.

Posttest

1 A client presents with suspected chest and spinal injuries after a motor vehicle accident. On receipt of the client from ambulance personnel, which of the following should take precedence in interventions?

(1) Preparaing spinal traction to align the head and spinal cord
(2) Clearing and maintaining a patent airway
(3) Applying pressure to areas of gross hemorrhaging
(4) Auscultating and inspecting the chest for the presence of pneumothorax or tamponade

2 Serial hematocrit and hemoglobin measurements are necessary to gauge treatment associated most commonly with which of the following shock states?

(1) Hypovolemic
(2) Cardiogenic
(3) Anaphylactic
(4) Distributive

3 Hemodynamic stability is maintained through a delicate balance between several factors. Mean arterial pressure (MAP) is increased through which of the following?

(1) An increase in intravascular volume
(2) A decrease in atrial volume
(3) An increase in pulmonary tension
(4) A decrease in peripheral vasoconstriction

4 A client has suffered from hypovolemic shock. Understanding the effects that a shock state has on multiple systems within the body, which indicator would prioritize the ongoing plan of care?

(1) Urinary output
(2) Skin turgor
(3) Range of mobility
(4) Temperature

5 A client involved in a motor vehicle accident is brought by ambulance to the trauma unit. She was thrown against the left side of her car, which has standard hand cranks for the window. Her abdomen is distended and painful to touch, her hematocrit and hemoglobin (H&H) are low, and BP 80/50. Which of the following would be the nurse's major concern?

(1) Head injury.
(2) Spontaneous pneumothorax.
(3) Ruptured liver or spleen.
(4) Ruptured kidney.

6 Which of the following forms of hemorrhaging within the brain tissue is generally caused by venous system damage and is more common?

(1) Intracerebral hematoma
(2) Epidural hematoma
(3) Subdural hematoma
(4) Brain stem hematoma

7 A client presents to the emergency department with a gunshot wound to the upper anterior left chest. The assessment performed after stabilization of life-threatening injuries would be known as the:

(1) Primary assessment.
(2) Secondary assessment.
(3) Life function assessment.
(4) Vital function assessment.

8 When evaluating the status of a client who is recovering from hypovolemic shock that was treated by the administration of colloids, which indicators would show the best outcome?

(1) Vital signs, hematocrit and hemoglobin (H&H), and coagulation tests within normal limits
(2) Vital signs and a hematocrit and hemoglobin (H&H) level within normal limits and a urinalysis without hematuria
(3) Vital signs and a hematocrit and hemoglobin (H&H) level within normal limits and a negative C-spine x-ray
(4) Vital signs and neurological exam within normal limits

9   A client suffering from a fracture of a long bone such as the femur is at greater risk for suffering which of the following complications?

(1) Disuse syndrome
(2) Fat embolism syndrome
(3) Reflex sympathetic dystrophy
(4) Infection

10   Successful outcome measurements for a client suffering from an open trauma to the head includes the:

(1) Recall of the actual event of injury.
(2) Loss of consciousness of no greater than 24 hours.
(3) Absence of signs of meningitis.
(4) Absence of pain.

See pages 553–554 for Answers and Rationales.

Answers and Rationales

Pretest

1   **Answer: 2** *Rationale:* All forms of pneumothoraces may progress to the extent that tension develops within the affected lung space and exerts pressure on the unaffected lung. A deviated trachea is a classic sign of tension pneumothorax.
Cognitive Level: Application
Nursing Process: Assessment; *Test Plan:* PHYS

2   **Answer: 4** *Rationale:* Aspiration of any liquid into the lungs places the client at risk for development of ARDS. Assessments to evaluate the onset of this syndrome should focus on the respiratory system and diminishing oxygen saturation despite increasing supplemental oxygen.
Cognitive Level: Analysis
Nursing Process: Assessment; *Test Plan:* PHYS

3   **Answer: 2** *Rationale:* During the compensatory phase of shock, the body attempts to correct the progression of a decrease in intravascular volume through an increase in pulse and respiration and the subjective sensation of thirst. Shunting of blood begins to occur from organs not vital for immediate survival. Renal blood flow is diminished and urinary output falls. Blood pressure is decreasing but adequate for current homeostasis.
Cognitive Level: Analysis
Nursing Process: Analysis; *Test Plan:* PHYS

4   **Answer: 4** *Rationale:* The presenting signs and symptoms are associated with the compensatory phase of shock. Myocardial infarction is the most common cause of cardiac damage resulting in cardiac insufficiency or "pump failure." Jugular venous dis-

tention and pulmonary congestion are consistent with heart failure.
Cognitive Level: Analysis
Nursing Process: Assessment; *Test Plan:* PHYS

5   **Answer: 2** *Rationale:* The client is exhibiting the standard immunological reaction to the administration of an antibiotic. Sensitizing dosages have already occurred as reported by the client. Anaphylactic shock is a form of distributive shock. More information is needed to determine that this client is developing septicemia.
Cognitive Level: Application
Nursing Process: Analysis; *Test Plan:* PHYS

6   **Answer: 3** *Rationale:* Cervical and spinal injuries are often associated with trauma to the head, chest, and upper back, as well as falls and deceleration incidents.
Cognitive Level: Analysis
Nursing Process: Analysis; *Test Plan:* PHYS

7   **Answer: 2** *Rationale:* Paradoxical pulses, or pulsus paradoxus, is a hallmark symptom of cardiac tamponade. As pressure is exerted on the left ventricle from fluid, the natural increase in pressure from the right ventricle during inspiration creates even more pressure, diminishing cardiac output. A deviated trachea is a sign of a tension pneumothorax, and a narrowing pulse pressure would be seen in tamponade (option 4). Atelectasis is not associated with tamponade.
Cognitive Level: Analysis
Nursing Process: Analysis; *Test Plan:* PHYS

8   **Answer: 2** *Rationale:* Penetrating injury to the bowel releases intracolonic material into the peritoneal cavity, predisposing the individual to a serious

infection that may progress to septicemia. While a paralytic ileus is of concern any time the abdominal cavity has been accessed through surgery or injury or with the administration of certain medications, it is not of the life-threatening nature that is found with the diagnosis of peritonitis. Peritonitis may cause the occurrence of a paralytic ileus.
Cognitive Level: Application
Nursing Process: Analysis; *Test Plan:* PHYS

9 **Answer: 3** *Rationale:* Many traumatic injuries occur as a result of the slowed responses and judgement associated with alcohol intoxication. Hyperglycemia may exhibit similar signs and symptoms of intoxication so it is necessary to assess both values. Skull x-rays are noncontributory for brain injuries unless there is an obvious or highly suspected fracture. CAT scans are reserved for obvious or highly suspected injuries to the brain itself that are generally accompanied by some alteration in consciousness surrounding the incident. An EEG measures the electrical brain waves to determine brain death or some type of seizure and abnormal cerebral activity.
Cognitive Level: Application
Nursing Process: Assessment; *Test Plan:* PHYS

10 **Answer: 4** *Rationale:* Compartment syndrome is a result of swelling or pressure that constricts blood flow to musculature and nerves. Hemorrhaging and loss of intravascular fluid to the interstitial spaces creates a tourniquet effect, compromising the circulation at the site of injury and distally.
Cognitive Level: Application
Nursing Process: Assessment; *Test Plan:* PHYS

Posttest

1 **Answer: 2** *Rationale:* The client's airway is priority in all phases of life support. Remember, a trauma team usually consists of many people and others can be assessing less critical areas.
Cognitive Level: Application
Nursing Process: Implementation; *Test Plan:* SECE

2 **Answer: 1** *Rationale:* Hematocrit and hemoglobin levels will continue to decrease with ongoing hemorrhaging indicating the aggressiveness of interventions to replace intravascular volume.
Cognitive Level: Application
Nursing Process: Assessment; *Test Plan:* PHYS

3 **Answer: 1** *Rationale:* Mean arterial pressure (MAP) elevates with any increase in cardiac output, systemic vascular resistance, or blood volume. Va-

sodilation decreases resistance, thereby diminishing MAP.
Cognitive Level: Application
Nursing Process: Analysis; *Test Plan:* PHYS

4 **Answer: 1** *Rationale:* All forms of shock diminish perfusion to the renal system. A decreasing output is indicative that the kidneys may be losing function as a result of significant tubular necrosis.
Cognitive Level: Application
Nursing Process: Planning; *Test Plan:* PHYS

5 **Answer: 3** *Rationale:* A distended, painful abdomen with signs of hypovolemic shock should trigger the nurse to consider a ruptured liver or spleen. Although a ruptured kidney could also occur, the major concern would be the liver because of its vascular nature. A head injury or pneumothorax should be assessed next.
Cognitive Level: Analysis
Nursing Process: Assessment; *Test Plan:* PHYS

6 **Answer: 3** *Rationale:* Subdural hematomas are formed most often from venous tissue bleeding and are more common than other forms of brain injury. They may occur without direct trauma. Epidural hematomas are more associated with arterial bleeding above the dural space.
Cognitive Level: Application
Nursing Process: Assessment; *Test Plan:* PHYS

7 **Answer: 2** *Rationale:* A secondary assessment occurs once the airway, breathing and circulation (primary) are assessed and interventions begun. Life-threatening injuries located during the primary assessment must be stabilized prior to reviewing for additional injuries or wounds.
Cognitive Level: Application
Nursing Process: Assessment; *Test Plan:* PHYS

8 **Answer: 1** *Rationale:* Administering colloidal solutions may diminish the blood's ability to coagulate by reducing platelet adhesion while expanding the intravascular volume needed in severe shock states. Vital signs within established parameters indicates support of vital functions. Acceptable hematocrit and hemoglobin levels substantiate and support perfusion at a cellular level as well as resolution of volume loss. The presence or lack of hematuria is not a viable indicator of the level of shock states or their resolution.
Cognitive Level: Analysis
Nursing Process: Evaluation; *Test Plan:* PHYS

9 **Answer: 2** *Rationale:* Fat is more easily expressed from the larger bones such as the hip and femur when they are fractured. Other answers are not associated with a specific bone group.
Cognitive Level: Application
Nursing Process: Analysis; *Test Plan:* PHYS

10 **Answer: 3** *Rationale:* An injury to the protective tissues of the brain poses a risk for infection in that bacterium can be introduced, especially with an open injury. Meningitis would be the manifestation exhibited.
Cognitive Level: Analysis
Nursing Process: Evaluation; *Test Plan:* PHYS

References

Bullock, B. A. & Henze, R. L. (2000). *Focus on pathophysiology*. Philadelphia: Lippincott, pp. 503–517, 938–962.

Kee, J. L. (1999). *Laboratory and diagnostic tests* (5th ed.). Stamford, CT: Appleton & Lange.

LeMone, P. & Burke, K. (2000). *Medical-surgical nursing: Critical thinking in client care* (2nd ed.). Upper Saddle River, NJ: Prentice Hall, pp. 163–179, 377–390, 799–801, 1166, 1295–1297, 1472–1502, 1583–1599, 1737–1793.

Porth, C. (1998). *Pathophysiology: Concepts of altered health states* (5th ed.). Philadelphia: Lippincott, pp. 291, 442–450.

Thomas, C. (1999). *Taber's cyclopedic medical dictionary* (19th ed.). Philadelphia: F.A. Davis Co.

Appendix

➤ **Practice to Pass Suggested Answers**

Chapter 1

Page 10: *Solution*—Beclomethasone (Vanceril) is a steroid; a common as well as concerning side effect in children is growth retardation. A child's asthma may require a medication on a daily basis as strong as the steroids. A decline in height and weight has been documented while children are on continuous doses of steroid therapy and these should be monitored monthly.

Page 10: *Solution*—Steroids such as prednisone are often used for exacerbations of COPD with effective results. A side effect of steroids, however, is fluid retention, which could easily occur in a cardiac client with a history of CHF. Careful monitoring of intake and output, weight, presence of edema, and lung sounds should be implemented in order to identify early signs of CHF should they occur.

Page 15: *Solution*—ARDS often occurs suddenly and is extremely fatiguing for the client. A client already stressed because of an acute MI doesn't need the additional respiratory stress, nor can their body tolerate extreme respiratory difficulty for long periods. Insufficient oxygenation coupled with a heart that has impaired circulation could be fatal. Treatment should be quick in order to prevent further complications.

Page 18: *Solution*—Either the antibiotic is not the correct treatment for the type of organism causing the pneumonia or the pneumonia is viral in nature. A culture and sensitivity should be obtained to identify the organism causing the problem and to ensure sensitivity of the antibiotic to the organism. If the problem is viral pneumonia, antibiotics will not usually help anyway. Any time fever persists after an individual has been on an antibiotic for at least 72 hours, additional considerations should be made.

Page 20: *Solution*—Remember that two groups at risk for tuberculosis are the disadvantaged and HIV-positive individuals. This client carries those risk factors and could be HIV-positive without knowing at this time. Also, females with sexually transmitted diseases (STDs) often test positive for resistant strains of TB.

Chapter 2

Page 46: *Solution*—The fact that she has CAD does not mean she has had damage (injury) to the heart muscle itself. CAD indicates blockage in the arteries that bring blood to the heart and supply the needed oxygen. She can live with coronary artery disease and never have a heart attack if she modifies her lifestyle and corrects the behaviors that lead to CAD. The symptoms of a heart attack need to be explained (nausea, vomiting, crushing chest pain, shortness of breath, diaphoresis) as well as the difference between angina and a myocardial infarction.

Page 48: *Solution*—The nurse should explain to the client that having stable angina does not mean that the client will have a heart attack. As long as the causes of the pain are known and it stops with rest or responds to nitroglycerin, it should not cause permanent injury to the heart. However, if the pain changes in duration or intensity, or if the number of attacks increases, a healthcare provider should be seen as soon as possible. During an angina attack, if the pain stays longer, is more intense, or does not respond to rest or nitroglycerin, call for emergency help.

Page 52: *Solution*—An example of an acceptable response might be: "I know you feel that way, but now that you are here we can help you. Try to take deep, even breaths. We will give you some medication to help with the pain." Explain the procedures that are being ordered and what appears to be happening. Also explain that the feeling is normal when someone is having chest discomfort and shortness of breath. Do not offer false reassurance that everything will be all right when it may not.

Page 60: *Solution*—The nurse should explain to the client that he has been very ill and it will take some time for his body to return to normal. The doctor should talk to him about follow-up care. It is important that he follow the directions and rehabilitation schedule and not try to return to work too soon or further problems or complications may develop. An appropriate explanation and comparison for clients with heart problems is to compare it to a broken leg. The broken bone cannot always be seen, but it's still there and takes 6 to 8 weeks to heal. The crutches are often the only reminder of the problem. The heart needs time to heal also and the signs and symptoms experienced are the only reminders of the problem. The client should check with the physician as to when the proper time is to return to work.

Page 74: *Solution*—The nurse should go immediately to the room and assess the client. If he is unresponsive and pulseless, call a code and call for the crash cart and defibrillator. If the client is awake, alert, and talking, check the monitor leads for proper connection. Chaotic activity could be caused by ventricular fibrillation, interference, a disconnected lead wire, a loose monitor pad, or activity such as bathing or respiratory percussion. Regardless, the client should always be assessed first.

Page 79: *Solution*—Inform the client that close follow-up care is needed. The disease progression must be monitored, as well as how well the client tolerates the progression. The client will have many tests done to determine the progression. If signs of congestive heart failure begin, the client will be treated with medication to help the heart beat more effectively. If angina occurs, clients often respond to beta blockers and nitroglycerin. Sometimes it is necessary to have a valve replaced. That is a decision that the client and the doctor must make together. The client must know that prior to any invasive procedure (including dental procedures), prophylactic antibiotics must be taken to prevent infection from getting to the valve and causing further problems or complications.

Chapter 3

Page 95: *Solution*—Discuss with the client what the client means by forgetting medicines and making up the dose at the next medication time. It would be very helpful to determine which medications the client is taking in this manner—prescription drugs, an over-the-counter medicine, or some alternative medicine. The nurse should review the medication schedule with the client. The primary outcome is to have the client's blood pressure reading be less than 140/90. Ask the client and family members if the medication schedule is convenient. Also, the purpose of each medication should be reviewed with the client and family members. The nurse should determine if the client is experiencing any side effects. If so, the nurse should ask which medications are involved, how long these problems have been present, and whether the client has notified the healthcare provider. Writing medication schedules on a card or pre-pouring the medicines for the client

on a weekly basis might take the confusion out of the schedule. Determine if the client can adequately read and see the medication labels in order to read the dosage and times. If the client cannot read, pictures or a video describing what is to be done and how should be provided. If the client cannot see to read the names of the medications, specific directions could be developed by the nurse and big numbers used to indicate the time of day the medicine is to be taken. In addition, a referral to a home health agency for supervisory visits focused on medication compliance might be helpful. Time for client questions should be provided.

Page 98: *Solution*—The focus of the plan of care is to assist the client in the prevention and reduction of risk factors. This may be accomplished by:

- Avoiding sitting or standing in one place for prolonged periods of time. Frequently, support hose will help manage venous congestion.
- Avoiding the use of round garters and the wearing of tight abdominal garments, which constrict blood flow.
- Elevating the legs while sitting if venous congestion is a problem.
- Encouraging the client to beginning walking and gradually increase distance up to 1 mile per day.
- Weight loss, if the client is obese. A referral to a weight reduction program within the community.
- Suggesting the adding of bulk to the diet to eliminate constipation to prevent straining and following a healthy-heart diet low in sodium, cholesterol, and fat.
- Discussing the cessation of smoking and limiting caffeine if these are present factors. Explain that cardiac disease such as congestive heart failure, myocardial infarction, and cardiomyopathy are risk factors for PVD and that PVD can lead to a thrombus or emboli.
- Educating the client on maintaining a normal blood pressure and having it monitored frequently if hypertension exists.

Page 101: *Solution*—The family should be commended on their concern and the nurse should identify that their concern is very important. Explain that surgery to repair an aneurysm is a serious operation and should not be considered lightly. The major complications are hemorrhage, stroke, and possibly death. Explain that an aneurysm that is not growing larger or leaking is often better left alone. The client should be compliant in having the MRIs every 6 months and keeping weight and blood pressure under control. Surgery is usually recommended when the aneurysm is at 5 cm (or greater) or shows signs of rapid growth or hemorrhage. Stress that the surgery will be a major operation for a 70-year-old individual; therefore, careful consideration should be made when the time is appropriate. The family should be instructed to seek medical advice if the back pain worsens or continues.

Page 107: *Solution*—Smoking is a primary cause of Buerger's disease, whereas genetics or unknown etiology is associated with Raynaud's disease. Raynaud's disease affects women more than men, while Buerger's affects mostly men. Raynaud's is usually triggered by stress or cold temperatures, while smoking triggers

Buerger's disease. Raynaud's involves the digits mostly and more commonly the hands, while Buerger's usually affects the lower extremities. The blue-white-red color changes in the hands are classic for Raynaud's. Intermittent claudication is associated with Buerger's disease. Clients with either disease should stop smoking to limit the events and protect the extremities from cold injury during an event.

Chapter 4

Page 129: *Solution*—Encourage discussion of concerns and major goals of rehabilitation based on the client goals. These may include improved mobility, maintenance of range-of-motion, self-care, bladder and bowel control, improved communication, optimal family functioning, and prevention of complications and repeated stroke. Stress that the goal of rehabilitation is to allow the client to learn his or her strengths and limitations and hopefully improve on the latter. The family should be encouraged to support the healthcare professionals and not to offer to "do things" for their loved one. Explain that an acute care setting usually offers a lot of assistance during the acute phase versus a rehabilitation facility that encourages the client to perform their own ADLs under supervision.

Page 140: *Solution*—Consult and follow the Infection Control Policies and Procedures recommended by the facility. Isolation is no longer recommended in most cases. Careful "standard precautions" are always important to protect the client and nurse with the exception of meningicoccal meningitis. Good handwashing, use of gloves, and proper disposal of waste products should be initiated. Small infants and pregnant women should always avoid any potential risk.

Page 145: *Solution*—Review the procedure with the client to assess understanding and emphasize that there is no pain involved; provide open-ended questions to encourage discussion; recommend washing hair to decrease oil and avoid gels or hairspray; no sedatives or hypnotics should be administered beforehand, except as part of the EEG study; do not allow client to fast before study or to use stimulants like caffinated drinks or coffee; clarify with physician if any routine medications are to be held; explain what the placement of the electrodes means.

Page 147: *Solution*—

- Ineffective airway clearance, ineffective breathing pattern, impaired gas exchange
- Impaired physical mobility
- Self-care deficit
- Altered nutrition: less than body requirements
- Elimination: constipation, diarrhea, urinary retention
- Risk for infection
- Risk for impaired skin integrity
- Impaired verbal communication (if tracheostomy)
- Pain
- Anxiety
- Powerlessness

Page 153: *Solution*—Assess the nature of the swallowing difficulty. Is the client having difficulty swallowing liquids and/or solids or chewing his food?

- Sit the client upright to eat and at least 30 to 45 minutes after eating.
- Observe the client swallow a sip of water; note coughing during and after eating.
- Observe as the client projects the tongue and moves it back and forth; refer to speech therapist for thorough evaluation; assist client to erect sitting position.
- Stay with the client while eating; cut food in small bites.
- Teach the client to think through the act of swallowing: close lips with teeth together, move the tongue up to the roof of the mouth with food on it; swallow with head bent forward.
- Try soft foods and thickened liquids.
- Massage client's face and neck muscles before eating.

Chapter 5

Page 175: *Solution*—The most effective way to increase joint mobility and maintain joint function is to participate in a regular exercise program and implement measures that decrease joint stress. The regular exercise program should be developed in collaboration with a physical therapist and include isometric exercises, PROM, and AROM. Some examples of measures that will decrease joint stress include: pacing activities, performing activities when sitting if possible, using a splint for hands and wrists, and relaxation techniques. Water aerobics are significantly helpful, especially to elderly clients.

Page 177: *Solution*—To determine the appropriate pharmacological therapy in the client diagnosed with gouty arthritis it is important to know if elevated levels of uric acid are related to an increase in the production of uric acid or a decrease in the excretion of uric acid. A 24-hour urine specimen is collected to determine if the client is excreting normal levels of uric acid, 200 to 750 cc/ 24 hrs. A level that exceeds 750 cc/24 hrs indicates that the production of uric acid is increased, levels below 200 cc/24 hrs indicate that the excretion of uric acid is impaired.

Page 180: *Solution*—Bone deformities occur in Paget's disease as a result of excessive bone remodeling. Normal bone marrow is replaced with vascular, fibrous connective tissue and bones eventually enlarge. Often one of the first symptoms of Paget's disease is of increased head size.

Page 186: *Solution*—The following factors differentiate these bone tumors; growth rate, age of onset, tissue origin, and location. All three bone tumors are classified as primary bone tumors: chondrosarcomas are characterized by slow growth; Ewing's sarcomas and osteosarcomas are characterized by rapid growth; Ewing's sarcomas metastasize to the lung tissue. Chondrosarcomas occur more frequently in adult males, the other two primary bone tumors occur more frequently in young males during periods of optimal growth, 10 to 25 years of age. The tissue of origin for osteosarcomas is the metaphysis of long bones and they are usually found in the distal femur, proximal tibia, and proximal humerus following an injury. The tissue of origin for chondrosarcomas is cartilage located in the pelvis, femur, and humerus. Ewing's sarcomas originate in the nerve tissue within the bone marrow, located in the pelvis, humerus, ribs, and femur.

Page 192: *Solution—*

Nursing diagnosis: Knowledge deficit related to cast care

Goal: Client and significant other will care for cast correctly and report problems to healthcare provider for early intervention.

Interventions: Instruct client and caregiver on the following:

* Keep cast supported on pillows while drying.
* Report increase in pain, decrease in movement, changes in color, coolness of fingers, loss of sensation, and/ or increased swelling.
* Apply ice directly over fracture for first 24 hours.
* Elevate the cast on pillows and expose to air while drying.
* Check areas of skin at cast edges for skin breakdown, provide padding as needed.
* Do not place any objects in the cast; use a blowdryer on cool setting for itching.
* Report drainage or odor from cast.
* Wear a sling to support the arm.
* Keep cast dry; cover with a plastic bag during bathing.

Chapter 6

Page 206: *Solution—*Explain to the client that open-angle glaucoma is a treatable condition and that blindness is not an inevitable result. Careful physician monitoring of intraocular pressure along with strict compliance to the medical regimen (i.e., use of prescribed beta adrenergic eye drops, miotics, and/or carbonic anhydrase inhibitors) will preserve sight.

Page 208: *Solution—*Postoperative instructions should include the importance of strict compliance with the administration of prescribed eye drops, the need to leave the eye covered between administration of eye drops, the need to avoid bending over, and the importance of sleeping on the non-operative side.

Page 212: *Solution—*The macula is an area in the center of the retina that receives light from the center of the visual field. It is the center of greatest visual acuity. Degeneration of the macula occurs when the outer layer of the retina deteriorates or "fails" and waste products build up. These wastes products cause death of retinal cells and loss of vision.

Page 213: *Solution—*Retinal detachment occurs when the retina (the inner layer of the eye) pulls away from the choroid (the middle layer of the eye). The retina is the sensory part of the eye that is essential for sight. When it separates, damage and/or death occurs to the nerve cells and loss of vision occurs. Retinal detachment is a medical emergency and requires surgical correction. However, surgical procedures like scleral buckling along with photocoagulation can reattach the retina and preserve sight.

Page 218: *Solution—*The nurse should urge the mother to avoid allowing the child to lie down while drinking from a bottle since

this position increases the risk of acute otitis media. In addition, the mother should be advised that exposure to tobacco smoke in the home poses risks for otitis media.

Page 226: *Solution—*The nurse should discuss with the client the availability of various types of speech generators as well as the possibility of learning esophageal speech. Surgical procedures to restore speech such as tracheoesophageal puncture (TEP) in conjunction with a prosthesis are also available.

Chapter 7

Page 237: *Solution—*Although the indigestion of GERD and that associated with a heart attack can feel very similar, angina usually feels like a tightness or heaviness, associated with shortness of breath, sweating, lightheadedness, and sometimes nausea. The discomfort of GERD will be centered more around meal time with stress and other factors increasing the acidity in the stomach. Instruct the client not to let indigestion unrelieved by medicine continue without seeking medical attention.

Page 239: *Solution—*Prevention of a peptic ulcer includes caution in the use of nonsteroidal anti-inflammatory drugs (NSAIDs), including acetylsalicylic acid (aspirin); avoiding excessive physiologic and psychologic stress; and avoiding cigarettes and too much caffeine. Additional risk factors are a positive family history for ulcers as well as type O blood. Clients should always know the side effects of any over-the-counter (OTC) and prescription medications, which could cause ulcers also. Consumption of spicy, hot foods in excess along with high stress levels add to the risk.

Page 243: *Solution—*Assessment criteria used for any client with possible dehydration are appropriate, including checking for skin turgor and sunken eyeballs, as well as observation for dryness of skin; dry mucous membranes; dark, amber urine with decreased output; and complaints of thirst. Lab data would include a high hematocrit level, increased blood urea nitrogen (BUN), increased specific gravity of urine, hypernatremia, and hypokalemia.

Page 246: *Solution—*An unrelieved obstruction that is accompanied by such significant symptoms needs immediate attention. The condition could worsen with increased distention, change in level of consciousness, electrolyte imbalances, and increased pain, especially if the bowel ruptures or peritonitis occurs.

Page 247: *Solution—*The lack of fever and normal WBC would help in determining a diagnosis of appendicitis. Rebound tenderness should be checked and an IV started. Without any further symptoms and no rebound tenderness, the condition may be only a stomach virus and the IV fluids will cause improvement in the pain within 24 hours. Remember, however, if appendicitis is an appropriate diagnosis, sudden cessation of the pain could mean the appendix ruptured.

Chapter 8

Page 262: *Solution*—Determination of ascites can be made through objective observation of the size and contour of the abdomen, weight gain, firmness to the abdomen, taunt skin over the abdomen, distant, low-pitched bowel sounds, intake greater than output, and daily increase in the measurement of the abdominal girth. Subjectively, the client may complain of fullness or back pain. Lab data should include: serum albumin, protein, electrolytes, and tests specific to the cause such as liver function tests for cirrhosis or hepatitis.

Page 262: *Solution*—In Laënnec's cirrhosis, scarring of the liver occurs such as in biliary cirrhosis but there is also fat accumulation. Both of these (scarring and fat accumulation) cause a decrease in the function of the liver. The alcohol is transformed to acetaldehyde, which begins the process of altering hepatic function. The acetaldehyde inhibits the removal of proteins from the liver and alters metabolism of vitamins and minerals. Ammonia is unable to be metabolized, therefore a serum level is high in an alcoholic (hence the odor). Failure of the liver to work properly can lead to a GI bleed. An alcoholic often forfeits good meals for drinking either because of lack of appetite, lack of money (money spent on alcohol instead of food), or remaining in a stuporous state and failure to eat. Blood pressure (BP) elevates in the client because of portal hypertension and can often reach stroke range.

Page 266: *Solution*—Hepatitis A and E can be prevented by avoiding contaminated food and water, by avoiding situations in which one might come in contact with food handlers who do not use the necessary precautions. The client also should avoid contact with possibly contaminated shellfish. Hepatitis B, C, and D may be avoided by preventing contact with contaminated blood and body fluids. This includes needles, syringes, pooled blood, and unprotected sexual activity. A vaccine for hepatitis A and B is available for prophylaxis. Immunoglobulin may be given after exposure to hepatitis A, B, and D.

Page 269: *Solution*—Nursing diagnoses would include Pain; Altered nutrition: less than body requirements; Risk for fluid volume deficit; and Altered elimination. If cholecystitis occurs and surgery is necessary, additional diagnoses would be: Risk for infection; Altered skin integrity; and Risk for impaired gas exchange. Nursing interventions would include keeping the client NPO, administering pain medication as needed, administering oral bile acids or dissolvers, monitoring lab work, assessing for pain, stool characteristics, GI complaints, and nutritional status. Teaching should be instituted when appropriate about eating less fat-containing foods and losing weight.

Page 273: *Solution*—Because these three diagnosis have similar elevated lab work, the nurse should be able to differentiate specific symptoms and lab work related to each.

Cholecystitis: A classic symptom is pain radiating to the back or right shoulder, intolerance to fat-containing foods, and fever. Remember, *itis* signifies inflammation, and fever is usually present.

Lab work specific for cholecystitis is elevated direct bilirubin and alkaline phosphatase with a normal serum amylase.

Pancreatitis: A classic symptom is pain that radiates to the back and is relieved by sitting up, leaning forward, flexing the left leg, or by walking, and fever. Classic lab work is an elevated amylase and lipase level.

Cirrhosis: Pain is usually not present, but ascites is characteristic as is spider angiomas, palmar erythema, and hepatomegaly. Specific lab work indicating cirrhosis is elevated liver function tests (alanine aminotransferase (ALT), aspartate aminotransferase (AST), alkaline phosphatase, gamma-glutamyl transpeptidase (GGT).

The symptoms of jaundice and clay-colored stools can be present in all three as well as an elevated bilirubin level.

Chapter 9

Page 291: *Solution*—Essential information to provide the client newly diagnosed with hypothyroidism includes the following:

- Take thyroid medications as prescribed; do not abruptly discontinue.
- Take medications 1 hour before or 2 hours after meals for optimal absorption.
- Monitor weight and report changes as instructed.
- Do not use iodized salt or drugs containing iodine.
- Avoid excessive intake of foods such as cabbage, turnips, spinach, and carrots because these foods inhibit the thyroid hormone (TH) utilization.
- Consume adequate fluids, at least 2000 mL, or as prescribed.
- Consume a high-fiber diet to avoid constipation.
- Obtain adequate rest.
- Maintain skin integrity by proper care of dry skin.

Page 293: *Solution*—Because there is a high risk of damage to the parathyroid glands during a thyroidectomy, the client should be monitored for hypoparathyroidism. Manifestations are attributed to hypocalcemia and include tetany, muscle spasms, positive Chvostek's sign, positive Trousseau's sign, a decreased serum calcium level, and increased serum phosphorus level.

Page 297: *Solution*—Fluid volume excess is a complication of Cushing's syndrome as a result of excess cortisol which leads to sodium and water reabsorption. Interventions would include the following actions:

- Weigh client daily at the same time, using the same scale.
- Measure and record intake and output every 8 hours; compare with previous 72 hour totals to identify trends.
- Monitor heart rate, blood pressure, respirations, lung sounds.
- Assess for jugular vein distention and peripheral edema.
- Educate client about fluid restriction as prescribed.

Page 298: *Solution*—In Addison's disease, an insufficient amount of glucocorticoids and mineralocorticoids leads to fluid volume deficit, hyperkalemia, and hyponatremia. Instructions on nutritional management of Addison's disease would include the following:

- Consume a diet high in sodium and low in potassium; high-potassium foods to avoid include fruits, vegetables, chicken, liver, tuna, turkey.
- Consume at least 3000 mL of fluid daily, or as prescribed.
- Do not skip meals.
- Weigh self daily and report changes as instructed.

Page 304: *Solution*—Chronic diabetes insipidus will require life-long replacement of antidiuretic hormone (ADH). Failure to replace the water loss can result in severe hypovolemia and hypernatremia. Instructions would include the following information:

- Treatment is lifelong.
- Take antidiuretic hormone as prescribed.
- Consume fluids as prescribed.
- Wear Medic-Alert bracelet.
- Signs and symptoms of diabetes insipidus.

Chapter 10

Page 319: *Solution*—Obtain history of present illness: duration of symptoms, history of kidney stones, previous UTI, kidney or bladder disease; past history of diabetes, hypertension, allergies, pregnancy; last menstrual period, use of birth control methods, date of last sexual contact, history of new sex partner; assess recent medication use including antibiotics; family history of kidney disorders; inquire about diet: caffeine or carbonated drinks and water intake. Instructions should include the following: take medication as prescribed; explain indications of medications and side effects; increase water intake to at least 8 glasses of water per day; avoid food or beverages that contribute to urine acidity, which may promote bacterial growth; explain the importance of follow up urinalysis to assure resolution of infection; and teach women hygiene measures to prevent contamination or irritation.

Page 321: *Solution*—Teach the client what factors increase the risk of stone formation (male, Caucasian race, prior or family history, medications such as vitamins A, C, and D, antacids with calcium, gout) and what they can do to minimize this risk; emphasize increasing fluid intake and dietary restrictions (such as limiting foods high in vitamin D, calcium, purines, oxalate, acidic and alkaline foods) to prevent further stone formation; teach the client regarding signs and symptoms of urinary tract infection; demonstrate how to strain all urine and save any stones for further analysis.

Page 323: *Solution*—Polycystic kidney disease is a hereditary disease and causes cysts to form in the kidney thereby causing the kidney to enlarge; these cysts may form a blockage of the kidney causing destruction of the kidney tissue; common symptoms include flank pain, blood in the urine, infection, and stones.

Page 325: *Solution*—Glomerular filtration rate is the amount of fluid filtered from the blood into the capsule per minute; this rate is influenced by three factors: total surface area available for filtration, permeability of the filtration membrane and the net filtration pressure; the normal GFR in both kidneys is 120 to 125 mL/min in adults; one advantage of a high GFR is that it allows the kidneys to rapidly filter waste products from the body and it allows the body fluid to be filtered and processed by the kidney many times a day; glomerulonephritis causes a decreased GFR which leads to azotemia and activation of the RAA system; this in turn causes sodium and water retention and edema.

Page 332: *Solution*—Fluids are usually limited in CRF, especially if dialysis is being done; the more fluid consumed, the sooner dialysis will be needed and edema will be evident; the client should be educated on the amount of fluid allowed in a 24-hour period and plan with the client how this will be distributed, accounting for medicine administration; provide an explanation that fluids are usually offered based on total allowance rather than randomly with each meal; explain that research has indicated that lowering protein in CRF slows the progression of the disease and decreases common signs of uremia such as anorexia, nausea, and vomiting.

Chapter 11

Page 344: *Solution*—There is a familial tendency to develop hypospadias, but no gene has yet been identified. Therefore, the client's sons may, but the risk is less than 50 percent. Assurance should be given to the parents that if the son does have the condition, surgery can be performed to correct the situation.

Page 346: *Solution*—Nonsteroidal anti-inflammatory drugs (NSAIDs) medications should have been discontinued at 10 days preoperatively. Additionally, clients with BPH should avoid taking OTC allergy medications, as they can induce urinary retention from spasm of the bladder sphincter.

Page 349: *Solution*—Testicles are comprised of tiny tube-like structures (seminal vesicles and vas deferens). If a lumpectomy were performed, any cancer present would escape into the tube systems and begin growing there, thus spreading the cancer. The inguinal route of surgery allows the testicle to be removed intact and prevent cancer seeding into the tissues surrounding the tumor.

Page 353: *Solution*—Primary dysmenorrhea is the condition where menses are painful from menarche. This condition is caused by an excessive production of prostaglandins. Although fairly common, not every woman has this condition. Familial tendencies exists, therefore asking the client whether her mother and sisters have always had painful periods would be a better predictor.

Page 360: *Solution*—The first mammogram should be performed between the ages of 35 and 40, with yearly mammograms beginning at 40 according to the American Cancer Society's recommendations. She should have a mammogram now and yearly from this point on.

Page 362: *Solution*—Doxycycline is a tetracycline and therefore contraindicated during pregnancy (Pregnancy Category D drug). Tetracycline is known to cause discoloration of tooth enamel. A pregnancy test must be performed. If the client is pregnant, withhold the doxycycline and notify the provider of the client's pregnancy. Expect the provider to order a different medication such as azithromycin (Zithromax).

Chapter 12

Page 382: *Solution*—The nurse should know that allergies to dust, mold, grasses, pollens, and spores trigger a type I hypersensitivity response that is localized rather than systemic. Systemic type I hypersensitivity would lead to anaphylaxis. In a localized type I hypersensitivity, cell-bound IgE in the bronchial tree, nasal mucosa, and conjunctival tissues come in contact with the allergen and releases histamine and chemical mediators that produce the symptoms of asthma, rhinitis, and conjunctivitis. A good explanation for the mother is to inform her that small doses of the agent the child is allergic to will be given in order to help the body develop antibodies. These antibodies will then build the immune system so that her child will react less or perhaps not at all when the allergen is introduced. Calm her fears about a severe reaction by explaining that the dose is usually diluted and will be slowly increased in strength to prevent major complications. Also inform her that the child will be monitored during the time immediately after receiving the injection for any complications.

Page 383: *Solution*—An autoimmune disease is when the body no longer recognizes self as self, but instead identifies and targets self as non-self. The basis of the immune system is that it has the ability to recognize self vs. non-self in order to target any foreign cell or particle. In essence, the body turns on itself in an autoimmune disease. In rejection of an organ tissue, the body recognizes the tissue as foreign and the immune system responds as it should to any foreign particle, rejecting its presence in the body. Although the desired outcome is for the body not to reject the tissue, the immune system is working correctly in this situation. Immunosuppressant drugs are given to stop the body from rejecting the donor organ tissue.

Page 384: *Solution*—The presence of antihistamines would prevent the test from producing true positive or negative results. When an allergen comes in contact with the individual, the response is for the immune system to release histamine and other chemicals (inflammatory symptoms). If an antihistamine is on board, the release of histamine will be blocked and a reaction may not occur.

Page 385: *Solution*—The mildest and most common symptoms would be dry, itchy, red rash on the back of the hands and fingers. Blistering and weeping may occur along with swelling. These symptoms constitute an irritant contact dermatitis. A true type I immediate hypersensitivity reaction would occur within 5 to 30 minutes and stop when the gloves were removed. Immediate itching and swelling of the fingers or hand occurs. The gloves should not be snapped because the latex can adhere to the particles of starch powder inside the gloves and the inhalation of the powder aerosol may provoke symptoms also.

Page 386: *Solution*—Individuals exhibiting a true anaphylaxis are usually highly sensitive individuals and the reactions, which may be mild or severe develop in minutes, are almost instantaneous. Second, anaphylactic shock is always a potential concern for anyone exhibiting anaphylactic symptoms. The effects may involve the respiratory or cardiac system along with vasodilation and fluid loss from the vascular system.

Page 392: *Solution*—In a client who has been exposed to HIV, antibodies may not be produced for 6 weeks to 6 months after the initial infection (known as seroconversion). The ELISA test identifies HIV antibodies. Therefore, depending on the timing of infection and antibody production, an ELISA may return negative initially but return positive later on. Hence, a second ELISA is often conducted to confirm a suspicion of positive HIV results. To actually confirm the diagnosis of positive HIV, a Western blot antibody test, which is more reliable than ELISA, is conducted once a positive ELISA has been obtained.

Chapter 13

Page 403: *Solution*—Clients with immune deficiency disorders, clients receiving chemotherapy, or clients receiving long-term corticosteroid therapy are often those who contract opportunistic infections. In all of these states, the immune system, which normally defends against pathogens, is suppressed and unable to perform normally.

Page 409: *Solution*—Some viruses enter the host cell and insert their genome into the chromosome of the host, remaining in a latent, non-replicative state for long periods of time. A virus can remain communicable during recurrence. Stress increases the recurrence of latent or recurrent viruses. The lack of symptoms may be problematic in that the client is contagious and does not know it. Also, a virus can reoccur and be more virulent than the first time, without a cure.

Page 415: *Solution*—Bacteria may be described as cocci (spherical), bacilli (rod-shaped), clavate (club-shaped), or spirochetal (corkscrew-shaped). Staining characteristics include gram-positive or gram-negative characteristics. Typically, Gram-negative organisms are more virulent. Bacteria may also be classified as aerobic (requiring oxygen) or anaerobic (not needing oxygen).

Page 417: *Solution*—Corticosteroids are immunosuppressant and therefore enhance the growth of fungal skin infections. A fungal infection as well as tuberculosis will be exacerbated if a corticosteroid is used.

Page 424: *Solution*—Intestinal obstruction can occur with helminth infestation and can be a life-threatening event. The organisms may also affect other organs: cestodes (brain), nematodes (alveoli), trematodes (blood vessels, intestines, liver, or lungs)

Chapter 14

Page 438: *Solution*—Sunburn is a minor burn injury of the superficial layer of the skin. Sporadic, intense sunburns are more damaging to the skin than everyday exposure with use of a sunscreen. Use of sunscreens and limiting sun exposure to the less hazardous hours of the day (before 10:00 A.M. and after 3:00 P.M.) can prevent sunburn. Recurrent sunburn can lead to other skin disorders such as early skin aging, seborrheic keratosis, basal and squamous cell carcinoma, and malignant melanoma.

Page 442: *Solution*—Instruct the client to wash the skin with a mild soap and water at least twice a day to remove accumulated oils. Eat a regular, well-balanced diet. Exposing the skin to sun may help but sunburns should be avoided; get regular exercise and sleep. Do not squeeze the pimple; this causes the material to go deeper into the skin and usually the pimple gets larger and infected. The client should be instructed to be patient because treatment for acne can take months for a noticeable difference.

Page 443: *Solution*—Stress the importance of good nutrition and cleanliness through good handwashing and proper disposal of dressings. Teach the client never to squeeze or try to open the infected area. Teach the client signs and symptoms that should be reported to a healthcare provider such as fever, swelling, redness, pain, and drainage. Teach the importance of taking the full course of medication that has been prescribed.

Page 447: *Solution*—HSV2 is a herpes simplex virus that usually involves the genitalia and skin below the waist in sexually active individuals. Explain the natural history of the disease with emphasis on recurrent episodes, asymptomatic viral shedding, and sexual transmission. Antiviral therapy can be used on an episodic basis or as suppressive therapy. Stress the importance of use of condoms during sexual intercourse, but the need to abstain from all sexual activity when lesions or prodromal symptoms are present.

Page 449: *Solution*—Do not share linens; use a clean towel and washcloth daily. Carefully dry between the toes. Do not wear the same pair of shoes every day, and avoid wearing rubber or plastic-soled shoes. Wear cotton socks that are changed frequently. Educate on the use of talcum powder and that over-the-counter fungal powder/spray should be used twice daily or prescribed medication for at least 2 weeks even though the symptoms have disappeared. Inquire if others in the family have the same symptoms. Educate on cleaning bathing surfaces after each bath/shower.

Chapter 15

Page 468: *Solution*—Since the client is in his nadir period, he is experiencing pancytopenia with all of his blood counts being affected. He is at high risk for infection and will require education on a neutropenic diet, limiting exposure to others, taking his temperature orally every four hours, and the importance of handwashing, especially after toileting. The client is also at risk for hemorrhage, secondary to a low platelet count. The client should be educated to avoid aspirin and aspirin-containing products, avoid straining to have a bowel movement, and use electric razors while shaving. He can expect frequent lab work, transfusions with red cells and platelets, as well as possible antibiotic and antifungal administration.

Page 472: *Solution*—Both Hodgkin's and non-Hodgkin's arise from the lymph nodes and then disseminate throughout the body. Hodgkin's disease usually affects younger people, while non-Hodgkin's lymphoma occurs in the middle to later years. The causative etiology for both is unknown, however chemical exposure may be a causative agent. Hodgkin's disease is classified by the presence of Reed-Sternberg cells, which don't occur in non-Hodgkin's lymphoma. Both clients are diagnosed by lymph node biopsy. Depending on bone marrow invasion, both clients are at risk for infection and bleeding. Depending on the stage of the disease, the client may need surgery only, surgery and radiation, therapy, or surgery, radiation, and chemotherapy. The chemotherapeutic protocols are unique for each of the diagnoses.

Page 473: *Solution*—Breast cancer often metastasizes to the bone in the late stages of the disease. With bone involvement the client is at risk for developing hypercalcemia. The family needs to be educated on the importance of maintaining mobility and to ensure the client ambulates with assistance due to her increased risk for falling. The role of hydration also needs to be emphasized, and the family needs to be educated on the importance of an intake and output record. The family should understand the signs and symptoms of hypercalcemia, and the importance of reporting these to the client's physician. Finally, the family should be educated on the administration of long-acting morphine and the importance of administering it on a specific schedule to avoid breakthrough pain.

Page 477: *Solution*—Both platelets and factor VIII play an important role in clot formation, therefore, the client with a decreased platelet count is just as susceptible to hemorrhage as the client with a factor VIII deficiency. The client with thrombocytopenia is at greater risk for spontaneous hemorrhage, and the problem is usually treated with platelet transfusions, except in idiopathic thrombocytopenia papura (ITP), when the treatment of choice is steroid therapy. The client with factor VIII deficiency usually receives scheduled factor VIII infusions and is at greater risk of bleeding into the joints. Both clients need to be educated on bleeding and safety precautions.

Page 480: *Solution*—Both pernicious anemia and folic acid deficiency are macrocytic (megaloblastic) anemia. Pernicious anemia is caused by a deficiency in vitamin B_{12}, usually caused by a lack of intrinsic factor, while folic acid deficiency is caused by a deficiency of folic acid. Both present with a smooth, sore, beefy, red tongue, while pernicious anemia presents with paresthesias and prioception, which delineates it from folic acid deficiency.

Page 482: *Solution*—The nurse should educate the client and his parents about the importance of adequate hydration during their vacation since dehydration will increase intravenous viscosity, triggering a crisis. The client should also be encouraged to take rest breaks while at any water or amusement parks, since extreme body heat and excessive exercise can trigger an event. Since high altitude can trigger a sickling episode, the nurse should discuss the feasibility of using ground transportation to get to the vacation destination.

Chapter 16

Page 492: *Solution*—The pedigree can demonstrate the risk for congenital defects in future offspring. The pedigree can also establish patterns of inheritance and what diseases the family is prone to develop.

Page 495: *Solution*—The child with Down syndrome is following the same pattern of development as peers of a similar age, but at a slower pace. The family needs anticipatory guidance as the child nears each phase of development. Erickson's stages of development can still be identified and need the same attention. Helping the client deal with social concerns as well as sexual questions should consist of fair treatment.

Page 496: *Solution*—There are three known types of chromosome 21 abnormalities; nondisjunction, translocation, and mosaicism. Translocation has a 5 to 15 percent chance of reoccurrence and should be considered in future family planning. Prevention of another child with trisomy 21 may be an option.

Page 497: *Solution*—The adolescent with Turner syndrome has no development of secondary sex characteristics and growth is below standard level. Because these clinical manifestations don't occur until adolescence, the diagnosis and treatment may be delayed.

Page 499: *Solution*—Nondisjunction is an abnormal separation during meiosis. This can lead to interference with fetal development. In nondisjunction, one zygote receives too many alleles and the other too few. Examples are trisomy 21, monosomy in Turner's syndrome, and Klinefelter's syndrome (which can be trisomy or multiple additions of X and possibly Y). In particular, Klinefelter's syndrome is an X-linked defect with one or more extra X chromosomes in a genotype; e.g., XXY, XXXY.

Page 501: *Solution*—Refer to Table 16-1 (p. 499) for autosomal recessive patterns. The risk of having children with PKU is 1:4, 2:4 risk of being carriers, and 1:4 risk being normal.

Page 504: *Solution*—At present there is no cure for Huntington's and no predictor of when symptoms will begin. If a client knows he or she has a disease, but no control over when and how it will develop, it can be an overwhelming piece of information. Yet a client has the right in family planning to know what might potentially be passed along to his or her children.

Page 512: *Solution*—The newborn with biuvula has a cleft palate that could possibly go undetected. The child with a cleft needs to be referred for treatment and prevent complications such as otitis media, aspiration, and speech impairment. Sometimes the biuvula is the only obvious physical characteristic.

Chapter 17

Page 528: *Solution*—In the absence of illness or injury, a woman in the childbearing years would have the pre-disposing risk factor of utilizing tampons for menstruation. A thorough assessment of recent menstruation and sanitary product utilization would be indicated. The concern for toxic shock syndrome is high in light of her age.

Page 533: *Solution*—Arterial blood gases (ABGs) are the most accurate measure of progressing shock. All forms of shock are a syndrome that result in inadequate perfusion and oxygenation of tissues. As shock progresses, anaerobic respiration replaces aerobic. Lactic acid production builds, causing metabolic acidosis. ABGs measure the pH of the blood. Other tests that may be ordered are creatinine phospholinase (CPK) and CPK isoenzymes, but these determine heart damage, not shock.

Page 536: *Solution*—A broad-spectrum antibiotic is usually begun initially as soon as the diagnosis is made. A narrow-spectrum antibiotic cannot be initiated until the culture and sensitivity returns, which then confirms the actual diagnosis. It is imperative to collect all cultures prior to the start of any antibiotic. Failure to collect all specimens can and most likely will result in improper treatment or incorrect diagnosis.

Page 544: *Solution*—An open hemothorax is suspected. A bullet wound provides an opening to the outside atmosphere so the development of a tension pneumothorax is possible. A tension pneumothorax is a life-threatening medical emergency. Bleeding within the pleural space could provide a significant source of hemorrhage so the shock state is hypovolemic in nature.

Page 546: *Solution*—Swelling from edema and bleeding may create a tourniquet-like effect, creating compartment syndrome. The nurse should assess circulation to the lower arm: pulses, capillary refill, color of extremities, and have client rank his or her pain. The physician should be notified immediately so that the casts can be removed or the client may need surgery.

Page 547: *Solution*—Necessary staff should be summoned including additional nursing support, as well as respiratory and radiology personnel. In a smaller institution or one that has on-call personnel, a representative from neurology and perhaps radiology should be made available. Resuscitative equipment should be ready including airway management equipment; an intravenous line should be primed and ready to infuse; cardiac monitor readied; suction available; a catheterization tray on hand; and typical wound care supplies available. Although most trauma rooms will be stocked with these supplies, a quick survey decreases time once the client arrives.

Page 549: *Solution*—A D-dimer test is indicated for a differential diagnosis. This test measures fragments, which elevate in response to clot breakdown. A steady increase in these values indicates ongoing clot breakdown rather than a lack of clotting factors.

➤ *Case Study Suggested Answers*

Chapter 1

1. The mother should be given an explanation as to what each drug does and any specific side effects. The montelukast (Singulair) carries few side effects, headaches being the most common. Stress to the mother that this medication should be taken every day regardless of the event of an asthma attack. Explain the difference between the maintenance inhaler nedocromil (Tilade) and the rescue inhaler albuterol (Ventolin). Be sure the mother understands that the maintenance drug is given every day and the albuterol is given only if an attack occurs and should be used immediately. If the attack does not stop within 30 to 60 minutes, the albuterol drops plus saline can be used via nebulization. Specific instructions on using a nebulizer and mixing the saline with albuterol should be given to the mother before discharge. The rescue inhaler as well as the nebulizer can cause extreme nervousness in clients. An explanation should be given on how to use the inhaler (complete exhalation; administering the correct number of puffs while inhaling to the count of 10), correctly cleaning the mouthpiece, and checking for fullness of the canister (if empty, the canister will float; if half full, it will sink half way; if full, it will sink completely).

2. Explain to the mother that asthma is an inflammation of the airways that leads to constriction (or closing) of the bronchi, but this constriction is reversible with medications. The closing of the bronchi causes clients to feel like they cannot get enough air, which can be very frightening. The wheezing that can be heard when these clients breathe is also due to the closing of the bronchi; the air is trying to pass through a smaller opening than usual.

3. Usually the physician will give specific instructions on when to seek medical attention. However, standard protocol is to seek treatment when first the rescue inhaler and then the nebulizer have been used without any results. If the physician allows more than one nebulizer treatment, encourage the mother to give the allowed number of treatments before seeking immediate attention; explain that some attacks may take longer to stop than others. However, any time the child is having more frequent or more severe attacks, a physician should examine the child. Also, if attacks are occurring right after another or an attack is prolonged (status asthmaticus), immediate attention is necessary.

4. The child should be given a brief explanation of what asthma is in terms they can understand. If the child is extremely anxious during an attack, assurance should be given that they will always be able to breathe, but may not be able to get a good, deep breath. Address the child's fears and allow the child to voice his concerns. Explain that the higher the anxiety level, the more difficult it is to breathe.

5. Triggers are stimuli that produce the initial inflammatory response that proceeds to the asthma attack, causing mucosal edema, mucus secretion, and inflammation of the airways. Triggers cause the bronchospasm and can be specific allergies (mold, dust, pollen, etc.) or such things as cold air, strong odors, high altitude, intense exercise, and emotional stress. An individual may also find other unusual triggers that are not common to all people with asthma.

Chapter 2

1. Begin by assessing the ABCs—airway, breathing, and circulation. He has an open airway and is breathing adequately. Assess his circulation by checking his pulse (apical and radial) and blood pressure and placing him on the monitor to assess his heart rhythm. Assess the level of pain on a pain scale of 1 to 10, with 10 being the worst pain. Assess the duration and location of the pain (does it radiate?) and have the client describe the pain in his own words. Listen to his heart sounds; note any abnormal sounds such as murmur, friction rub, or S_3 or S_4 gallops. Assess his skin color and temperature; note capillary refill (should be less than 3 seconds). Listen to his lung fields anteriorly and posteriorly for crackle, rhonchi, or wheezes. Note any labored respirations or use of accessory muscles and ask whether he feels short of breath. Assess his abdomen and extremities for signs of swelling. Assess distal pulses.

2. The nurse would ask if he has had prior history of cardiac disease or episodes of angina, any previous heart attack, or history of coronary artery disease. Does he have a history of hypertension, hypercholesterolemia, or hyperlipidemia? The nurse needs to assess if he has a strong family history of cardiac problems. Is he diabetic? Has he ever had previous ECGs done and where? Who is his family doctor and does he have a cardiologist?

3. Laboratory data would include Troponin I, CK-MB, LDH with isoenzymes, CBC with differential, complete chemistries (electrolytes, glucose, BUN/Cr, liver functions), PT and PTT, as well as a chest x-ray and 12-lead ECG at bedside. If necessary, ABGs or continuous pulse oxymetry may be ordered.

4. Possible medications ordered include nitroglycerin (Nitrostat, NTG) sublingual 0.4 mg or nitroglycerin IV drip, titrated to pain and/or systolic blood pressure of 100 mmHg; nitrol paste (Nitro-Dur) 1 or 2 inches to chest wall; acetylsalicylic acid (aspirin) as an antiplatelet drug to prevent clots; morphine sulfate 2 to 5 mg IV push if nitroglycerin is not effective in relieving chest pain or if BP is too low; lidocaine (Xylocaine) IV if cardiac irritability is noted. After the initial chest pains are relieved, a beta blocker, ni-

trate, and/or calcium channel blocker would probably be ordered.

5. The nurse should look for inverted T waves and depressed S-T segments as a sign of ischemia; elevated S-T segments as a sign of injury; Q waves in two contiguous leads as a sign of infarct of undetermined age; tachycardia that may be present because of the effects of pain and anxiety; any abnormal rhythm or ectopic beats such as PVCs as a sign of irritability.

Chapter 3

1. Since the client has had several colds, the healthcare provider should assess what medications, both prescription and over-the-counter (OTC), the client took during these periods of illness and whether they are still being taken. Many OTC products can cause an increase in blood pressure. Second, data should be collected on whether the client has ever had a sudden increase in BP before; if so, what was the reason (if known), and what was done about it? It is always suggested to verify that the client is indeed compliant with medicine administration and diet. It would be helpful to know if a family member has been visiting the healthcare provider with the client in order to relay accurate information. Lastly, verify that the instructions about correct dose and time of administration are being followed by the client.

2. The family and client should be counseled on what is meant by a high blood pressure value and the possible complications (stroke, death, etc.). If medications are not being taken correctly, educate on each medication—what it is for, how much should be taken, and setting up a dosing schedule that meets the needs of the client. Explain what side effects can occur and the consequences of skipping a dose. If diet is a concern, educate the client on low-sodium foods and the relationship of sodium to blood pressure. Using the readings from the Council on Aging, establish a normal range of blood pressure that is safe for the client. Be sure the family knows how to monitor the BP as well as when to report to a healthcare professional.

3. Essential information includes drug name, dosage and time for administration, need to assess pulse and/or blood pressure prior to taking the medication, reason for taking the medication, and side effects that need to be reported to the healthcare provider. Report any chest pain or problems with respirations. Some medications require the client to move slowly when changing positions to avoid lightheadedness. Emphasis should be placed on not "making up" a missed medication; rather wait until the next time the medicine is due to take the dose prescribed unless instructed otherwise. Parameters for low pulse and blood pressure reading should be provided as well.

4. Priority of care is decreasing the blood pressure to a range acceptable for the client. Once this is established, priorities include:

- Teaching the client and family about the medication regime.
- Awareness of the possibility of compliance issues.
- Assisting the client in maintaining compliance through clear instructions; make accomodations for clients with poor eyesight and those who are unable to read or speak English.
- Implementing the plan to form a partnership with the client, the significant others, and the health team for support, information, and care.

5. Essential hypertension is usually from an unknown cause and is also termed primary hypertension. It occurs in a majority of hypertensive clients (about 95 percent). Secondary hypertension, on the other hand, is usually related to a disease process. Secondary hypertension is often easier to control because control of the disease will often regulate the blood pressure (BP). It is important to understand that in essential hypertension the left ventricle (the power chamber of the heart) must work harder to overcome the resistance it encounters when blood is pumped out. When the ventricle must continuously work hard, the muscle will hypertrophy (or stiffen); this can cause heart problems later on. When the heart is unable to adjust to the hypertension, the kidneys become involved in an effort to regulate the pressure. One of the serious concerns is that there are rarely obvious symptoms, and often there are no symptoms at all. A headache or nosebleed may occur when the pressure rises extremely high.

Chapter 4

1. Anticipated signs and symptoms of Parkinson's include resting tremors, stooped posture, mask-like face, soft monotone voice, drooling, poor balance, shuffling propulsive gait, rigidity, insomnia, weight loss, constipation, depression, and dementia. In addition, the client might be withdrawn, uncooperative, and noncompliant because of his reluctance to be at the facility.

2. A priority nursing diagnosis for the client is Impaired physical mobility, as well as High risk for injury. The client with Parkinson's disease has difficulty initiating ambulation, is unsteady, and often has difficulty stopping and righting himself if he begins to fall. Safety should be a primary goal in the care of this client. Other diagnoses would include Self-care deficit; Altered nutrition: less than body requirements; Potential for constipation; Noncompliance; and Altered thought processes.

3. It would be best to schedule his physical therapy to coincide with peak drug action. Planned rest periods should be a part of his daily routine to allow him to prevent fatigue and frustration during physical therapy. An explanation should be given to the client as to the importance of the physical therapy.

4. A good approach to handling the client with Parkinson's disease who has become upset would be to:

- Acknowledge to him that you recognize he is frustrated and upset.
- State that you are sorry if it seemed you were trying to rush him.
- Encourage and praise him for his efforts to maintain independence. Stress that you recognize it is important for him.
- Allow him as much time as he needs to dress.
5. Some specific instructions to assist with mobility problems are:
   - Daily exercise to maintain function: walking, swimming, stretching.
   - Stretching and posture exercises as suggested by physical therapy.
   - Take big steps and lift legs.
   - Think about stepping over an object for episodes of "freezing."

Chapter 5

1. Emergency nursing care for the client with a fracture includes:
   - Immobilizing the fracture: Anything sturdy can be used to immobilize the fractured area; belts can be used to secure the fracture to the hard surface. The extremity or limb should be placed in the same position on the area where it is to be immobilized.
   - Controlling any bleeding: Pressure should be held to control bleeding. If clean linens are available, these can be applied to the area. Firm pressure should be held constantly if an artery has been severed.
   - Cleaning the wound if there is an open fracture: Open fractures should be cleaned if possible and a moist, clean towel applied to keep the bone from drying.
2. The nurse should assess the 5 Ps: pain, paresthesia, pulses, pallor, and paralysis; elevate the extremity and apply ice during the first 24 hours; keep the cast open to air and supported on pillow to allow for drying; assess for signs and symptoms of compartment syndrome during the first 48 hours.
3. Provide instructions to client and caregivers regarding cast care and complications to report.
   - Keep cast supported on pillows while drying.
   - Report increase in pain, decrease in movement, changes in color, coolness of fingers, loss of sensation, and/ or increased swelling.
   - Apply ice directly over fracture for first 24 hours.
   - Elevate the cast on pillows and expose to air while drying.
   - Check areas of skin at cast edges for skin breakdown, provide padding as needed.
   - Do not place any objects in the cast; use a blow dryer on cool setting for itching.
   - Report drainage or odor from cast.
   - Wear a sling to support the arm.
   - Keep cast dry; cover with a plastic bag during bathing.

- Instruct the client to expect pain, especially during the first 24 to 48 hours. The client should also be instructed to use pain medicine at the first sign of pain and avoid waiting since this makes pain control more difficult.
4. Compartment syndrome is usually the reason for excruciating pain after 48 hours. Even with a crushing fracture, pain will begin to decrease within 48 hours if a cast has been applied and the area is immobilized. Swelling and pressure accounts for the excruciating pain and should be relieved immediately.
5. Notify the physician immediately. The cast will need to be removed to assess the limb. Then elevate the extremity and apply ice to relieve the edema. Next, assist with bivalving the cast or prepare client for fasciotomy as indicated. Usually, the relief of the edema and pressure relieves the pain. If not, analgesics should be administered. Remember to obtain a surgical permit before medication is administered in the event of surgery. An explanation of the problem should be given to the client and family, especially if pain medicine is being held.

Chapter 6

1. Assessment findings in acute Meniere's disease include the symptoms outlined in the case study as well as hypotension, diaphoresis, and nystagmus. The vertigo may be so severe that the client becomes immobilized and may even fall to the floor.
2. Medical interventions for acute attacks may include the use of anticholinergics (i.e., scopolamine [Isopto Hyoscine], atropine [Isopto Atropine]), antiemetics (i.e., prochlorperazine [Compazine], meclizine [Antivert]), and central nervous system (CNS) depressants (i.e., diazepam [Valium]) to control the nausea, vomiting, and symptoms of motion sickness. Bedrest should be initiated as well as fluid and electrolyte replacement if necessary.
3. Diagnostic tests include audiometry, x-rays, and computed tomography (CT) scans of the vestible, and an electronystagmography (ENG) test battery including caloric ice water testing. In addition, an auditory dehydration test that uses glycerine or fast-acting diuretics to dehydrate the inner ear is often used. Acute, temporary improvement in symptoms following this test is considered diagnostic of Meniere's disease.
4. Meniere's disease is a chronic disorder of the inner ear that presents with three major symptoms: dizziness (vertigo), ringing in the ears (tinnitus), and hearing loss. The cause of the disorder is unknown and usually affects only one ear. The symptoms appear to be caused by the accumulation of fluid in a part of the inner ear known as the membranous labyrinth. Factors that cause acute symptoms include increased sodium intake, stress, allergies, and premenstrual fluid retention.
5. Discharge instructions for clients with Meniere's disease should include:

- The signs of impending attacks (i.e., feeling of fullness in the ear, increasing tinnitus, dizziness, nausea, and/or vomiting).
- Avoidance of attack triggers (i.e., stress, fatigue, blinking lights, loud noises, and/or quick or jerky body movements).
- The need for adequate rest and sleep as well as relaxation techniques.
- Safety measures to utilize if attacks occur while driving.
- Sodium-restricted diets.
- The avoidance of substances causing vasoconstriction (i.e., tobacco, alcohol, and caffeine).

Chapter 7

1. Questions would include the following:
   - What caused you to come to the health facility?
   - Have you been vomiting? What other symptoms have you had? When did these start?
   - How many bowel movements do you usually have a day?
   - Have you had this problem before?
   - What are your usual dietary habits?
   - How much weight have you lost? Over what period of time?
   - Are you able to care for yourself?
   - Have you noticed blood or mucus in your bowel movements?
2. Objective data should include observation of color, consistency, and character of stools; level of pain; relationship between diarrhea and meal time; abdominal palpation to determine areas of tenderness, check for rebound tenderness as an indication of peritonitis or appendicitis; monitor hemoglobin, hematocrit, WBC, serum Na, K, and Cl.
3. Social history information that would assist in her plan of care would be identification of job or family stress; use of cigarettes or alcohol; and presence of family or support systems. Stress factors have been known to aggravate the exacerbation of symptoms. Cigarettes and alcohol also are aggravating symptoms. The client will need to depend on family and/or social support systems as a part of her adjustment to home care.
4. Nursing measures would include administering anti-diarrheal medications as ordered, teaching good skin care, monitoring and encouraging fluid intake, being sure the client has easy access to the bedpan or bathroom, supplying room deodorizers as necessary, and weighing the client daily.
5. Other nursing measures include administering corticosteroid or immunosuppressive drugs as ordered, implementing a low-fiber diet, promoting rest, using antianxiety measures (planned rest periods, decreasing excess stimuli if pain medicine is administered, allowing privacy if diarrhea occurs), and preparing for surgery if indicated. In addition, client education should be given on what the illness is, com-

plications that can occur and prevention techniques, type of medications used and possible side effects, and how to lower stress.

Chapter 8

1. The risk factors present for pancreatic cancer in this client are age and cigarette smoking. Other risk factors include industrial chemicals, environmental toxin exposure, high-fat diet, pancreatitis, and diabetes mellitus.
2. The likely location of the pancreatic tumor based upon the symptoms of pain when supine, jaundice and weight loss, is the body of the pancreas. The jaundice could be significant of cancer of the head of the pancreas, but the pain when supine does not correlate. There are usually no symptoms if the cancer is in the tail of the pancreas.
3. The primary preoperative nursing interventions are:
   - Evaluate physical and psychological status. Create a collaborative care plan, which includes physical, psychological, and spiritual interventions
   - Determine client's acuity level
   - Provide a teaching plan for client and family for postoperative care
   - Explain that client may be cared for in the intensive care unit for a period of time
   - Provide comfort measures through proper positioning and administration of pain medication as needed; avoid the use of morphine because it can cause spasms of the pancreatic duct
   - Monitor and maintain nausea and vomiting
   - Assess lab work as ordered
4. The primary postoperative nursing interventions are:
   - Monitor respiratory status
   - Monitor renal output
   - Monitor cardiac status
   - Prevent wound infections
   - Maintain patency of the gastric suction
   - Administer pain medications at regular intervals; avoid the use of morphine because it can cause spasms of the pancreatic duct
   - Monitor blood chemistries
   - Watch for complications of hemorrhage, hypovolemic shock, and hepatorenal failure
5. The prognosis for this client is poor—nearly all pancreatic cancer is fatal within the first year. 85 percent of cases are not diagnosed until too late because the symptoms are not specific and the onset is slow. Although this type of cancer is rare (3 to 4 percent of the cancers in United States), it is more likely to occur in adults between 50 and 70 years of age.

Chapter 9

1. Diabetes mellitus at a young age occurs when beta cells in the pancreas fail to work properly and do not control glucose (sugar) correctly. The glucose builds up in the blood-

stream; this is called hyperglycemia. Normally, a certain amount of glucose is produced by the beta cells, then the body uses what glucose it needs and gets rid of what it doesn't need. With diabetes, the increased level of glucose spills into the urine. Glucose acts to draw fluid with it, resulting in increased urination and thirst. A third problem is hunger. The body needs insulin to use the carbohydrates, which our body needs for energy. The body finds other things for energy, like protein and fat and often any other stored nutrients, which causes the hungry feeling.

2. The most important symptoms are the 3 Ps (polyphagia, polyuria, polydipsia), the signs of hypoglycemia (nervousness, weakness, faint feeling, and possible coma), and the signs and symptoms of diabetic ketoacidosis (fruity breath, a change in respirations, extreme fatigue, nausea, and vomiting).

3. Although DM is often familial, it is considered an autoimmune disease and may occur without any family history. Explain what an autoimmune disease is and that diabetes at age 16 may be from genetics, environmental, or immunological factors. Calm the mother by including her in the teaching sessions and allowing her to ask questions and share concerns.

4. Explain what peak time means and what the time is for each type of insulin. Explain that the most likely time for a hypoglycemic reaction is 2 to 4 hours after taking regular insulin and 8 to 12 hours after taking NPH insulin. Be sure she understands that she has to consider both peak times if the medications are mixed in the morning.

5. The client will most likely experience symptoms of hyperglycemia. The goal of maintaining her glucose values within a normal range should be emphasized, especially since teenagers do not always eat healthy foods. Without scaring her, stress the long-term consequences of DM. At the same time, factors that affect her glucose level, such as exercise, over- or under-eating, and stress, could cause her glucose to drop and therefore she should know the symptoms of hypoglycemia. Instructions should be given to her about taking candy, fruit, or a regular cola if her glucose level does drop, especially during school hours.

Chapter 10

1. L. J. is experiencing metabolic acidosis, which is common in ARF. Hydrogen ions, which are high in acidosis, are unable to be eliminated along with other metabolic wastes. Remember, if the pH is low, H^+ ions are high. The pH and bicarbonate are both low and the carbon dioxide is normal, which indicates metabolic acidosis.

2. The hyperkalemia could cause cardiac arrhythmias. The normal potassium level is 3.5 to 5.0 mEq/L and the heart does not tolerate values too low or too high.

3. L. J. is in the maintenance phase of ARF. Most of the signs and symptoms presented by L. J. are typical of this phase. The initial phase has very few manifestations and hopefully

the recovery phase shows renal improvement. This phase should lasts from 1 to 2 weeks.

4. L. J. could possibly experience CHF or pulmonary edema. The edema, rales, and low urinary output are suggestive of these disorders. The strain placed on the heart by the ARF episode could also trigger a cardiovascular event.

5. The diet should not be high in sodium because of the retention of fluid being experienced by the client. The low sodium is of least concern in his present state. Sodium supplements may be used to exchange potassium, thereby increasing sodium and lowering potassium levels. The main dietary restriction is protein and high carbohydrates should be given to accommodate for the low proteins.

Chapter 11

1. General anesthesia is usually used. A low abdominal incision is made. The prostate is resected and lymph nodes are also obtained. If it appears that the prostate capsule has been invaded with cancer, additional tissue around the prostate may be removed. Postoperative pain medication is provided. An indwelling urinary catheter will be in place.

2. The pathology report of the tissue removed (the prostate gland, surrounding tissue if taken, and lymph nodes) reveals the extent of the disease. Additional scans may also be utilized to stage the disease.

3. Prostate cancer in the elderly is a very slow-growing cancer, and conservative treatment is utilized because of the expectation that the client's eventual demise will result from a cause other than the prostate cancer. The younger the client is at diagnosis, the more likely it is that the cancer is an aggressive form that will require more aggressive treatment. Another factor in determining what type of anesthesia to use is based on the surgical procedure and the age of the client.

4. Radiation therapy and chemotherapy will most likely be required after the surgery.

5. Stage 3 prostate cancer indicates that the cancer is outside the capsule of the prostate, and may also be in the seminal vesicles. It has not spread to the lymph nodes or other organs.

Chapter 12

1. Immediate assessment should focus on airway patency (respiratory rate, depth, lung sounds, any dyspnea or stridor). The client is exhibiting initial signs of possible anaphylaxis (type I hypersensitivity reaction). Although his blood pressure (BP) is within normal limits (WNL), it is on the lower side and with tachycardia, the nurse should be proactive at this time. The welts definitely indicate a localized reaction and his anxiety may or may not be related to anaphylaxis. If the airway is not patent, oxygen should be administered and an oropharyngeal of nasopharyngeal airway instituted immediately.

2. The nurse should first determine what the client's normal BP range is and then identify how he reacted to bee stings in the past for comparison. If the client runs a much higher BP than this, the nurse may be concerned that hypotension is developing. Individuals allergic to a specific insect often react similarly when bitten or stung by other insects. This reaction may be typical for this client when venom is injected. If this response is exaggerated, the nurse should again be proactive and monitor the client closely. The reaction may be caused by the multiple stings of the hornets.

3. Drug therapy would involve topical and oral antihistamines and possibly corticosteroids. Epinephrine should be on hand for administration if airway management or severe edema presents.

4. The wife should be informed that her husband apparently has a type I hypersensitivity reaction to insect bites and stings (if he has presented with similar symptoms to bees) and that he probably always will respond in this fashion. Explain that each subsequent episode may be more exaggerated because the body has become sensitized to the allergen. Emphasize that the massive amount of welts is probably caused by the number of hornet stings, as hornets swarm and attack in large numbers. Calm the wife by explaining that the antihistamines will help with his symptoms and that he may be sleepy because of the antihistamines.

5. This client needs to be instructed on the following:
   - Have a "bee sting kit" available at all times, which includes a prefilled syringe of epinephrine (Epi-pen). The wife should be taught how to administer the Epi-pen. If the kit contains an inhaler, teach her on the use of the inhaler also.
   - Have antihistamine lotion and tablets available.
   - Have corticosteroid lotion available.
   - Teach her the symptoms of a true anaphylactic reaction and when to bring the client in by ambulance versus trying to drive him.
   - Discuss strategies to avoid allergens as much as possible.
   - Purchase a Medic-alert bracelet that should be worn at all times.
   - Encourage the wife to have an alternate plan if a local ambulance service is not available where she lives.
   - Demonstrate and have her return demonstrate steps to take when an anaphylactic reaction occurs: open the airway, place the client in high Fowler's position, count the respirations, calm the victim.

Chapter 13

1. This is classified as a nosocomial infection, hospital-acquired and is probably related to the surgical procedure. Good handwashing and use of aseptic technique in changing the dressing are the best interventions.

2. A culture and sensitivity of the wound is the diagnostic test. If this is positive, an antibiotic showing sensitivity will be ordered. If this is negative, other tests will be ordered. Complete blood count (CBC), blood culture, and sensitivity, chest x-ray (CXR) to rule-out sepsis or pneumonia are recommended.

3. A white blood count (WBC) and differential should be analyzed. If an infection as described here is present, bacteria are the most likely cause. The WBC will probably be elevated with elevated neutrophils (since the onset is new).

4. vancomycin (Vancocin) is the recommended treatment because it has bactericidal and bacteriostatic action. It interferes with cell membrane synthesis in multiplying organisms. It is active against both Gram positive and Gram negative organisms.

5. Neurotoxicity, ototoxicity, nephrotoxicity, fever, and chills are adverse effects. "Red neck syndrome" can be reduced by slowing the infusion.

6. Quinupristin and dalfopristin (Synercid); linezolid (Zyvox), or the synergistic effect of vancomycin (Vancocin) and gentamycin (Garamycin) are effective against vancomycin-resistant staphylococcus aureus (VRSA).

Chapter 14

1. The nurse should inquire as to when the eruption began, the appearance, and where the rash is located. Questions should be asked about any pain, itching, or burning around the area before the blisters appeared. The nurse should inquire about a history of chickenpox and any other medical diagnoses that may have compromised her immune status. A thorough review of all medications she is currently taking would be indicated, as some drugs also depress the immune system.

2. The nurse should thoroughly examine the skin for characteristic lesions and distribution. A determination should be made as to whether the involvement is dermatomal or unilateral and whether there is opthalmic involvement. If the eyes are involved, emergency treatment and referral is indicated. Assessment for pain management is also essential as this can be very painful, especially for an elderly client.

3. Herpes zoster is caused by a reactivation of the varicella virus (chickenpox) that remained dormant in the basal ganglia after an episode of chickenpox. It is a viral infection usually involving the skin of a single dermatome and usually resolves within about 2 weeks. An antiviral medication will be necessary to shorten the duration of the disease, help lessen the itching, and control the pain.

4. The goal of therapy is suppression of pain, inflammation, and infection. Use of over-the-counter nonsteroidal antiinflammatory drugs (NSAIDs) is recommended for pain and fever. Oral antiviral medications are available: valacyclovir HCL (Valtrex) 1 gm, 3 times a day for 7 days; famiciclovir (Famvir) 500 mg, three times a day for 7 days; and aysyekloever (Acyclovir) 800 mg, 5 times a day for 7 days. Antipruritic medications such as corticosteroids or antihistamines will decrease itching and scratching.

5. Wet compresses using Burow's solution or cool tap water can be used for a soothing effect. Avoid scratching the area to prevent secondary infection. Stress keeping follow-up appointments in 3 days and again a week later to monitor the disease. Fever, chills, increased pain, or drainage should be reported promptly. The client needs to isolate herself from neonates, pregnant women, and immunosuppressed persons. Explain that she is contagious to those persons who have never had chickenpox. The disease usually resolves, but there may be scarring at the site of the lesions.

Chapter 15

1. Nursing diagnoses should be prioritized as follows:
   - Risk for infection related to decreased circulating granulocytes secondary to acute lymphocytic leukemia and decreased ability to heal properly secondary to diabetes mellitus
   - Risk for injury: bleeding related to decreased circulating platelets secondary to acute lymphocytic leukemia
   - Ineffective airway clearance related to increased phlegm, decreased secondary defenses, prolonged bed rest, and age
   - Altered nutrition: less than body requirements related to increased metabolism secondary to acute lymphocytic leukemia
   - Altered oral mucus membranes related to the effect of chemotherapeutic medications and neutropenia
   - Altered role performance related to recent cancer diagnosis
   - Anticipatory grieving related to fear of impending death secondary to recent cancer diagnosis

   Since infection is the number one cause of death in these clients and the client's circulating granulocytes are decreased (Absolute granulocyte count [AGC] = 990), the risk for infection is more life threatening than the other diagnoses and therefore is listed first. Since she is already experiencing petechiae and her platelet count is decreased (12,000/mm^3), bleeding becomes the second most life-threatening complication and should be considered second. Her weight loss of 10 pounds makes Altered nutrition an important diagnosis.

2. The client's absolute granulocytes/neutrophil count (AGC or ANC) is extremely low. The AGC is calculated by taking the WBC (% bands + % segs) and normally should be greater than 1,000. In this case: 9,000 (0.01 + 0.10) = 990, makes the client extremely susceptible to opportunistic infection. When the client's granulocytes are decreased, the client will lose first line of defense against infection. Neutrophils are the first cells to arrive at a site of infection; they engulf the invading organism and trigger the inflammation response. These clients are highly susceptible to life-threatening infections and often don't produce the normal response to infection. Fever may be the only sign of infection in these clients.

3. Monitor for manifestations of infection, which include elevated temperature, chills, throat pain, chest pain, cough, burning on urination, rectal or vaginal itching or irritation. Monitor vital signs and oxygenation every four hours. Assess for temperature spikes with chills, tachypnea, tachycardia, restlessness, change in PaO$_2$, and hypotension. Although the body temperature is usually elevated in infection, clients with leukemia may have an altered response and sepsis may be present before abnormal vital signs occur. Hypotension is usually a late symptom of sepsis. The presence of yellow-colored sputum and redness to the Hickman catheter are concerning since these are significant signs of infection.

4. Part of the client's treatment protocol includes prednisone. Steroid therapy will cause an increase release of glycogen from the liver thereby increasing the glucose level in the blood. As a result, the client will require frequent glucose monitoring and sliding scale insulin to regulate her diabetes. This will create an increase in the number of invasive procedures, since both capillary blood glucose monitoring and insulin injects will require a needle stick. Because of the underlying leukemia diagnosis, the client is more susceptible to infection, and with her diabetes diagnosis, she is susceptible to delayed healing. The nurse should use meticulous skin preparation for this client, and keep capillary blood glucose testing to a minimum. The nurse may consider discussing accessing a blood sample from the Hickman, but due to the small sample required, the risk may outweigh the benefit.

5. Primary caregiver support and place of discharge needs to be determined early in the hospital stay. Many clients are discharged at the completion of their chemotherapy induction to nadir at home. Because this client's children are dispersed all over the country and her spouse travels a good deal with his job, the nurse should discuss how the family plans to assist the client after discharge. The nurse also needs to begin teaching the primary caregiver about Hickman catheter maintenance as well as preparation of the home to decrease infection exposure. Subcutaneous injection technique also needs to be assessed since the client will be discharged on insulin as well as other medications such as filgrastim (Neupogen), epoetin alfa (Procrit), and methotrexate (MTX).

Chapter 16

1. Cystic fibrosis is a multi-system disease. Respiratory compromise, recurrent pneumonia, and failure to thrive (FTT) are all symptoms of cystic fibrosis. The client with cystic fibrosis has thick, increased viscosity of secretions, decreased ciliary function, decreased alveolar function and alveolar plugs that lead to repeat infections and long-term chronic obstructive pulmonary disease (COPD). *Pseudomonas* and *staphylococcus* are the most common organisims and are often resistant to antibiotics. The gastrointestinal tract is also involved and malabsorption occurs due to blockage of the ducts leading from the pancreas to the duodenum. Fats and fat-soluble vitamins are not absorbed and malnutrition

can occur. In an infant, this is manifested as failure to thrive.

2. The test most commonly performed to confirm cystic fibrosis is the sweat chloride test revealing an elevated sodium chloride level. The defective protein inhibits transport of sodium chloride and these electrolytes are excreated in the sweat. The nurse could also refer to pulmonary function tests to determine the level of respiratory compromise. Hypoxia is chronic because of the COPD and can lead to Cor pulmonale (right-sided congestive heart failure from a respiratory cause). Arterial blood gases (ABGs) or pulse oximetry are usually also conducted. In the newborn screen, a decreased trypsin in the stool indicates pancreatic insufficiency or cystic fibrosis.

3. Medications the nurse may administer would be albuterol (Ventolin), beclomethasone (Vanceril), and dornase alfa (Dnase). The Ventolin and Vanceril should aid in opening the lungs and improving respirations. The Dnase alters the mucous viscosity, which should allow greater ease in expectorating any secretions. Antibiotics may also be ordered. Other interventions include administering low dose oxygen, chest physiotherapy (CPT), and suctioning as needed.

4. The client with cystic fibrosis has plugging of the pancreatic duct, which leads to decrease in absorption of fats, carbohydrates, and protein. The malabsorption leads to failure to thrive.

5. The family needs to be able to perform CPT, respiratory aerosol treatments, and know the potential side effects of those treatments. The family also must be able to recognize the signs and symptoms of infection and respiratory distress. Teaching the client concerning signs of hypoxia and use of a pulse oximetry is useful to avoid frequent visits to a healthcare provider. The nurse should also stress the need to keep the child current on immunizations in order to avoid other diseases that may be exaggerated in cystic fibrosis. The nurse can review with the family what an autosomal recessive pattern is and if both parents are carriers what is the chance of reoccurrence. The family can also have the disease diagnosed in the prenatal and perinatal period.

Chapter 17

1. Fundamental interventions would include maintaining spinal alignment, providing supplemental oxygen and maintaining the airway. Initiation of two large bore cannulas, control of scalp hemorrhage, and laboratory/radiology testing to include arterial blood gases, complete blood count, chemistry panel (glucose), urinalysis, blood alcohol, type and crossmatch for donor specific blood and cervical spine, chest, hip, and pelvic x-rays. Further assessment of the client would include heart sounds, respiratory status, cardiac monitoring, peripheral pulses, complaints voiced by the client, especially chest or leg pain. A thorough head-to-toe assessment would then need to be made.

2. A thoracostomy (chest tube) may be inserted for the diagnosis of pneumothorax. A CT scan or MRI may be performed for possible brain injuries. A urinary catheter would also need to be inserted unless contraindicated.

3. The client is in the compensatory phase of shock. The rise in pulse and respiration, along with the change in level of consciousness are indications. ABGs indicate the level of cellular perfusion and acid-base balance that is affected by respiration at the cellular level. Hematocrit and hemoglobin levels are also useful in determining active blood loss for hypovolemic shock.

4. While the scalp is very vascular and will bleed profusely depending on the size of the laceration, the potential for pelvic and hip fractures constitute the greatest threat of hemorrhage from both the bone itself and the possible injury to great vessels in the femoral area. With a diagnosis of flail chest, the potential for a pneumothorax or hemothorax could contribute to the overall volume loss. The client could also suffer a cardiac contusion or a hematoma.

5. It is vitally important to maintain an accurate output recording, however, in the presence of pelvic or hip injury there may also be penetrating damage to the bladder. Bleeding from the meatus would indicate bladder trauma or actual urethral damage that would contraindicate the insertion of a urinary catheter.

Credits

Chapter 1

Figure 01-01 Art, © Prentice Hall Health, Upper Saddle River, New Jersey.

Figure 01-02 Art, From Medical Surgical Nursing: Critical Thinking in Client Care, by Priscilla LeMone, Karen M. Burke, Edition 2, © 2000 by Prentice-Hall, Inc., Upper Saddle River, New Jersey; Page 1473, Fig. 34-19; Artist: Kristin N. Mount

Figure 01-03 Art, From Medical Surgical Nursing: Critical Thinking in Client Care, by Priscilla LeMone, Karen M. Burke, Edition 2, © 2000 by Prentice-Hall, Inc., Upper Saddle River, New Jersey; Page 1485, Fig. 34-24; Artist: Nea Hanscomb

Chapter 2

Figure 02-01 Art, From Medical Surgical Nursing: Critical Thinking in Client Care, by Priscilla LeMone, Karen M. Burke, Edition 2, © 2000 by Prentice-Hall, Inc., Upper Saddle River, New Jersey; Page 1075, Fig. 28-12; Artist: Kristin N. Mount

Figure 02-02 Art, From Medical Surgical Nursing: Critical Thinking in Client Care, by Priscilla LeMone, Karen M. Burke, Edition 2, © 2000 by Prentice-Hall, Inc., Upper Saddle River, New Jersey; Page 1106, Fig. 28-17; Artist: Kristin N. Mount

Figure 02-03 Art, From Medical Surgical Nursing: Critical Thinking in Client Care, by Priscilla LeMone, Karen M. Burke, Edition 2, © 2000 by Prentice-Hall, Inc., Upper Saddle River, New Jersey; Page 1123, Fig. 28-19; Artist: Kristin N. Mount

Figure 02-04 Art, From Medical Surgical Nursing: Critical Thinking in Client Care, by Priscilla LeMone, Karen M. Burke, Edition 2, © 2000 by Prentice-Hall, Inc., Upper Saddle River, New Jersey; Page 1124, Fig. 28-20; Artist: Kristin N. Mount

Table 02-06 Art, From Medical Surgical Nursing: Critical Thinking in Client Care, by Priscilla LeMone, Karen M. Burke, Edition 2, © 2000 by Prentice-Hall, Inc., Upper Saddle River, New Jersey; Page 1039-1041, Table 28-01; Artist: GTS Graphics/Kristin N. Mount.

Chapter 3

Figure 03-01 Art, From Medical Surgical Nursing: Critical Thinking in Client Care, by Priscilla LeMone, Karen M. Burke, Edition 2, © 2000 by Prentice-Hall, Inc., Upper Saddle River, New Jersey; Page 1233, Fig. 30-01; Artist: Christopher Burke

Chapter 4

Figure 04-01 Art, From Medical Surgical Nursing: Critical Thinking in Client Care, by Priscilla LeMone, Karen M. Burke, Edition 2, © 2000 by Prentice-Hall, Inc., Upper Saddle River, New Jersey; Page 1696, Fig. 39-17,18; Artist: Precision Graphics

Figure 04-02 Art, From Medical Surgical Nursing: Critical Thinking in Client Care, by Priscilla LeMone, Karen M. Burke, Edition 2, © 2000 by Prentice-Hall, Inc., Upper Saddle River, New Jersey; Page 1696, Fig. 39-16; Artist: Precision Graphics

Figure 04-03 Art, From Medical Surgical Nursing: Critical Thinking in Client Care, by Priscilla LeMone, Karen M. Burke, Edition 2, © 2000 by Prentice-Hall, Inc., Upper Saddle River, New Jersey; Page 1696, Fig. 39-15; Artist: Precision Graphics

Chapter 5

Figure 05-01 Art, © Prentice Hall Health, Upper Saddle River, New Jersey.

Chapter 6

Figure 06-01 Art, From Medical Surgical Nursing: Critical Thinking in Client Care, by Priscilla LeMone, Karen M. Burke, Edition 2, © 2000 by Prentice-Hall, Inc., Upper Saddle River, New Jersey; Page 1879, Fig. 43-03; Artist: Barbara Cousins/Nea Hanscomb.

Figure 06-02 Art, From Medical Surgical Nursing: Critical Thinking in Client Care, by Priscilla LeMone, Karen M. Burke, Edition 2, © 2000 by Prentice-Hall, Inc., Upper Saddle River, New Jersey; Page 1881, Fig. 43-05; Artist: Todd A. Buck/Nea Hanscomb.

Figure 06-03 Art, From Medical Surgical Nursing: Critical Thinking in Client Care, by Priscilla LeMone, Karen M. Burke, Edition 2, © 2000 by Prentice-Hall, Inc., Upper Saddle River, New Jersey; Page 1369, Fig. 33–5; Artist: Christopher Burke.

Chapter 7

Figure 07-01 Art, From Medical Surgical Nursing: Critical Thinking in Client Care, by Priscilla LeMone, Karen M. Burke, Edition 2, © 2000 by Prentice-Hall, Inc., Upper Saddle River, New Jersey; Page 498, Fig. 14-08; Artist: Precision Graphics

Figure 07-02 Art, From Medical Surgical Nursing: Critical Thinking in Client Care, by Priscilla LeMone, Karen M. Burke, Edition 2, © 2000 by Prentice-Hall, Inc., Upper Saddle River, New Jersey; Page 471, Fig. 13-07 A&B; Artist: Kristin N. Mount

Figure 07-03 Art, From Medical Surgical Nursing: Critical Thinking in Client Care, by Priscilla LeMone, Karen M. Burke, Edition 2, © 2000 by Prentice-Hall, Inc., Upper Saddle River, New Jersey; Page 833 Fig. 23-10; Artist: Nea Hanscomb

Chapter 8

Figure 08-01 Art, From Medical Surgical Nursing: Critical Thinking in Client Care, by Priscilla LeMone, Karen M. Burke, Edition 2. © 2000 by Prentice-Hall, Inc., Upper Saddle River, New Jersey, Page 512, Fig. 15-01; Artist: Kristin N. Mount

Chapter 9

Figure 09-01 Art, From Medical Surgical Nursing: Critical Thinking in Client Care, by Priscilla LeMone, Karen M. Burke, Edition 2, © 2000 by Prentice-Hall, Inc., Upper Saddle River, New Jersey; Page 685, Fig. 20-01; Artist: Biomed Arts Associates/Wendy Hiller Gee/Kristin N. Mount

Figure 09-02 Art, From Medical Surgical Nursing: Critical Thinking in Client Care, by Priscilla LeMone, Karen M. Burke, Edition 2, © 2000 by Prentice-Hall, Inc., Upper Saddle River, New Jersey; Page 695, Fig. 20-04; Artist: Biomed Arts Associates/Wendy Hiller Gee/Kristin N. Mount

Figure 09-03 Art, From Medical Surgical Nursing: Critical Thinking in Client Care, by Priscilla LeMone, Karen M. Burke, Edition 2, © 2000 by Prentice-Hall, Inc., Upper Saddle River, New Jersey; Page 726, Fig. 21-03; Artist: Biomed Arts Associates/Wendy Hiller Gee/Kristin N. Mount

Chapter 10

Figure 10-01 Art, From Medical Surgical Nursing: Critical Thinking in Client Care, by Priscilla LeMone, Karen M. Burke, Edition 2, © 2000 by Prentice-Hall, Inc., Upper Saddle River, New Jersey; Page 954, Fig. 26-02; Artist: Nea Hanscomb

Figure 10-02 Art, From Medical Surgical Nursing: Critical Thinking in Client Care, by Priscilla LeMone, Karen M. Burke, Edition 2, © 2000 by Prentice-Hall, Inc., Upper Saddle River, New Jersey; Page 981, Fig. 26-05; Artist: Kristin N. Mount

Figure 10-03 Art, From Medical Surgical Nursing: Critical Thinking in Client Care, by Priscilla LeMone, Karen M. Burke, Edition 2, © 2000 by Prentice-Hall, Inc., Upper Saddle River, New Jersey; Page 994, Fig. 26-09, Artist: Biomed Arts Associates/Wendy Hiller Gee/Kristin N. Mount

Chapter 11

Figure 11-01 Art, From Medical Surgical Nursing: Critical Thinking in Client Care, by Priscilla LeMone, Karen M. Burke, Edition 2, © 2000 by Prentice-Hall, Inc., Upper Saddle River, New Jersey; Page 1953, Fig. 45-01; Artist: Barbara Cousins/Nea Hanscomb

Figure 11-02 Art, From Medical Surgical Nursing: Critical Thinking in Client Care, by Priscilla LeMone, Karen M. Burke, Edition 2, © 2000 by Prentice-Hall, Inc., Upper Saddle River, New Jersey; Page 1973, Fig. 46-01; Artist: Christopher Burke

Figure 11-03 Art, © Prentice Hall Health, Upper Saddle River, New Jersey.

Chapter 12

Figure 12-01 Art, From Medical Surgical Nursing: Critical Thinking in Client Care, by Priscilla LeMone, Karen M. Burke, Edition 2, © 2000 by Prentice-Hall, Inc., Upper Saddle River, New Jersey; Page 221, Fig. 08-01; Artist: Christopher Burke

Figure 12-02 Art, From Medical Surgical Nursing: Critical Thinking in Client Care, by Priscilla LeMone, Karen M. Burke, Edition 2, © 2000 by Prentice-Hall, Inc., Upper Saddle River, New Jersey; Page 223, Fig. 08-02; Artist: Christopher Burke

Figure 12-03 Art, From Medical Surgical Nursing: Critical Thinking in Client Care, by Priscilla LeMone, Karen M. Burke, Edition 2, © 2000 by Prentice-Hall, Inc., Upper Saddle River, New Jersey; Page 293, Fig. 08-19; Artist: Christopher Burke

Chapter 13

Figure 13-01 Art, From Medical Surgical Nursing: Critical Thinking in Client Care, by Priscilla LeMone, Karen M. Burke, Edition 2, © 2000 by Prentice-Hall, Inc., Upper Saddle River, New Jersey; Page 253, Fig. 08-12; Artist: Nea Hanscomb

Chapter 14

Figure 14-01 Art, From Medical Surgical Nursing: Critical Thinking in Client Care, by Priscilla LeMone, Karen M. Burke, Edition 2, © 2000 by Prentice-Hall, Inc., Upper Saddle River, New Jersey; Page 234, Fig. 08-10; Artist: Christopher Burke

Figure 14-02 Art, From Medical Surgical Nursing: Critical Thinking in Client Care, by Priscilla LeMone, Karen M. Burke, Edition 2, © 2000 by Prentice-Hall, Inc., Upper Saddle River, New Jersey; Page 649, Fig. 18-06; Artist: Precision Graphics

Chapter 15

Figure 15-01 Art, From Medical Surgical Nursing: Critical Thinking in Client Care, by Priscilla LeMone, Karen M. Burke, Edition 2, © 2000 by Prentice-Hall, Inc., Upper Saddle River, New Jersey; Page 1297, Fig. 31-11; Artist: Nea Hanscomb

Figure 15-02 Art, From Medical Surgical Nursing: Critical Thinking in Client Care, by Priscilla LeMone, Karen M. Burke, Edition 2, © 2000 by Prentice-Hall, Inc., Upper Saddle River, New Jersey; Page 1272, Fig. 31-06; Artist: Nea Hanscomb

Chapter 16

Figure 16-01 Art, From Maternal-Newborn Nursing: A Family and Community-Based Approach, by Sally B. Olds, Marcia L. London, Patricia Wieland Ladewig, Edition 6, © 2000 by Prentice-Hall, Inc., Upper Saddle River, New Jersey; Page 207, Fig. 08-19, Artist: Christopher Burke

Chapter 17

Figure 17-01 Art, © Prentice Hall Health, Upper Saddle River, New Jersey.

Figure 17-02 Art, From Medical Surgical Nursing: Critical Thinking in Client Care, by Priscilla LeMone, Karen M. Burke, Edition 2, © 2000 by Prentice-Hall, Inc., Upper Saddle River, New Jersey; Page 167, Fig. 06-01; Artist: Biomed Arts Associates/Wendy Hiller Gee/Kristin N. Mount

Figure 17-03 Art, From Medical Surgical Nursing: Critical Thinking in Client Care, by Priscilla LeMone, Karen M. Burke, Edition 2, © 2000 by Prentice-Hall, Inc., Upper Saddle River, New Jersey; Page 1789, Fig. 41-06; Artist: Kristin N. Mount

Index